Senior Trauma Patients

Hans-Christoph Pape
Stephen L. Kates
Christian Hierholzer
Heike A. Bischoff-Ferrari
Editors

Senior Trauma Patients

An Integrated Approach

Springer

Editors
Hans-Christoph Pape
Department of Trauma Surgery
University Hospital Zurich
Zürich, Switzerland

Stephen L. Kates
Department of Orthopaedic Surgery
Virginia Commonwealth University
Richmond, VA, USA

Christian Hierholzer
Department of Trauma Surgery
University Hospital Zurich
Zürich, Switzerland

Heike A. Bischoff-Ferrari
Department of Aging Medicine
and Aging Research
City Hospital Zurich-Waid
Zurich University
Zürich, Switzerland

ISBN 978-3-030-91482-0 ISBN 978-3-030-91483-7 (eBook)
https://doi.org/10.1007/978-3-030-91483-7

This Springer imprint is published by the registered company Springer Nature Switzerland AG
The registered company address is: Gewerbestrasse 11, 6330 Cham, Switzerland

We would like to dedicate this book to Prof. Dr. Hans-Peter Simmen, Prof. emeritus, Department of Trauma, University of Zurich, Switzerland, for his accomplishments in regard to orchestrating the first certified Geriatric Trauma Center in Switzerland.

Foreword

It is well known that people are getting older in all industrialized countries offering good quality of life as well as modern medical treatment. For instance, statistical mean age is as high as 86 years for women and 82 years for men in Switzerland, respectively. Similar figures are reported from other European nations. To provide optimal treatment for aged persons, many hospitals established specialized geriatric departments in the last years. Even congresses with tailored programs are held to fit the scientific needs for treating elderly people.

A femur fracture in 80-year-old person may not only be a broken bone. In the presence of comorbidities, it is an "attack on the entire organism." Identical surgical principles are applied. However, impaired bone quality and comorbidities make the healing process much more complicated. The follow-up care requires the advice of many specialists; the rehabilitation procedures have to be adapted.

The people 70+ suffer more severe injuries. According to publicly available data from the "German Trauma Registry," 25% of the polytraumatized patients are over 70 years old. These injuries include not only high velocity trauma such as road traffic accidents but rather low impact trauma resulting from a fall on stairs. It is not unusual that frail patients present with head injury (intracerebral hematoma), serial rib fractures with lung contusions in addition to a hip fracture. Many persons 70+ are on anticoagulant or antiplatelet agents which aggravate their condition.

How to go on if you are called to an aged patient suffering from fractures in addition to many comorbidities such as an insulin-dependent diabetes and bleeding disorders due to antiplatelet agents following stent implantation ? Please, consult this textbook.

This textbook *Senior Trauma Patients: An Integrated Approach* is designed to improve diagnostics and treatments of patients 70+, who belong to the most difficult ones, a doctor has to deal with. The editors are to be congratulated: They realized a comprehensive overview on geriatric trauma. I am sure that this reference work will help to better understand and treat the sickest patients.

Hans-Peter Simmen
Professor Emeritus of Surgery, Former Chairman
of the Department of Traumatology
University Hospital Zurich
Zurich, Switzerland

Preface

The world's aging population is rapidly growing, and many older adults will suffer low energy trauma due to falls or accidents. Over the past decade, many initiatives have been developed to improve the management of older adults with such injuries.

The two most popular approaches include efforts to improve the aftercare provided by orthopedic trauma surgeons and the interdisciplinary comanagement approach that involves both geriatricians and surgeons. The latter approach has been adopted widely and involves care in the hospital, including medication management, peri-surgical care, and prevention of secondary fractures by standardized protocols.

Among these initiatives are Orthogeriatric Management with the Fragility Fracture Network (FFN) and the AO, the Geriatric Trauma Center certification initiative by the German Trauma Association and the German Geriatric Association, and the "Own the Bone" by the American Orthopaedic Association (AOA).

This book covers the essential aspects of geriatric fracture management, perioperative care, postoperative ICU management, and follow-up care. Because the number of geriatric (poly-) trauma cases will rise significantly, it includes a new standard operating procedure (SOP) for these and other patients. Outcome differences (compared with younger patients) are explained for major fracture types along with physiological compensation mechanisms, frailty, and nutrition. We hope that this comprehensive text will add to the general knowledge of this important topic.

Zürich, Switzerland	Hans-Christoph Pape
Richmond, VA, USA	Stephen L. Kates
Zürich, Switzerland	Christian Hierholzer
Zürich, Switzerland	Heike A. Bischoff-Ferrari

Contents

Part VIII Rehabilitation and Outcomes

Part I

Introduction: Physiology of Ageing

Epidemiology

1

Marianne Comeau-Gauthier, Daniel Axelrod, and Mohit Bhandari

1.1 Introduction

Geriatric patients may pose unique and significant challenges in the trauma setting with regard to injury severity assessment, resuscitation, and treatment, when compared to patients under the age of 65 years. Apart from the substantially higher morbidity and mortality [8, 9], one must recognize the critical and unique psychosocial components in the care of the elderly [10]. While special considerations should be made for the geriatric polytraumatized patient, current evidence-based recommendations are founded primarily on retrospective studies including a significant portion of registry-based cohort studies and a limited number of prospective studies [7, 11, 12]. To date, no randomized controlled trials have been performed to guide best practice and improve outcomes.

The geriatric trauma population is commonly defined as patients aged 65 and older [12], although trauma mortality increases significantly from the age of 55 [13–19], independently from the degree of injury. Additionally, some authors have reported specific predictive factors that may apply for patients aged 80 years and older only [14, 20]. The National Trauma Data Bank (NTDB) reports the first peak in the number of trauma-related injuries leading to admission to a trauma center between ages of 14–29 years old, primarily from motor vehicle-related accidents, and reports a second peak starting after the age of 50 years, when falls begin to increase [1]. Males account for 70% of all incidents up to age 70, while after 71 years, most patients are female [1].

1.2 Clinical Significance of the Aging Process on the Polytraumatized Patient

1.2.1 Age-Related Physiologic Decline

Despite defining the elderly as aged above 65 years, the impact of aging on trauma has been found to be as early as 40 years [21]. The combination of age-related immunosenescence and trauma-related immune dysregulation likely contributes to a higher mortality and morbidity rate in older adults [22]. It was found that elderly victims had increased tissue inhibitor of metalloproteinases-2 (TIMP-2) levels [23], an indicator of

M. Comeau-Gauthier · D. Axelrod (✉)
Division of Orthopedic Surgery, McMaster University, Hamilton, ON, Canada
e-mail: marianne.comeaugauthier@medportal.ca; daniel.axelrod@medportal.ca

M. Bhandari
Division of Orthopedic Surgery, McMaster University, Hamilton, ON, Canada

Department of Health Research Methods, Evidence and Impact (HEI), McMaster University, Hamilton, ON, Canada
e-mail: bhandam@mcmaster.ca

H.-C. Pape et al. (eds.), *Senior Trauma Patients*, https://doi.org/10.1007/978-3-030-91483-7_1

the severity of pathologic immune activation, and polytraumatized geriatric patients more often develop SIRS compared with younger patients [24].

Decreased myocardial pumping efficacy [25–27], decline in myocardial conducting system responsiveness to demands on the cardiovascular system [28, 29], hypertension [30], and accumulation of atherosclerotic plaque [26] lead to a narrower range of end diastolic volumes required to preserve and optimize cardiac function/output. These changes in the cardiovascular system translate into a reduced ability to respond to hypovolemia and shock and challenges during resuscitation, as both under-resuscitation and over-resuscitation are harmful [31], which is why some authors advocate for a lower threshold in implementing invasive monitoring in this population [12, 32, 33]. The loss of functional respiratory reserve, decreased lung compliance, loss of alveolar surface, and increased ventilation/perfusion mismatch [34] added with higher rates of multiple rib fractures with a seemingly lower transfer of energy [35–37] could partially account for a higher number of days on ventilators [3] and a higher risk of pulmonary infection [37] associated with elderly victims. Increased prevalence of osteoporosis in this population [38] leads to higher severity fractures compared to younger patients with a similar mechanism of injury. Increased intracranial space due to brain atrophy and greater stretching of intracranial vessels directly increase the rate of intracranial bleedings [18, 39].

1.2.2 Effect on Triage

In a 10-year retrospective review (1994–2004) of the Maryland Ambulance Information System by Chang et al. [40], elderly victims were three times more likely to be under-triaged compared with younger patients, which remained significant on multivariate analysis (controlling for year, sex, injury, mechanism, transport reasons, emergency medical service provider level training, jurisdictional region). These results were corroborated by two subsequent large registry-based cohort studies [41, 42]. These findings are highly significant as under-triage of an elderly victim leads to fourfold the mortality and discharge disability rate as compared to their younger counterparts [43].

Several factors have been reported to impair adequate triage of elderly patients, including healthcare provider bias, unrecognized comorbidities, communication impairment, inaccuracy of Glasgow Coma Scale (GCS) scoring in geriatric patients, and lack of reliable parameters indicator of injury severity and sufficient resuscitation. Elderly victims are found to be less likely to trigger a trauma team activation, despite a similar percentage of ISS above 15 and the higher need for urgent craniotomy and orthopedic procedures [43]. A noisy and chaotic trauma bay is certainly not favorable to doctor-patient communication and history taking in a "hard of hearing" elderly, which is often assumed as intellectual impairment [10]. Mental status examinations and GCS scoring can be particularly difficult in geriatric patients with preexisting cognitive decline, hearing impairment, or sequelae of previous strokes [44]. Furthermore, heart rate and blood pressure were not found to be predictive of severe impending mortality and inadequate resuscitation in patients aged above 65 years old [43]. Increased mortality has been reported among the elderly with heart rates greater than 90 beats per minute and systolic blood pressure less than 110 mmHg, while the same increase in mortality is not seen in younger patients [45].

Current guidelines from the America Trauma Life Support (ATLS) recommend transporting any patient older than 55 years old to a trauma center [46], while the Eastern Association from the Surgery of Trauma (EAST) guidelines recommend geriatric-specific care for any patient older than 65 years old [12]. Recent evidence-based review from EAST has shown decreased mortality in severely injured geriatric patients treated in trauma care centers as compared to non-trauma centers, and therefore, recommend initial assessment and care in a certified trauma center [7].

1.3 Mechanisms of Injury

While trauma is the fifth cause of death in the elderly, blunt trauma secondary to a fall from any height is the leading cause of high-energy injuries in the geriatric patient [1, 3, 47–50], representing nearly three-quarters of all traumas in this population [3], followed by traffic-related accidents, either as the driver or as a pedestrian hit by a car [1, 49, 50]. Penetrating trauma, firearm injuries, assault, and burns are much less common. Adults aged over 65 are almost two to three times more likely to die of their injuries, even after controlling for race, sex, injury mechanism, and ISS [3, 50, 51] Geriatric status was found to be one of the main independent factors for mortality across all mechanisms of injury [49].

A 10-year retrospective review found that nearly 60% of trauma admission in the geriatric population are secondary to high-energy mechanism [3]. However, elderly presented following low or high-energy injury mechanism are nearly seven times more likely to have higher Abbreviated Injury Score (AIS) to any body region [2] and usually present with a higher ISS [3] as compared with younger patients.

Traumatic brain injuries (TBI) are the leading cause of trauma-related mortality and morbidity in the elderly, with falls as the leading causative mechanism (51%), followed by motor vehicle traffic crashes (9%) [4]. Independently of the mechanism of injury, subdural hematomas are three times more likely in the elderly population [3, 5]. Extensive guidelines on primary assessment, imaging indications, and normalization of the lowering of the International Normalized Radio (INR) have been published in an attempt to prevent the disastrous outcomes associated with severe TBIs [52–54].

A 6-year retrospective chart review (2004–2010) from a level I trauma center reported the frequency of fracture location in high-energy (ISS ≥ 16) geriatric traumas. Elderly most often sustained a fracture to the spine (74%), followed by the pelvis (35%), femur (31%), forearm (24%), clavicle (23%), scapula (21%), tibia/fibula (19%), ankle (17%), acetabulum (10%), humerus shaft (7%), hand (7%), proximal humerus (5%), and foot (4%) [55]. Of all the spine injuries, only 13% required surgery [55]. Injuries to the odontoid and the C1–C2 level are the most frequent spinal injuries [5, 6] and can result from a seemingly trivial mechanism of injuries such as a fall from standing or seating height. Around 95% of the pelvis fractures did not require surgical management from which lateral compression injury types are most frequently encountered [56], whereas 10% of the acetabulum fracture were treated operatively [55]. Long bones, pelvic, rib, and sternal fractures are most commonly seen due to osteoporosis. These fractures are usually more complex secondary to bone osteoporosis, making it more fragile or the presence of prosthesis/implants. Adults aged 70 years old are less likely to have solid organ injuries compared with younger patients [57]. Although abdominal traumas are rare, they, much like other injuries, have four times higher mortality compared to the younger trauma patients [5, 58] and are significantly more frequent in the non-survivors [59].

1.3.1 Falls

In the largest aggregation of U.S./Canadian trauma registry data, NTDB reports falls as the leading cause of admission in a trauma center, while the largest number of deaths are caused by fall-related injuries [1]. Elderly patients presented with an ISS ≥ 16 were more likely to have sustained a fall from any height [48, 60] and less likely to have sustained a firearm injury [60]. When comparing younger and older groups, same-level falls resulted in serious injury 30% of the time in the elderly group compared with 4% in the younger patients [48]. In the same study, falls from standing height were also responsible for an ISS above 15, approximately 30-fold more in the elderly group [48].

Low energy falls are responsible for more than 50% of traumatic-related deaths in patients over 65 years old, while they account for only 9–11% of injury-related deaths in younger individuals [61, 62]. Additionally, the elderly are up to 4 times more likely to die from a fall compared with patients under the age of 65 years old [3, 49]. Traumatic brain injury [4, 63, 64] and long bone fractures [4] are the leading cause of mortality and morbidity following a fall. Other injuries that commonly occur to the elderly following ground-level falls are cervical spine fractures, rib fractures, and pelvis fractures, which are most frequently lateral compression injuries, while abdominal injuries are rare [64]. Death-related falls from a low height (≤3 m) are most commonly associated with fractures of the skull, cervical spine, and thoracic injuries and are more likely to occur as the height of the fall increases, whereas fracturing of the lower extremities is more likely to occur as the height of the fall decreases [65]. In the same study, postmortem skeletal analysis reports only a rare incidence of upper extremity fractures in cases of fatal low free falls [65]. Growing evidence supports the promotion of ground-level falls as high-energy mechanism of injury in geriatric trauma.

1.3.2 Traffic-Related Injuries

Traffic-related injuries account for 10–25% of trauma admission in the elderly population [3]. Although this particular population does not necessarily have a higher incidence of traffic-related accidents [35], they have twice the mortality rate as compared to their younger counterpart [3, 35–37, 66, 67], either as a driver, a passenger, or a pedestrian. Patients aged more than 55 years old are more likely to sustain severe (ISS ≥ 16) or critical injuries (ISS ≥25) with a higher rate of severe head injuries (AIS head/neck score ≥ 3) [18, 36], spinal injuries [18], pelvis fractures [18], and chest injuries [18, 35–37], from which the three most common include rib fractures [35–37], flail chest [35], and sternum fractures [35]. While younger patients have a higher rate of abdominal, solid organ (spleen, liver, kidney), and facial injuries [18, 35], operative rates for chest, abdomen, and musculoskeletal injuries are similar for both group ages [35]. Moreover, the number of rib fractures has been correlated with increased mortality and risk of pneumonia [37]. As such, healthcare providers should maintain a high suspicion index for chest injuries in this population and scrutinize radiographs for chest wall fractures that are easily missed on plain, low-quality, radiographs taken in the trauma bay [35].

1.3.3 Pedestrian Injuries

In regard to pedestrian injuries, tibia and combined tibia and femur fractures are more common in adults and the elderly, whereas femur fractures are more common in children [15, 17]. This propensity for femur fracture is likely related to the patient's height and location of the first impact. In general, patients older than 55 years will have more intracranial injuries [15, 17, 68], upper [68] and lower extremity fractures [15, 17, 68], and more pelvic fracture [15, 68], but similar rate of solid organ injury [17, 68], abdomen [17, 68], and GI injuries [17, 68]. The seriousness of the injuries also showed a significant linear increase with increasing age [15, 17] along with mortality rate [3, 15, 17, 68]. While spinal injuries are uncommon in children and young adults, the risk of spinal injuries increases significantly with age [15, 17], demonstrating the importance to have a high index of suspicion when evaluating the spine in elderly patients.

1.3.4 Other Mechanism of Injuries

Other mechanisms of injuries include penetrating trauma, abuse and assaults, and burns. They are less frequent in the elderly compared with their younger counterparts; nevertheless, they are associated with higher mortality, longer ICU stay [69], higher morbidity [69], more complications [69], and longer length of hospital stay [69] and less likely to be discharged home [69]. Geriatric patients have the highest suicide risk among all age group [70] and constitute the third leading cause of injury in this population [71]. Patients older than 75 years were significantly more likely than patients 55–74 years old to suffer self-inflicted injuries [72]. The most common methods used are firearms and jumping from height [73, 74], both of which are associated with the highest case-fatality rate [1].

1.4 Outcomes

1.4.1 Comorbidities and Mortality

The in-hospital death rate in geriatric trauma victims has been estimated from 15% to 30%, whereas mortality in younger patients has been estimated at 4–8% [8, 75–78]. One explanation is the higher comorbidity rate compared with younger patients [49, 50, 79], longer Intensive Care Unit (ICU) stay [3, 35], and higher rate of overall complications [3, 80, 81], which increase the likelihood of death or severe disability [50]. In a meta-analysis by Hashmi et al. [8], combined odds of dying in those older than 74 years was 1.67 (96% CI, 1.34–2.08) compared with patients aged 65–74 years old, while no significant difference was observed between those aged 75–84 years old compared with those older than 84 years old. However, registry-based cohort reported a linear relationship between age and mortality rate [47, 82, 83]. Among all injuries, head traumas, spinal cord, and extremity injuries have the highest risk of in-hospital mortality, with severe head injury correlating with mortality the most [4].

Geriatric status [80, 81, 84], ISS (≥9 and ≥16) [47, 63, 76, 80–85], GCS (≤8) [20, 47, 63, 76, 81–83, 85], intubation [20, 47], coagulopathy and blood thinners [20, 63], anemia [63, 85], fluid requirements [76, 82, 84], dementia [86], and pre-existing pulmonary conditions [86], cardiovascular [80, 81, 86] or liver disease [80, 81, 86], and chronic renal failure [20, 81, 86] have been shown to be predictors of mortality. Similarly, the development of cardiovascular complications [76, 80], ARDS [76], renal failure [80] or infections [47, 76, 80], and geriatric status [80, 81, 84] also contribute to a higher mortality rate. A retrospective review comparing mortality and outcomes in the early decade vs late decade could not report a significant decrease in hospital mortality or ICU length of stay [87]. Others have reported a slight, but barely significant, improvement in mortality rates over the past 10 years [83, 88].

1.4.2 Discharge Status

Elderly trauma patients are more likely to be discharged into a care facility compared with younger patients with similar injuries [36]. Grossman et al. [78] examined long-term survival and functional status in geriatric trauma patients 5 years after previous study completion; nearly half of the patients were still alive, with 22% of geriatric patients still living at home. The authors report that although it was not possible to determine the true cost-effectiveness of this outcome, it is likely considered as a desirable outcome following trauma and appreciable long-term survival with a reasonable functional status can be anticipated for some [78]. In another study, recorded discharge disposition demonstrated that 45% of patients were ultimately discharged home, and 76% returned to baseline independence with activities of daily living or returned to the baseline level of activity [89].

The ISS and comorbidities appear to play a role in predicting mortality, but not necessarily functional outcome and discharge status [11, 32, 89]. Geriatric patients older than 80 years have poorer functional outcomes than those aged 65–80 years [90]. Furthermore, geriatric patients who do not respond to aggressive resuscitation efforts within a timely fashion are more likely to have poorer outcomes [11]. The EAST guidelines propose to consider less aggressive resuscitation measures in "non-responders" or without improvement within 72 h in patients with initial GCS score less than 8 [11, 12]. Although elderly victims are at higher risk of mortality and morbidity than younger patients, we are not able to accurately predict functional outcomes based on initial presentation, with the exception of severe head injury [11]. This requires prompt and aggressive treatment program to allow geriatric patients to regain their preinjury functional level.

1.4.3 Palliative Care and Withdrawal of Care

A recent evidence-based review by EAST has not shown a definitive and solid evidence to justify the use of routine palliative care in the geriatric population, while no studies have effectively assessed the impact on discharge disposition, quality of life, pain, and long-term functional status [7]. The argument for routine palliative care in geriatric trauma patients is driven by the decreased length of stay [91–93] and hospital costs [91] without negatively impacting mortality in the ICU [94, 95]. However, Kupensky et al. [93] compared geriatric trauma patients who had received a palliative medicine consultation compared with those who had not; patients receiving palliative care were significantly older, had higher mean ISS, and higher mortality rate than patients who did not receive palliative care.

Withdrawal of support remains more common in the very old patient. There remains a paucity of documentation in regard to advance directives and code status [96, 97]. Patients receiving palliative medicine care were significantly more likely to discuss advanced directives and resulted in consensus around goals of care [93].

1.5 Conclusion

The geriatric population is expected to live longer, with more comorbidities, while having more active lives much more later in life, thereby engaging in activities that increase the risk of high-energy trauma [3]. One must recognize one's own bias regarding treatment of the geriatric patient as well as the increased mortality rate associated with this specific population even in instances of low energy traumas. Evidence suggests very little, if any, improvement in incidence rates of fall-related injuries and death and the need for much-needed investment in preventive measures. No specific factors have been found to be predictive of functional outcomes, and aggressive management is warranted as there remains a substantial potential to retain the elderly as active and productive members of society, even after a significant trauma [50].

References

1. (COT) ACoSACoT. National Trauma Data Bank Annual Report 2016. 2016 [cited 2020 August 21]; Available from: https://www.facs.org/quality-programs/trauma/tqp/center-programs/ntdb/docpub.
2. Henary BY, Ivarsson J, Crandall JR. The influence of age on the morbidity and mortality of pedestrian victims. Traffic Inj Prev. 2006;7(2):182–90.
3. Lowe JA, Pearson J, Leslie M, Griffin R. Ten-year incidence of high-energy geriatric trauma at a level 1 trauma center. J Orthop Trauma. 2018;32(3):129–33.
4. Thompson HJ, McCormick WC, Kagan SH. Traumatic brain injury in older adults: epidemiology, outcomes, and future implications. J Am Geriatr Soc. 2006;54(10):1590–5.
5. Mandavia D, Newton K. Geriatric trauma. Emerg Med Clin North Am. 1998;16(1):257–74.
6. Lomoschitz FM, Blackmore CC, Mirza SK, Mann FA. Cervical spine injuries in patients 65 years old and older: epidemiologic analysis regarding the effects of age and injury mechanism on distribution, type, and stability of injuries. Am J Roentgenol. 2002;178(3):573–7.
7. Aziz HA, Lunde J, Barraco R, Como JJ, Cooper Z, Hayward Iii T, et al. Evidence-based review of trauma center care and routine palliative care processes for geriatric trauma patients; A collaboration from the American Association for the Surgery of Trauma Patient Assessment Committee, the American Association for the Surgery of Trauma Geriatric Trauma Committee, and the Eastern Association for the Surgery of Trauma Guidelines Committee. J Trauma Acute Care Surg. 2019;86(4):737–43.
8. Hashmi A, Ibrahim-Zada I, Rhee P, Aziz H, Fain MJ, Friese RS, et al. Predictors of mortality in geriatric trauma patients: a systematic review and meta-analysis. J Trauma Acute Care Surg. 2014;76(3):894–901.
9. McCoy GF, Johnstone RA, Duthie RB. Injury to the elderly in road traffic accidents. J Trauma Acute Care Surg. 1989;29(4):494–7.
10. Marciani RD. Critical systemic and psychosocial considerations in management of trauma in the elderly. Oral Surg Oral Med Oral Pathol Oral Radiol Endodontol. 1999;87(3):272–80.
11. Jacobs DG, Plaisier BR, Barie PS, Hammond JS, Holevar MR, Sinclair KE, et al. Practice management guidelines for geriatric trauma: the EAST Practice Management Guidelines Work Group. J Trauma Acute Care Surg. 2003;54(2):391–416.
12. Calland JF, Ingraham AM, Martin N, Marshall GT, Schulman CI, Stapleton T, et al. Evaluation and management of geriatric trauma: an Eastern

Association for the Surgery of Trauma practice management guideline. J Trauma Acute Care Surg. 2012;73(5):S345–S50.
13. Kuhne CA, Ruchholtz S, Kaiser GM, Nast-Kolb D. Mortality in severely injured elderly trauma patients—when does age become a risk factor? World J Surg. 2005;29(11):1476–82.
14. Campbell-Furtick M, Moore BJ, Overton TL, Phillips JL, Simon KJ, Gandhi RR, et al. Post-trauma mortality increase at age 60: a cutoff for defining elderly? Am J Surg. 2016;212(4):781–5.
15. Demetriades D, Murray J, Martin M, Velmahos G, Salim A, Alo K, et al. Pedestrians injured by automobiles: relationship of age to injury type and severity. J Am Coll Surg. 2004;199(3):382–7.
16. Davis JW, Kaups KL. Base deficit in the elderly: a marker of severe injury and death. J Trauma Acute Care Surg. 1998;45(5):873–7.
17. Hannon M, Hadjizacharia P, Chan L, Plurad D, Demetriades D. Prognostic significance of lower extremity long bone fractures after automobile versus pedestrian injuries. J Trauma Acute Care Surg. 2009;67(6):1384–8.
18. Talving P, Teixeira PGR, Barmparas G, DuBose J, Preston C, Inaba K, et al. Motorcycle-related injuries: effect of age on type and severity of injuries and mortality. J Trauma Acute Care Surg. 2010;68(2):441–6.
19. Vollmer DG, Torner JC, Jane JA, Sadovnic B, Charlebois D, Eisenberg HM, et al. Age and outcome following traumatic coma: why do older patients fare worse? J Neurosurg. 1991;75(Supplement):S37–49.
20. Bala M, Willner D, Klauzni D, Bdolah-Abram T, Rivkind AI, Gazala MA, et al. Pre-hospital and admission parameters predict in-hospital mortality among patients 60 years and older following severe trauma. Scand J Trauma Resusc Emerg Med. 2013;21(1):91.
21. Morris JA, Mackenzie EJ, Damiano AM, Bass SM. Mortality in trauma patients: the interaction between host factors and severity. J Trauma Acute Care Surg. 1990;30(12):1476–82.
22. Lineberry C, Stein DE. Infection, sepsis, and immune function in the older adult receiving critical care. Crit Care Nurs Clin. 2014;26(1):47–60.
23. Braunstein M, Kusmenkov T, Mutschler W, Kammerlander C, Böcker W, Bogner-Flatz V. Polytrauma in older adults leads to significantly increased TIMP-1 levels in the early posttraumatic period. J Immunol Res. 2020;2020
24. Baltazar GA, Bassett P, Pate AJ, Chendrasekhar A. Older patients have increased risk of poor outcomes after low-velocity pedestrian–motor vehicle collisions. Pragmatic Observ Res. 2017;8:43.
25. Boss GR, Seegmiller JE. Age-related physiological changes and their clinical significance. West J Med. 1981;135(6):434.
26. Weisfeldt M. Aging, changes in the cardiovascular system, and responses to stress. Am J Hypertens. 1998;11(S2):41S–5S.
27. Hossack KF, Bruce RA. Maximal cardiac function in sedentary normal men and women: comparison of age-related changes. J Appl Physiol. 1982;53(4):799–804.
28. Davies MJ, Lye M. Pathology of the aging heart. In: Textbook of geriatric medicine and gerontology. Edinburgh: Churchill Livingstone; 1992. p. 181–5.
29. Feldman RD, editor. Physiological and molecular correlates of age-related changes in the human beta-adrenergic receptor system; 1986.
30. Rommens PM, Kuhn S. Principles of damage control in the elderly. In: Damage control management in the polytrauma patient. Springer; 2017. p. 249–61.
31. Demarest GB, Osler TM, Clevenger FW. Injuries in the elderly: evaluation and initial response. Geriatrics. 1990;45(8)
32. McMahon DJ, Shapiro MB, Kauder DR. The injured elderly in the trauma intensive care unit. Surg Clin. 2000;80(3):1005–19.
33. Sartorelli KH, Rogers FB, Osler TM, Shackford SR, Cohen M, Vane DW. Financial aspects of providing trauma care at the extremes of life. J Trauma Acute Care Surg. 1999;46(3):483–7.
34. Fairman R, Rombeau JL, Miller TA. Physiologic problems in the elderly surgical patient. Physiologic basis of modern surgical care. St Louis: CV Mosby; 1988. p. 1108–17.
35. Yee WY, Cameron PA, Bailey MJ. Road traffic injuries in the elderly. Emerg Med J. 2006;23(1):42–6.
36. Bauzá G, LaMorte WW, Burke PA, Hirsch EF. High mortality in elderly drivers is associated with distinct injury patterns: analysis of 187,869 injured drivers. J Trauma Acute Care Surg. 2008;64(2):304–10.
37. Bulger EM, Arneson MA, Mock CN, Jurkovich GJ. Rib fractures in the elderly. J Trauma Acute Care Surg. 2000;48(6):1040–7.
38. Lyles KW. Osteoporosis: pathophysiology, clinical presentation, and management. Textb Internal Med. 1997:2536–41.
39. Gowing R, Jain MK. Injury patterns and outcomes associated with elderly trauma victims in Kingston, Ontario. Can J Surg. 2007;50(6):437.
40. Chang DC, Bass RR, Cornwell EE, MacKenzie EJ. Undertriage of elderly trauma patients to state-designated trauma centers. Arch Surg. 2008;143(8):776–81.
41. Xiang H, Wheeler KK, Groner JI, Shi J, Haley KJ. Undertriage of major trauma patients in the US emergency departments. Am J Emerg Med. 2014;32(9):997–1004.
42. Garwe T, Stewart K, Stoner J, Newgard CD, Scott M, Zhang Y, et al. Out-of-hospital and inter-hospital under-triage to designated tertiary trauma centers among injured older adults: a 10-year statewide geospatial-adjusted analysis. Prehosp Emerg Care. 2017;21(6):734–43.
43. Lehmann R, Beekley A, Casey L, Salim A, Martin M. The impact of advanced age on trauma triage decisions and outcomes: a statewide analysis. Am J Surg. 2009;197(5):571–5.

44. Zuercher M, Ummenhofer W, Baltussen A, Walder B. The use of Glasgow Coma Scale in injury assessment: a critical review. Brain Inj. 2009;23(5):371–84.
45. Heffernan DS, Thakkar RK, Monaghan SF, Ravindran R, Adams CA Jr, Kozloff MS, et al. Normal presenting vital signs are unreliable in geriatric blunt trauma victims. J Trauma Acute Care Surg. 2010;69(4):813–20.
46. Chapleau W, Haskin D, LeBlanc P, Cardenas G, Borum S, Torres N, et al. Advanced trauma life support (ATLS®): the ninth editio; 2013.
47. Labib N, Nouh T, Winocour S, Deckelbaum D, Banici L, Fata P, et al. Severely injured geriatric population: morbidity, mortality, and risk factors. J Trauma Acute Care Surg. 2011;71(6):1908–14.
48. Sterling DA, O'connor JA, Bonadies J. Geriatric falls: injury severity is high and disproportionate to mechanism. J Trauma Acute Care Surg. 2001;50(1):116–9.
49. Brown CVR, Rix K, Klein AL, Ford B, Teixeira PGR, Aydelotte J, et al. A comprehensive investigation of comorbidities, mechanisms, injury patterns, and outcomes in geriatric blunt trauma patients. Am Surg. 2016;82(11):1055–62.
50. Keller JM, Sciadini MF, Sinclair E, O'Toole RV. Geriatric trauma: demographics, injuries, and mortality. J Orthop Trauma. 2012;26(9):e161–e5.
51. Shifflette VK, Lorenzo M, Mangram AJ, Truitt MS, Amos JD, Dunn EL. Should age be a factor to change from a level II to a level I trauma activation? J Trauma Acute Care Surg. 2010;69(1):88–92.
52. Docimo S Jr, Demin A, Vinces F. Patients with blunt head trauma on anticoagulation and antiplatelet medications: can they be safely discharged after a normal initial cranial computed tomography scan? Am Surg. 2014;80(6):610–3. Epub 2014/06/03
53. Ivascu FA, Howells GA, Junn FS, Bair HA, Bendick PJ, Janczyk RJ. Rapid warfarin reversal in anticoagulated patients with traumatic intracranial hemorrhage reduces hemorrhage progression and mortality. J Trauma Acute Care Surg. 2005;59(5):1131–9.
54. Ivascu FA, Janczyk RJ, Junn FS, Bair HA, Bendick PJ, Howells GA. Treatment of trauma patients with intracranial hemorrhage on preinjury warfarin. J Trauma Acute Care Surg. 2006;61(2):318–21.
55. Abdelfattah A, Core MD, Cannada LK, Watson JT. Geriatric high-energy polytrauma with orthopedic injuries: clinical predictors of mortality. Geriatr Orthop Surg Rehab. 2014;5(4):173–7.
56. Henry SM, Pollak AN, Jones AL, Boswell S, Scalea TM. Pelvic fracture in geriatric patients: a distinct clinical entity. J Trauma Acute Care Surg. 2002;53(1):15–20.
57. Peterson BE, Jiwanlal A, Della Rocca GJ, Crist BD. Orthopedic trauma and aging: it isn't just about mortality. Geriatr Orthop Surg Rehab. 2015;6(1):33–6.
58. Young L, Ahmad H. Trauma in the elderly: a new epidemic? Aust N Z J Surg. 1999;69(8):584–6.
59. Akköse Aydýn Þ, Bulut M, Fedakar R, Özgürer A, Özdemir F. Trauma in the elderly patients in Bursa. Turkish J Trauma Emerg Surg. 2006;12(3):230–4.
60. Reich MS, Dolenc AJ, Moore TA, Vallier HA. Is early appropriate care of axial and femoral fractures appropriate in multiply-injured elderly trauma patients? J Orthop Surg Res 2016;11(1):1–6.
61. Baker SP, Harvey AH. Fall injuries in the elderly. Clin Geriatr Med. 1985;1(3):501–12.
62. Hogue CC. Injury in late life: Part I. Epidemiology. J Am Geriatr Soc. 1982;30(3):183–90.
63. Schoeneberg C, Probst T, Schilling M, Wegner A, Hussmann B, Lendemans S. Mortality in severely injured elderly patients: a retrospective analysis of a German level 1 trauma center (2002–2011). Scand J Trauma Resusc Emerg Med. 2014;22(1):45.
64. Bhattacharya B, Maung A, Schuster K, Davis KA. The older they are the harder they fall: injury patterns and outcomes by age after ground level falls. Injury. 2016;47(9):1955–9.
65. Rowbotham SK, Blau S, Hislop-Jambrich J, Francis V. Skeletal trauma resulting from fatal low (≤3 m) free falls: an analysis of fracture patterns and morphologies. J Forensic Sci. 2018;63(4):1010–20.
66. Azami-Aghdash S, Aghaei MH, Sadeghi-Bazarghani H. Epidemiology of road traffic injuries among elderly people; a systematic review and meta-analysis. Bull Emerg Trauma. 2018;6(4):279.
67. Etehad H, Yousefzadeh-Chabok SH, Davoudi-Kiakalaye A, Moghadam DA, Hemati H, Mohtasham-Amiri Z. Impact of road traffic accidents on the elderly. Arch Gerontol Geriatr. 2015;61(3):489–93.
68. Siram SM, Sonaike V, Bolorunduro OB, Greene WR, Gerald SZ, Chang DC, et al. Does the pattern of injury in elderly pedestrian trauma mirror that of the younger pedestrian? J Surg Res. 2011;167(1):14–8.
69. Nagy KK, Smith RF, Roberts RR, Joseph KT, An GC, Bokhari F, et al. Prognosis of penetrating trauma in elderly patients: a comparison with younger patients. J Trauma. 2000;49(2):190–3.
70. Baker S, Baker SP, Ginsburg MJ, Li GG, O'Neill B. The injury fact book. USA: Oxford University Press; 1992.
71. Binder S. Injuries among older adults: the challenge of optimizing safety and minimizing unintended consequences. Injury Prev. 2002;8(Suppl. 4):iv2–4.
72. Lustenberger T, Inaba K, Schnüriger B, Barmparas G, Eberle BM, Lam L, et al. Gunshot injuries in the elderly: patterns and outcomes. A national trauma databank analysis. World J Surg. 2011;35(3):528–34.
73. Stevens JA, Hasbrouck LM, Durant TM, Dellinger AM, Batabyal PK, Crosby AE, et al. Surveillance for injuries and violence among older adults. Morb Mortal Wkly Rep: CDC Surveillance Summaries. 1999:27–50.
74. Abrams RC, Marzuk PM, Tardiff K, Leon AC. Preference for fall from height as a method of suicide by elderly residents of New York City. Am J Public Health. 2005;95(6):1000–2.
75. MacKenzie EJ, Rivara FP, Jurkovich GJ, Nathens AB, Frey KP, Egleston BL, et al. A national evaluation of the effect of trauma-center care on mortality. N Engl J Med. 2006;354(4):366–78.

76. Tornetta P, Mostafavi H, Riina J, Turen C, Reimer B, Levine R, et al. Morbidity and mortality in elderly trauma patients. J Trauma Acute Care Surg. 1999;46(4):702–6.
77. Dimitriou R, Calori GM, Giannoudis PV. Polytrauma in the elderly: specific considerations and current concepts of management. Eur J Trauma Emerg Surg. 2011;37(6):539–48.
78. Grossman MD, Ofurum U, Stehly CD, Stoltzfus J. Long-term survival after major trauma in geriatric trauma patients: the glass is half full. J Trauma Acute Care Surg. 2012;72(5):1181–5.
79. Bergeron E, Clement J, Lavoie A, Ratte S, Bamvita J-M, Aumont F, et al. A simple fall in the elderly: not so simple. J Trauma Acute Care Surg. 2006;60(2):268–73.
80. Perdue PW, Watts DD, Kaufmann CR, Trask AL. Differences in mortality between elderly and younger adult trauma patients: geriatric status increases risk of delayed death. J Trauma Acute Care Surg. 1998;45(4):805–10.
81. Grossman MD, Miller D, Scaff DW, Arcona S. When is an elder old? Effect of preexisting conditions on mortality in geriatric trauma. J Trauma Acute Care Surg. 2002;52(2):242–6.
82. Ley EJ, Clond MA, Srour MK, Barnajian M, Mirocha J, Margulies DR, et al. Emergency department crystalloid resuscitation of 1.5 L or more is associated with increased mortality in elderly and non-elderly trauma patients. J Trauma Acute Care Surg. 2011;70(2):398–400.
83. Ringen AH, Gaski IA, Rustad H, Skaga NO, Gaarder C, Naess PA. Improvement in geriatric trauma outcomes in an evolving trauma system. Trauma Surg Acute Care Open. 2019;4(1):e000282.
84. Hammer PM, Storey AC, Bell T, Bayt D, Hockaday MS, Zarzaur BL Jr, et al. Improving geriatric trauma outcomes: a small step toward a big problem. J Trauma Acute Care Surg. 2016;81(1):162–7.
85. Ross SW, Adeyemi FM, Zhou M, Minhajuddin AT, Porembka MR, Cripps MW, et al. One-year mortality in geriatric trauma patients: improving upon the geriatric trauma outcomes score utilizing the social security death index. J Trauma Acute Care Surg. 2019;87(5):1148–55.
86. Camilloni L, Farchi S, Rossi PG, Chini F, Borgia P. Mortality in elderly injured patients: the role of comorbidities. Int J Injury Control Safety Promotion. 2008;15(1):25–31.
87. Samayoa AX, Vu T, Olszewski T, Bova M, Yan Q, Kirton O. Have outcomes improved in trauma patients age 90 years and older over the past decade: experience at a level II trauma center. Am J Surg. 2018;215(6):1000–3.
88. Maxwell CA, Miller RS, Dietrich MS, Mion LC, Minnick A. The aging of America: a comprehensive look at over 25,000 geriatric trauma admissions to United States hospitals. Am Surg. 2015;81(6):630–6.
89. Ferrera PC, Bartfield JM, D'Andrea CC. Outcomes of admitted geriatric trauma. Am J Emerg Med. 2000;18(5):575–80.
90. Grossman M, Scaff DW, Miller D, Reed Iii J, Hoey B, Anderson Iii HL. Functional outcomes in octogenarian trauma. J Trauma Acute Care Surg. 2003;55(1):26–32.
91. Khandelwal N, Benkeser D, Coe NB, Engelberg RA, Teno JM, Curtis JR. Patterns of cost for patients dying in the intensive care unit and implications for cost savings of palliative care interventions. J Palliat Med. 2016;19(11):1171–8.
92. Katrancha ED, Zipf J. Evaluation of a virtual geriatric trauma institute. J Trauma Nurs. 2014;21(6):278–81.
93. Kupensky D, Hileman BM, Emerick ES, Chance EA. Palliative medicine consultation reduces length of stay, improves symptom management, and clarifies advance directives in the geriatric trauma population. J Trauma Nurs. 2015;22(5):261–5.
94. Mosenthal AC, Murphy PA, Barker LK, Lavery R, Retano A, Livingston DH. Changing the culture around end-of-life care in the trauma intensive care unit. J Trauma Acute Care Surg. 2008;64(6):1587–93.
95. Matsushima K, Schaefer EW, Won EJ, Armen SB. The outcome of trauma patients with do-not-resuscitate orders. J Surg Res. 2016;200(2):631–6.
96. McBrien ME, Kavanagh A, Heyburn G, Elliott JRM. 'Do Not Attempt Resuscitation'(DNAR) decisions in patients with femoral fractures: modification, clinical management and outcome. Age Ageing. 2013;42(2):246–9.
97. Trunkey DD, Cahn RM, Lenfesty B, Mullins R. Management of the geriatric trauma patient at risk of death: therapy withdrawal decision making. Arch Surg. 2000;135(1):34–8.

2 Cardiovascular Ageing

Marco Luciani, Frank Ruschitzka, and Giovanni G. Camici

2.1 Epidemiology

According to the World Health Organization, cardiovascular diseases (CVD) are the leading causes of morbidity and mortality in industrialized nations, and they are expected to become the first cause of mortality also in low- and middle-income countries in the near future.

Incidence of CVD has reached pandemic proportions in light of combined social changes and medical improvements occurred in the last decades, resulting in a significant demographic shift that will lead by 2040 to a 22% prevalence of subjects older than 65 [1]. Owing to numerous preventive, diagnostic, and therapeutic means implemented on a global scale, life expectancy has dramatically increased over the course of the last 50 years, resulting in a 16.5 year gain in life expectancy within this timeframe and reaching a life expectancy of 71.9 years worldwide.

M. Luciani (✉)
Department of Internal Medicine, Cantonal Hospital of Baden, Baden, Switzerland

F. Ruschitzka
Department of Cardiology, University Heart Center, University Hospital Zurich, Zurich, Switzerland
e-mail: frank.ruschitzka@usz.ch

G. G. Camici
Department of Cardiology, University Heart Center, University Hospital Zurich, Zurich, Switzerland

Center for Molecular Cardiology, University of Zurich, Schlieren, Switzerland
e-mail: giovanni.camici@uzh.ch

Increased life expectancy has, particularly in high-income areas, expanded the terminal phase of life which is characterized by a series of different disabilities affecting the quality of life itself where non-mutually exclusive CVD lead to a final stage of cardiac impairment called heart failure [2]. Concomitantly, the clinical picture and therefore the general population outlook is heterogeneous with non-cardiovascular diseases also playing a role. Together with intrinsic risk factors, environmental ones such as nutrition [3], alcohol abuse [4], lack of physical exercise [5], and pollution [6] can determine the morphofunctional phenotype of cardiac impairment.

A recent population study in the UK showed that, despite a reduction in the annual incidence of heart failure diagnosis (−7%), its prevalence increased (+12%) in light of adequate public health policies and effective therapeutic strategies [7].

These numbers are translated into a public healthcare system challenge with an annual expenditure of nearly $125,000 per heart failure patient, a sum that is doomed to increase in the near future [8].

2.2 Features

With ageing, the cardiovascular system undergoes a series of structural and functional changes dictated by molecular and cellular mechanisms affecting different anatomical structures such as

H.-C. Pape et al. (eds.), *Senior Trauma Patients*, https://doi.org/10.1007/978-3-030-91483-7_2

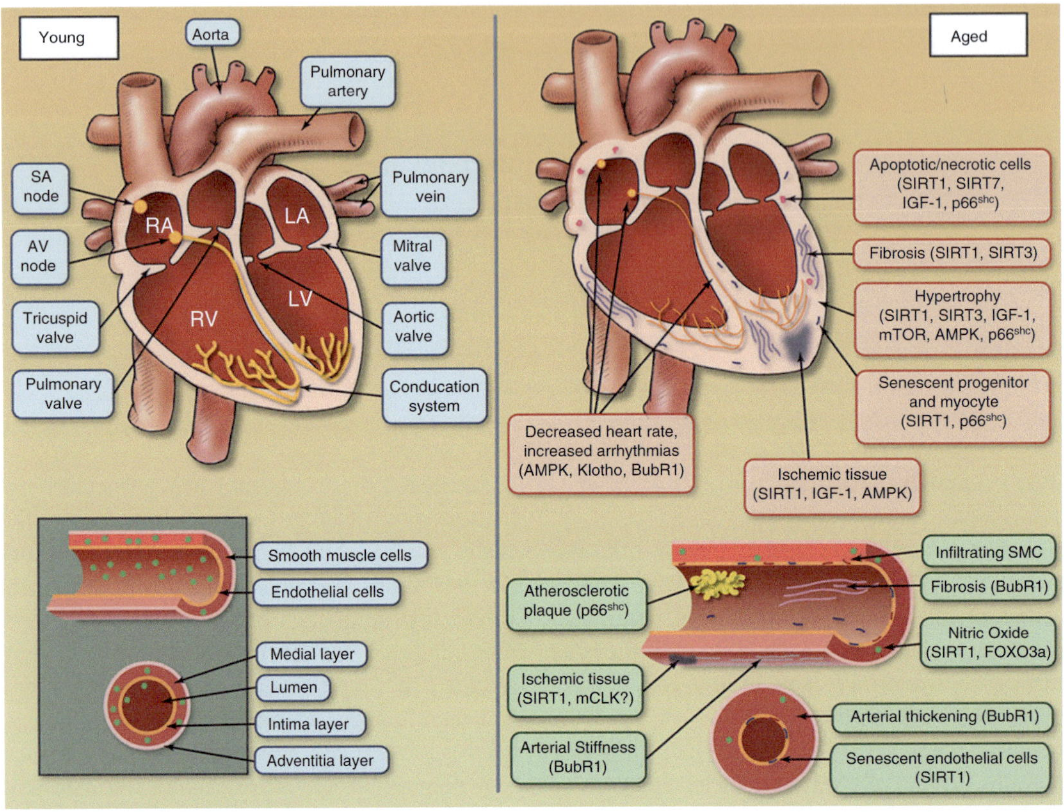

Fig. 2.1 Age-dependent changes to cardiovascular tissues. Molecular, cellular, and tissue changes occurring with time ultimately altering morphology and function of the heart and vessels. (North BJ, Sinclair DA, *The Intersection between Aging and Cardiovascular Disease,* Circulation Research 2012;110:1097–1108)

the myocardium, the valve apparatus, the conduction system, and the vasculature as shown in Fig. 2.1.

The indisputable evidence connecting CVD with age notwithstanding, it still remains elusive whether ageing per se should be considered as an independent risk factor, a process, or rather an epiphenomenon of accumulated stochastic molecular events exhausting compensatory defensive response and ultimately yielding to reduced homeostasis and therefore morbid conditions.

2.3 Arterial Ageing

Over time, significant peripheral and coronary vascular changes occur leading to the two most common forms of CVD observed in the elderly: arterial hypertension and coronary artery disease (CAD). A key early step in the development of these diseases is represented by endothelial dysfunction where the bioavailability of nitric oxide (NO)—a key protective factor with vasodilatory, anti-adhesion, and anti-aggregation properties—is drastically reduced.

2.3.1 Arterial Ageing: Arterial Hypertension

Starting from the age of 50, arterial hypertension in elderly patients is principally characterized by isolated, elevated systolic pressure with a progressive decline in diastolic pressure, intuitively leading to widened pulse pressure and an increased pulse wave velocity (PWV). Such condition is primarily driven by concomitant endothelial dysfunction and central arterial stiffness, which are intimately interconnected within a self-sustaining vicious cycle of hemodynamic load, endothelial activation, inflammation, and persistent damage. Endothelial dysfunction includes reduced vasodilatatory capability determined by reduced NO bioavailability [9], impaired endothelial-dependent responsiveness to prostaglandins [10], increased levels of the vasoconstrictor endothelin-1, and systemic molecular signature changes towards pro-inflammatory molecules, i.e. TNF-alpha, IL-6. Such changes are associated with altered vascular homeostasis, favouring a prooxidant and pro-inflammatory milieu with a tendency to cardiovascular adverse events [11]. On the other hand, arterial stiffness is due to altered proteolytic activities by metalloproteinases (MMPs), cathepsins, and neutrophil elastase as well as an age-related increased production of TGF-β favouring abnormal elastin fragmentation, fibers calcification, augmented collagen deposition, endothelial senescence, and tissue invasion by inflammatory cells and smooth muscle cells overgrowth [12]. This process is macroscopically translated into luminal enlargement and wall thickening as well as wall stiffening with reduced arterial distensibility yielding an increased PWV.

In order to compensate these changes and preserve sufficient peripheral perfusion, the myocardium undergoes a series of cellular, structural, and functional ploys which in the long run predispose to irreversible chronic cardiac dysfunction. As shown in Fig. 2.2, increased aortic impedance and ventricular loading are counteracted by increased wall tension featuring augmented wall thickness and prolonged systole.

A longer systolic interval is possible when time from diastole is borrowed. In order to preserve contractile activity, this physiological compromise causes an incomplete relaxation and thus forces the heart to increase its cavities as well as filling pressures.

2.3.2 Arterial Ageing: Coronary Artery Disease

Among CVD, CAD is the most common cause of morbidity and mortality in elderly patients responsible for nearly one-fifth of death cases and representing the first aetiology of heart failure [13] as illustrated in Fig. 2.3.

In comparison to the general population, elderly patients are usually more difficult to diagnose in light of the concomitant comorbidities and of atypical clinical presentation; this still holds true despite this subpopulation being more frequently affected and with extended involvement of the coronary tree.

Pathogenesis of *CAD* is based on a plethora of interconnected factors determining atherosclerosis. Despite being initially considered solely as a cholesterol storage disease, it is now accepted that inflammation plays a central role in atherosclerotic plaque formation, progression, and rupture. Initiation sites are usually localized in peculiar sectors where laminar blood flow is disturbed (branches); lack of luminal elastin coupled with proteoglycans exposure favours subendothelial low-density lipoproteins' (LDL) deposition. In the presence of inflammatory cells, LDLs are a vulnerable substrate to a number of posttranslational modifications as well as to oxidative stress caused by myeloperoxidase or lypoxygenases release. LDL oxidation triggers endothelial adhesion molecules overexpression (CCL5, CXCR3, CCL2, CCR5, CCR2, CXCR1), promoting further cellular invasion. Over time, plaques evolve from fatty streaks where T-cells and monocytes-derived foam cells load are predominant towards more complex histological lesions [14–16].

The natural history of CAD is strongly affected by age: in fact, CAD is more commonly diagnosed in aged individuals and a positive direct correlation between age and number and size of lesions is present. As later discussed, compensatory myocardial hypertrophy represents an additional metabolic challenge for coronary cir-

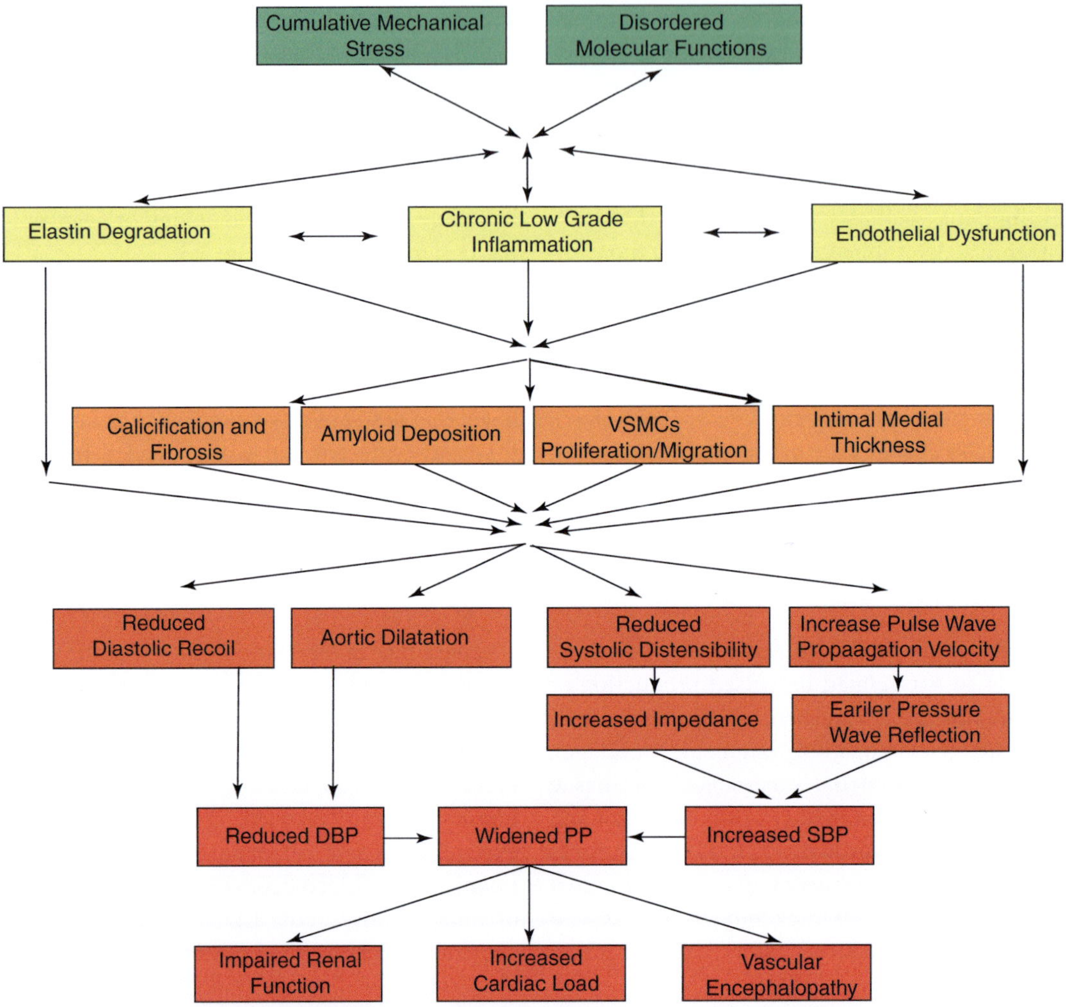

Fig. 2.2 Conceptual model of arterial ageing and arterial decline. Herein are reported the intertwined, compensating mechanisms which will eventually lead to the well-characterized vascular dysfunction of the elderly (Lakatta EG. So! What's Ageing? Is Cardiovascular Ageing a Disease? Journal of Molecular and Cellular Cardiology;83:1–13)

culation. With prolonged systolic time, reduced luminal diameter, and decreased vascular density, chronic and/or acute ischemic damage can occur more frequently.

Specific histological features distinguish atherosclerotic lesions that are more prone to rupture and thus cause acute coronary syndromes. Such lesions are usually larger, presenting a bigger necrotic core (cell debris and cholesterol crystals) and a protective fibrous cap invaded by pro-inflammatory cells and less smooth muscle cells [17].

2.3.3 Arterial Ageing: Cardiac Microvascular Disease

Microcirculation is defined as blood vessels with a diameter inferior to 100 mm and its role is particularly important in regulating tissue perfusion and cell function in response to the release of a multitude of dilating and constricting factors [18].

Even in the absence of image-detectable and clinically significant coronary lesions, dysfunc-

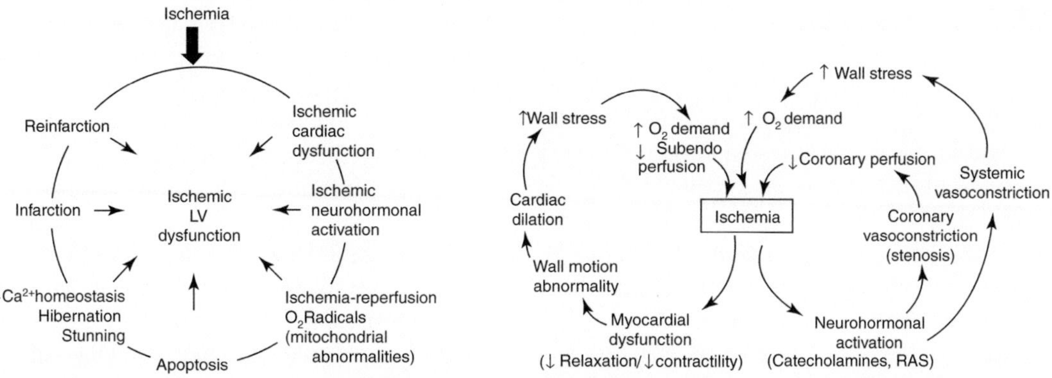

Fig. 2.3 The vicious cycle of myocardial ischemia—Ischemic damage, independently of magnitude and extension, leads to ventricular dysfunction which is temporarily compensated by a number of physiological ploys (autonomic, neurohormonal, etc.) preserving myocardial function. Over time, these ploys exhaust their compensatory capabilities yielding to a decompensated myocardium. (Remme WJ, *Overview of the relationship between ischemia and congestive heart failure*, Clinical Cardiology 2000;23 (Suppl. IV):1–13)

tional microcirculation can dramatically change patients' prognosis. Microcirculation can be affected in a wide range of chronic and acute conditions (ischemia, hypertension, diabetes, obesity, tobacco use, renal impairment, and with age per se). As previously mentioned, senescent endothelium as well as smooth muscle cells, in low calibre arterioles, tend to lose their capability to regulate vascular resistance and match energy request with blood flow, ultimately affecting cardiac performance itself and increasing the chances of myocardial ischemia. In fact, myocardial oxygen extraction tends already to maximal capabilities in resting conditions, and therefore its delivery heavily relies on blood flow. In case of increased oxygen demand, a proportional increase in coronary blood flow must be matched with metabolic requests [19, 20].

2.4 Myocardial Hypertrophy

Pathological myocardial hypertrophy as frequently observed in the elderly is an irreversible process governed by different yet intertwined molecular pathways in contrast to the physiological reversible hypertrophy observed in other conditions such as in athletes. Hypertrophy in the failing ageing heart is characterized by cellular loss, partially compensated with survived hypertrophic cardiomyocytes, and due to the aforementioned ischemic burden, progressively replaced with nonfunctional fibroblasts.

Such structural changes can be regarded as a maladaptation of cardiomyocytes to mechanical and chemical stress events, reactivating the so-called "fetal gene program" by promoting chromatin remodelling, transcriptional, and posttranscriptional upregulation for specific genes transcription factors such as the myocyte enhancer factor 2 (MEF2A-C), erythroid transcription factor (GATA4).

Upon reactivation, a series of common fetal isoforms genes are accessed for transcription such as muscle creatine kinase (Ckm), alpha myosin chain (Myh-6), myosin light chain (Myl1), and Troponins C and I (Tnnc1, Tnni3). It is now widely accepted that the aberrant expression of fetal genes in the postnatal heart involved in contractility, calcium handling, and myocardial energetics has only a temporary beneficial effect as it bears a negative prognostic significance [21].

2.5 Amyloidosis

An additional, yet underestimated, cause of myocardial hypertrophy is represented by amyloidosis caused by the extracellular deposition of insoluble fibrils. This is an autoptic finding; in nearly 20% of subjects older than 80, it is the amyloid deposition within the myocardium.

Amyloid plaques are stable, extracellular aggregates derived from proteinaceous by-products yielding to histological changes and organ dysfunction. All amyloidoses have a common pathogenic mechanism consisting of erroneous protein folding. In fact, each protein sequence undergoes a number of quality control systems in order to acquire a correct tridimensional structure and therefore fulfil the physiological function, localization, and interactions. In the unfortunate, yet not uncommon, case of combined adverse events (genetic mutation, protein overproduction, age per se, concomitant comorbidities, iatrogenic factors), proteins can acquire aberrant conformations. Once a single protein is abnormally arranged (monomer) and has overwhelmed additional cellular control systems, it aggregates into larger and more complex structures called oligomers, and further on into fibers and finally deposit into stable and pathognomonic structures called amyloid plaques [22].

With the term cardiac amyloidosis, we engulf a heterogenous group of medical conditions affecting the heart muscle which can have variable degrees of severity, prevalence, and evolution.

Light chain immunoglobulins can affect the heart in 50% of cases depending on the type of cell dyscrasia and median age of presentation can vary for the same reason. Of note, heart failure represents the worst prognostic factor in these patients [23].

Transthyretin, whether wild-type or mutated, is the biological precursor of systemic senile and systemic familial amyloidosis, respectively. In the absence of mutations, the mean age of presentation is around 75 years and cardiac involvement prevalence increases with age. Nowadays, nearly 100 different transthyretin mutations have been reported, each with their peculiar physicochemical properties determining their noxious properties and natural progression. Cardiac involvement greatly varies in terms of age presentation and concomitant nervous involvement based on the type of mutation [24].

Other proteins of cardiac and noncardiac origins can deposit within the myocardium such as Atrial Natriuretic Peptide giving rise to isolated atrial amyloidosis, serum amyloid A to amyloid A amyloidosis, and β_2-microglobulin which tends to deposit in patients with long-standing dialytic treatment [25].

At early stages when typical signs of prominent cardiac involvement such as thickened myocardial walls with reduced electrical voltages on ECG tracings are not apparent yet, cardiac amyloidosis can represent a challenging diagnosis. While endomyocardial biopsy represents the definitive mean for confirming the diagnostic hypothesis [26, 27], Technetium 99 m pyrophosphate (Tc 99 m PYP) cardiac imaging has emerged as a highly sensitive and specific technique for detecting ATTR cardiac amyloidosis and capable of distinguishing it from AL cardiac amyloidosis [28].

2.6 Atrial Fibrillation

AF is already the most commonly occurring dysrhythmia with a lifetime risk for AF of around 25%, indicating that one out of four women or men over age 40 will experience AF.

The estimated global prevalence of AF of 33 million in 2010 is expected to double by 2050 because of population ageing, the rising prevalence of cardiometabolic risk factors, and the improved survival from cardiovascular events [29, 30]. Importantly, prevalence, both of the global incidence and the age-adjusted mortality rates, is also rising [29]. The most important modifiable risk factors, particularly elevated blood pressure and obesity, explain about 50% of the population's attributable risk for AF development.

While AF is associated with a five-fold increase in the risk of ischemic stroke and up to 20% of all strokes are attributable to AF, the lack of temporal relationship between arrhythmia episodes and adverse outcomes has questioned the causal role of AF in the development of stroke.

Characterized by the presence of rapid, irregular, and fibrillatory waves that vary in magnitude, shape, and timing, possibly affecting hemodynamic cardiac performance itself [31], atrial fibrillation usually develops in the context of a diseased left atrium due to the hemodynamical challenges of high filling pressures, as in hypertension and/or heart failure with preserved or reduced ejection and fraction, and altered histological substrates that predispose to arrhythmic event or increased vulnerability. Indeed, on top of structural abnormalities, AF normally requires a trigger event of cardiac or noncardiac origin such as autonomic tone change, neurohormonal activation, inflammation, or other stimuli.

2.7 Valvular Diseases

Cardiac valve diseases are of remarkable importance in the general population; over the last decades, they have changed aetiology and demographic patterns transitioning from prevalent rheumatologic sequelae of the adult to a typical degenerative process of the elderly with increasing prevalence starting from the sixth and seventh decade of life.

As shown in Fig. 2.4, heart valve diseases of any severity rapidly increase from 0.5% before the age of 55 and they reach at least a 12% prevalence in subjects older than 75, with mitral regurgitation being the most common (from 10.9% to 7.1%) form followed by aortic stenosis (4.6–2.8%), aortic regurgitation (2–1.7%), and mitral stenosis (0.2%) [32].

Each type of valve disease challenges the myocardium with peculiar combinations of pressure and/or volume overload determining temporary compensatory responses, ultimately exhausting the morphofunctional reserve of the heart itself and becoming a significant determinant of mortality.

Mitral regurgitation provokes left ventricular cavities enlargement without compensatory wall hypertrophy; on the other hand, aortic insufficiency predisposes to ventricular enlargement coupled to hypertrophy. Patients with aortic stenosis have hypertrophic hearts without cavities dilatation, whereas mitral stenosis presents with significant left atrial enlargement leaving the left ventricle unaffected.

Mitral insufficiency can be divided into two distinct nosocomial entities: a primary degeneration of the valve called organic and a function regurgitation due to altered surrounding structures. Organic mitral valve degeneration can have two major pathogenic mechanisms: myxomatous degeneration or fibroelastic deficiency. The former is believed to be driven by myofibroblast activation secreting MMPs and altering extracellular matrix turnover as well as TGF-β sustaining

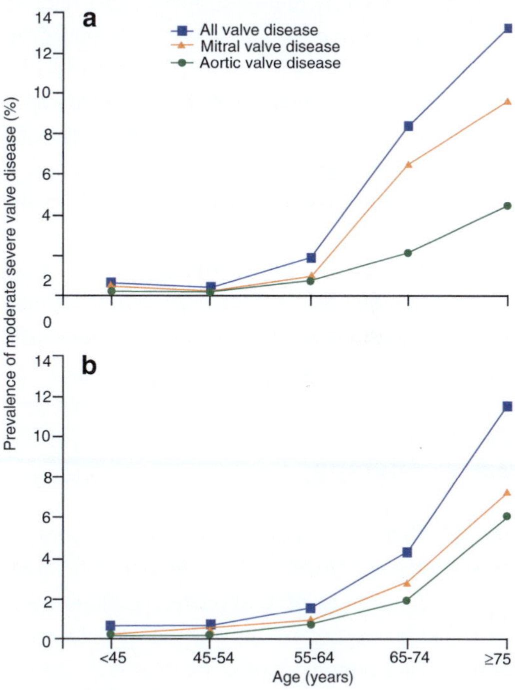

Fig. 2.4 Prevalence of valve heart disease per age**.** Both aortic and mitral valves undergo a series of herein described histological changes that are clinically translated into stenosis and insufficiency. Prevalence increases over the course of three decades from nearly 1% (45–54 years of age) to 12% (>75 years of age) representing a common finding in this population. (Nkomo VT, Gardin JM, Skelton TN, Gottidiner JC, Scott GC, Enrriquez-Sarano M. *Burden of valvular heart diseases: a population-based study*, Lancet. 2006;368: 1005–1011)

myofibroblast proliferation and differentiation. The latter is still not well-understood, but it is characterized by an age-dependent impairment of connective tissue fiber synthesis. Myxomatous mitral valves feature redundant prolapsing tissue, leaflet, and annulus calcification as well as annular dilatation in contrast to the other form which usually tends to tether chordae and eventually rupture them [33, 34]. Patients may remain symptomatic over the vast majority of the natural history of the disease until an irreversible stage characterized by preserved systolic function with pulmonary hypertension or atrial fibrillation begins.

Concerning aortic stenosis, the sclerotic process (with or without stenosis) represents a classic echocardiographic finding of the elderly being detectable in nearly half of subjects older than 85 [35]. Aortic valve calcification is believed to progress with the same cellular and molecular mechanisms of atherosclerosis; nevertheless, such hypothesis remains *open* in light of the lack of benefit from statin therapy.

After a long asymptomatic phase where the myocardium can counteract flow obstruction with compensatory hypertrophy, patients with severe aortic stenosis rapidly complain of angina, syncope, and fatigue and mortality rate abruptly rises to 25% per year [36].

2.8 Therapy

Medical therapeutic mainstays of the various cardiovascular conditions rely on judicious evaluation in the setting of polymorbic patients who most likely require multidrug therapy. In addition, renal function should be regularly monitored in order to correctly provide dose medication and to avoid expectable, adverse, and overdosing effects. Unfortunately, the elderly population is underrepresented in the vast majority of clinical trials in spite of the unmet need for tailored medical therapy for this subpopulation. The above-mentioned complex clinical scenario poses an additional challenge in the decision making process since classic, clinical hard endpoints should be coupled with the quality of life and frailty scoring systems. In fact, life expectancy might not be perceived as a pivotal determinant by senior patients who are more concerned in preserving their daily activity independence.

Conflict of Interest *Prof. Ruschitzka has not received personal payments by pharmaceutical companies or device manufacturers in the last 3 years (remuneration for the time spent in activities, such as participation as steering committee member of clinical trials and member of the Pfizer Research Award selection committee in Switzerland, were made directly to the University of Zurich). The Department of Cardiology (University Hospital of Zurich/University of Zurich) reports research-, educational-, and/or travel grants from Abbott, Amgen, Astra Zeneca, Bayer, Berlin Heart, B. Braun, Biosense Webster, Biosensors Europe AG, Biotronik, BMS, Boehringer Ingelheim, Boston Scientific, Bracco, Cardinal Health Switzerland, Corteria, Daiichi, Diatools AG, Edwards Lifesciences, Guidant Europe NV (BS), Hamilton Health Sciences, Kaneka Corporation, Kantar, Labormedizinisches Zentrum, Medtronic, MSD, Mundipharma Medical Company, Novartis, Novo Nordisk, Orion, Pfizer, Quintiles Switzerland Sarl, Sahajanand IN, Sanofi, Sarstedt AG, Servier, SIS Medical, SSS International Clinical Research, Terumo Deutschland, Trama Solutions, V-Wave, Vascular Medical, Vifor, Wissens Plus, and ZOLL. The research and educational grants do not impact on Prof. Ruschitzka's personal remuneration.*

References

1. Heidenreich PA, Trogdon JG, Khavjou OA, et al. Forecasting the future of cardiovascular disease in the United States: a policy statement from the American Heart Association. Circulation. 2011;123:933–44.
2. Braunwald E. Heart failure. JACC Heart Fail. 2013;1:1–20.
3. Miller V, Mente A, Dehghan M, et al. Fruit, vegetable, and legume intake, and cardiovascular disease and deaths in 18 countries (PURE): a prospective cohort study. Lancet. 2017;390:2037–49.
4. Whitman IR, Agarwal V, Nah G, et al. Alcohol abuse and cardiac disease. J Am Coll Cardiol. 2017;69:13–24.
5. Lear SA, Hu W, Rangarajan S, et al. The effect of physical activity on mortality and cardiovascular disease in 130,000 people from 17 high-income, middle-income, and low-income countries: the PURE study. Lancet. 2017;390:2643–54.
6. Aung N, Sanghvi MM, Zemrak F, et al. Association between ambient air pollution and cardiac morpho-functional phenotypes: insights from the UK Biobank Population Imaging Study. Circulation. 2018;138:2175–86.
7. Conrad N, Judge A, Tran J, et al. Temporal trends and patterns in heart failure incidence: a population-

based study of 4 million individuals. Lancet. 2018;391:572–80.
8. Lesyuk W, Kriza C, Kolominsky-Rabas P. Cost-of-illness studies in heart failure: a systematic review 2004–2016. BMC Cardiovasc Disord. 2018;18:74.
9. Donato AJ, Eskurza I, Silver AE, et al. Direct evidence of endothelial oxidative stress with aging in humans: relation to impaired endothelium-dependent dilation and upregulation of nuclear factor-kappaB. Circ Res. 2007;100:1659–66.
10. Singh N, Prasad S, Singer DR, MacAllister RJ. Ageing is associated with impairment of nitric oxide and prostanoid dilator pathways in the human forearm. Clin Sci (Lond). 2002;102:595–600.
11. Camici GG, Sudano I, Noll G, Tanner FC, Luscher TF. Molecular pathways of aging and hypertension. Curr Opin Nephrol Hypertens. 2009;18:134–7.
12. Chung HY, Sung B, Jung KJ, Zou Y, Yu BP. The molecular inflammatory process in aging. Antioxid Redox Signal. 2006;8:572–81.
13. Remme WJ. Overview of the relationship between ischemia and congestive heart failure. Clin Cardiol. 2000;23:IV4–8.
14. Libby P, Theroux P. Pathophysiology of coronary artery disease. Circulation. 2005;111:3481–8.
15. Libby P. Inflammation in atherosclerosis. Nature. 2002;420:868–74.
16. Weber C, Noels H. Atherosclerosis: current pathogenesis and therapeutic options. Nat Med. 2011;17:1410–22.
17. Virmani R, Burke AP, Farb A, Kolodgie FD. Pathology of the vulnerable plaque. J Am Coll Cardiol. 2006;47:C13–8.
18. Gutterman DD, Chabowski DS, Kadlec AO, et al. The human microcirculation: regulation of flow and beyond. Circ Res. 2016;118:157–72.
19. Taqueti VR, Di Carli MF. Coronary microvascular disease pathogenic mechanisms and therapeutic options: JACC State-of-the-Art Review. J Am Coll Cardiol. 2018;72:2625–41.
20. Camici PG, Crea F. Coronary microvascular dysfunction. N Engl J Med. 2007;356:830–40.
21. Dirkx E, da Costa Martins PA, De Windt LJ. Regulation of fetal gene expression in heart failure. Biochim Biophys Acta. 2013;1832:2414–24.
22. Merlini G, Bellotti V. Molecular mechanisms of amyloidosis. N Engl J Med. 2003;349:583–96.
23. Falk RH, Alexander KM, Liao R, Dorbala S. AL (Light-chain) cardiac amyloidosis: a review of diagnosis and therapy. J Am Coll Cardiol. 2016;68:1323–41.
24. Gertz MA, Dispenzieri A, Sher T. Pathophysiology and treatment of cardiac amyloidosis. Nat Rev Cardiol. 2015;12:91–102.
25. Banypersad SM, Moon JC, Whelan C, Hawkins PN, Wechalekar AD. Updates in cardiac amyloidosis: a review. J Am Heart Assoc. 2012;1:e000364.
26. Rapezzi C, Lorenzini M, Longhi S, et al. Cardiac amyloidosis: the great pretender. Heart Fail Rev. 2015;20:117–24.
27. Rapezzi C, Merlini G, Quarta CC, et al. Systemic cardiac amyloidoses: disease profiles and clinical courses of the 3 main types. Circulation. 2009;120:1203–12.
28. Castano A, Haq M, Narotsky DL, et al. Multicenter study of planar technetium 99m pyrophosphate cardiac imaging: predicting survival for patients with ATTR cardiac amyloidosis. JAMA Cardiol. 2016;1:880–9.
29. Chugh SS, Havmoeller R, Narayanan K, et al. Worldwide epidemiology of atrial fibrillation: a Global Burden of Disease 2010 Study. Circulation. 2014;129:837–47.
30. Schnabel RB, Yin X, Gona P, et al. 50 year trends in atrial fibrillation prevalence, incidence, risk factors, and mortality in the Framingham Heart Study: a cohort study. Lancet. 2015;386:154–62.
31. Falk RH. Atrial fibrillation. N Engl J Med. 2001;344:1067–78.
32. Nkomo VT, Gardin JM, Skelton TN, Gottdiener JS, Scott CG, Enriquez-Sarano M. Burden of valvular heart diseases: a population-based study. Lancet. 2006;368:1005–11.
33. Levine RA, Hagege AA, Judge DP, et al. Mitral valve disease--morphology and mechanisms. Nat Rev Cardiol. 2015;12:689–710.
34. Anyanwu AC, Adams DH. Etiologic classification of degenerative mitral valve disease: Barlow's disease and fibroelastic deficiency. Semin Thorac Cardiovasc Surg. 2007;19:90–6.
35. Supino PG, Borer JS, Preibisz J, Bornstein A. The epidemiology of valvular heart disease: a growing public health problem. Heart Fail Clin. 2006;2:379–93.
36. Ross J Jr, Braunwald E. Aortic stenosis. Circulation. 1968;38:61–7.

3 Bone Mineralization and Osteoporotic Changes

Enrique Guerado, Juan Ramón Cano, Vicente Crespo, and Antonio Campos

3.1 Introduction

The human skeleton comprises bones, which are organs that are connected by joints. These joints allow the bones—with the exception of the cranium bones—to move, thanks to the contractions of the muscles inserted on them. This muscle action is regulated by the peripheral nerves, which conduct electrical impulses that originate in the spinal cord. This set of elements is called the locomotor system. It makes it possible to move the lower limbs in order to travel and the upper limbs in order to grasp objects. An adequately developed musculature of the lower limbs allows for normal standing and walking while minimizing falls and the upper limbs also play a role in both actions by providing stability.

There are other soft tissues in this system, including several varieties of connective tissue as well as the skin, which serves as a covering. The entirety of the system is supplied with blood by the vascular system. In addition to movement, the skeleton serves to protect the organs and is also involved in cellular regulation of the hematopoietic system, which is contained within it, and mineral metabolism.

Bone tissue, the substrate that forms the skeleton, is organized into a hierarchical structure called building blocks (BB) [1], which consist of collagen fibers and other proteins configured in intertwined lamellae, osteons, and trabecular as well as cortical bone. This structure is interconnected by molecular links that mechanically join the BBs. Significant changes in bone quantity and quality occur in the structure throughout the lifespan, leading to a decrease in both.

The bone, as an organ, is composed of a compact external structure called cortical bone which encloses another less compact, spongier structure called cancellous bone. The cortical bone is responsible for 80% of the organ's weight. Its function is fundamentally mechanical and protective, although it also plays a role in regulating mineral metabolism when there is a prolonged severe deficiency, as it is affected by the hormonal changes that reach it through the blood supply. For example, in cases of postmenopausal osteoporosis, the cortical bone grows thinner with the passing of the years, especially in the long bones (Fig. 3.1).

Trabecular bone forms both ends of the organ in long bones and is surrounded by cortical bone that is thinner than diaphyseal cortical bone. While trabecular bone is much more active in metabolic processes than cortical bone, it also plays a role in mechanical support, though not for its hardness but rather for the architectural

E. Guerado (✉) · J. R. Cano · A. Campos
Department of Orthopedic Surgery and Traumatology, Costa del Sol University Hospital, University of Málaga, Marbella, Málaga, Spain
e-mail: acampos@ugr.es

V. Crespo
Department of Histology, School of Medicine, University of Granada, Granada, Spain
e-mail: pvcrespo@ugr.es

H.-C. Pape et al. (eds.), *Senior Trauma Patients*, https://doi.org/10.1007/978-3-030-91483-7_3

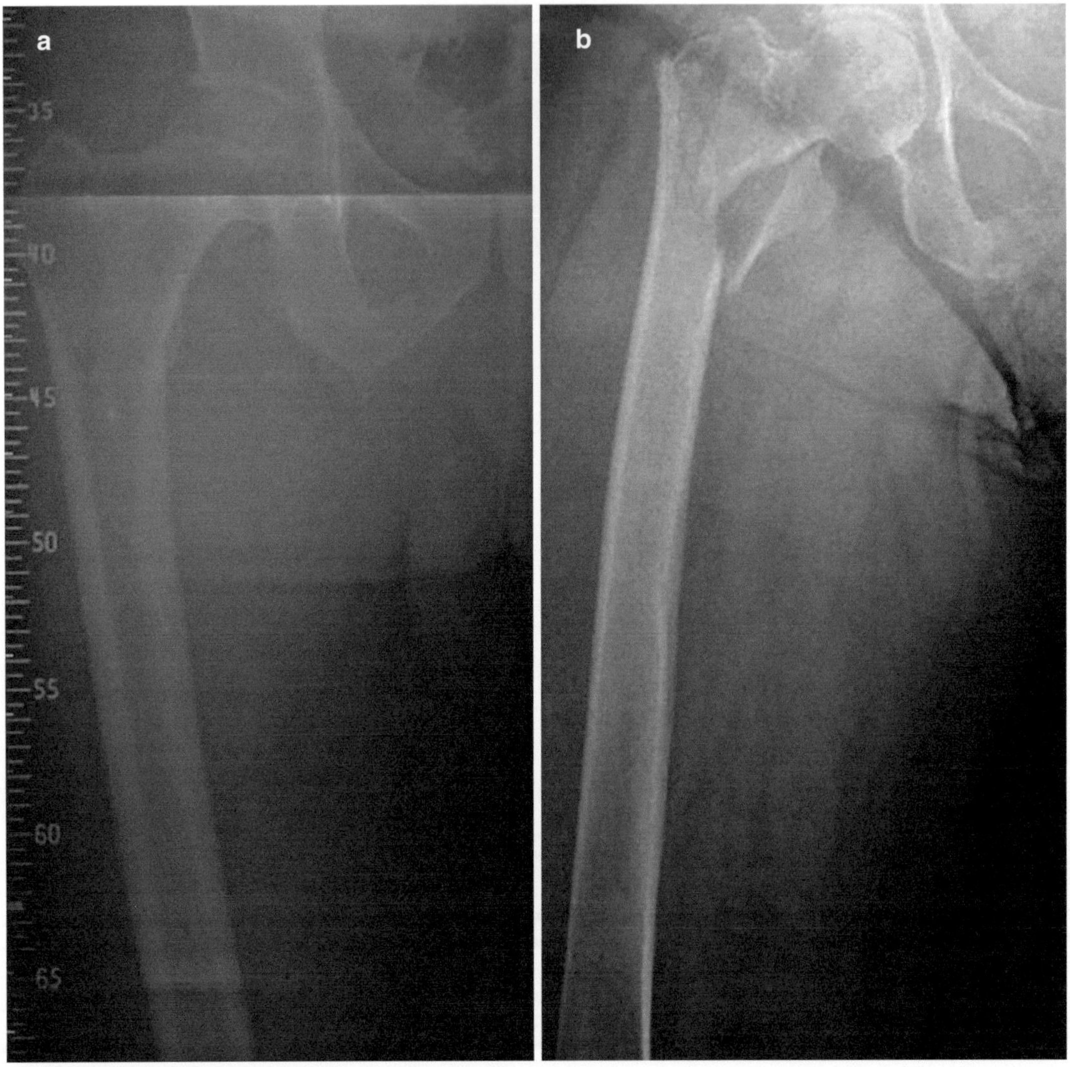

Fig. 3.1 With menopause, the cortical bone is observed to thin considerably, especially the long bones. (**a**) X-ray of a 31-year-old patient. (**b**) X-ray of an 81-year-old patient

arrangement of its trabeculae. This is much more important in short bones, like the vertebrae. However, with age and especially after menopause, bone trabeculae grow fewer and thinner (Fig. 3.2) [2, 3]; as such, the trabeculae structure is less resistant to mechanical stress. This can lead to vertebral fractures due to a low-energy mechanism. These are most common in postmenopausal ages, as the vertebral bodies have a very thin cortical layer, and the trabeculae, due to their decreasing number and thinning, are not able to maintain the height of the vertebrae (Fig. 3.3).

When on a diagnostic imaging test such as an x-ray, it is observed that the cortical bone is thinner and the trabeculae are less numerous and thinner, it is affirmed that the bone is osteoporotic. Although this is a judgment based on anatomical pathology, it is the image of the bone which indicates porosis. That is to say, the pores in the trabeculae are observed to be larger on the diagnostic test. The bone tissue whose image is used to diagnose osteoporosis would have osteopenia, if its matrix is diminished, or osteomalacia, if its matrix is less calcified. If the density analysis is performed via x-ray—on which a loss of 15-30% of bone mass is necessary for the image to be significantly different—osteoporosis will be diagnosed later than if the analyses were performed via a biopsy [4].

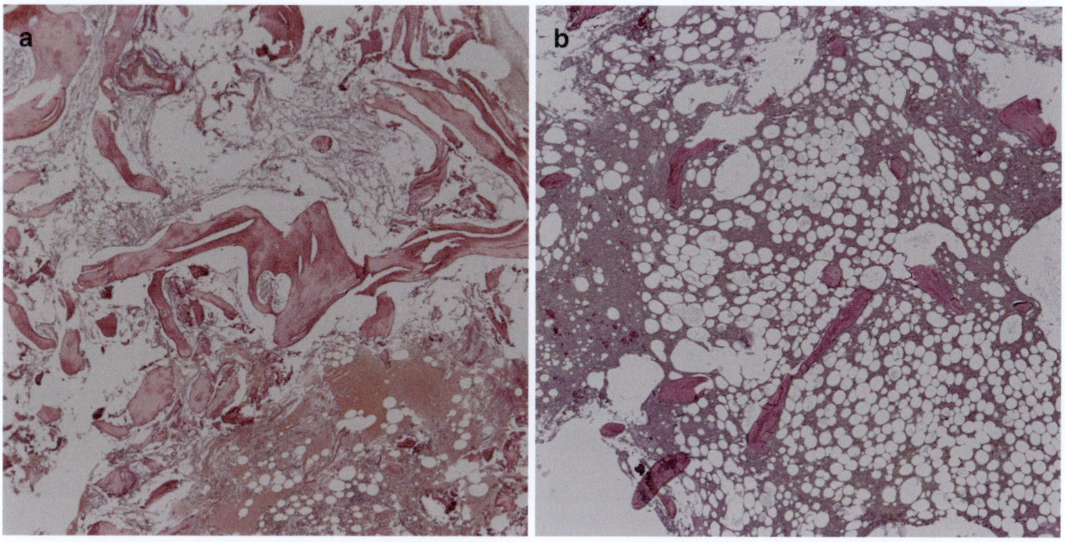

Fig. 3.2 With age, bone trabeculae are thinner and fewer in number, making the trabecular structure less resistant to mechanical stress. (**a**) Image of a bone from a patient with coxarthrosis (obtained via 4× optical microscopy). (**b**) Image of a bone from a patient with osteoporosis (obtained via 4× optical microscopy)

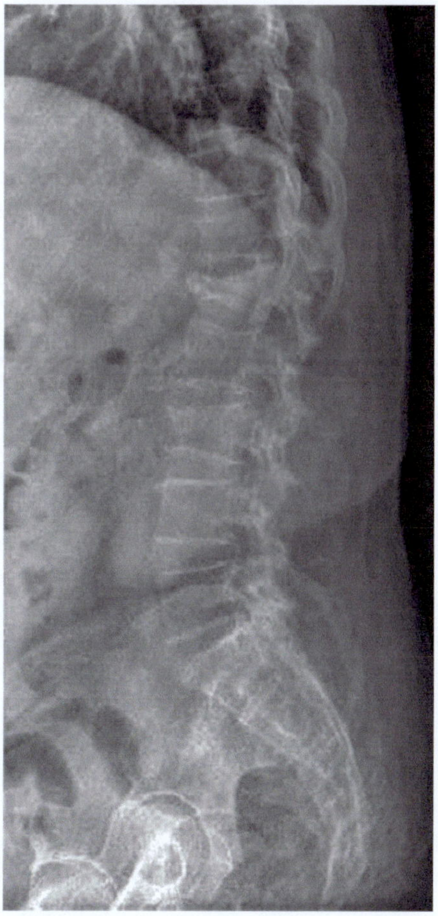

Fig. 3.3 Vertebral fractures due to a low-energy mechanism

Therefore, the concept of osteoporosis is quantitative and based on an image of osteopenia or osteomalacia. Thus, the term osteoporotic fracture is erroneous because osteoporosis is a variable defined based on the image of an osteopenic or osteomalacic bone. Indeed, other variables such as age or sarcopenia, which are also independent variables and which cause falls, do not define a fracture and the use of the terms sarcopenic or senile fracture is not common [4–6]. It would therefore be more correct to use the term fracture in an osteopenic or osteomalacic bone. A fracture in an osteopenic bone thus includes everything from fractures in children who have osteogenesis imperfecta to those in the elderly who have "osteoporosis."

However, usage has made it so that the visual opinion of the anatomy-pathology is inferred and it is understood that osteoporosis is characterized by loss of bone mass, changes in trabecular microstructure, and, as a consequence, skeletal fragility. This leads to a greater risk of fracture as a result of low-energy trauma and greater difficulty in achieving stable osteosynthesis (Fig. 3.4). Nevertheless, there is a more objective definition that differentiates between the concepts of osteoporosis and osteopenia based on the bone mineral density (BMD) T-score [7]. This definition, however, is very controversial [8–13].

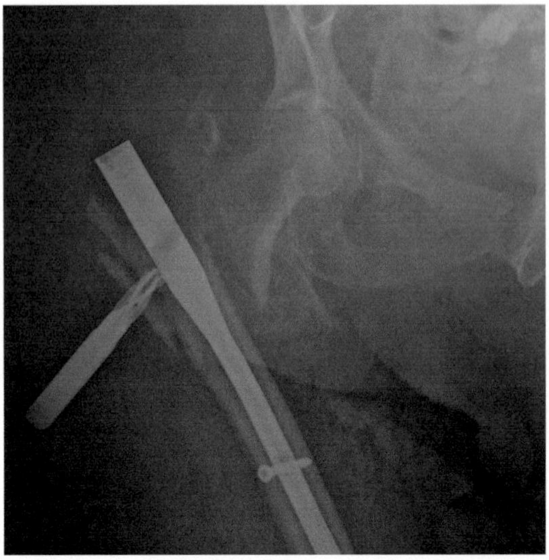

Fig. 3.4 Skeletal fragility leads to greater difficulty in achieving stable osteosynthesis. Loss of reduction and failure of osteosynthesis in a hip fracture

A BMD T-score that is equal to or less than 2.5 standard deviations (SD), after having ruled out other causes of low BMD, is defined as osteoporosis. When the T-score is less than 1-2.5 SD, it is defined as osteopenia. When it is within 1 SD of the value for young adults, BMD is considered normal. Although values below 2.5 SDs tend to indicate a greater risk of fracture, these are more frequent in the 1-2.5 SD range due to the greater number of people in this category. This WHO categorization [7], which has been adopted by patients' associations, has been called into question [9–11, 13] and systematically distorts both the evidence and the evidence-based medicine and indications [8, 12]. As a result, osteopathies that present with fragility are divided into different types, including non-osteopenic (normal bone mass), simple osteopenia (decreased bone mass), or osteopenic disorders that lead to fragility, such as osteoporosis. In clinical practice, however, this classification is not as categorical.

3.2 Bone Cells

Bone tissue is composed of a calcified protein matrix and the cells that regulate it: osteoblasts synthesize the matrix and osteoclasts digest it. In addition, it includes the precursor cells of both as well as other cells related to hematopoiesis and the immune system that are precursors to osteoclasts. When osteoblasts are surrounded by the protein matrix, they differentiate into osteocytes and their functions shift more toward the regulation of bone metabolism than the synthesis of the osteoid matrix.

3.2.1 Osteoblasts

Osteoblasts are cells that secrete the bone matrix protein that is later mineralized. They arise from the differentiation of multipotent mesenchymal stem cells (MSCs) [14] located in the bone marrow, such as stromal cells or pericytes, which are the MSCs adhered to the vascular endothelium and are also fundamental to the formation of blood vessels [15, 16].

The Runx2 protein, also known as core-binding factor alpha-1 (CBFA1), a member of the runt homology domain transcription factor family, is fundamental to the differentiation of MSCs into osteoblasts [17]. Runx2 is the earliest differentiation marker of osteogenic lineage and, along with Runx3, acts in the maturation of hypertrophic chondrocytes [18]. The Sp7 transcription factor (Osterix) and a zinc-finger protein act after Rnx2 and are responsible for the specialization of osteoprogenitor cells into preosteoblasts. The nuclear receptor peroxisome proliferator-activated receptor (PPAR)-gamma also acts, spurring the commitment process of multipotent osteoprogenitor cells [19, 20]. The differentiated osteoblasts express genes for these three proteins as well as for others such as osteopontin, or bone sialoprotein [21, 22]. Runx2 inhibits osteocalcin, halting the cells in differentiation [23]. Osterix controls the transcription of specific genes of osteoblasts, such as osteocalcin, osteopontin, and type I collagen [19].

Wnt proteins are also important. They form part of a group of signaling molecules for skeletal and bone mass development and are mobilized through stimulation of genetic expression of Runx2. Activation of the canonical Wnt pathway gives rise to the formation of a complex of Wnt proteins, low-density lipoprotein receptor-related protein 5 (LRP5), or LRP6, which leads to the phosphorylation and inactivation of glycogen synthase kinase (GSK)-3 beta, inhibition of beta-catenin degradation, and the subsequent accumulation of this metabolite in the osteoblast nucleus [24, 25]. Nuclear beta-catenin binds to the family of TCF/LEF transcription factors and induces expression in the target genes [26]. Therefore, beta-catenin is essential for the differentiation of precursor cells into osteoblasts, preventing differentiation into chondrocytes or adipocytes. The action of beta-catenin in later stages can eliminate or activate osteoclastogenesis through regulation of osteoprotegerin as well as abnormalities in Wnt signaling, which may lead to defects in skeletal homeostasis that can lead to early-onset hereditary osteoporosis or osteogenesis imperfecta, as also occurs with loss of function or mutation in LRP5 [27, 28].

Osteoblasts are arranged lengthwise, increasing their surface area in order to deposit the secreted matrix protein (Fig. 3.5).

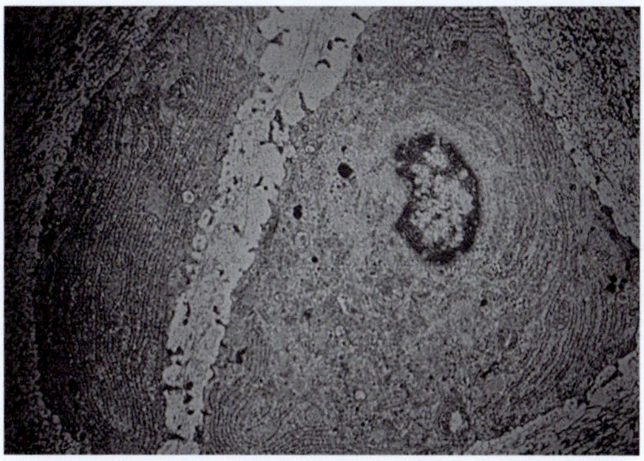

Fig. 3.5 Image of osteoblasts depositing osteoid substance (obtained via electron microscope)

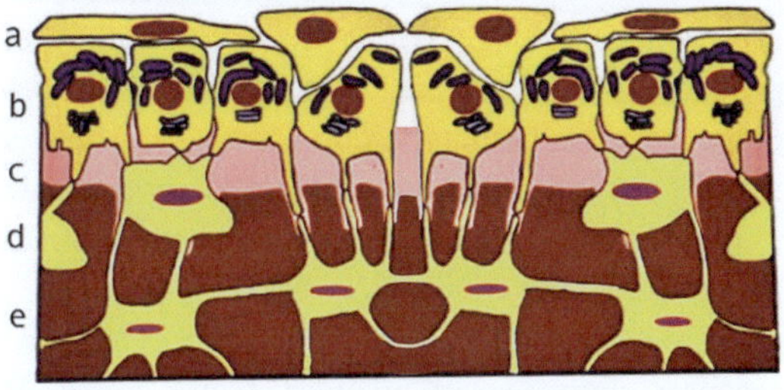

Fig. 3.6 Long cytoplasmic elongations that connect osteocytes to one another. (**a**) Osteoblast precursor cells, (**b**) Osteoblasts. (**c**) Noncalcified extracellular matrix. (**d**) Calcified extracellular matrix. (**e**) Osteocytes with cytoplasmic elongations in the canaliculi

3.2.2 Osteocytes

When osteoblasts are surrounded by osteoid, they differentiate into osteocytes, transforming their phenotype through the development of long cytoplasmic extensions that connect to other osteocytes, surrounded by a gelatinous matrix linked through the bone tissue canaliculi (Fig. 3.6). Osteocytes are the last step in the cellular differentiation of MSCs into the osteogenic line and, therefore, as they are highly differentiated cells, they do not multiply [29]. Many osteoblasts do not differentiate into osteocytes, but rather die by apoptosis [30]. This differentiation is an active process in which the cell develops long cytoplasmic extensions thanks to the action of a protein called podoplanin [31]. Mature osteocytes also express high levels of SOST, an inhibitor of the canonical Wnt/β-catenin pathway. They also intervene in bone regulation through the secretion of sclerostin, a product of the *SOST* gene, which can antagonize LRP5 and LRP6. In fact, the absence of the *SOST* gene leads to a pathological increase in bone mass [27].

Osteocytes express different proteins related to mineral metabolism. These proteins include fibroblast growth factor (FGF), which regulates renal excretion of phosphorus, or matrix extracellular phosphoglycoprotein (MEPE), which inhibits mineralization [32].

Osteocytes, through their cytoplasmic extensions, play a very active role in bone mechanics. The transport of solutes through the canaliculi system that the osteocytic cytoplasmic extensions pass through is regulated by blood pressure and diffusion and convection induced by mechanical stress. This physical and chemical process is called mechanotransduction, a phenomenon by which mechanical stimuli are translated into molecular variations that lead to changes in cellular multiplication and differentiation [33, 34]. Cytoplasmic extensions bind the osteocytes to the collagen, which allows them to note changes in fluids, modulating secretion of sclerostin in order to stimulate bone formation or absorption [35, 36]. This distinctive response of the connective tissue to mechanical stimuli (mechanotransduction) characterizes Wolff's law [37]. This is the reason why physical exercise is so important before and after menopause in order to preserve bone and muscle mass.

3.2.3 Osteoclasts

Osteoclasts are multinucleated cells formed by the fusion of monocytes from the monocyte-macrophage lineage which dissolves bone and produce resorption [38, 39]. The macrophages come from the hematopoietic lineage and have a function in inflammation, although they are now known to also have a role in bone metabolism itself.

Osteoclasts are stimulated by two cytokines: receptor activator of nuclear factor-kappa B ligand (RANKL) and macrophage colony-stimulating factor (M-CSF). They are differentiated from monocytes by the nuclear factor of activated T cells 1 (NAFATc1), the master regulator transcription factor responsible for this differentiation [40–43]. Osteoblasts and osteocytes, whether apoptotic or alive, are the main source of RANKL and osteoprotegerin, the signaling proteins which stimulate bone resorption in osteoclasts, although they are also produced by other cells, such as T lymphocytes [44–46].

The RANKL protein interacts with an osteoclast precursor cell receptor called RANK, which is identical to that of the T-cells and dendritic cells [42]. NFATc1 is induced by RANKL and coactivated by immunoglobulin-like receptors [39, 42, 47]. RANKL also binds to osteoprotegerin or osteoclastogenesis inhibitory factor [39, 42, 47]; as such, when osteoprotegerin or a RANKL antibody is administered to postmenopausal women, bone turnover markers (BTMs) reduce drastically, indicating increasing bone mass.

Bone resorption is carried out by osteoclasts, which have phosphatase acid in their cellular membrane and other hydrolytic enzymes that act on the calcified osteoid, releasing collagen fragments and minerals deposited in the reticular structure that collagen forms together with pyridinoline and deoxypyridinoline. These molecules are also released, circulating freely in the blood until they are excreted in urine [48]. Some of these molecules are digested incompletely and circulate, such as pyridinoline cross-links bound to alpha-1 and alpha-2 chains, which also circulate and are excreted in the same manner [49]. Some diseases, such as diabetes, can interfere with this metabolism [50, 51].

Both acid phosphatase and alkaline phosphate activity take place in other locations, but activities that occur there are fundamentally different from what occur in bone cells in regards to insensitivity to tartrate-tartrate-resistant acid phosphate (TRAP) inhibition, in the case of osteoclastic activity [52], and in regards to hepatic and pancreatic antigenic characterization, in the case of osteoblastic activity.

Therefore, osteocytes, their precursor osteoblasts, osteoclasts, and monocyte-origin cells are molecularly connected so that the bone formation-resorption balance is appropriate [45, 46, 53, 54].

3.3 Osteogenesis and Mineralization

3.3.1 Osteoid Synthesis

Bone formation is initiated by osteoblasts, which synthesize the triple-helix type I collagen of the bone tissue [55, 56] as well as other proteins—including osteocalcin—which combine extracellularly to form the osteoid on which mineralization occurs [57, 58].

This collagen is deposited in layers and strengthened by multiple intra- and intermolecular cross-links, interconnected with an alpha 2 polypeptide chain with two alpha 1 chains. This structure, known as procollagen, goes through a cleavage process in its aminoterminal and carboxyterminal peptides in order to form tropocollagen. In addition to a helicoidal structure, it also has a nonhelicoidal area in the aforementioned terminal peptides called N-telopeptide (NTX) and C-telopeptide (CTX), respectively. [59, 60].

The hydroxylysine side chains of different tropocollagen molecules condense to form a pyridinium ring, thus creating the pyridinoline cross-links that connect three different tropocollagen molecules. A deoxypyridinoline (D-PYR) cross-link is a variant of a pyridinoline cross-link that is formed when two hydroxylysine side chains condense with a lysine side chain. Pyridinoline cross-links are also present in many types of collagen in other tissues, except for in the skin [59, 61, 62]. There are three types of pyridinoline cross-links that are characteristic of bone collagen: D-PYR, which is only found in large amounts in the bone and dentin; N-telopeptide, which is the pyridinoline cross-link in the N-telopeptide region that binds to the alpha 1 and alpha 2 chains; and C-telopeptide, which is a fragment of alpha 1 peptide with an isomerized bond between the aspartate and the glycine of the C-telopeptide region [63, 64].

Immature collagen fibers do not have the necessary tensile strength until they are connected by these covalent bonds, which are resistant to degradation. Noncollagenous proteins in the bone matrix are fundamental in regulating mineralization and strengthening the collagen structure, forming a protein lattice which calcium and phosphate are deposited on in the form of hydroxyapatite crystals [60, 65, 66] (Fig. 3.7).

3.3.2 Mineralization

Noncollagenous proteins that bind calcium include vitamin K-dependent carboxylation/gamma-carboxyglutamic (Gla) proteins—including osteocalcin, which is secreted by osteoblasts—which contain gamma-carboxyglutamic acid and, like many coagulation factors, are vitamin K-dependent [67–69]. Some of these proteins, such as the calcification-inhibiting matrix Gla protein (MGP), can delay mineralization and allow for the bone matrix to mature. In this manner, secondary bone mineralization in humans does not cease suddenly, but rather slowly continues until a calcium content of around 30% of the bone's weight is reached [70].

Although osteocalcin is the most specific protein product of osteoblasts, eliminating the osteocalcin gene does not alter growth or skeletal mineralization [68, 71] due to the concurrence of other proteins. Osteopontin—bone sialopro-

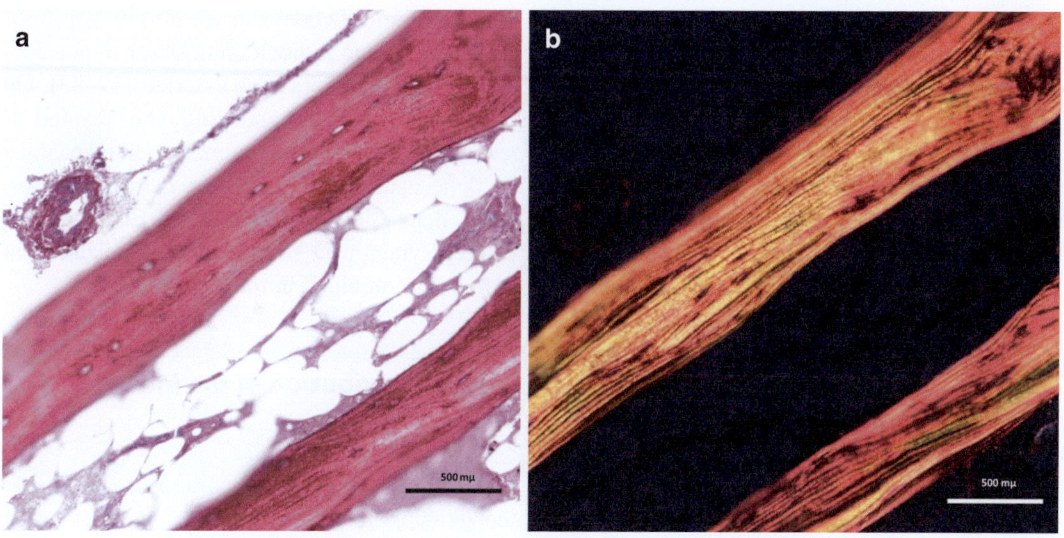

Fig. 3.7 Microscopic images. (**a**) bone trabeculae of a larger size in a patient with coxarthrosis. Picrosirius staining that allows for identification of fibrillar collagens in red on bright-field microscopy. The same staining observed via polarized light microscopy in image (**b**) shows zones in which collagen has a parallel structure, which is seen with positive birefringence (between green, orange, and red). 40×

tein—binds both to calcium and to collagen and can also play a role in the adherence of osteoclasts to the bone surface [22, 72].

Phosphorylated osteopontin (OPN) inhibits the formation of hydroxyapatite crystals, whereas bone alkaline phosphatase (BALP) promotes extracellular mineralization through the release of inorganic phosphate from inorganic pyrophosphate (PPi), which inhibits mineralization. Tartrate-resistant acid phosphatase (TRAP) produced by osteoclasts, osteoblasts, and osteocytes exhibits potent phosphate activity toward osteopontin, though its potential effect on mineralization regulation is unknown. Therefore, osteopontin is important for mineralization inhibition regulated by TRAP, but not by BALP. In conclusion, BALP and TRAP appear to be able to improve the effect of osteopontin on mineralization, suggesting a potential role of TRAP in skeletal mineralization [52, 73].

Crystallized hydroxyapatite that is deposited on the aforementioned protein lattice—collagen or noncollagenous—represents approximately one-fourth of the volume and half of the mass of normal adult bones. The Ca and P (inorganic phosphate) components of these crystals are produced from blood plasma and, in turn, from nutritional sources. Amorphous Ca phosphate matures through various intermediate stages in order to form hydroxyapatite, with the vitamin D metabolites acting as important mediators of Ca regulation. Therefore, vitamin D deficiency will lead to the depletion of bone minerals [74–76]. Likewise, insufficient intake of Ca and P will lead to mineralization defects. Hydroxyapatite crystals may also contain carbonate, fluoride, and a variety of trace minerals, depending on the environment in which the skeleton grows. These crystals are relatively small, which is appropriate for a structure which may be subjected to tension, and thus suffer minor microdamage. However, despite the plasmatic and nutritional origin of the Ca and P that form hydroxyapatite crystals, in a study on bone extracted from the metaphysis of the proximal end of the femur in patients with hip fracture treated surgically with arthroplasty, our group found lower levels of Ca, P, and vitamin D in the blood, but not in bone concentration, when compared to a control group of patients without hip fracture, despite the fact that the patients with hip fracture were malnourished [3]. All results of the samples from both groups were calculated according to the weight of Ca and P [77]. The differences were not statistically significant for Ca, P, or the Ca:P ratio, revealing that bone mineral composition, measured by quantitative microanalysis of trabecular bone obtained from patients with hip fracture, is similar to the bone of patients with hip osteoarthrosis. This finding, associated with abnormal serum Ca and P concentrations (serum/bone levels with a correlation coefficient of -0.197 for Ca and -0.274 for P), refutes the idea of increasing Ca intake or administering medications to increase mineralization in patients with osteoporosis with the objective of preventing hip fractures. Therefore, it is to follow that some authors recommend measuring Ca and P fractions in BMD measurements in order to improve the evaluation of fracture risk and determine more specific therapies [78].

In the literature, there is little evidence of a relationship between bone density and calcium intake, but there is evidence of the occurrence of adverse effects such as gastrointestinal problems, kidney stones, or even cardiovascular problems [79]. Therefore, treatment of osteoporosis with Ca and vitamin D does not seem to be appropriate if there is no hypovitaminosis or hypocalcemia, as many authors have asserted [79–83]. On the other hand, extrapolating the results of research on vitamin D in animals to humans must be done cautiously, given that there are differences depending on the species. For example, whereas vitamin D stimulates mineralization in humans, it inhibits it in rodents [76].

3.3.3 Distribution of the Mineral Phase

In addition to the mineral composition of bone, the geographical distribution of mineralization within the proximal end of the femur is also important. In studies of the nanostructure, composition, and microarchitecture of the superolateral area of the femoral neck in elderly patients with hip fracture compared to healthy control subjects, it was observed that mineral crystals on the external cortical bone surfaces of the fracture group were larger and had a greater mineral content and a more homogeneous mineralization profile. Samples from the patients with hip fracture showed cortical porosity values that were nearly 35% higher [84]. In general, the Ca:P ratio did not appear to differ between the hypermineralized osteocytic lacunae (micropetrosis) and the bone matrix in the osteoporosis and osteoarthrosis groups, though the micropetrosis was greater in the group of patients with hip fractures [84]. Although the role of hypermineralized osteocyte lacunae in bone remodeling and the biomechanical properties of the bone requires more research, these findings are very interesting in regard to the relationship between hypermineralization and susceptibility to femoral neck fracture [85].

3.4 Contribution to Biochemical Homeostasis of the Mineral Phase

3.4.1 Calcium

In addition to its biomechanical function, the mineral fraction of the bone also plays an important role in the regulation of mineral metabolism in the human body. More than 98% of the body's Ca is found in the bone, where in addition to acting as a mechanical support, it serves as an endogenous reservoir. One percent of bone Ca is exchangeable with extracellular fluid in order to maintain a stable Ca equilibrium. The Ca in the extracellular fluid, which, in turn, is 1% of total Ca, is found in various forms: as free ions (active form), ions bound to plasma proteins (predominantly albumin), and in compounds (phosphate, sulfate) [86]. Intestinal absorption of Ca is poor (<50%) and decreases in the elderly [87]. It is eliminated in urine, sweat, and feces. Kidney losses vary little even if the quantity consumed varies greatly. In cases of negative Ca balances, with greater losses than the Ca absorbed in the intestines, calcium levels will remain within normal ranges as a result of reabsorption of bone Ca. Normal total plasma Ca values in healthy adults range from 8.8 to 10.4 mg/dl [88]. Serum calcium levels in patients with hip fracture are lower with respect to patients with coxarthrosis, although this could be an effect of the malnutrition that the majority of these patients present with [3].

3.4.2 Phosphorus

The most important location of phosphorus is in the bone, where 80–85% of phosphorus in the human body is found. The remaining phosphorus is distributed in extracellular fluid and soft tissues. Phosphorus intervenes in a multitude of metabolic processes as an energy store. It acts as a cellular intermediary in membrane transport and is a component of ribonucleic acid (RNA) and deoxyribonucleic acid (DNA) [86]. Normal plasma concentration of phosphorus in an adult is between 2.5 and 4.5 mg/dl. This range is maintained thanks to intestinal absorption, renal tube reabsorption, and intracellular and bone exchanges [88]. Our group found phosphorus levels within normal range in both the group of patients with hip fracture and the control group. However, in the case of the fracture group, phosphorus levels were on the lower limit of normal [3].

3.4.3 Other Ions

Sodium balance regulation within the human body is very complex. Appropriate sodium content in the body is necessary in order to maintain central blood volume and renal perfusion. Therefore, it is closely regulated by homeostatic defense mechanisms mediated by the renin-angiotensin-aldosterone (RAAS) system [89]. The role of elevated sodium intake in health problems has been the subject of controversy [90, 91]. The World Health Organization recommends limiting sodium intake to less than 2 g per day [92]. In the United States of America, it is recommended that sodium intake should not exceed 2300 mg per day or 1500 mg per day or less for certain populations. Sodium increases calcium excretion, which is associated with lower BMD that, in turn, is a predictor of bone fragility risk [89]. Consequently, a hypothesis has been posed that high sodium intake may also be a risk factor for developing osteoporosis [93, 94]. Our group found that the patients with hip fracture presented with lower serum sodium levels than the patients with coxarthrosis [3]. These low serum sodium levels must theoretically be a "protective" mechanism against calcium deficit, but serum calcium was also lower in this group of patients.

A high intake of potassium increases the absorption of calcium, but studies in this regard are not unanimous. Therefore, this could mean that the relationship between sodium intake and osteoporosis may depend on calcium and potassium intake [89, 95]. Our group found that potassium levels in the group of patients with fractures were significantly lower than in the coxarthrosis group [3].

3.5 Age- and Disease-Related Changes in Mineralization

There are other interactions in bone mineralization that in large part are related to age and diseases [62, 96–98].

Whereas gender and bone mass are not associated with bone mineralization, age is indeed related to the populations' average increased calcium concentration spikes, the percentage of highly mineralized bone areas, and mean bone calcium content. Both the bone volume fraction and trabecular thickness are inversely correlated with mean calcium. Trabecular thickness is associated with calcium spikes, high calcium levels, and the quantity of poorly mineralized bone. It is the only structural parameter which can predict bone mineralization independently of age. Variables associated with the osteoid correlate with mineralization parameters and are the only predictor of its heterogeneity. Although elevated trabecular mineralization correlates with age and bone loss, these associations are attributed to the thinning of the bone trabeculae which occurs with high mineralization due to the loss of poorly mineralized bone surfaces. Therefore, it appears that the degree of bone mineral reabsorption is primarily associated with the quantity of osteoid that is physiologically present and the thickness of the mineralized trabecular bone [99].

Menopause is a physiological phenomenon in women that begins at varying ages which tend to range from 45 to 55 years. In menopause, in addition to various clinical symptoms due to hormones, some histological changes in bone also occur; these changes are generally asymptomatic. The mineralized bone matrix appears to be preserved during the first year post-menopause; its density does not change [100]. In young postmenopausal women with vitamin D deficiency, isolated supplementation with 1000 IU of vitamin D3 for 9 months is associated with a reduction in BTMs. However, no differences in BTMs were observed between the group that was supplemented with vitamin D and the group that was not [101].

Inorganic calcium and phosphate are also critically important for many body functions. Consequently, regulation of their plasma concentration is strictly controlled by renal absorption-reabsorption, intestinal absorption, and bone exchange, as bone is a reservoir of calcium and phosphate. Parathyroid hormone and 1,25-dihydroxyvitamin D control calcium homeostasis, whereas these hormones and FGF 23 are derived from bone control phosphate homeostasis [74, 75, 102–105]. As a result, hypoparathyroidism can cause hypocalcemia and hyperphosphatasemia, whereas deficient vitamin D action can cause osteomalacia in adults and rickets in children. On the contrary, hyperparathyroidism can cause hypercalcemia and hypophosphatasemia. In order to diagnose these abnormalities associated with calcium and phosphate metabolism, a laboratory diagnostic test for calcium, phosphate, PTH, and 25-hydroxyvitamin D is very important [74, 75, 102–105].

On the other hand, the combination of elevated mean calcium concentration in the bone and low mineralization heterogeneity in adults with type 2 diabetes can have detrimental effects on the biomechanical properties of the bone. These microscopic abnormalities in bone mineralization, which may be obstructed by suppression of bone remodeling, provoke a higher risk of fracture in adults with type 2 diabetes [50].

3.6 Bone Turnover Markers

Continuous bone remodeling is important because it allows for a bone to adapt to physical requirements, such as load, through the formation of more bone (mechanotransduction) or as a result of chemical stimulants produced by signaling molecules that are released in fractures [33, 34, 37]. Modulation of sclerotin secretion is important in order to stimulate bone formation or bone absorption that occurs based on the cytoplasmic extensions of osteocytes into the collagen, which capture changes [35, 36].

The nature of this continuous replacement of bone tissue can be determined thanks to the measurement of molecules released by osteoblasts and osteoclasts in the bone formation and resorption processes. These BTMs can be measured in blood or urine.

The amino acids that form the cross-link between collagen molecules are released during bone resorption as free forms or as peptides that can be measured in serum or urine. Although cross-links are not exclusive to the bone, given that bone tissue is the largest reservoir of type 1 collagen in the entire human body and is remodeled more quickly than the rest of the connective tissues, it is believed that the majority of cross-links present in the urine of an adult come from the bone resorption process. In this process, collagen begins to break down, releasing free forms of cross-links (40%) and peptide-bound cross-links (60%), both of which are excreted in the urine. Measurement of BTMs is very useful for detecting bone metabolism abnormalities [98].

BMTs are predictive of loss of bone mass and in some studies are used as a fracture risk test [106–109]. However, they must be measured over time because a single measurement is meaningless. Measured over time, progressive bone mass loss does seem to correlate to fracture risk. Therefore, although BMTs are useful when they are measured over time, their variability makes it so that they do not form part of the majority of osteoporosis diagnostic and treatment guidelines, despite their usefulness in detecting lack of response to treatment.

For bone formation, serum measurements of bone-specific alkaline phosphatase (BSAP)—which requires normal liver functioning, given that on the contrary, they may appear abnormal—, osteocalcin, and aminoterminal propeptide of type I procollagen (PINP) are highly clinically useful. The serum concentration of BSAP and osteocalcin shows osteoblastic activity [71]. The serum concentration of carboxyterminal and aminoterminal propeptides of type I collagen (PICP and PINP, respectively) shows changes in the synthesis of new collagen; measuring PINP is more specific than measuring PICP. For bone resorption, the N-telopeptide (NTX) cross-link in urine and the C-terminal telopeptide of type I collagen (ICTX) and the pyridinoline cross-link can be measured in blood [63, 97].

Urine and serum measurements of collagen cross-link concentrations show bone resorption. Therefore, these substances are better indicators of bone resorption than calcium in urine or excretion of hydroxyproline. What is more, as D-PYR and the peptide binding alpha 1 to alpha 2 NTX and ICTX are almost exclusively derived from bone collagen, measurement of these substances specifically shows bone resorption.

The measurement of these metabolites (BTMs) can vary depending on the measurement method as well as patient variables. The circadian rhythm, which peaks at dawn and decreases in the afternoon; a high body mass index; tobacco use; ovulation; and the first 4–6 months following a fracture increase BTMs. Use of contraception, the postprandial period, and physical exercise decrease BTMs. Therefore, urine collection must always be done at the same time mid-morning and in the same laboratory. Likewise, dietary intake also influences these measurements [110].

The validity of BTM measurements must comply with some requirements. Changes in the metabolite must correspond to real changes in turnover measured by means of histomorphometry and calcium kinematics. Serum and urine concentrations of these metabolites must correspond to the appearance of metabolic bone diseases such as those related to the thyroids and parathyroids or to the administration of certain drugs.

Nevertheless, although these markers are useful for understanding a drug's mechanism of action, their role in each patient is unclear; indeed, they are not important for the selection of candidates for osteoporosis treatment. In addition, there is significant variability between individuals, which in some instances may lead to poor clinical interpretation. Furthermore, it is important to note that the predictive validity of variations in BTM values varies according to which BTM is measured. For example, a variation by a factor of more than 2.8 is considered abnormal, whereas for a lower value of NTX to be predictive of improvement in mineral density and decrease of fracture risk, it must be 50% or 30% of serum values of ICTX, PINP, or BSAP [97, 111–113]. (Table 3.1)

3.7 Osteoporosis

Osteoporosis is a generalized skeletal disease classified as an osteopenic fragilizing osteopathy that predisposes individuals to a greater risk of fracture. Therefore, it is called fragilizing because fracture can occur with low-energy trauma. One of the etiopathogenic problems related to these fractures is establishing the limit from which trauma is considered of low- or high-energy. Though it seems clear that vertebral fractures spontaneously appear in patients with osteoporosis, hip fractures require a fall, even if it is from standing, for them to be considered significant trauma. Even a young individual who is not wearing protective gear whose trochanteric area impacts directly on the ground has a high probability of fracturing the hip [114]. However, unlike an elderly person, a young person has reflexes and the protection of the upper limbs to avoid this impact.

Generally speaking, the literature offers diverse classifications of osteoporosis. Five types can be distinguished: Type I: primary or due to a decrease in estrogen; type 2: due to aging; type 3: secondary or due to a genetic or acquired disease excluding menopause or aging, most often metabolic or rheumatic diseases; type IV: idiopathic juvenile; type V: regional due to immobility.

3.7.1 Symptoms and Diagnosis of Postmenopausal Osteoporosis

The majority of postmenopausal women present with osteoporosis due to estrogen deficiency. Medical records show the osteoporosis risk-related medical history, and thus, the indication for the imaging and laboratory tests that should be performed (Table 3.2). Early diagnosis offers the possibility of slowing disease progression, especially in cases of osteoporosis secondary to endocrinologic or rheumatic disease.

In general, there are no symptoms of osteoporosis unless a fracture occurs which reveals the disease. This, among other circumstances, differentiates it from osteomalacia, in which there is pain even if a fracture does not occur. Therefore, it is very common to incidentally observe vertebral fractures as well as a progressive decrease in height in osteoporotic women.

A diagnosis of osteoporosis is usually made when a fracture occurs. These fractures are generally located in the vertebral body, hip, wrist, humerus, rib, or pelvis. Many of them, except for hip and wrist fractures, occur without clinical episodes of pain or trauma. Therefore, the concept of clinical onset of osteoporosis is related to the occurrence of a fracture [2, 87, 114, 115].

Nevertheless, it is believed that a more objective diagnosis of osteoporosis, especially if there has not been a fracture due to fragility, would be when the T-score is less than or equal to 2.5 SD of BMD measured via dual-energy x-ray absorciometry (DXA) and after ruling out other causes of low BMD. The T-score is a comparison of a patient's mean bone density with that of a healthy 30-year-old person of the same sex and ethnicity. This value is used in men and postmenopausal women older than 50 years of age as it better pre-

Table 3.1 Utility of bone turnover markers

Metabolic indicators of bone formation and resorption			
Bone formation	Indicator	Activity	Specificity
Serum	Bone-specific alkaline phosphatase (BSAP)	Osteoblastic activity	High
	Osteocalcin (OC)	Osteoblastic activity	Medium
	Aminoterminal propeptides of type I procollagen (PINP)	Changes in the synthesis of new collagen	High
	Carboxyterminal propeptides of type I collagen (PICP)	Changes in the synthesis of new collagen	Medium
Bone resorption	**Indicator**	**Activity**	**Specificity**
Serum	Cross-links of C-telopeptide of type I collagen (ICTP)	Changes in collagen degeneration	Low
	Tartrate-resistant acid phosphatase (TRAP)	Osteoclastic activity	High
Urine	N-telopeptide of collagen cross-links (NTx)	Osteoclastic activity	High
	C-telopeptide of collagen cross-links (CTx)	Osteoclastic activity	High
	Total and free deoxypyridinoline (Dpd)	Osteoclastic activity	Medium
	Total and free pyridinoline (Pyd)	Osteoclastic activity	Low
	Hydroxyproline	Changes in collagen degeneration	Low

Table 3.2 Osteoporosis risk factors

Osteoporosis risk factors
– Age.
– Female sex.
– Caucasian or Asian race.
– Primary or secondary hypogonadism.
– Primary or secondary amenorrhea.
– Weight (BMI).
– Alcohol/tobacco/caffeine consumption.
– Medical history of fracture due to fragility.
– Use of glucocorticoids.
– Type I diabetes.
– Untreated hyperthyroidism
– Hyperparathyroidism
– Chronic liver disease
– Malnutrition-malabsorption
– Low dietary calcium intake, or vitamin D deficiency
– Low physical activity, prolonged immobilization

dicts the risk of future fractures. Another measurement, the *Z*-score, is the number of SD of a patient with a mean bone density different from the mean bone density that corresponds to a person of their age, sex, and ethnicity. This value is used in premenopausal women, men younger than 50 years of age, and children. It also serves to establish whether a patient has a mean bone density that is so low with respect to his/her age group that it leads the physician to suspect a secondary cause [7].

According to the pharmaceutical industry, all people who present with these abnormalities must have pharmaceutical treatment, even if the clinical situation does not indicate illness [7]. Moreover, the industry claims that people older than an unspecified age should receive pharmaceuticals to increase and preserve their bone mass. Consequently, to the majority of physicians, the elderly population is in large part undertreated. Nevertheless, there is not enough evidence to support these assertions, according to reports from assessment agencies [5, 10, 11, 116]. It is also important to highlight that although all elderly people present with osteopenia, only a small percentage suffer a fall and less than half sustain a lesion as a consequence of trauma. People older than 65 years of age who suffer a fall may have another within 1 year without this necessarily entailing a fracture [117].

Various epidemiological studies have attempted to identify osteoporosis early in order to prevent complex fracture patterns. However, only a better understanding of the molecular pathways, gene expression regulators, and gene expression profiles related to osteoporosis can allow for personalized treatments to be introduced [118–120]. Given that osteoporosis is caused by changes in the number or activities of osteoblasts and osteoclasts, by monitoring the biomarkers of these cells' activities, trends in osteoporosis risk can be identified. However, the majority of osteoporotic fractures occur not in individuals with osteoporosis, but rather in individuals with osteopenic BMD. While osteopenic patients (T-score of BMD −1 to −2.5 SD according to DXA testing) have an individual risk of fracture that is lower than osteoporotic patients (T-score <−2.5 SD), the larger overall number of osteopenic patients means that the majority of fractures will occur in this subset of the total population [121].

Therefore, the positive predictive value of abnormal BTM levels for accelerated bone loss in elderly white women is modest [122]. Due to the low efficiency and cost-effectiveness of detection programs, use of BTMs as a public health measure for identifying patients at increased risk of rapid bone loss is not currently recommendable [116].

The bone equilibrium index is a creative solution to this problem. It is based on a regression to determine the relative quantities of osteocalcin (OC) versus urine NTX observed in a cohort of patients with stable bone mass [123]. Patients are then evaluated in relation to this regression standard in order to determine if their quantity of NTX in relation to osteocalcin is greater than or less than the expected quantity that corresponds to stable bone mass.

It is necessary to distinguish between the capacity of BTMs to predict bone loss, as discussed above, and their capacity to predict fracture risk, as patients may have markedly different fracture risks but the same general level of bone mass due to demographic variations, clinical factors, and bone microarchitecture.

In general, prospective studies that analyze the relationship between bone formation markers and posterior fracture risk have not demonstrated a clear utility for anabolic BTMs for this purpose [122]. On the contrary, many studies have demonstrated that an increase in bone resorption markers is predictive of fracture due to posterior fragility [124].

Comorbid clinical conditions can alter the relationship among BTMs for predicting fracture risk. One of the better studied examples is that measurements of BMD underestimate fracture risk in people with diabetes [125]. ROC analyses have not been able to demonstrate that a combination of low BMD and an increase in BTMs detects more women at risk of fracture than low BMD alone [126].

In conclusion, though BTMs are powerful research tools for epidemiologists who study populations' fracture risks, the current evidence is insufficient for recommending their routine use for identifying individual patients who would optimally benefit from pharmaceutical therapies for osteoporosis. However, a distinction must be made for patients with "secondary" bone loss for reasons such as hyperparathyroidism, hyperthyroidism, vitamin D deficiency, and paraproteinemia, as BTMs may be useful for these subgroups of higher-risk patients.

Furthermore, unlike the limitations of the use of BTMs to identify patients at risk for rapid bone loss, their use in guiding osteoporosis therapy has a clearer potential utility. The pattern of change in BTMs in response to treatment is well-described. These changes have been used to predict both increases in bone density and therapeutic efficiency for reducing fracture risk.

References

1. Bala Y, Seeman E. Bone's material constituents and their contribution to bone strength in health, disease, and treatment. Calcif Tissue Int. 2015;97:308–26. https://doi.org/10.1007/s00223-015-9971-y.
2. Guerado E, Cruz E, Cano JR, Crespo PV, Alaminos M, del Carmen Sánchez-Quevedo M, et al. Bone mineral density aspects in the femoral neck of hip fracture patients. Injury. 2016;47(Suppl. 1):S21–4. https://doi.org/10.1016/S0020-1383(16)30005-5.
3. Cano JR, Crespo PV, Cruz E, Rivas-Ruiz F, Sanchez-Quevedo MC, Guerado E, Campos A. In patients with hip fracture, is the bone tissue of the femoral neck demineralised? Injury. 2019; In editorial process
4. Etxebarria-Foronda I, Caeiro-Rey JR, Larrainzar-Garijo R, Vaquero-Cervino E, Roca-Ruiz L, Mesa-Ramos M, et al. SECOT-GEIOS guidelines in osteoporosis and fragility fracture. An update. Rev Esp Cir Ortop Traumatol. 2015;59:373–93. https://doi.org/10.1016/j.recot.2015.05.007.
5. Guerado E, Sandalio RM, Caracuel Z, Caso E. Understanding the pathogenesis of hip fracture in the elderly, osteoporotic theory is not reflected in the outcome of prevention programmes. World J Orthop. 2016;7:218. https://doi.org/10.5312/wjo.v7.i4.218.
6. Chenbhanich J, Thongprayoon C, Atsawarungruangkit A, Phupitakphol T, Cheungpasitporn W. Osteoporosis and bone mineral density in patients with Wilson's disease: a systematic review and meta-analysis. Osteoporos Int. 2018;29(2):315–22. https://doi.org/10.1007/s00198-017-4295-6.
7. The World Health Organization (WHO). Assessment of fracture risk and its application to screening for postmenopausal osteoporosis. Report of a WHO Study Group. World Health Organ Tech Rep Se. 1994;843:1–129.
8. Upshur REG, Tracy CS. Is evidence-based medicine overrated in family medicine? Yes. Can Fam Physician. 2013;59:1160–1.
9. Tiner R. The pharmaceutical industry and disease mongering. The industry works to develop drugs, not diseases. BMJ. 2002;325:216. author reply 216
10. Moynihan R, Cassels A. Selling sickness: how the world's biggest pharmaceutical companies are turning us all into patients. New York, NY: NationBooks; 2005.
11. Gotzsche PC. Deadly medicines and organised crime. how big pharma has corrupted healthcare. London: Radcliffe Publishing; 2013.
12. Spencer D. Evidence based medicine is broken. Br Med J. 2014;348:g22.
13. Morgan DJ, Wright SM, Dhruva S. Update on medical overuse. JAMA Intern Med. 2015;175:120–4. https://doi.org/10.1001/jamainternmed.2014.5444.
14. Shyh-Chang N, Ng HH. The metabolic programming of stem cells. Genes Dev. 2017;31(4):336–46. https://doi.org/10.1101/gad.293167.116. Epub 2017 Mar 17
15. Thomas H, Cowin AJ, Mills SJ. The importance of pericytes in healing: wounds and other pathologies. Int J Mol Sci. 2017;18(6) pii: E1129 https://doi.org/10.3390/ijms18061129.
16. Fang J, Hirschi K. Molecular regulation of arteriovenous endothelial cell specification. F1000Res. 2019;8. pii: F1000 Faculty Rev-1208; eCollection 2019 https://doi.org/10.12688/f1000research.16701.1.

17. Komori T. Regulation of bone development and extracellular matrix protein genes by RUNX2. Cell Tissue Res. 2010;339:189–95. https://doi.org/10.1007/s00441-009-0832-8.
18. Balogh P, Adelman ER, Pluvinage JV, Capaldo BJ, Freeman KC, Singh S, et al. RUNX3 levels in human hematopoietic progenitors are regulated by aging and dictate erythroid-myeloid balance. Haematologica. 2019. pii: haematol.2018.208918 [Epub ahead of print]; https://doi.org/10.3324/haematol.2018.208918.
19. Nakashima K, Zhou X, Kunkel G, Zhang Z, Deng JM, Behringer RR, et al. The novel zinc finger-containing transcription factor osterix is required for osteoblast differentiation and bone formation. Cell. 2002;108:17–29. https://doi.org/10.1016/s0092-8674(01)00622-5.
20. Seenprachawong K, Tawornsawutruk T, Nantasenamat C, Nuchnoi P, Hongeng S, Supokawej A. miR-130a and miR-27b Enhance osteogenesis in human bone marrow mesenchymal stem cells via specific down-regulation of peroxisome proliferator-activated receptor γ. Front Genet. 2018;9:543. https://doi.org/10.3389/fgene.2018.00543. eCollection 2018
21. Hoac B, Susan-Resiga D, Essalmani R, Marcinkiweicz E, Seidah NG, McKee MD. Osteopontin as a novel substrate for the proprotein convertase 5/6 (PCSK5) in bone. Bone. 2018;107:45–55. https://doi.org/10.1016/j.bone.2017.11.002. Epub 2017 Nov 7
22. Singh A, Gill G, Kaur H, Amhmed M, Jakhu H. Role of osteopontin in bone remodeling and orthodontic tooth movement: a review. Prog Orthod. 2018;19(1):18. https://doi.org/10.1186/s40510-018-0216-2.
23. Ducy P, Zhang R, Geoffroy V, Ridall AL, Karsenty G. Osf2/Cbfa1: a transcriptional activator of osteoblast differentiation. Cell. 1997;89:747–54. https://doi.org/10.1016/s0092-8674(00)80257-3.
24. Xia Z, Wu S, Wei X, Liao Y, Yi P, Liu Y, et al. Hypoxic ER stress suppresses beta-catenin expression and promotes cooperation between the transcription factors XBP1 and HIF1alpha for cell survival. J Biol Chem. 2019;294:13811–21. pii: jbc.RA119.008353. https://doi.org/10.1074/jbc.RA119.008353.
25. Wang J, Yang J, Cheng X, Yin F, Zhao Y, Zhu Y, et al. Influence of calcium supplementation against fluoride-mediated osteoblast impairment in vitro: involvement of the canonical Wnt/beta-catenin signaling pathway. J Agric Food Chem. 2019;67:10285–95. https://doi.org/10.1021/acs.jafc.9b03835.
26. Salazar VS, Zarkadis N, Huang L, Watkins M, Kading J, Bonar S, et al. Postnatal ablation of osteoblast Smad4 enhances proliferative responses to canonical Wnt signaling through interactions with beta-catenin. J Cell Sci. 2013;126:5598–609. https://doi.org/10.1242/jcs.132233.
27. Baron R, Kneissel M. WNT signaling in bone homeostasis and disease: from human mutations to treatments. Nat Med. 2013;19(2):179–92. https://doi.org/10.1038/nm.3074.
28. Laine CM, Joeng KS, Campeau PM, Kiviranta R, Tarkkonen K, Grover M, et al. WNT1 mutations in early-onset osteoporosis and osteogenesis imperfecta. N Engl J Med. 2013;368:1809–16. https://doi.org/10.1056/NEJMoa1215458.
29. Balaian E, Wobus M, Weidner H, Baschant U, Stiehler M, Ehninger G, et al. Erythropoietin inhibits osteoblast function in myelodysplastic syndromes via the canonical Wnt pathway. Haematologica. 2018;103(1):61–8. https://doi.org/10.3324/haematol.2017.172726.
30. Manolagas SC, Parfitt AM. What old means to bone. Trends Endocrinol Metab. 2010;21:369–74. https://doi.org/10.1016/j.tem.2010.01.010.
31. Zhang K, Barragan-Adjemian C, Ye L, Kotha S, Dallas M, Lu Y, et al. E11/gp38 Selective expression in osteocytes: regulation by mechanical strain and role in dendrite elongation. Mol Cell Biol. 2006;26:4539–52. https://doi.org/10.1128/mcb.02120-05.
32. Plotkin LI, Bellido T. Osteocytic signalling pathways as therapeutic targets for bone fragility. Nat Rev Endocrinol. 2016;12:593–605. https://doi.org/10.1038/nrendo.2016.71.
33. Guerado E, Andrist T, Andrades JA, Santos L, Cervan A, Guerado G, et al. Spinal arthrodesis. basic science. Rev Esp Cir Ortop Traumatol. 2012;56:227–44. https://doi.org/10.1016/j.recot.2012.01.003.
34. Winkler DG, Sutherland MK, Geoghegan JC, Yu C, Hayes T, Skonier JE, et al. Osteocyte control of bone formation via sclerostin, a novel BMP antagonist. EMBO J. 2003;22:6267–76. https://doi.org/10.1093/emboj/cdg599.
35. Ellies DL, Viviano B, McCarthy J, Rey J, Itasaki N, Saunders S, et al. Bone density ligand, sclerostin, directly interacts with LRP5 but Not LRP5G171V to modulate Wnt activity. J Bone Miner Res. 2006;21:1738–49. https://doi.org/10.1359/jbmr.060810.
36. Delgado-Calle J, Sato AY, Bellido T. Role and mechanism of action of sclerostin in bone. Bone. 2017;96:29–37. https://doi.org/10.1016/j.bone.2016.10.007.
37. Frost HM. Wolff's Law and bone's structural adaptations to mechanical usage: an overview for clinicians. Angle Orthod. 1994;64:175–88. https://doi.org/10.1043/0003-3219(1994)064<0175:WLABSA>2.0.CO;2.
38. Miyamoto T. Regulators of osteoclast differentiation and cell-cell fusion. Keio J Med. 2011;60:101–5. https://doi.org/10.2302/kjm.60.101.
39. Ikeda K, Takeshita S. The role of osteoclast differentiation and function in skeletal homeostasis. J Biochem. 2016 Jan;159(1):1–8. https://doi.org/10.1093/jb/mvv112.
40. Boyle WJ, Simonet WS, Lacey DL. Osteoclast differentiation and activation. Nature.

2003;423(6937):337–42. https://doi.org/10.1038/nature01658.
41. Teitelbaum SL. Bone resorption by osteoclasts. Science. 2000;289:1504–8. https://doi.org/10.1126/science.289.5484.1504.
42. Park JH, Lee NK, Lee SY. Current understanding of RANK signaling in osteoclast differentiation and maturation. Mol Cells. 2017;40(10):706–13. https://doi.org/10.14348/molcells.2017.0225.
43. Tanaka S, Tanaka Y, Ishiguro N, Yamanaka H, Takeuchi T. RANKL: a therapeutic target for bone destruction in rheumatoid arthritis. Mod Rheumatol. 2018 Jan;28(1):9–16. https://doi.org/10.1080/14397595.2017.1369491.
44. Boyce BF. Advances in the regulation of osteoclasts and osteoclast functions. J Dent Res. 2013;92(10):860–77. https://doi.org/10.1177/0022034513500306.
45. Drissi H, Sanjay A. The multifaceted osteoclast; far and beyond bone resorption. J Cell Biochem. 2016 Aug;117(8):1753–6. https://doi.org/10.1002/jcb.25560.
46. Chen X, Wang Z, Duan N, Zhu G, Schwarz EM, Xie C. Osteoblast–osteoclast interactions. Connect Tissue Res. 2018 Mar;59(2):99–107. https://doi.org/10.1080/03008207.2017.1290085.
47. Takahashi N, Maeda K, Ishihara A, Uehara S, Kobayashi Y. Regulatory mechanism of osteoclastogenesis by RANKL and Wnt signals. Front Biosci (Landmark Ed.). 2011 Jan;1(16):21–30. https://doi.org/10.2741/3673.
48. Naffa R, Watanabe S, Zhang W, Maidment C, Singh P, Chamber P, et al. Rapid analysis of pyridinoline and deoxypyridinoline in biological samples by liquid chromatography with mass spectrometry and a silica hydride column. J Sep Sci. 2019 Apr;42(8):1482–8. https://doi.org/10.1002/jssc.201801292.
49. Camozzi V, Tossi A, Simoni E, Pagani F, Francucci CM, Moro L. Role of biochemical markers of bone remodeling in clinical practice. J Endocrinol Invest. 2007;30(6 suppl):13–7.
50. Pritchard JM, Papaioannou A, Tomowich C, Giangregorio LM, Atkinson SA, Beattie KA, et al. Bone mineralization is elevated and less heterogeneous in adults with type 2 diabetes and osteoarthritis compared to controls with osteoarthritis alone. Bone. 2013;54(1):76–82. https://doi.org/10.1016/j.bone.2013.01.032.
51. Sav NM, Kendirci M, Akin L, Kurtoglu S. Urinary levels of pyridinoline and deoxypyridinoline and bone mineral density in children with type 1 diabetes mellitus. Endocr Res. 2017 Nov;42(4):281–6. https://doi.org/10.1080/07435800.2017.1295982.
52. Halling Linder C, Ek-Rylander B, Krumpel M, Norgård M, Narisawa S, Millán JL, Andersson G, Magnusson P. Bone alkaline phosphatase and tartrate-resistant acid phosphatase: potential co-regulators of bone mineralization. Calcif Tissue Int. 2017 Jul;101(1):92–101. https://doi.org/10.1007/s00223-017-0259-2.
53. Charles JF, Aliprantis AO. Osteoclasts: more than "bone eaters". Trends Mol Med. 2014 Aug;20(8):449–59. https://doi.org/10.1016/j.molmed.2014.06.001.
54. Kylmaoja E, Nakamura M, Tuukkanen J. Osteoclasts and remodeling based bone formation. Curr Stem Cell Res Ther. 2016;11(8):626–33. https://doi.org/10.2174/1574888x10666151019115724.
55. Loro E, Ramaswamy G, Chandra A, Tseng W-J, Mishra MK, Shore EM, et al. IL15RA is required for osteoblast function and bone mineralization. Bone. 2017 Oct;103:20–30. https://doi.org/10.1016/j.bone.2017.06.003.
56. Unal M, Creecy A, Nyman JS. The role of matrix composition in the mechanical behavior of bone. Curr Osteoporos Rep. 2018 Jun;16(3):205–15. https://doi.org/10.1007/s11914-018-0433-0.
57. Wei J, Karsenty G. An overview of the metabolic functions of osteocalcin. Rev Endocr Metab Disord. 2015 Jun;16(2):93–8. https://doi.org/10.1007/s11154-014-9307-7.
58. Moser SC, van der Eerden BCJ. Osteocalcin—a versatile bone-derived hormone. Front Endocrinol (Lausanne). 9:794. https://doi.org/10.3389/fendo.2018.00794.
59. Saito M, Marumo K. Collagen cross-links as a determinant of bone quality: a possible explanation for bone fragility in aging, osteoporosis, and diabetes mellitus. Osteoporos Int. 2010;21(2):195–214. https://doi.org/10.1007/s00198-009-1066-z.
60. Oftadeh R, Perez-Viloria M, Villa-Camacho JC, Vaziri A, Nazarian A. Biomechanics and mechanobiology of trabecular bone: a review. J Biomech Eng. 2015;137:1–15. https://doi.org/10.1115/1.4029176.
61. Knott L, Bailey AJ. Collagen cross-links in mineralizing tissues: a review of their chemistry, function, and clinical relevance. Bone. 1998;22(3):181–7. https://doi.org/10.1016/s8756-3282(97)00279-2.
62. Shankar S, Hosking DJ. Biochemical assessment of Paget's disease of bone. J Bone Miner Res. 2006;21(Suppl. 2):P22–7. https://doi.org/10.1359/JBMR.06S204.
63. Hanson DA, Weis MA, Bollen AM, Maslan SL, Singer FR, Eyre DR. A specific immunoassay for monitoring human bone resorption: quantitation of type I collagen cross-linked N-telopeptides in urine. J Bone Miner Res. 1992;7:1251–8. https://doi.org/10.1002/jbmr.5650071119.
64. Enciso R, Keaton J, Saleh N, Ahmadieh A, Clark GT, Sedghizadeh PP. Assessing the utility of serum C-telopeptide cross-link of type 1 collagen as a predictor of bisphosphonate-related osteonecrosis of the jaw: a systematic review and meta-analysis. J Am Dent Assoc. 2016;147(7):551–560.e11. https://doi.org/10.1016/j.adaj.2016.02.011.
65. Fonseca H, Moreira-Goncalves D, Coriolano H-JA, Duarte JA. Bone quality: the determinants of bone strength and fragility. Sports Med. 2014;44(1):37–53. https://doi.org/10.1007/s40279-013-0100-7.

66. Main RP. Osteocytes and the bone lacunar-canalicular system: insights into bone biology and skeletal function using bone tissue microstructure. Int J Paleopathol. 2017;18:44–6. https://doi.org/10.1016/j.ijpp.2017.05.002.
67. Villa JKD, Diaz MAN, Pizziolo VR, Martino HSD. Effect of vitamin K in bone metabolism and vascular calcification: a review of mechanisms of action and evidences. Crit Rev Food Sci Nutr. 2017;57(18):3959–70. https://doi.org/10.1080/10408398.2016.1211616.
68. Mizokami A, Kawakubo-Yasukochi T, Hirata M. Osteocalcin and its endocrine functions. Biochem Pharmacol. 2017;132:1–8. https://doi.org/10.1016/j.bcp.2017.02.001.
69. Myneni VD, Mezey E. Regulation of bone remodeling by vitamin K2. Oral Dis. 2017;23(8):1021–8. https://doi.org/10.1111/odi.12624.
70. Buenzli PR, Lerebours C, Roschger A, Roschger P, Weinkamer R. Late stages of mineralization and their signature on the bone mineral density distribution. Connect Tissue Res. 2018 Dec;59(Suppl. 1):74–80. https://doi.org/10.1080/03008207.2018.1424149.
71. Karsenty G. Update on the biology of osteocalcin. Endocr Pract. 2017;23(10):1270–4. https://doi.org/10.4158/EP171966.RA.
72. Hao C, Cui Y, Owen S, Li W, Cheng S, Jiang WG. Human osteopontin: potential clinical applications in cancer (review). Int J Mol Med. 2017;39(6):1327–37. https://doi.org/10.3892/ijmm.2017.2964.
73. Hayman AR. Tartrate-resistant acid phosphatase (TRAP) and the osteoclast/immune cell dichotomy. Autoimmunity. 2008;41(3):218–23. https://doi.org/10.1080/08916930701694667.
74. Priemel M, Von Domarus C, Klatte TO, Kessler S, Schlie J, Meier S, et al. Bone mineralization defects and vitamin D deficiency: histomorphometric analysis of iliac crest bone biopsies and circulating 25-Hydroxyvitamin D in 675 patients. J Bone Miner Res. 2010 Feb;25(2):305–12. https://doi.org/10.1359/jbmr.090728.
75. Fogelman I, Van Der Wall H, Gnanasegaran G. Radionuclide and hybrid bone imaging. Radionucl Hybrid Bone Imaging. 2012;9783642024:1–1046. https://doi.org/10.1007/978-3-642-02400-9.
76. Van Driel M, Van Leeuwen JPTM. Vitamin D endocrinology of bone mineralization. Mol Cell Endocrinol. 2017 Sep;15(453):46–51. https://doi.org/10.1016/j.mce.2017.06.008.
77. Sanchez-Quevedo MC, Nieto-Albano OH, Garcia JM, Gomez de Ferraris ME, Campos A. Electron probe microanalysis of permanent human enamel and dentine. A methodological and quantitative study. Histol Histopathol. 1998;13:109–13. https://doi.org/10.14670/HH-13.109.
78. Zoehrer R, Perilli E, Kuliwaba JS, Shapter JG, Fazzalari NL, Voelcker NH. Human bone material characterization: integrated imaging surface investigation of male fragility fractures. Osteoporos Int. 2012;23:1297–309. https://doi.org/10.1007/s00198-011-1688-9.
79. Reid IR, Bristow SM, Bolland MJ. Calcium supplements: benefits and risks. J Intern Med. 2015;278:354–68. https://doi.org/10.1111/joim.12394.
80. Winzenberg T, Powell S, Shaw KA, Jones G. Effects of vitamin D supplementation on bone density in healthy children: systematic review and meta-analysis. BMJ. 2011;342:c7254. https://doi.org/10.1136/bmj.c7254.
81. Bolland MJ, Grey A, Reid IR. Should we prescribe calcium or vitamin D supplements to treat or prevent osteoporosis? Climacteric. 2015;18 https://doi.org/10.3109/13697137.2015.1098266.
82. Reid IR, Bolland MJ, Grey A. Effects of vitamin D supplements on bone mineral density: a systematic review and meta-analysis. Lancet. 2014;383:146–55. https://doi.org/10.1016/S0140-6736(13)61647-5.
83. Bolland MJ, Leung W, Tai V, Bastin S, Gamble GD, Grey A, et al. Calcium intake and risk of fracture: systematic review. BMJ. 2015;351:h4580. https://doi.org/10.1136/bmj.h4580.
84. Milovanovic P, Rakocevic Z, Djonic D, Zivkovic V, Hahn M, Nikolic S, et al. Nano-structural, compositional and micro-architectural signs of cortical bone fragility at the superolateral femoral neck in elderly hip fracture patients vs. healthy aged controls. Exp Gerontol. 2014;55:19–28. https://doi.org/10.1016/j.exger.2014.03.001.
85. Carpentier VT, Wong J, Yeap Y, Gan C, Sutton-Smith P, Badiei A, et al. Increased proportion of hypermineralized osteocyte lacunae in osteoporotic and osteoarthritic human trabecular bone: implications for bone remodeling. Bone. 2012;50:688–94. https://doi.org/10.1016/j.bone.2011.11.021.
86. Cabezas Agrícola JM. Hipocalcemia. Med Programa Form Médica Contin Acreditado. 2004;9:1045–54. https://doi.org/10.1016/S0211-3449(04)70157-5.
87. NIH Consensus Development Panel on Osteoporosis Prevention, Diagnosis, T. Osteoporosis prevention, diagnosis, and therapy. JAMA. 2001;285:785–95.
88. Domínguez López O, De La M, Almazán EM, Muñoz C, Araceli R, Martín Á, et al. Intepretación de las pruebas del metabolismo calcio-fósforo y magnesio. Tratado Geriatr Para Resid. 2014:615–26.
89. Carbone L, Johnson KC, Huang Y, Pettinger M, Thomas F, Cauley J, et al. Sodium intake and osteoporosis. J Clin Endocrinol Metab. 2016;101:1414–21. https://doi.org/10.1210/jc.2015-4017.
90. Mente A, O'Donnell MJ, Rangarajan S, McQueen MJ, Poirier P, Wielgosz A, et al. Association of urinary sodium and potassium excretion with blood pressure. N Engl J Med. 2014;371:601–11. https://doi.org/10.1056/NEJMoa1311989.
91. O'Donnell M, Mente A, Rangarajan S, McQueen MJ, Wang X, Liu L, et al. Urinary sodium and potassium excretion, mortality, and cardiovascular

events. N Engl J Med. 2014;371:612–23. https://doi.org/10.1056/NEJMoa1311889.
92. Buring JE, Hennekens CH. Prevention of cardiovascular disease. J Gen Intern Med. 2007;5:S54–7. https://doi.org/10.1007/bf02600843.
93. Jones G, Beard T, Parameswaran V, Greenaway T, von Witt R. A population-based study of the relationship between salt intake, bone resorption and bone mass. Eur J Clin Nutr. 1997;51:561–5.
94. Heaney RP. Role of dietary sodium in osteoporosis. J Am Coll Nutr. 2006;25:271S–6S.
95. Kim Y, Kim H-Y, Kim JH. Associations between reported dietary sodium intake and osteoporosis in Korean Postmenopausal Women: the 2008–2011 Korea National Health and Nutrition Examination Survey. Asia-Pacific J Public Heal. 2017;29:430–9. https://doi.org/10.1177/1010539517712759.
96. D'Oronzo S, Brown J, Coleman R. The role of biomarkers in the management of bone-homing malignancies. J Bone Oncol. 2017 Sep;11(9):1–9. https://doi.org/10.1016/j.jbo.2017.09.001.
97. Greenblatt MB, Tsai JN, Wein MN. Bone turnover markers in the diagnosis and monitoring of metabolic bone disease. Clin Chem. 2017 Feb;63(2):464–74. https://doi.org/10.1373/clinchem.2016.259085.
98. Vlot MC, den Heijer M, de Jongh RT, Vervloet MG, Lems WF, de Jonge R, et al. Clinical utility of bone markers in various diseases. Bone. 2018;114:215–25. https://doi.org/10.1016/j.bone.2018.06.011.
99. Koehne T, Vettorazzi E, Kusters N, Luneburg R, Kahl-Nieke B, Puschel K, et al. Trends in trabecular architecture and bone mineral density distribution in 152 individuals aged 30–90 years. Bone. 2014;66:31–8. https://doi.org/10.1016/j.bone.2014.05.010.
100. Misof BM, Roschger P, Blouin S, Recker R, Klaushofer K. Bone matrix mineralization is preserved during early perimenopausal stage in healthy women: a paired biopsy study. Osteoporos Int. 2016;27(5):1795–803. https://doi.org/10.1007/s00198-015-3446-x.
101. Nahas-Neto J, Cangussu LM, Orsatti CL, Bueloni-Dias FN, Poloni PF, Schmitt EB, et al. Effect of isolated vitamin D supplementation on bone turnover markers in younger postmenopausal women: a randomized, double-blind, placebo-controlled trial. Osteoporos Int. 2018;29(5):1125–33. https://doi.org/10.1007/s00198-018-4395-y.
102. Silva BC, Bilezikian JP. Parathyroid hormone: anabolic and catabolic actions on the skeleton. Curr Opin Pharmacol. 2015;22:41–50. https://doi.org/10.1016/j.coph.2015.03.005.
103. Khundmiri SJ, Murray RD, Lederer E. PTH and vitamin D. Compr Physiol. 2016;6(2):561–601. https://doi.org/10.1002/cphy.c140071.
104. Van Driel M, Van Leeuwen JP. Vitamin D endocrine system and osteoblasts. Bonekey Rep. 2014;3:493. https://doi.org/10.1038/bonekey.2013.227. PMID: 24605210; PMCID: PMC3944124
105. Corbetta S, Mantovani G, Spada A. Metabolic syndrome in parathyroid diseases. Front Horm Res. 2018;49:67–84. https://doi.org/10.1159/000486003.
106. Garnero P, Sornay-Rendu E, Chapuy MC, Delmas PD. Increased bone turnover in late postmenopausal women is a major determinant of osteoporosis. J Bone Miner Res. 1996;11:337–49. https://doi.org/10.1002/jbmr.5650110307.
107. Garnero P. Biomarkers for osteoporosis management: utility in diagnosis, fracture risk prediction and therapy monitoring. Mol Diagn Ther. 2008;12:157–70. https://doi.org/10.1007/BF03256280.
108. Bauer DC, Sklarin PM, Stone KL, Black DM, Nevitt MC, Ensrud KE, et al. Biochemical markers of bone turnover and prediction of hip bone loss in older women: the study of osteoporotic fractures. J Bone Miner Res. 1999;14:1404–10. https://doi.org/10.1359/jbmr.1999.14.8.1404.
109. Mohamed Y, Haifa H, Datel O, Fadoua HN, Smeh BH, Mahbouba J, et al. The role of biochemical markers of bone turnover in the diagnosis of osteoporosis and predicting fracture risk. Tunis Med. 2014;92:304–10.
110. Song L. Calcium and bone metabolism indices. Adv Clin Chem. 2017;82:1–46. https://doi.org/10.1016/bs.acc.2017.06.005.
111. Christgau S, Rosenquist C, Alexandersen P, Bjarnason NH, Ravn P, Fledelius C, et al. Clinical evaluation of the Serum CrossLaps One Step ELISA, a new assay measuring the serum concentration of bone-derived degradation products of type I collagen C-telopeptides. Clin Chem. 1998;44:2290–300.
112. Bauer DC, Black DM, Garnero P, Hochberg M, Ott S, Orloff J, et al. Change in bone turnover and hip, non-spine, and vertebral fracture in alendronate-treated women: the fracture intervention trial. J Bone Miner Res. 2004;19:1250–8. https://doi.org/10.1359/JBMR.040512.
113. Rosen HN. Use of biochemical markers of bone turnover in osteoporosis UpToDate.www.uptodate.com 2019. Last Accessed June 2019.
114. Guerado E, Cruz E, Cano JR, Crespo PV, Alaminos M, Sánchez-Quevedo MC, Campos A. Mineralization: effectson hip fractures. Injury. 2015;47(Suppl. 1):S21–4.
115. Rachner T, Khosla S, Hofbauer L, Manuscript A. New horizons in osteoporosis. Lancet. 2011;377:1276–87. https://doi.org/10.1016/S0140--6736(10)62349-5.New.
116. Burch J, Rice S, Yang H, Neilson A, Stirk L, Francis R, et al. Systematic review of the use of bone turnover markers for monitoring the response to osteoporosis treatment: The secondary prevention of fractures, and primary prevention of fractures in high-risk groups. Health Technol Assess (Rockv). 2014;18:1–180. https://doi.org/10.3310/hta18110.
117. To KG, Meuleners LB, Fraser ML, Van DD, Van DD, Huynh V-AN, et al. Prevalence and visual risk factors for falls in bilateral cataract patients in Ho Chi Minh City, Vietnam. Ophthalmic Epidemiol.

2014;21:79–85. https://doi.org/10.3109/09286586.2014.885058.
118. Rivadeneira F, Makitie O. Osteoporosis and bone mass disorders: from gene pathways to treatments. Trends Endocrinol Metab. 2016;27:262–81. https://doi.org/10.1016/j.tem.2016.03.006.
119. Nishi E, Masuda K, Arakawa M, Kawame H, Kosho T, Kitahara M, et al. Exome sequencing-based identification of mutations in non-syndromic genes among individuals with apparently syndromic features. Am J Med Genet A. 2016;170:2889–94. https://doi.org/10.1002/ajmg.a.37826.
120. Zheng H-F, Forgetta V, Hsu Y-H, Estrada K, Rosello-Diez A, Leo PJ, et al. Whole-genome sequencing identifies EN1 as a determinant of bone density and fracture. Nature. 2015;526:112–7. https://doi.org/10.1038/nature14878.
121. Sornay-Rendu E, Munoz F, Garnero P, Duboeuf F, Delmas PD. Identification of osteopenic women at high risk of fracture: The OFELY study. J Bone Miner Res. 2005;20:1813–9. https://doi.org/10.1359/JBMR.050609.
122. Garnero P, Hausherr E, Chapuy MC, Marcelli C, Grandjean H, Muller C, et al. Markers of bone resorption predict hip fracture in elderly women: the EPIDOS Prospective Study. J Bone Miner Res. 1996;11:1531–8. https://doi.org/10.1002/jbmr.5650111021.
123. Shieh A, Han W, Ishii S, Greendale GA, Crandall CJ, Karlamangla AS. Quantifying the balance between total bone formation and total bone resorption: an index of net bone formation. J Clin Endocrinol Metab. 2016;101:2802–9. https://doi.org/10.1210/jc.2015-4262.
124. Gerdhem P, Ivaska KK, Alatalo SL, Halleen JM, Hellman J, Isaksson A, et al. Biochemical markers of bone metabolism and prediction of fracture in elderly women. J Bone Miner Res. 2003;19:386–93. https://doi.org/10.1359/JBMR.0301244.
125. Vestergaard P, Rejnmark L, Mosekilde L. Diabetes and its complications and their relationship with risk of fractures in type 1 and 2 diabetes. Calcif Tissue Int. 2009;84:45–55. https://doi.org/10.1007/s00223-008-9195-5.
126. Szulc P, Bauer DC. Biochemical markers of bone turnover in osteoporosis. In: Marcus R, Feldman D, Dempster DW, Luckey M, Cauley JA, editors. Osteoporosis, vol. 4. San Diego (CA): Academic Press; 2013. p. 1573–610.

The Concept of Sarcopenia and Frailty

4

Heike A. Bischoff-Ferrari

4.1 Introduction

The European population is aging rapidly. By 2030, the number of adults aged 75 and older is predicted to double [1], as is the number of older adults with physical frailty [2]. Physical frailty [2] is defined by a decline in multiple body systems [3] causing increased vulnerability that has been linked to multiple negative health outcomes, including extended length of stay in acute care due to complications [4, 5], hospital readmissions [6], and mortality [7, 8] among older patients [9]. Therefore, frailty causes an enormous challenge to the individual, to medical care, and the society as a whole.

A condition that is considered central to the development of physical frailty and its consequences is sarcopenia [10–25] and the loss of muscle mass and strength. Notably, to date, both frailty and sarcopenia are underdiagnosed in clinical care, although effective treatments for these conditions (i.e., exercise, vitamin D, protein) have been proposed especially for older adults at risk for or after fragility fractures [11, 17, 26–31]. This textbook is addressing diagnostic options of sarcopenia and frailty and treatment options for these conditions, among the target population of older adults seen in senior trauma centers, in individual chapters.

H. A. Bischoff-Ferrari (✉)
Department of Aging Medicine and Aging Research, City Hospital Zurich-Waid, Zurich University, Zürich, Switzerland
e-mail: heike.bischoff@usz.ch

4.2 Overlap Between Sarcopenia and Frailty

Muscle mass is reduced by as much as 40% from age 20 to age 80, most pronounced in the lower limb [32]. It has been estimated that 5–13% of adults aged 60–70 and 11–50% of adults aged 80+ years are affected by sarcopenia [26–28, 33, 34]. Conceptually, while sarcopenia is central to the development of frailty [35–38], not all patients with sarcopenia are frail. In fact, it has been suggested that sarcopenia is about twice as common as frailty [14, 28, 35, 36].

4.3 Relevance of Frailty

About 10–30% of community-dwelling older adults are considered frail [39], with an additional 40% being at risk for the condition (pre-frailty [40–42]). Frail older adults consume 3-times more health care resources than their robust counterparts [43]. Thus, the health economic impact of frailty is expected to be enormous [44] and a call to action has been posed [2]. Relevant to outcomes in acute care settings, frailty is considered a better predictor of adverse outcomes than chronological age alone [45]. Therefore, several medical specialties have

H.-C. Pape et al. (eds.), *Senior Trauma Patients*, https://doi.org/10.1007/978-3-030-91483-7_4

started to assess frailty in older trauma patients [46–48], in cancer patients [49, 50], and in heart surgery candidates [51–53].

4.4 Relevance of Sarcopenia

As described above, sarcopenia is a driver frailty [13, 54–56], plus causes mobility disability, falls, fractures, and loss of autonomy [13, 54–56]. Based on a representative sample of U.S. adults aged 60 and older, the estimated direct healthcare cost attributable to sarcopenia in 2000 was $18.5 billion, which represented about 1.5% of total healthcare expenditures for that year [24]. According to Janssen et al., the assessment of 10% reduction in sarcopenia prevalence would result in savings of $1.1 billion (dollars adjusted to 2000 rate) per year in U.S. healthcare costs [24].

4.5 Summary

The importance of diagnosing and treating sarcopenia and frailty among older patients, at risk for or treated in acute care for a fall-related injury such as a fragility fracture, cannot be overestimated for their overt and independent link to adverse outcomes after surgery and regaining autonomy [4–8]. The close collaboration between trauma surgeons and geriatricians, as well as expert teams in physiotherapy and nursing trained within senior trauma centers, will allow these conditions to be addressed most effectively [46–48].

References

1. Ogura S, Jakovljevic MM. Editorial: global population aging—health care, social and economic consequences. Front Public Health. 2018;6:335.
2. Cesari M, et al. Frailty: an emerging public health priority. J Am Med Dir Assoc. 2016;17(3):188–92.
3. Lipsitz LA. Dynamics of stability: the physiologic basis of functional health and frailty. J Gerontol A Biol Sci Med Sci. 2002;57(3):B115–25.
4. Assmann P, et al. Frailty is associated with delirium and mortality after transcatheter aortic valve implantation. Open Heart. 2016;3(2):e000478.
5. Jung, P., et al., The impact of frailty on postoperative delirium in cardiac surgery patients. J Thorac Cardiovasc Surg 2015; 149(3): 869–75 e1–2.
6. Wou F, et al. The predictive properties of frailty-rating scales in the acute medical unit. Age Ageing. 2013;42(6):776–81.
7. Fried LP, et al. Frailty in older adults: evidence for a phenotype. J Gerontol A Biol Sci Med Sci. 2001;56(3):M146–56.
8. Avila-Funes JA, et al. Frailty among community-dwelling elderly people in France: the three-city study. J Gerontol A Biol Sci Med Sci. 2008;63(10):1089–96.
9. Zekry D, et al. High levels of comorbidity and disability cancel out the dementia effect in predictions of long-term mortality after discharge in the very old. Dement Geriatr Cogn Disord. 2011;32(2):103–10.
10. Fried LP, et al. Frailty in older adults: evidence for a phenotype. J Gerontol A Biol Sci Med Sci. 2001;56(3):M146–56.
11. Abellan van Kan G, et al. Carla Task Force on Sarcopenia: propositions for clinical trials. J Nutr Health Aging. 2009;13(8):700–7.
12. Visser M. Towards a definition of sarcopenia--results from epidemiologic studies. J Nutr Health Aging. 2009;13(8):713–6.
13. Visser M, Schaap LA. Consequences of sarcopenia. Clin Geriatr Med. 2011;27(3):387–99.
14. Cruz-Jentoft AJ, et al. Sarcopenia: European consensus on definition and diagnosis: Report of the European Working Group on Sarcopenia in Older People. Age Ageing. 2010;39(4):412–23.
15. Fielding RA, et al. Sarcopenia: an undiagnosed condition in older adults. Current consensus definition: prevalence, etiology, and consequences. International Working Group on Sarcopenia. J Am Med Dir Assoc. 2011;12(4):249–56.
16. Morley JE, et al. Sarcopenia with limited mobility: an international consensus. J Am Med Dir Assoc. 2011;12(6):403–9.
17. Vellas B, et al. Designing pharmaceutical trials for sarcopenia in frail older adults: EU/US Task Force Recommendations. J Nutr Health Aging. 2013;17(7):612–8.
18. Studenski S. What are the outcomes of treatment among patients with sarcopenia? J Nutr Health Aging. 2009;13(8):733–6.
19. Morley JE, et al. Sarcopenia. J Lab Clin Med. 2001;137(4):231–43.
20. Baumgartner RN, et al. Epidemiology of sarcopenia among the elderly in New Mexico. Am J Epidemiol. 1998;147(8):755–63.
21. Delmonico MJ, et al. Alternative definitions of sarcopenia, lower extremity performance, and functional impairment with aging in older men and women. J Am Geriatr Soc. 2007;55(5):769–74.

22. Delmonico MJ, et al. Longitudinal study of muscle strength, quality, and adipose tissue infiltration. Am J Clin Nutr. 2009;90(6):1579–85.
23. Motion AI. Aging in Motion: the facts about sarcopenia. http://www.aginginmotion.org/wp-content/uploads/2011/04/sarcopenia_fact_sheet.pdf, 2013.
24. Janssen I, et al. The healthcare costs of sarcopenia in the United States. J Am Geriatr Soc. 2004;52(1):80–5.
25. Sayer AA. Sarcopenia. BMJ. 2010;341:c4097.
26. Bischoff-Ferrari HA, et al. Comparative performance of current definitions of sarcopenia against the prospective incidence of falls among community-dwelling seniors age 65 and older. Osteoporos Int. 2015;
27. Rizzoli R, et al. Quality of life in sarcopenia and frailty. Calcif Tissue Int. 2013;93(2):101–20.
28. von Haehling S, Morley JE, Anker SD. An overview of sarcopenia: facts and numbers on prevalence and clinical impact. J Cachexia Sarcopenia Muscle. 2010;1(2):129–33.
29. Morley JE, et al. Nutritional recommendations for the management of sarcopenia. J Am Med Dir Assoc. 2010;11(6):391–6.
30. Morley JE, et al. Frailty consensus: a call to action. J Am Med Dir Assoc. 2013;14(6):392–7.
31. Cesari M, et al. Pharmacological interventions in frailty and sarcopenia: report by the International Conference on Frailty and Sarcopenia Research Task Force. J Frailty Aging. 2015;4(3):114–20.
32. Koopman, R., L.J. van Loon, Aging, exercise, and muscle protein metabolism. J Appl Physiol (1985), 2009; 106(6): 2040–2048.
33. Perez-Zepeda MU, Gutierrez-Robledo LM, Arango-Lopera VE. Sarcopenia prevalence. Osteoporos Int. 2013;24(3):797.
34. Cruz-Jentoft, A.J., et al., Prevalence of and interventions for sarcopenia in ageing adults: a systematic review. Report of the International Sarcopenia Initiative (EWGSOP and IWGS). Age Ageing 2014.
35. Cesari M, et al. Sarcopenia and physical frailty: two sides of the same coin. Front Aging Neurosci. 2014;6:192.
36. Cooper C, et al. Frailty and sarcopenia: definitions and outcome parameters. Osteoporos Int. 2012;23(7):1839–48.
37. Landi F, et al. Sarcopenia as the biological substrate of physical frailty. Clin Geriatr Med. 2015;31(3):367–74.
38. Roubenoff R. Sarcopenia: a major modifiable cause of frailty in the elderly. J Nutr Health Aging. 2000;4(3):140–2.
39. Santos-Eggimann B, et al. Prevalence of frailty in middle-aged and older community-dwelling Europeans living in 10 countries. J Gerontol A Biol Sci Med Sci. 2009;64(6):675–81.
40. Choi J, et al. Global prevalence of physical frailty by Fried's criteria in community-dwelling elderly with national population-based surveys. J Am Med Dir Assoc. 2015;16(7):548–50.
41. Collard RM, et al. Prevalence of frailty in community-dwelling older persons: a systematic review. J Am Geriatr Soc. 2012;60(8):1487–92.
42. Nguyen TN, Cumming RG, Hilmer SN. A review of frailty in developing countries. J Nutr Health Aging. 2015;19(9):941–6.
43. Ilinca S, Calciolari S. The patterns of health care utilization by elderly Europeans: frailty and its implications for health systems. Health Serv Res. 2015;50(1):305–20.
44. Fried LP, et al. Untangling the concepts of disability, frailty, and comorbidity: implications for improved targeting and care. J Gerontol A Biol Sci Med Sci. 2004;59(3):255–63.
45. Joseph B, et al. Superiority of frailty over age in predicting outcomes among geriatric trauma patients: a prospective analysis. JAMA Surg. 2014;149(8):766–72.
46. Muller FS, et al. Impaired nutritional status in geriatric trauma patients. Eur J Clin Nutr. 2017;71(5):602–6.
47. Wilson JM, et al. Frailty and malnutrition are associated with inpatient postoperative complications and mortality in hip fracture patients. J Orthop Trauma. 2019;33(3):143–8.
48. Vasu BK, et al. Geriatric patients with hip fracture: frailty and other risk factors affecting the outcome. Anesth Essays Res. 2018;12(2):546–51.
49. Puts MT, et al. Are frailty markers useful for predicting treatment toxicity and mortality in older newly diagnosed cancer patients? Results from a prospective pilot study. Crit Rev Oncol Hematol. 2011;78(2):138–49.
50. Stauder R, et al. Management of Chronic Lymphocytic Leukemia (CLL) in the elderly: a position paper from an International Society of Geriatric Oncology (SIOG) task force. Ann Oncol. 2016;
51. Schoenenberger AW, et al. Predictors of functional decline in elderly patients undergoing transcatheter aortic valve implantation (TAVI). Eur Heart J. 2013;34(9):684–92.
52. Chauhan D, et al. Quantitative increase in frailty is associated with diminished survival after transcatheter aortic valve replacement. Am Heart J. 2016;182:146–54.
53. Kim DH, et al. Preoperative frailty assessment and outcomes at 6 months or later in older adults undergoing cardiac surgical procedures: a systematic review. Ann Intern Med. 2016;165(9):650–60.
54. Book, S. Alliance for aging research. http://www.agingresearch.org, 2013.
55. Commission, E. Healthy ageing: a keystone of a sustainable Europe. http://ec.europa.eu/health/ph_information/indicators/docs/healthy_ageing_en.pdf, 2007.
56. Romero-Ortuno R, Kenny RA. The frailty index in Europeans: association with age and mortality. Age Ageing. 2012;41(5):684–9.

Applied Fall and Fracture Epidemiology 70+

5

Heike A. Bischoff-Ferrari

5.1 Introduction

Over 90% of fragility fractures occur after a fall and fall rates increase with age [1] and poor muscle strength or function [1]. Mechanistically, the circumstances [2] and the direction [3] of a fall determine the type of fracture, whereas bone density and factors that attenuate a fall, such as better strength or better padding, critically determine whether a fracture will take place when the faller lands on a certain bone [4]. Moreover, falling may also affect bone density through increased immobility from self-restriction of activities [5]. Notably, after their first fall, about 30% of persons develop a fear of falling resulting in self-restriction of activities, decreased quality of life, and a high risk of sustaining another fall or fracture [5]. Therefore, relevant to clinical care of older trauma patients with fall-related injuries, the implementation of integrated care concepts that include early rehabilitation and nutritional concepts that target both fall and fracture prevention is of significant importance [6, 7].

H. A. Bischoff-Ferrari (✉)
Department of Aging Medicine and Aging Research, City Hospital Zurich-Waid, Zurich University, Zürich, Switzerland
e-mail: heike.bischoff@usz.ch

5.2 Epidemiology of Falls

Each year, one out of three persons aged 65 and older and one out of two aged 80 and older experience at least one fall [7–10]. Serious injuries occur with 10–15% of falls, 9% of these falls require an emergency room visit and 5–6% result in a fracture [11]. Fall injuries are among the 20 most expensive medical conditions [12] amounting to $34 billion annually of direct medical costs for fall injuries [13].

As an independent determinant of functional decline [14], falls lead to 40% of all nursing home admissions [15]. The primary risk factor for a hip fracture is a fall, and over 90% of all fractures occur after a fall [16]. Recurrent fallers may have close to a fourfold increased odds of sustaining a fall-related fracture compared to individuals with a single fall [17]. As the number of adults aged 65 and older is predicted to double by 2030 [18], the number of fall-related fractures will increase substantially. Notably, even today, 75% of fractures occur among seniors aged 65 and older [19]. Because of the increasing proportion of older adults, annual costs from all fall-related injuries in the US in persons aged 65 years or older were projected to increase from $20.3 billion in 1994 to $32.4 billion in 2020, including medical, rehabilitation, hospital costs, and the costs of morbidity and mortality [20].

H.-C. Pape et al. (eds.), *Senior Trauma Patients*, https://doi.org/10.1007/978-3-030-91483-7_5

5.3 Fall Definition and Ascertainment Methods

Buchner and colleagues created a useful fall definition for the common database of the FICSIT (Frailty and Injuries: Cooperative Studies of Intervention Techniques) trials [21]. Falls were defined as "unintentionally coming to rest on the ground, floor, or other lower level." Coming to rest against furniture or a wall was not accounted as a fall [21].

Challenging for their ascertainment is that falls tend to be forgotten if not associated with significant injury [22], requiring short periods of follow-up. Thus, high quality fall assessment in older adults requires a prospective ascertainment of falls and their circumstances, ideally in short periods of time (<3 months) [22].

Useful fall ascertainment methods include postcards, phone calls, or diary/calendar [23]. Only recently, the usefulness and comprehensiveness of different ascertainment methods have been compared directly for 704 falls recorded with the same fall protocol among pre-frail and frail older adults [23]. The authors concluded that most falls were reported by active-asking by monthly phone calls: 81% of total falls in pre-frail, and 78% in frail older adults. Among pre-frail older adults, diaries captured additional 19% falls, while a telephone hotline added none. Among frail older adults, the hotline added 16% falls, while diaries added 6%. Further, the authors found that while monthly active-asking by phone calls captures most falls in both groups, this method alone missed 19% of falls in pre-frail and 22% in frail seniors. Thus, a combination of active-asking and diaries for pre-frail and active-asking and the hotline for frail older adults was recommended by the authors [23].

5.4 Epidemiology of the Four Most Common Fragility Fractures

Hip fractures are the most serious and most frequent fragility fractures occurring among adults aged 75 and older [24, 25]. In fact, an estimated one in three women and one in six men will have sustained a hip fracture by their 90th decade [26]. Notably, by 2050, the worldwide incidence of hip fractures is expected to increase by 240% among women and 310% among men [27]. Critical for the understanding of fragility fractures at the hip is their close relationship with muscle weakness[16] and falling [28].

Apart from hip fractures, **the other two most common fragility fractures at non-vertebral sites** are distal forearm and proximal humerus fractures, and similar to hip fractures, distal forearm and proximal humerus fractures show a steep increase with age [24]. Notably, the circumstances of these fractures are strikingly different. Hip fractures tend to occur in less active individuals falling indoors from a standing height with little forward momentum, and they tend to fall sideways or straight down on their hip [29–31]. On the other hand, distal forearm or humerus fractures tend to occur among more active older individuals who are correspondingly more likely to be outdoors and have a greater forward momentum when they fall [32–34]. This may also explain why hip fracture incidence shows little to no seasonal change, while the winter/summer seasonal swing is pronounced in the distal forearm and humerus fractures, and more so in men than in women [35]. Men aged 65 and older have a 51% greater risk to sustain a distal forearm and 23% greater risk to sustain a proximal humerus fracture in the winter compared with the summer season [35]. Women aged 65 and older have a 15% greater risk to sustain a distal forearm and 19% greater risk to sustain a proximal humerus fracture in the winter compared with the summer season [35]. In the same study, in winter, total snowfall was associated with a reduced risk of hip fracture (−5% per 20 in./51 cm), but an increased risk of distal forearm and proximal humerus fractures (6–12%; $p < 0.05$ at all sites) [35].

Compared to the three most common fragility fractures at non-vertebral sites (hip, distal forearm, and proximal humerus), the epidemiology of vertebral fractures is challenging with less than 30% of vertebral fractures coming to clinical attention [25]. Similar to the three non-vertebral fragility fractures, vertebral fractures increase exponentially after age 65 among men and women, and incidence rates for vertebral fractures project between hip and radius fractures for both genders after age 75 [25]. Women with a first vertebral fracture have a more than 19% risk of developing a second vertebral fracture in the subsequent year [36], a 2.5-fold increased risk for any subsequent fracture [37], and a 2.8-fold increased mortality rate within the following 10 years [38].

Notably **in** men, after age 80, vertebral fracture rates have been reported to be similar to those in women [39]. However, mechanistically there are gender-specific differences: more than 90% of vertebral fractures in women result from mild to moderate trauma, while among men, this proportion is only 55% [40]. Severe vertebral deformities in both genders appear to have a predilection between T10 and L1 [40].

5.5 Risk of Repeat Fragility Fractures

For a future perspective on the fragility fracture epidemic, it is important to note that often the first fragility fracture is followed by a second fragility fracture, and drawing attention to that first fracture and the need for secondary prevention is key in fragility fracture care [6]. Based on a 16-year follow-up of one large population-based study in Australia [37], the absolute risk for a repeat fracture increases steeply and equally in men and women with age, despite a lower absolute risk for the first fracture among men. The relative risk for a repeat fracture among women aged 60–69, 70–79, and 80+ is 1.65 (95% CI: 1.18–2.32), 2.36 (1.91–2.92), and 1.80 (1.45–2.25), respectively [37]. The relative risk for a repeat fracture among men aged 60–69, 70–79, and 80+ is 3.75 (2.19–6.43), 4.32 (3.00–6.21), and 2.77 (1.69–4.54), respectively [37].

5.6 Summary

We will see many more falls and fall-related fragility fractures in the coming 20 years and an integrated care approach as implemented in senior trauma centers, including an interprofessional team of traumatologists, geriatricians, physiotherapist, nutritionists, and nursing experts will be needed to face this challenge. One integrated care concept developed at the University Hospital in Zurich (Zurich-POPS) that includes both a novel communication tool and a comprehensive research agenda is described in a chapter of this textbook.

References

1. Tinetti ME. Risk factors for falls among elderly persons living in the community. N Engl J Med. 1988;319:1701–7.
2. Cummings SR, Nevitt MC. Non-skeletal determinants of fractures: the potential importance of the mechanics of falls. Study of Osteoporotic Fractures Research Group. Osteoporos Int. 1994;4(Suppl. 1):67–70.
3. Nguyen ND, et al. Development of a nomogram for individualizing hip fracture risk in men and women. Osteoporos Int. 2007;17:17.
4. Nevitt MC, Cummings SR. Type of fall and risk of hip and wrist fractures: the study of osteoporotic fractures. The Study of Osteoporotic Fractures Research Group. J Am Geriatr Soc. 1993;41(11):1226–34.
5. Vellas BJ, et al. Fear of falling and restriction of mobility in elderly fallers. Age Ageing. 1997;26(3):189–93.
6. Pape HC, Bischoff-Ferrari HA. How can we influence the incidence of secondary fragility fractures? A review on current approaches. Injury. 2017;48(Suppl. 7):S24–6.
7. Bischoff-Ferrari HA. Chapter: fall prevention. In: ASBMR; 2018. https://doi.org/10.1002/9781119266594.ch68.
8. Blake AJ, et al. Falls by elderly people at home: prevalence and associated factors. Age Ageing. 1988;17(6):365–72.
9. Graafmans WC, et al. Falls in the elderly: a prospective study of risk factors and risk profiles. Am J Epidemiol. 1996;143(11):1129–36.
10. Tinetti ME, Speechley M, Ginter SF. Risk factors for falls among elderly persons living in the community. N Engl J Med. 1988;319(26):1701–7.
11. Bischoff HA, et al. Effects of vitamin D and calcium supplementation on falls: a randomized controlled trial. J Bone Miner Res. 2003;18(2):343–51.
12. Carroll NV, Slattum PW, Cox FM. The cost of falls among the community-dwelling elderly. J Manag Care Pharm. 2005;11(4):307–16.
13. Stevens JA, et al. The costs of fatal and nonfatal falls among older adults. Inj Prev. 2006;12(290–5)
14. Tinetti ME, Williams CS. The effect of falls and fall injuries on functioning in community-dwelling older persons. J Gerontol A Biol Sci Med Sci. 1998;53(2):M112–9.
15. Tinetti ME, Williams CS. Falls, injuries due to falls, and the risk of admission to a nursing home. N Engl J Med. 1997;337(18):1279–84.

16. Cummings SR, et al. Risk factors for hip fracture in white women. Study of Osteoporotic Fractures Research Group. N Engl J Med. 1995;332(12):767–73.
17. Pluijm SM, et al. A risk profile for identifying community-dwelling elderly with a high risk of recurrent falling: results of a 3-year prospective study. Osteoporos Int. 2006;17(3):417–25. Epub 2006 Jan 17
18. Ogura S, Jakovljevic MM. Editorial: global population aging—health care, social and economic consequences. Front Public Health. 2018;6:335.
19. Melton LJ 3rd, Crowson CS, O'Fallon WM. Fracture incidence in Olmsted County, Minnesota: comparison of urban with rural rates and changes in urban rates over time. Osteoporos Int. 1999;9(1):29–37.
20. Englander F, Hodson TJ, Terregrossa RA. Economic dimensions of slip and fall injuries. J Forensic Sci. 1996;41(5):733–46.
21. Buchner DM, et al. Development of the common data base for the FICSIT trials. J Am Geriatr Soc. 1993;41(3):297–308.
22. Cummings SR, Nevitt MC, Kidd S. Forgetting falls. The limited accuracy of recall of falls in the elderly. J Am Geriatr Soc. 1988;36(7):613–6.
23. Teister CJ, et al. Which method of fall ascertainment captures the most falls in prefrail and frail seniors? Am J Epidemiol. 2018;187(10):2243–51.
24. Barrett JA, et al. Fracture risk in the U.S. Medicare population. J Clin Epidemiol. 1999;52(3):243–9.
25. Cooper C, Melton LJ 3rd. Epidemiology of osteoporosis. Trends Endokrin Metab. 1992;314:224–9.
26. Birge SJ, Morrow-Howell N, Proctor EK. Hip fracture. Clin Geriatr Med. 1994;10(4):589–609.
27. Gullberg B, Johnell O, Kanis JA. World-wide projections for hip fracture. Osteoporos Int. 1997;7(5):407–13.
28. Fatalities and Injuries from Falls Among Older Adults--United States. 1993–2003 and 2001–2005. MMWR Morb Mortal Wkly Rep. 2006;55(45):1221–4.
29. Nevitt MC, Cummings SR. Type of fall and risk of hip and wrist fractures: the study of osteoporotic fractures. J Am Geriatr Soc. 1994;42(8):909.
30. Carter SE, et al. Accidents in older people living at home: a community-based study assessing prevalence, type, location and injuries. Aust N Z J Public Health. 2000;24(6):633–6.
31. Campbell AJ, et al. Circumstances and consequences of falls experienced by a community population 70 years and over during a prospective study. Age Ageing. 1990;19(2):136–41.
32. O'Neill TW, et al. Risk factors, falls, and fracture of the distal forearm in Manchester. UK J Epidemiol Commun Health. 1996;50(3):288–92.
33. Graafmans WC, et al. Different risk profiles for hip fractures and distal forearm fractures: a prospective study. Osteoporos Int. 1996;6(6):427–31.
34. Keegan TH, et al. Characteristics of fallers who fracture at the foot, distal forearm, proximal humerus, pelvis, and shaft of the tibia/fibula compared with fallers who do not fracture. Am J Epidemiol. 2004;159(2):192–203.
35. Bischoff-Ferrari HA, et al. Effect of seasonality and weather on fracture risk in individuals 65 years and older. Osteoporos Int. 2007;18(9):1225–33.
36. Lindsay R, et al. Risk of new vertebral fracture in the year following a fracture. JAMA. 2001;285(3):320–3.
37. Center JR, et al. Risk of subsequent fracture after low-trauma fracture in men and women. JAMA. 2007;297(4):387–94.
38. Hasserius R, et al. Long-term morbidity and mortality after a clinically diagnosed vertebral fracture in the elderly—a 12- and 22-year follow-up of 257 patients. Calcif Tissue Int. 2005;76(4):235–42.
39. Praemer A, Furner S, Rice DP. Musculoskeletal conditions in the United States. Rosemont, IL: American Academy of Orthopedic Surgeons; 1992. p. 145–70.
40. Melton LJ 3rd, et al. Prevalence and incidence of vertebral deformities. Osteoporos Int. 1993;3(3):113–9.

Part II

Prevention of Complications Related to Ageing

6 Protein Malnutrition, Falls, and Fractures in Older Trauma Patients

Patricia Lanz and Heike A. Bischoff-Ferrari

6.1 Introduction

People with higher muscle strength fall less, have stronger bones, and suffer significantly fewer fractures [1]. Therefore, the prevention of fragility fractures in older adults should focus not only on bone healths but also muscle health and fall prevention (as illustrated in Fig. 6.1). Both mechanically and biologically, the bone is linked to the muscular system. The prevention of vitamin D deficiency and a diet rich in calcium and protein combined with regular physical activity are key strategies to fall and fracture prevention [2]. In this chapter, we will summarize the available evidence on the amount and quality of protein intake from diet and supplements relevant to fall and fracture prevention among older adults.

6.2 Fragility Fracture: Osteoporosis, Sarcopenia, and Falls

The risk of suffering a fragility fracture, such as a hip fracture, increases exponentially with age [3]. Important drivers of this risk are the presence of reduced bone density (osteoporosis) and reduced muscle mass and function (sarcopenia) and thus increased risk of falling [2] (as illustrated in Fig. 6.1). Fragility fractures have been associated with permanent functional disability, loss of quality of life, and loss of autonomy and increased mortality [3]. The socioeconomic burden caused by fragility fractures and their consequences are enormous and will continue to increase in view of demographic developments [4].

Risk factors of both increased bone loss (osteoporosis) and sarcopenia plus increased risk of falling are listed in Table 6.1.

6.2.1 Sarcopenia

The term sarcopenia (Greek "sarx" meat and "penia" loss) was proposed by Rosenberg in 1989 and describes the age-associated decrease in skeletal muscle mass and strength that exceeds the average [5]. While the diagnostic crieteria of sarcopenia is still under debate [6], there is increasing international consensus that sarcopenia should be diagnosed both by the presence of reduced appendicular muscle mass (ALM) and functional decline assessed by reduced muscle strength or gait speed, as proposed by the EWGSOP (European-working group on Sarcopenia in Older People) in 2010 [7, 8] and updated in 2019 [9]. Further, and relevant to clinical care, since 2017 the ICD-10-CM M62.84 exists for sarcopenia [10]. Notably, the prevalence of sarcopenia among

P. Lanz (✉)
Department of Geriatrics, University Hospital of Zurich, Zürich, Switzerland
e-mail: patricia.lanz@usz.ch

H. A. Bischoff-Ferrari
Department of Aging Medicine and Aging Research, City Hospital Zurich-Waid, Zurich University, Zürich, Switzerland

H.-C. Pape et al. (eds.), *Senior Trauma Patients*, https://doi.org/10.1007/978-3-030-91483-7_6

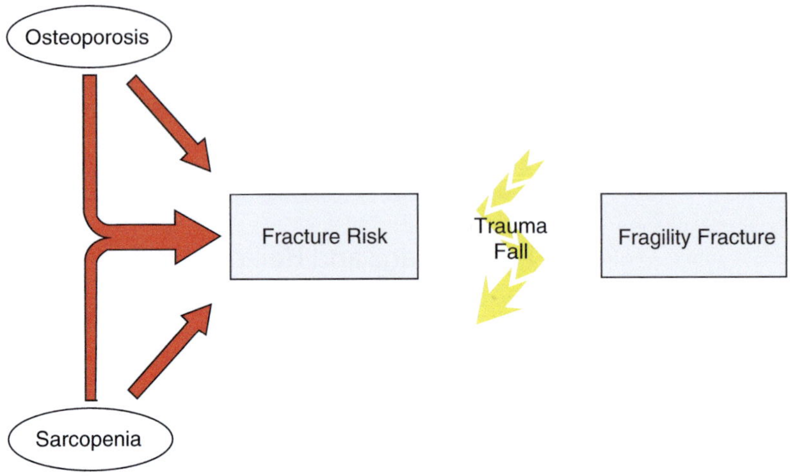

Fig. 6.1 Relationship between osteoporosis, sarcopenia, and fracture

Table 6.1 Risk factors for increased bone loss and sarcopenia and increased risk of falling

Osteoporosis [61]	Sarcopenia [9]	Increased risk of falling [16, 62]
• Previous fracture • Parent Fractured Hip • Current smoking • Intake of glucocorticoids (>5 mg prednisolone daily for three months or equivalent steroid dose) • Rheumatoid arthritis • Excessive alcohol consumption (three or more standard units/day) • Other secondary causes of Osteoporosis (e.g., diabetes mellitus, untreated hyperthyroidism and hypothyroidism, hypogonadism, malabsorption in the context of inflammatory bowel disease)	• Age-associated muscle loss • Diseases – Inflammatory conditions (e.g., organ failure, malignancy) – Osteoarthritis – Neurological disorders • Inactivity – Sedentary behavior (e.g., limited mobility or bedrest) – Physical inactivity • Malnutrition – Undernutrition or malabsorption – Medication-related anorexia – Overnutrition/obesity	• Previous falls • Balance impairment • Decreased muscle strength • Sensual impairment (visual, presbyacusis) • Medication (>4 or psychoactive medication) • Gait and impairment or walking difficulty (e. g., due to underlying neurological and/or orthopedic disease) • Depression • Dizziness or orthostasis • Functional limitations, ADL disabilities • Age > 80 y • Female • Low body mass index (BMI) • Urinary incontinence • Cognitive impairment • Arthritis • Diabetes • Pain • Vitamin D deficiency • Fear of falling

adults aged 70 years and older with a prior fall event may vary between 2.5–27.2% depending on sarcopenia definition [6].

Muscle mass reaches its maximum in humans between the age of 20 and 30 and accounts for about 44% of body weight among young men and about 37% among young women. Between the age of 20 and 80, muscle mass decreases by about 40%, especially on the lower limbs [11]. An accelerated decrease in muscle mass occurs in both sexes after the age of 50 (decrease: 1–2%/year) [11]. This decline is explained by an increasing metabolic resistance of muscle with age [12].

Muscle is comprised of two basic fiber types and a loss of these fibers has been described with age [13]. With aging, there is preferential loss of

Type II fibers, related to a decline in the Type II fiber stem cell or satellite cell population [14]. Type II fibers have fast contraction time, high force production, and low resistance to fatigue (<5 min) and are needed for fast reactions in the prevention of a fall. Type I fibers decline less with age and have a slow contraction time, low force production, and high resistance to fatigue (hours) and are needed for endurance tasks [13]. In addition, the number of innervating motoneurons decreases with age, and as a consequence, fat is deposited in the atrophied muscle [7].

6.2.2 Falls

More than 90% of all fragility fractures occur as a result of a fall [15]. Further, falls are frequent and are regarded as "Hallmark of Frailty". Every third person aged 65 and every second person aged 80 fall at least once a year [16, 17]. Risk factors of both increased bone loss (osteoporosis) and sarcopenia plus increased risk of falling are listed in Table 6.1.

6.3 Risk Factors for the Development of Malnutrition at Older Age

Malnutrition is a broad term used to define any deviation from normal nutritional status. The imbalance between food intake and demand can lead to malnutrition with associated deficiency of one or more essential nutrients or obesity with an excess of nutrients [18]. Malnutrition in older adults has been linked to chronic diseases, infections, frailty, loss of autonomy, and mortality risk [19]. It is favored by a decrease in energy demand with age and the associated reduction in energy intake [20]. The term "anorexia of aging" (AA) was coined in 1988 by Morley and Silver [21]. It attributes AA to changes in appetite regulation and the prolonged absence of hunger [22]. Contributing physiological changes include reduced sensory impressions (smell, taste, and visual stimuli), changes in secretion and peripheral effect of regulatory hormones for appetite, hunger, and saturation, and changes in the gastrointestinal tract (reduced motility) [22]. Further aggravating factors are the presence of comorbidities, polypharmacy, psychosocial factors (isolation, depression, cognitive disorders, poverty in old age), a reduced functional status (reduced mobility that impairs shopping and cooking activities), as well as a poor condition of oral health [19].

In addition to regular weight monitoring and the calculation of the Body Mass Index (BMI), the uses of validated questionnaires such as the Nutritional Risk Screening Tool [23] and the Mini Nutritional Assessment [24] are recommended tools in clinical care to identify older adults at risk of malnutrition. Protein Energy Malnutrition (PEM) is a special form of malnutrition in which the body has too little energy in the form of calories and too little protein. This can be caused by reduced nutrient intake, insufficient absorption and assimilation, increased energy requirements, or a combination of these [25, 26].

6.3.1 Protein

Proteins are essential macronutrients and can be of both animal and plant-based origin. They provide structural and functional building blocks for bones and muscles. The amino acids contained in dietary proteins are required for the synthesis of bone matrix and muscle proteins [27]. Consequently, inadequate protein intake contributes to bone [28–30] and muscle mass [31, 32] loss, frailty, and increased risk of falls [33] and fractures [34].

Notably, the development of protein malnutrition may be caused by inadequate protein intake (in anorexia, inappetence, due to gatrointestinal disorders), reduced ability to utilize ingested protein (insulin resistance, anabolic resistance, high splanchnic extraction, immobility), and increased protein requirement in chronic inflammatory conditions [35].

The recommended daily intake of protein by the WHO for adults irrespective of age and gender is 0.8 g/kg body weight/d [36]. In contrast, the PROT-AGE Group recommends a daily protein intake for individuals over 65 years of age to be higher, namely of at least 1.0–1.2 g/kg body weight/d, and 1.2–1.5 g/kg body weight/d for active older adults and geriatric patients with acute or chronic diseases [35].

The Swiss SEMOF study showed in 2006 that 26.2% of women over 75 years of age take in less than 0.8 g/kg body weight/d and only 29.9% more than 1.2 g/kg body weight/d protein [37]. A survey from the U.S. showed that 15–38% of older men and 27–41% of older women could not even cover the minimal recommendation of 0.8 g/kg body weight/d of protein with food [38].

6.4 Effects of Dietary Proteins on Bones and Muscles

A meta-analysis by Komar et al. published in 2015 found that protein supplementation tested in 16 small clinical intervention studies with a total of 999 participants aged 65+ led to an increase in body weight with an almost exclusive increase in lean body mass [39]. This increase was particularly pronounced in relatively sarcopenic individuals and was not linked to additional muscle training. Also, with regard to large cohort studies, a protein intake of 1 g/kg body weight/d or more was associated with a significant reduction in hip fracture incidence in the Framingham study [34], confirmed by a more recent meta-analysis of 12 cohort studies including 407,104 individuals [40]. One clinical trial among older patients with acute hip fracture found that patients receiving a protein supplement compared to placebo had a 40% shorter rehabilitation time[30] and a higher probability of remaining independent [41].

A more recent meta-analysis of five randomized clinical trials in healthy adults concluded that a higher (1.4 g/kg body weight/d) compared to a lower protein intake (0.8 g/kg body weight/d) has a positive effect on lumbar bone mineral density [42].

Mechanistically, next to the fact that proteins are building blocks of bone matrix and muscle, it has been found that a higher protein intake increases insulin growth factor-1 (IGF-1) [30, 43]. IGF-1 is synthesized in the liver and has an anabolic effect on bone and muscle plus supports the conversion of vitamin D into its active form (1, 25 dihydroxyvitamin D) [44].

The same randomized controlled trial conducted in geriatric patients with acute hip fracture found a 40% reduction on rehabilitation time, also documented a significantly higher IGF-1 levels in the blood at six months with an oral milk-based protein supplement of 20 g/day compared to an isocaloric placebo (85.5 ± 14.8% versus 34.1 ± 7.2%, $p = 0.003$ [30].

Studies of whey protein, naturally rich in leucine, also support a direct anabolic effect on muscle protein synthesis [45]. With regard to large cohort studies, the Health ABC Study showed that a higher protein intake over 3 years in 70–79-year-old adults was associated with a decreased loss of muscle mass [31].

With regard to clinical trials, as mentioned above, the 2015 meta-analysis by Komar et al. including 16 trials with 999 participants found that protein supplementation led to an increase in lean body mass among older adults at risk of sarcopenia [39]. Conversely, a meta-analysis of five clinical trials (n = 557) published in 2017 by Tieland et al. found no evidence that protein or amino acid supplementation increases muscle mass or function in healthy older adults [46].

6.5 What Protein Supplement Is Recommended and How Should It Be Ingested?

The definition of protein quality is used to be based on the composition and content of essential amino acids [47]. Newer concepts also take into consideration the digestibility of the protein, the intestinal absorption (slow vs. fast), and the presence of branch-chained anabolic amino acids (BCAA) like leucine [48–50]. Based on these criteria, in comparison to casein or soy protein, whey protein seems to be superior [51]. Based on current literature, for the anabolic effect on muscle, the target dose of whey protein appears to be a minimum of 20 g per day [52]. For optimal benefits of protein supplementation, a temporal link to exercise has been recommended [52, 53]. Also, giving a large amount of protein as a bolus (defined as taking 50% or more of the daily amount of protein in a meal or as a single supplement) has been suggested beneficial to overcome anabolic resistance of muscle among older adults [52]. Also, even distribution of protein intake for all meals has been shown to be advantageous: a study of 481 nursing home residents in Australia found that an even distribution of the amount of protein over several meals, in contrast to pulse administration, led to an overall increase in protein intake (RDI of 0.8 g/kg body weight/d achieved: 96.2 ± 30% against 87.3 ± 30.5%) [54]. Therefore, regardless of dose, ensuring protein sources at each meal is an essential basic strategy also in clinical care of older patients [35].

6.6 Negative Effects of an Increased Protein Intake

In contrast to earlier beliefs, a high protein intake does not promote bone loss but improves bone health [55]. In fact, a higher protein intake has been found to increase intestinal calcium absorption and improve bone mineral density and reduced risk of hip fracture [56].

While it has been long suspected that high protein intake may affect kidney function, results from large cohorts (WHI and NHS) suggest that high protein intakes do not affect kidney function [57, 58].

However, it has been suggested that among patients with severe renal insufficiency grade 3 and 4 (GFR < 30 ml/min), it may be warranted to limit protein intake to 0.8 g/kg/d [59, 60]. Patients requiring dialysis, on the other hand, should follow a protein-rich diet (REF).

6.7 Summary

The declines in bone and muscle mass are drivers of fragility fractures in older adults. Effective preventive strategies that address both bone and muscle health are therefore of great clinical value. In this chapter, we summarize available evidence in the literature that a protein-rich diet has positive effects on both bone and muscle health in older adults at risk for or with a fragility fracture. A uniform recommendation as to how much dietary protein is optimal in this risk situation is still under investigation. However, there is increasing consensus that a higher protein intake than currently recommended would be advantageous in senior adults, especially among those at increased risk for falls and fractures. The newer recommendations by the Prot-AGE group support an increase from the current 0.8 g/kg body weight/d to 1.2–1.5 g/kg body weight/d for active older adults and geriatric patients with an acute or chronic disease [35]. Further evidence is expected by ongoing research. The results of one Investigator initiated and independently funded trial (Swiss National Foundations) investigating a 40 g whey protein supplement with and without exercise among 800 older adults who sustained a fall injury (STRONG study) are expected in the near future. In the meantime, based on evidence reviewed in this chapter, we believe that for enhancing protein intake in patients with fragility fractures protein supplementation is warranted, especially among those with malnutrition and sarcopenia.

Key Messages

- Nutritional proteins have a positive effect on muscle and bone health.
- There is increasing consensus that the recommended protein intake for older adults needs to be increased for optimal muscle and bone health.
- The PROT-AGE study group recommends a daily protein intake of at least 1.0–1.2 g/kg body weight/d and 1.2–1.5 g/kg body weight/d for active older adults and those with an acute or chronic disease, respectively.
- There is evidence that whey protein supplements may be superior to other protein types due to their composition and higher leucine content.

References

1. Nguyen ND, et al. Development of a nomogram for individualizing hip fracture risk in men and women. Osteoporos Int. 2007;18(8):1109–17.
2. Bischoff-Ferrari, H.A., Three steps to unbreakable bones: the 2011 World Osteoporosis Day Report https://www.iofbonehealth.org/news/three-steps-unbreakable-bones-world-osteoporosis-day (access November 6th 2016), 2011.
3. Bischoff-Ferrari H. Fragility fractures: the future epidemic and its challenges. Skeletal Radiol. 2013;42(2):161–3.
4. Nations, U., D.O.E.A.S. Affairs, P. Division. World Population Prospects 2019: Highlights. 2019; Available from: https://population.un.org/wpp/Publications/Files/WPP2019_10KeyFindings.pdf.
5. Rosenberg IH, Roubenoff R. Stalking sarcopenia. Ann Intern Med. 1995;123(9):727–8.
6. Bischoff-Ferrari HA, et al. Comparative performance of current definitions of sarcopenia against the prospective incidence of falls among community-dwelling seniors age 65 and older. Osteoporos Int. 2015;
7. Dawson-Hughes B, Bischoff-Ferrari H. Considerations concerning the definition of sarcopenia. Osteoporos Int. 2016;27(11):3139–44.
8. Cruz-Jentoft AJ, et al. Sarcopenia: European consensus on definition and diagnosis. Report of the European Working Group on Sarcopenia in Older People A. J. Cruz-Gentoft et al. Age Ageing. 2010;39(4):412–23.
9. Cruz-Jentoft AJ, et al. Sarcopenia: revised European consensus on definition and diagnosis. Age Ageing. 2019;
10. Anker SD, Morley JE, von Haehling S. Welcome to the ICD-10 code for sarcopenia. J Cachexia Sarcopenia Muscle. 2016;7(5):512–4.
11. Lexell J, Taylor CC, Sjostrom M. What is the cause of the ageing atrophy? Total number, size and proportion of different fiber types studied in whole vastus lateralis muscle from 15- to 83-year-old men. J Neurol Sci. 1988;84(2–3):275–94.
12. Wolfe RR. The underappreciated role of muscle in health and disease. Am J Clin Nutr. 2006;84(3):475–82.
13. Lexell J, Downham D. What is the effect of ageing on type 2 muscle fibres? J Neurol Sci. 1992;107(2):250–1.
14. Verdijk LB, et al. Satellite cell content is specifically reduced in type II skeletal muscle fibers in the elderly. Am J Physiol Endocrinol Metab. 2007;292(1):E151–7.
15. Bischoff-Ferrari HA. The role of falls in fracture prediction. Curr Osteoporos Rep. 2011;9(3):116–21.
16. Tinetti ME, Speechley M, Ginter SF. Risk factors for falls among elderly persons living in the community. N Engl J Med. 1988;319(26):1701–7.
17. Campbell AJ, et al. Falls in old age: a study of frequency and related clinical factors. Age Ageing. 1981;10(4):264–70.
18. Orlandoni P, et al. Malnutrition upon hospital admission in geriatric patients: why assess it? Front Nutr. 2017;4:50.
19. Bischoff HA, Staehelin HB, Willett WC. The effect of undernutrition in the development of frailty in older persons. J Gerontol A Biol Sci Med Sci. 2006;61(6):585–9.
20. Wakimoto P, Block G. Dietary intake, dietary patterns, and changes with age: an epidemiological perspective. J Gerontol A Biol Sci Med Sci. 2001;56 (Spec No. 2):65–80.
21. Morley JE, Silver AJ. Anorexia in the elderly. Neurobiol Aging. 1988;9(1):9–16.
22. Malafarina V, et al. The anorexia of ageing: physiopathology, prevalence, associated comorbidity and mortality. A systematic review. Maturitas. 2013;74(4):293–302.
23. Kondrup J, et al. Nutritional risk screening (NRS 2002): a new method based on an analysis of controlled clinical trials. Clin Nutr. 2003;22(3):321–36.
24. Vellas B, et al. Nutrition assessment in the elderly. Curr Opin Clin Nutr Metab Care. 2001;4(1):5–8.
25. Jeejeebhoy KN. Nutritional assessment. Nutrition. 2000;16(7–8):585–90.
26. Hoffer LJ. Clinical nutrition: 1. Protein-energy malnutrition in the inpatient. CMAJ. 2001;165(10):1345–9.
27. Bonjour JP. Dietary protein: an essential nutrient for bone health. J Am Coll Nutr. 2005;24(Suppl. 6):526S–36S.
28. Cooper C, et al. Dietary protein intake and bone mass in women. Calcif Tissue Int. 1996;58(5):320–5.
29. Jesudason D, Clifton P. The interaction between dietary protein and bone health. J Bone Miner Metab. 2011;29(1):1–14.
30. Schurch MA, et al. Protein supplements increase serum insulin-like growth factor-I levels and attenuate proximal femur bone loss in patients with recent hip fracture. A randomized, double-blind, placebo-controlled trial. Ann Intern Med. 1998;128(10):801–9.
31. Houston DK, et al. Dietary protein intake is associated with lean mass change in older, community-dwelling adults: the Health, Aging, and Body Composition (Health ABC) Study. Am J Clin Nutr. 2008;87(1):150–5.
32. Mangano KM, et al. Dietary protein is associated with musculoskeletal health independently of dietary pattern: the Framingham Third Generation Study. Am J Clin Nutr. 2017;105(3):714–22.
33. Zoltick ES, et al. Dietary protein intake and subsequent falls in older men and women: the Framingham Study. J Nutr Health Aging. 2011;15(2):147–52.
34. Misra D, et al. Does dietary protein reduce hip fracture risk in elders? The Framingham Osteoporosis Study. Osteoporos Int. 2011;22(1):345–9.
35. Bauer J, et al. Evidence-based recommendations for optimal dietary protein intake in older people: a position paper from the PROT-AGE Study Group. J Am Med Dir Assoc. 2013;14(8):542–59.

36. World Health Organization, F.a.A.O.o.t.U.N., United Nations University, Protein and amino acid requirements in human nutrition, W.H. Organization, Editor, 2007.
37. Dumartheray EW, et al. Energy and nutrient intake of Swiss women aged 75–87 years. J Hum Nutr Diet. 2006;19(6):431–5.
38. Campbell WW, et al. The recommended dietary allowance for protein may not be adequate for older people to maintain skeletal muscle. J Gerontol A Biol Sci Med Sci. 2001;56(6):M373–80.
39. Komar B, Schwingshackl L, Hoffmann G. Effects of leucine-rich protein supplements on anthropometric parameter and muscle strength in the elderly: a systematic review and meta-analysis. J Nutr Health Aging. 2015;19(4):437–46.
40. Wu AM, et al. The relationship between dietary protein consumption and risk of fracture: a subgroup and dose-response meta-analysis of prospective cohort studies. Sci Rep. 2015;5:9151.
41. Tkatch L, et al. Benefits of oral protein supplementation in elderly patients with fracture of the proximal femur. J Am Coll Nutr. 1992;11(5):519–25.
42. Shams-White MM, et al. Dietary protein and bone health: a systematic review and meta-analysis from the National Osteoporosis Foundation. Am J Clin Nutr. 2017;105(6):1528–43.
43. Zhu K, et al. The effects of a two-year randomized, controlled trial of whey protein supplementation on bone structure, IGF-1, and urinary calcium excretion in older postmenopausal women. J Bone Miner Res. 2011;26(9):2298–306.
44. Lombardi G, et al. Role of IGF-I on PTH effects on bone. J Endocrinol Invest. 2010;33(Suppl. 7):22–6.
45. Breen L, Churchward-Venne TA. Leucine: a nutrient 'trigger' for muscle anabolism, but what more? J Physiol. 2012;590(9):2065–6.
46. Tieland M, et al. The impact of dietary protein or amino acid supplementation on muscle mass and strength in elderly people: individual participant data and meta-analysis of RCT's. J Nutr Health Aging. 2017;21(9):994–1001.
47. Joint FAO/WHO Expert Consultation on Protein Quality Evaluation (1989: Bethesda, Maryland), World Health Organization & Food and Agriculture Organization of the United Nations. Protein quality evaluation: report of the Joint FAO/WHO Expert Consultation, Bethesda, MD, USA, 4–8 December 1989. Rome: FAO; 1991.
48. Tang JE, Phillips SM. Maximizing muscle protein anabolism: the role of protein quality. Curr Opin Clin Nutr Metab Care. 2009;12(1):66–71.
49. Millward DJ, et al. Protein quality assessment: impact of expanding understanding of protein and amino acid needs for optimal health. Am J Clin Nutr. 2008;87(5):1576S–81S.
50. Xu ZR, et al. The effectiveness of leucine on muscle protein synthesis, lean body mass and leg lean mass accretion in older people: a systematic review and meta-analysis. Br J Nutr. 2015;113(1):25–34.
51. Devries MC, Phillips SM. Supplemental protein in support of muscle mass and health: advantage whey. J Food Sci. 2015;80(Suppl. 1):A8–A15.
52. Yang Y, et al. Resistance exercise enhances myofibrillar protein synthesis with graded intakes of whey protein in older men. Br J Nutr. 2012;108(10):1780–8.
53. Wall BT, et al. Leucine co-ingestion improves postprandial muscle protein accretion in elderly men. Clin Nutr. 2013;32(3):412–9.
54. Tieland M, et al. An even distribution of protein intake daily promotes protein adequacy but does not influence nutritional status in institutionalized elderly. J Am Med Dir Assoc. 2018;19(1):33–9.
55. Fenton TR, et al. Meta-analysis of the effect of the acid-ash hypothesis of osteoporosis on calcium balance. J Bone Miner Res. 2009;24(11):1835–40.
56. Bonjour JP. Protein intake and bone health. Int J Vitam Nutr Res. 2011;81(2-3):134–42.
57. Beasley JM, et al. Higher biomarker-calibrated protein intake is not associated with impaired renal function in postmenopausal women. J Nutr. 2011;141(8):1502–7.
58. Knight EL, et al. The impact of protein intake on renal function decline in women with normal renal function or mild renal insufficiency. Ann Intern Med. 2003;138(6):460–7.
59. Eyre S, Attman PO. Protein restriction and body composition in renal disease. J Ren Nutr. 2008;18(2):167–86.
60. Brunori G, et al. Efficacy and safety of a very-low-protein diet when postponing dialysis in the elderly: a prospective randomized multicenter controlled study. Am J Kidney Dis. 2007;49(5):569–80.
61. Middleton RG, et al. FRAX and the assessment of the risk of developing a fragility fracture. J Bone Joint Surg Br. 2012;94(10):1313–20.
62. Tinetti ME, Kumar C. The patient who falls: "It's always a trade-off". JAMA. 2010;303(3):258–66.

7 Supplementation: Vitamin D, Calcium

Heike A. Bischoff-Ferrari

7.1 Introduction

Vitamin D deficiency remains prevalent in older adults aged 65 and older, with about 50% not reaching the threshold for a replete vitamin D status of 20 ng/mL [1]. Among older adults, the highest prevalence of vitamin D deficiency is seen in patients with fragility fractures, reaching 80% among hip fracture patients [2, 3]. This may be best explained as reduced mobility limiting sun exposure, but also the fact that aging reduces skin production of vitamin D four-fold compared with younger adults [4, 5].

Mechanistically, vitamin D deficiency contributes to the risk of sustaining a hip fracture in two ways: (1) vitamin D deficiency causes muscle weakness and thereby promotes the risk of falling [6, 7]; (2) and impairs calcium metabolism causing secondary hyperparathyroidism and thereby bone loss [1].

Notably and central to this chapter targeted to the care of older patients with fragility fractures [1], vitamin D deficiency has been linked to an increased risk of falls and fractures, as well as worse functional outcomes after hip fractures [8]. Further, based on meta-analyses of double-blind RCTs among vitamin D-deficient adults aged 65 and older, daily vitamin D supplementation of 800–1000 IU with or without calcium has been found to significantly reduce fall risk by 38% with a treatment duration of 2–5 months and a sustained significant effect of 17% with a treatment duration of 12–36 months [7, 9], and a 30% reduction of hip fractures [10]. Relevant to clinical care, this chapter will review the recent meta-analysis on vitamin D and fall plus fracture prevention that extended to adults without vitamin D deficiency and osteoporosis. Finally, this chapter will discuss daily versus large-dose bolus application of vitamin D, of which the latter has been consistently shown to increase the risk of falls and fractures among older adults.

7.2 Risk Factors for Vitamin D Deficiency and Its Prevalence

Most vulnerable to vitamin D deficiency are older adults [4, 5], individuals living in northern latitudes with prolonged winters and thus low UVB exposure [11, 12], obese individuals [13], and individuals of all ages with a dark skin tone [14–16]. Other risk factors include medical conditions such as malabsorption and the use of antiepileptic drugs [17]. The prevalence of vitamin D deficiency (serum levels below 20 ng/mL or 50 nmol/L) among older adults has been found to be about 50% in many countries around the world [18], with the highest prevalence (80%) in older women with hip fractures [2, 3]. As a first sign of

H. A. Bischoff-Ferrari (✉)
Department of Aging Medicine and Aging Research, City Hospital Zurich-Waid, Zurich University, Zürich, Switzerland
e-mail: heike.bischoff@usz.ch

H.-C. Pape et al. (eds.), *Senior Trauma Patients*, https://doi.org/10.1007/978-3-030-91483-7_7

toxicity, only serum 25(OH)D levels of above 220 nmol/L have been associated with hypercalcemia [19, 20].

7.3 Evidence Linking Vitamin D to Muscle Health

First, proximal muscle weakness is a prominent feature of the clinical syndrome of vitamin D deficiency [6]. Clinical findings in vitamin D deficiency myopathy include proximal muscle weakness, diffuse muscle pain, and gait impairments such as waddling way of walking [21]. *Second,* the vitamin D receptor (VDR) is expressed [7] in human muscle tissue, as documented in all [22–27] but one [28] investigation. Further, several studies among older individuals suggest that VDR activation in muscle promotes de novo protein synthesis preferentially in type II fast twitch muscle fibers relevant for fall prevention [29–31]. *Third,* several observational studies suggest a positive association between 25(OH)D and muscle strength or lower extremity function in older persons [32, 33]. *Fourth,* vitamin D supplementation in vitamin D-deficient older adults increased muscle strength and balance [34, 35] and reduced the risk of falling in community-dwelling individuals [35–37], as well as in institutionalized individuals [34, 38].

7.4 Vitamin D Supplementation and Fall Risk Reduction Among Vitamin D-Deficient Older Adults

Several meta-analyses of clinical trials that targeted older adults with vitamin D deficiency suggest a reduction in falls [7, 39–46] with vitamin D supplementation, although conclusions have varied by trial quality, dose, and bolus application. Notably, low dose vitamin D (<700 IU/day) did not reduce fall risk significantly, while high bolus doses (500,000 IU vitamin D3 annually [47], 100,000 IU monthly [48], and 60,000 IU monthly [49]) increased the risk of falling in older adults at risk of falling and are therefore not recommended in the care of older patients with fragility fractures.

On the other hand, based on a meta-analysis of double-blind RCTs among older adults at risk of falls and vitamin D deficiency [7, 9], a higher daily dose of 700–1000 IU vitamin D reduced the risk of falling by 38% with a treatment duration of 2–5 months and a sustained significant effect of 17% fall reduction with treatment duration of 12–36 months, and this benefit was independent of type of dwelling and age [7, 9].

7.5 Recent Recommendations by the USPSTF Regarding Vitamin D and Fall Prevention

In 2019 [50], the US Preventive Services Task Force (USPSTF) panel revised their earlier favorable assessment of vitamin D supplementation for fall prevention in 2012 [51] to a recommendation against supplementation with vitamin D for fall prevention among community-dwelling adults, 65 or older, who are not known to have osteoporosis or vitamin D deficiency, or to be at high risk of falling or fracture [52]. The latter conclusion was based on the inconsistent findings from 5 trials and strongly influenced by evidence from a single trial that tested a large bolus dose of 500,000 IU of vitamin D annually [47] and reported increased risks of both falls and fractures with this treatment among community-dwelling adults at increased risk of falling.

Notably, for patients at increased risk of osteoporosis and/or those with vitamin D deficiency, evidence from double-blind RCTs supports vitamin D supplementation (800–1000 IU/day), consistent with recommendations of other professional societies such as the U.S. Endocrine Society [17] and National Osteoporosis Foundation [53]. The literature is especially supportive of a benefit of vitamin D supplementation in most vulnerable populations, such as older adults living in institutions, or at high risk of fracture, and those with vitamin D deficiency [52, 54].

7.6 Vitamin D and Function and Strength and Frailty

In three double-blind RCTs among older adults with vitamin D deficiency and increased risk of falling, supplementation with 800 IU vitamin D3 resulted in a 4–11% gain in lower extremity strength or function [34, 35] and up to 28% improvement in body sway[35, 37] in older adults aged 65+ within 2–12 month of treatment. Extending to individuals better vitamin D status, a 2014 meta-analysis by Beaudart et al. included 30 randomized controlled trials (5615 individuals with mean age 61.1 years) and found a small but significant positive effect of vitamin D supplementation with or without calcium on global muscle strength with a standardized mean difference (SMD) of 0.17 ($P = 0.02$), while no significant effect was found on muscle mass and muscle power [55]. Results on muscle strength were most pronounced in individuals with 25-hydroxyvitamin D level below 30 nmol/L and were more effective in adults aged 65 years or older compared to younger subjects (SMD 0.25; 95% CI 0.01–0.48 vs. SMD 0.03; 95% CI −0.08 to 0.14) [55].

Regarding frailty, low levels of 25-hydroxavitamin D have been associated with a higher risk of frailty in the majority of cohort studies [56, 57]. However, insufficient evidence exists regarding the effectiveness of vitamin D supplementation for older adults preselected for frailty. However, frailty is very common in older adults at risk of hip fracture, where a daily median supplementation of 800 IU vitamin D reduced hip fracture risk by 30% [10].

7.7 Fracture Prevention with Vitamin D Supplementation Based on The Four Recent Meta-Analyses

From 2016 to 2018, four meta-analyses efforts were undertaken to review the benefit of vitamin D on fracture prevention. Two of these meta-analyses focused on primary prevention of fractures among adults aged 50 years and older, who are not at risk of fracture or vitamin D deficiency [58, 59], which has not been established before. One of these meta-analyses focused on the combination of vitamin D plus calcium only [60] and one on the individual effect of vitamin D without calcium [61]. Notably, only the meta-analysis that focused on the combined effects of vitamin D and calcium [60] targeted primarily adults aged 65 and older living in the community or in institutions.

The latter found a significant 15% reduction of total fractures (RR = 0.85; 95% CI 0.73–0.98) and a significant 30% reduction of hip fractures (RR = 0.70; 95% CI 0.56–0.87) for a daily combination of vitamin D plus calcium [60]. The other three meta-analyses suggested that there was no benefit of vitamin D. In order to transfer these findings to clinical care of older patients with fragility fractures, it is important to understand the goals and target groups of these recent meta-analyses.

Regarding the meta-analyses by Zhao et al. [58] and the US Preventive Task Force [59], both teams of authors state that their recommendations only apply to community-dwelling adults who are not known to have osteoporosis or vitamin D deficiency or are not at high risk of falling. Their results therefore do not apply to a large segment of older adults who have these risk factors.

The fourth meta-analysis by Bolland et al. [61] included trials of primary and secondary prevention among adults aged 50 years and older. Their findings regarding no benefit of vitamin D have been questioned based on the exclusion of about 40% of high-quality trials on the combined effect of vitamin D and calcium and their biased results by vitamin D dose [62] that combined 800 IU with any lower dose. In fact, a published reanalysis of the Bolland meta-analysis for trials that tested the currently recommended dose of 800–1000 IU vitamin D with more than 50% adherence, and excluding the large annual dosing trials, suggested a significant 14% reduction in total fractures (RR = 0.86; 95% CI 0.75–0.98) and a significant 12% reduction of falls (RR = 0.88; 95% CI 0.81–0.95) [62].

7.8 In Summary

For older adults at increased risk of falls and fragility fractures and/or vitamin D deficiency, evidence from double-blind RCTs supports supplementation with 800–1000 IU vitamin D per day to treat their high prevalence of vitamin D deficiency and reduce their risk of falls and fractures [63, 64].

This is consistent with the International Osteoporosis Foundation [65], the US Endocrine Society [17], and NOF [53] guidelines on vitamin D. In fact, reducing the risk of fractures among vulnerable older adults aged 65 and older, who sustain 75% of all osteoporotic fractures [66], remains an important public health target. At a public health level, in view of the small risk and cost, we believe that it is essential not to discourage older adults from receiving daily 800–1000 IU vitamin D.

References

1. Lips, P., et al., Management of endocrine disease: current vitamin D status in European and Middle East countries and strategies to prevent vitamin D deficiency; a position statement of the European Calcified Tissue Society. Eur J Endocrinol, 2019.
2. Bischoff-Ferrari HA, et al. Severe vitamin D deficiency in Swiss hip fracture patients. Bone. 2008;42(3):597–602.
3. LeBoff MS, et al. Occult vitamin D deficiency in postmenopausal US women with acute hip fracture. JAMA. 1999;281(16):1505–11.
4. McKenna MJ. Differences in vitamin D status between countries in young adults and the elderly. Am J Med. 1992;93(1):69–77.
5. Theiler R, et al. Calcidiol, calcitriol and parathyroid hormone serum concentrations in institutionalized and ambulatory elderly in Switzerland. Int J Vitam Nutr Res. 1999;69(2):96–105.
6. Al-Shoha A, et al. Osteomalacia with bone marrow fibrosis due to severe vitamin D deficiency after a gastrointestinal bypass operation for severe obesity. Endocr Pract. 2009;15(6):528–33.
7. Bischoff-Ferrari HA, et al. Fall prevention with supplemental and active forms of vitamin D: a meta-analysis of randomised controlled trials. BMJ. 2009;339(1):339:b3692.
8. LeBoff MS, et al. Vitamin D-deficiency and post-fracture changes in lower extremity function and falls in women with hip fractures. Osteoporos Int. 2008;19(9):1283–90.
9. Bischoff-Ferrari, H.A., et al., Re: Fall prevention with Vitamin D. Clarifications needed. http://www.bmj.com/content/339/bmj.b3692?tab=responses (accessed: Feb 13, 2012), 2011.
10. Bischoff-Ferrari, H.A., et al., A pooled analysis of vitamin D dose requirements for fracture prevention. N Engl J Med, 2012.
11. Webb AR, Kline L, Holick MF. Influence of season and latitude on the cutaneous synthesis of vitamin D3: exposure to winter sunlight in Boston and Edmonton will not promote vitamin D3 synthesis in human skin. J Clin Endocrinol Metab. 1988;67(2):373–8.
12. Dawson-Hughes B, Harris SS, Dallal GE. Plasma calcidiol, season, and serum parathyroid hormone concentrations in healthy elderly men and women. Am J Clin Nutr. 1997;65(1):67–71.
13. Parikh SJ, et al. The relationship between obesity and serum 1,25-dihydroxy vitamin D concentrations in healthy adults. J Clin Endocrinol Metab. 2004;89(3):1196–9.
14. Looker AC, et al. Serum 25-hydroxyvitamin D status of adolescents and adults in two seasonal subpopulations from NHANES III. Bone. 2002;30(5):771–7.
15. Bischoff-Ferrari HA, et al. Positive association between 25-hydroxy vitamin D levels and bone mineral density: a population-based study of younger and older adults. Am J Med. 2004;116(9):634–9.
16. Nesby-O'Dell S, et al. Hypovitaminosis D prevalence and determinants among African American and white women of reproductive age: third National Health and Nutrition Examination Survey, 1988–1994. Am J Clin Nutr. 2002;76(1):187–92.
17. Holick MF, et al. Evaluation, treatment, and prevention of vitamin D deficiency: an endocrine society clinical practice guideline. J Clin Endocrinol Metab. 2011;96(7):1911–30.
18. van Schoor NM, Lips P. Worldwide vitamin D status. Best Pract Res Clin Endocrinol Metab. 2011;25(4):671–80.
19. Gertner JM, Domenech M. 25-Hydroxyvitamin D levels in patients treated with high-dosage ergo- and cholecalciferol. J Clin Pathol. 1977;30(2):144–50.
20. Vieth R. Vitamin D supplementation, 25-hydroxyvitamin D concentrations, and safety. Am J Clin Nutr. 1999;69(5):842–56.
21. Schott GD, Wills MR. Muscle weakness in osteomalacia. Lancet. 1976;1(7960):626–9.
22. Bischoff HA, et al. In situ detection of 1,25-dihydroxyvitamin D3 receptor in human skeletal muscle tissue. Histochem J. 2001;33(1):19–24.
23. Bischoff-Ferrari HA, et al. Vitamin D receptor expression in human muscle tissue decreases with age. J Bone Miner Res. 2004;19(2):265–9.
24. Boland R. Role of vitamin D in skeletal muscle function. Endocr Rev. 1986;7(4):434–48.
25. Costa EM, Blau HM, Feldman D. 1,25-dihydroxyvitamin D3 receptors and hormonal responses in cloned human skeletal muscle cells. Endocrinology. 1986;119(5):2214–20.

26. Simpson RU, Thomas GA, Arnold AJ. Identification of 1,25-dihydroxyvitamin D3 receptors and activities in muscle. J Biol Chem. 1985;260(15):8882–91.
27. Ceglia L, et al. Multi-step immunofluorescent analysis of vitamin D receptor loci and myosin heavy chain isoforms in human skeletal muscle. J Mol Histol. 2010;41(2–3):137–42.
28. Wang Y, DeLuca HF. Is the vitamin d receptor found in muscle? Endocrinology. 2011;152(2):354–63.
29. Sorensen OH, et al. Myopathy in bone loss of ageing: improvement by treatment with 1 alpha-hydroxycholecalciferol and calcium. Clin Sci (Colch). 1979;56(2):157–61.
30. Freedman LP. Transcriptional targets of the vitamin D3 receptor-mediating cell cycle arrest and differentiation. J Nutr. 1999;129(Suppl. 2S):581S–6S.
31. Ceglia, L., et al., A randomized study on the effect of vitamin D3 supplementation on skeletal muscle morphology and vitamin D receptor concentration in older women. J Clin Endocrinol Metab, 2013.
32. Wicherts IS, et al. Vitamin D status predicts physical performance and its decline in older persons. J Clin Endocrinol Metab. 2007;6:6.
33. Bischoff-Ferrari HA, et al. Higher 25-hydroxyvitamin D concentrations are associated with better lower-extremity function in both active and inactive persons aged >=60 y. Am J Clin Nutr. 2004;80(3):752–8.
34. Bischoff HA, et al. Effects of vitamin D and calcium supplementation on falls: a randomized controlled trial. J Bone Miner Res. 2003;18(2):343–51.
35. Pfeifer M, et al. Effects of a long-term vitamin D and calcium supplementation on falls and parameters of muscle function in community-dwelling older individuals. Osteoporos Int. 2008;16:16.
36. Bischoff-Ferrari HA, Orav EJ, Dawson-Hughes B. Effect of cholecalciferol plus calcium on falling in ambulatory older men and women: a 3-year randomized controlled trial. Arch Intern Med. 2006;166(4):424–30.
37. Pfeifer M, et al. Effects of a short-term vitamin D and calcium supplementation on body sway and secondary hyperparathyroidism in elderly women. J Bone Miner Res. 2000;15(6):1113–8.
38. Broe KE, et al. A higher dose of vitamin d reduces the risk of falls in nursing home residents: a randomized, multiple-dose study. J Am Geriatr Soc. 2007;55(2):234–9.
39. Bischoff-Ferrari HA, et al. Effect of vitamin D on falls: a meta-analysis. JAMA. 2004;291(16):1999–2006.
40. Jackson C, et al. The effect of cholecalciferol (vitamin D3) on the risk of fall and fracture: a meta-analysis. QJM. 2007;100(4):185–92.
41. Kalyani RR, et al. Vitamin D treatment for the prevention of falls in older adults: systematic review and meta-analysis. J Am Geriatr Soc. 2010;58(7):1299–310.
42. O'Donnell S, et al. Systematic review of the benefits and harms of calcitriol and alfacalcidol for fractures and falls. J Bone Miner Metab. 2008;26(6):531–42.
43. Richy F, Dukas L, Schacht E. Differential effects of D-hormone analogs and native vitamin D on the risk of falls: a comparative meta-analysis. Calcif Tissue Int. 2008;82(2):102–7.
44. Michael, Y.L., et al., Interventions to prevent falls in older adults: an updated systematic review. US Preventive Services Task Force Evidence Syntheses, formerly Systematic Evidence Reviews, 2011.
45. Michael YL, et al. Primary care-relevant interventions to prevent falling in older adults: a systematic evidence review for the U.S. Preventive services task force. Ann Intern Med. 2011;153(12):815–25.
46. Cameron ID, et al. Interventions for preventing falls in older people in nursing care facilities and hospitals. Cochrane Database Syst Rev. 2010;1:CD005465.
47. Sanders KM, et al. Annual high-dose oral vitamin D and falls and fractures in older women: a randomized controlled trial. JAMA. 2010;303(18):1815–22.
48. Ginde AA, et al. High-dose monthly vitamin D for prevention of acute respiratory infection in older long-term care residents: a randomized clinical trial. J Am Geriatr Soc. 2017;65(3):496–503.
49. Bischoff-Ferrari HA, et al. Monthly high-dose Vitamin D treatment for the prevention of functional decline: a randomized clinical trial. JAMA Intern Med. 2016;176(2):175–83.
50. Force USPST, et al. Interventions to prevent falls in community-dwelling older adults: US Preventive Services Task Force Recommendation Statement. JAMA. 2018;319(16):1696–704.
51. Moyer VA, U.S.P.S.T. Force. Prevention of falls in community-dwelling older adults: U.S. Preventive Services Task Force recommendation statement. Ann Intern Med. 2012;157(3):197–204.
52. Bischoff-Ferrari HA, Bhasin S, Manson JE. Preventing fractures and falls: a limited role for calcium and vitamin D supplements? JAMA. 2018;319(15):1552–3.
53. Cosman F, et al. Clinician's guide to prevention and treatment of osteoporosis. Osteoporos Int. 2014;25(10):2359–81.
54. Bischoff-Ferrari HA, et al. Effect of high-dosage cholecalciferol and extended physiotherapy on complications after hip fracture: a randomized controlled trial. Arch Intern Med. 2010;170(9):813–20.
55. Beaudart C, et al. The effects of vitamin d on skeletal muscle strength, muscle mass, and muscle power: a systematic review and meta-analysis of randomized controlled trials. J Clin Endocrinol Metab. 2014;99(11):4336–45.
56. Morley JE, Malmstrom TK. Frailty, sarcopenia, and hormones. Endocrinol Metab Clin N Am. 2013;42(2):391–405.
57. Ju SY, Lee JY, Kim DH. Low 25-hydroxyvitamin D levels and the risk of frailty syndrome: a systematic review and dose-response meta-analysis. BMC Geriatr. 2018;18(1):206.
58. Zhao JG, et al. Association between calcium or vitamin D supplementation and fracture incidence in community-dwelling older adults: a systematic review and meta-analysis. JAMA. 2017;318(24):2466–82.
59. Force USPST, et al. Vitamin D, calcium, or combined supplementation for the primary prevention of frac-

tures in community-dwelling adults: US Preventive Services Task Force Recommendation Statement. JAMA. 2018;319(15):1592–9.
60. Weaver CM, et al. Calcium plus vitamin D supplementation and risk of fractures: an updated meta-analysis from the National Osteoporosis Foundation. Osteoporos Int. 2016;27(1):367–76.
61. Bolland MJ, Grey A, Avenell A. Effects of vitamin D supplementation on musculoskeletal health: a systematic review, meta-analysis, and trial sequential analysis. Lancet Diabetes Endocrinol. 2018;6(11):847–58.
62. Bischoff-Ferrari HA, et al. Vitamin D supplementation and musculoskeletal health. Lancet Diabetes Endocrinol. 2019;7(2):85.
63. Bischoff-Ferrari HA. Fall prevention, in primer on the metabolic bone diseases and disorders of mineral metabolism. In: ASBMR; 2018. p. 526–33.
64. Bischoff Ferrari, H.A.e.a., Vitamin D Summary Report BAG. http://www.blv.admin.ch/themen/04679/05108/05869/index.html, 2012.
65. Dawson-Hughes B, et al. IOF position statement: vitamin D recommendations for older adults. Osteoporos Int. 2010;21(7):1151–4.
66. Melton LJ 3rd, Crowson CS, O'Fallon WM. Fracture incidence in Olmsted County, Minnesota: comparison of urban with rural rates and changes in urban rates over time. Osteoporos Int. 1999;9(1):29–37.

8 Exercise Concepts for Fall Prevention

M. Mattle and R. Theiler

8.1 Introduction

Exercise is an established and effective concept in fall prevention among both community-dwelling and frail older adults [1]. Many studies demonstrate that simple balance and weight-bearing exercise programs improve gait speed, muscle strength, and balance in community-dwelling and frail older adults, which translates into fall reduction by 15–50% [2–6]. As falls are the primary risk factor for fractures, the rationale is that these interventions should also protect against fractures [1]. In this chapter, we review the currently available evidence concerning the effect of exercise on fall prevention among healthy community-dwelling older adults, as well as pre-frail and frail older adults with a history of previous falls or cognitive decline.

M. Mattle (✉)
Center on Aging and Mobility, University Hospital Zurich, Zurich City Hospital-Waid and University of Zurich, Zurich, Switzerland

Department of Aging Medicine and Aging Research, University Hospital Zurich and University of Zurich, Zurich, Switzerland
e-mail: michele.mattle@usz.ch

R. Theiler
Department of Aging Medicine and Aging Research, University Hospital Zurich and University of Zurich, Zurich, Switzerland

8.2 Physical Exercise Approaches to Prevent Falling in Older Adults

Older adults who engage regularly in physical exercise and reduce their time spent with sedentary behavior are more likely to maintain their health and stay independent [7, 8]. Moreover, physical exercise has been shown to be the most promising prevention strategy for falls and injurious falls, both as a single intervention component and as a part of a multifactorial approach, as, e.g., in combined behavioral, educational, and environmental adaption approaches [9].

8.2.1 Home- or Group-Based Multicomponent Exercise Interventions

Recently, Sherrington et al. published a Cochrane review evaluating exercise for falls prevention in older adults living in the community (average age of participants in included trials was 76) and confirmed the findings about exercise as an effective prevention strategy to reduce falls among older adults found earlier by Gillespie et al. [5]. This updated meta-analysis including 63 trials with a total of 13,518 participants showed that the number of persons experiencing one or more falls was reduced by 15% in the intervention groups, if taking into account all types of exercise programs (risk ratio (RR): 0.85; 95% Confidence Interval

H.-C. Pape et al. (eds.), *Senior Trauma Patients*, https://doi.org/10.1007/978-3-030-91483-7_8

(CI): 0.81–0.89) [6]. Further, the rate of falls was reduced by 23% for participants in exercise groups (all types) compared to controls (rate ratio (RaR): 0.77; 95% CI 0.71–0.83; 12,981 participants in 59 trials) [6]. Moreover, in this meta-analysis, exercise (all types) reduced the number of people experiencing at least one fall-related fracture by 27% (RR: 0.73; 95% CI 0.56–0.95; 10 trials including 4047 participants) compared to controls [6].

Exercise strategies incorporating the enhancement of more than one physical ability simultaneously (interventions that comprise balance, strength, and functional exercises at once) seem more effective than single-component exercise strategies [5, 6]. Specifically, for so-called multi-component exercise interventions, a subgroup analysis within the same Cochrane review by Sherrington et al. including 11 trials with a total of 1374 community-dwelling participants showed that the rate of falls was reduced by 34% (RaR: 0.66; 95% CI 0.50–0.88) for participants in intervention groups compared to controls [6].

8.2.2 Mind-Motor Exercise Interventions

Mind-motor exercise interventions (also known as cognitive-motor or cognitive-physical interventions) combine physical and cognitive tasks (e.g., dual-, or multitasking) and involve working memory and deliberate motor-control [10–12]. Classic examples of mind-motor exercises are Tai Chi, a form of exercise which emphasizes static and dynamic balance, incorporates specific weight transferences, and requires upright posture and subtle changes of head positioning and gaze direction [13]; dance, which involves a wide range of dynamic movement qualities, speeds, and step patterns [14]; and volitional and reactive stepping interventions, where participants stand on platforms or grids painted on the floor and need to place their feet into the accurate square in their front, in the back, or side wards timed onto visual or acoustic cues [15].

The Prevention of Falls Network Europe (ProFaNE) summarizes Tai Chi, Qi Gong, Yoga, and dance under "3D training" [16]. ProFaNE characterizes 3D training as "constant movements in a controlled, fluid, repetitive way through all three spatial planes or dimensions (forward and back, side to side, and up and down" [6]. This definition was used to classify exercise interventions in the Cochrane Reviews evaluating interventions to prevent falls [5, 6].

Huang et al. found in their meta-analysis a reduced risk of falling at least once (RR: 0.80; 95% CI 0.72–0.88; 16 trials including 3539 participants) and a reduction of the rate of falls (Incidence Rate Ratio (IRR): 0.69; 95% CI 0.60–0.80; 15 trials including 3470 events) for older adults aged 65 and older participating in a Tai Chi intervention group compared to participants in control groups. Notably, this meta-analysis included studies among healthy community-dwelling older adults, as well as participants with comorbidities such as stroke, frailty, or Parkinson's disease [17]. Nevertheless, the Cochrane review by Gillespie et al., which included trials with participants aged 60 and older living in the community and explicitly excluded trials among patients post-stroke or with Parkinson's disease, showed that Tai Chi reduced the risk of falling by 29% (RR: 0.71; 95% CI 0.57–0.87; 6 trials including 1625 participants), while the reduction in rate of falls bordered on statistical significance (RaR: 0.72; 95% CI 0.52–1.00; 5 trials including 1563 participants) [5].

The Cochrane Review by Sherrington et al. found only one trial with an intervention that classified as 3D-dance and reported on falls [18]. The latest available systematic review (7 trials including 354 participants) suggested that dance may improve balance, strength, and gait parameters [19].

Most recently, in a meta-analysis, dance-based mind-motor activities (defined as "coordinated upright mind-motor movements that emphasize dynamic balance, structured through music or an inner rhythm (e.g., breathing) and distinctive instructions or choreography, and that involve social interaction" which includes different styles of dance as well as Tai Chi) were reported to reduce risk of falling (RR: 0.63; 95% CI 0.49–

0.80; 8 trials including 1579 participants) and rate of falls (IRR: 0.69; 95% CI 0.53–0.89, 7 trials including 2012 participants) among community-dwelling older adults aged 65 and older—alongside statistically significantly improving balance, mobility, and lower-body strength [20].

Yoga, a form of exercise focusing on static balance, isometric strength, and stretching, seems to improve balance, physical function, and quality of life, but no meta-analysis has been published yet investigating the effect of Yoga on falls in older adults [21, 22].

A meta-analysis (7 trials including 660 participants) evaluating stepping exercises and exercise setups, which instruct the participant to place her feet within a given rhythm on target fields on a platform (so-called dance platforms), found a reduced risk of falling at least once (RR: 0.51; 95% CI 0.38–0.68) and a reduced rate of falls (RaR: 0.48; 95% CI 0.36–0.65) [15].

8.2.3 Perturbation-Based Balance Training and Active Video Games

New approaches to physical exercise modalities include perturbations-based balance training (PBT) or the use of modern devices and virtual realities (such as, e.g., the Nitendo *Wii exergame)*.

In PBT, participants are exposed to unexpected balance perturbations while exercising on a treadmill or performing tasks of daily living. Perturbations can be induced by a therapist or through the exercise device (e.g., treadmill shifts or accelerations). When performed with older adults at high risk of falling, participants may be supported by weight-bearing belts [23].

Preliminary randomized controlled trials using PBT were summarized in a meta-analysis by Mansfield et al. (2015) including participants within the age range of 50–96 years. In this meta-analysis, participants who completed PBT were less likely to report at least one fall (RaR 0.71; 95% CI 0.52–0.96) and had a lower number of falls compared to the control groups (RaR 0.54; 95% CI 0.34–0.85) [24]. However, this meta-analysis pooled studies including healthy participants as well as patients with Parkinson's disease or frailty (total 8 trials including 404 participants) [24].

In the last decade, home-based active video games (AVG) gained popularity. Examples of AVG used to enhance physical activity and train specific functions in rehabilitation settings are the *Wii exergames* (Nintendo Co. Ltd., Kyoto, Japan, 2006). A monitor displays a virtual reality and the players react on gaming commands given within this reality. Their movements are detected through cameras and accelerometers and then transmitted back to the computer program executing the game. Activities provided include different sports, such as tennis or soccer, as well as balance trainings and fun activities such as imaginary dance battles. The effects of interventions using virtual realities have been evaluated in several different populations, including healthy community-dwelling older adults, participants with Parkinson's disease, stroke survivors, and frail older adults [25, 26]. However, the trials published to date were small with a focus on balance and feasibility. None of these novel virtual reality approaches have been tested with regard to incident falls or number of fallers in older adults. Nevertheless, relevant to clinical care, the meta-analyses summarizing PBT, and AVG, suggest that these novel exercise interventions are feasible and potentially beneficial as well in frail older patients [24, 26].

8.3 Effect of Physical Exercise in Older Adults at High Risk of Falling

The most important risk factors for accidental falls encompass the experience of previous falls often promoted by muscle weakness, gait impairment, as well as decreased balance [27].

8.3.1 Exercise for Older Adults with Previous Falls (with or Without Fractures) and Frailty

Sherrington et al. report in their Cochrane Review that in trials where all participants were at increased risk of falling, exercise (all types) reduced the number of people experiencing at least one fall by 13% (RR: 0.87; 95% CI 0.83–0.91; 35 trials including 7171 participants) compared to controls. The rate of falls in the high-risk populations was reduced by 20% for participants in the exercise groups (all types) compared to controls (RaR: 0.80; 95% CI 0.72–0.88; 30 trials including 6858 participants). The same review, when evaluating the effect of multicomponent exercises specifically, found a reduction of the rate of falls of 30% for participants at high risk of falling in intervention groups compared to controls (RaR: 0.77; 95% CI 0.63–0.94; 5 trials including 618 participants) [6].

8.3.2 Home-Based Exercises Programs

Home-based exercise programs include safe and simple strength and balance exercises that focus on the functionality needed for daily life tasks. In general, a trained health care professional instructs the patient how to conduct home-based exercises, e.g., at discharge from the hospital or in a rehabilitation setting. In the following, the patients perform the exercises on their own at home. Regular control and adaptions by a trained health professional are crucial for the success of home-based exercise programs (adjust intensity, provide motivation, and enhance adherence).

A comprehensive home-based exercise program for older adults at high risk of falling is the Otago Exercise Program (OEP) [28]. Campbell and colleagues developed the OEP in New Zealand specifically to prevent falls [28]. The OEP is an extended, individually tailored, and expert-supported home exercise program with gradually increased intensity and a focus on strength and balance [28]. The program includes 17 exercises initially delivered by a physical therapist or trained health care professional [28]. Additionally, five home visits by the exercise instructor and monthly telephone calls to ensure adherence are part of the program [29]. In a meta-analysis of 7 trials including 1503 community-dwelling participants with a mean age of 81.6 years, a positive effect of OEP on reducing fall rates over 12 months was found (IRR: 0.68; 95% CI 0.56–0.79) [30]. Additionally, the authors found that OEP significantly reduced risk of death over 12 months (RR: 0.45; 95% CI 0.25–0.80) [30].

Significant limitations of individualized and complex home-based exercise programs such as the OEP are their high costs and implementation time and personnel burden. Before implementing such programs at a broader level within a health care system, these barriers need to be addressed in a cost-effectiveness analysis [1].

Notably, less complex interventions have been shown to be effective to prevent falls in patients at high risk as well. In a randomized controlled trial among 173 patients (mean age 84 years), a simple home exercise program instructed during acute care after hip fracture surgery reduced falls significantly by 25% over a 12 months follow-up compared to standard of care without the simple home exercise program (adjusted relative rate difference, −25%; 95% CI, −44% to −1%) [31]. Relevant to clinical care, this trial supports feasibility and effectiveness of unsupervised home exercise among older adult trauma patients [32, 33].

Clemson et al. developed an exercise program for patients at high risk for falling with an integrative approach: The LiFE training program (Lifestyle integrated Functional Exercise) [34]. Instead of performing prescribed exercises isolated from daily living activities, in the LiFE program, the participants learn how different activities of daily life can be converted to small exercise sessions themselves (e.g., balance training during tooth brushing, strength training while walking stairs) [34]. In an RCT with 317 participants who experienced either multiple falls or one injurious fall in the 12 months prior to study inclusion, the participants in the LiFE program group had a 31% reduction in the rate of falls compared to participants in the control group (IRR: 0.69; 95% CI 0.48–0.99) [34]. Life-style integrated exercise programs with approaches of behavioral change seem to be promising alternatives to structured home-based exercises for community-dwelling older adults with a history of falls or institutionalized older adults [35]. However, more research is needed to confirm the positive results in different target populations on rate of falls, physical function, and quality of life, as reported in the recent systematic review by Weber et al. (2018) [35].

De Labra et al. (2015) performed a systematic review about the effects of exercises interventions on frail older adults including only studies which provided an operational definition of frailty [36]. The included studies assessed very heterogeneous populations (community-dwelling, institutionalized, and hospitalized populations) and most of the reported exercise interventions were delivered in supervised group settings. Consequently, the results regarding the risk of falling were controversial among the studies and further research using state-of-the-art definitions of frailty, as well as evaluating standardized exercise programs, is needed [36]. As a precaution of exercise programs in frail older adults with poor balance, increased mobility may lead to an increased opportunity to fall and fracture [1]. Therefore, more complex exercise programs should preferably be supervised and include suitable and tailored adaptions of the common strength and balance exercises [1].

8.3.3 Mind-Motor Exercise Interventions

Tai Chi has been successful in reducing falls among healthy older individuals [3, 37] and physically inactive community-dwelling older individuals [38], while frail older individuals [13] and fallers [37] may not benefit as much [1, 5]. However, one trial by Tousignant et al. (2013) among community-dwelling frail older adults showed greater reduction of falls for Tai Chi compared to conventional physiotherapy (RR: 0.74; 95% CI 0.56–0.98) [39].

Dalcroze Eurhythmics, a music-based exercise including multitasking and balance exercise executed to improvised piano music, has been shown to reduce the risk of falls by 39% (RR: 0.61; 95% CI: 0.39–0.96) in community-dwelling older adults at high risk of falling [4].

A comprehensive meta-analysis summarizing the evidence of mind-motor interventions such as Tai Chi, dance, or Dalcroze Eurhythmics on the risk of falls in the frail population is missing.

8.3.4 Exercise for Older Adults with Cognitive Impairment

Prevalence of dementia increases with age: Among community-dwelling adults aged 65 and older, prevalence of dementia has been reported to be around 6–10% [40, 41] rising to around 43% among those aged 90 years [42]. Additionally, 16–20% of adults without dementia are affected by mild cognitive impairment, MCI—an intermediate stage within the trajectory of normal age-related cognitive decline to dementia, of whom 20–40% are expected to progress to dementia [43, 44]. Notably, the presence of dementia more than doubles an older person's risk of falling [45–47].

The decline of physical and cognitive function has been proposed to interrelate and has similar underlying mechanistic pathways [5, 48–51]. In particular, muscle weakness [50] and slow walking speed [52] were identified as shared risk factors for both, falls and dementia. Considering the interrelationship of cognitive and physical function, effective physical exercise strategies targeted to this population at high risk for falling are urgently needed. Randomized controlled trials evaluating the effects of exercise programs among this particular population often face challenges related to adherence, recruitment, sample size, and time of follow-up [53, 54]. Nevertheless, a meta-analysis of 7 trials including 781 participants with MCI and mean ages 80 or older showed that group-based exercise programs reduced the number of falls (RaR 0.68, 95% CI 0.51–0.91) [55].

Multimodal cognitive-physical exercises or multitasking mind-motor interventions (such as Dalcroze Eurhythmics or Tai Chi) showed most promising results on gait speed, balance, and global cognitive function [56, 57].

8.4 Motivation of Older Adults to Engage in and Adhere to Physical Exercise

Different factors are relevant for the motivation of older adults to implement physical exercise programs successfully into their lives. These factors include the availability and knowledge about the appropriate type of exercise, accessibility of the venue without transport needed, affordable costs, and options to tailor the program to their personal needs [58, 59]. Furthermore, the decision of health providers about which programs could be offered to a specific population needs to account for environmental conditions, cultural and individual preferences, available provider resources, and the amount of supervision needed [60].

Picorelli et al. (2014) found in their review that adherence to physical exercise programs among older adults was higher in supervised settings, although one trial of an unsupervised and simple home-based exercise program among frail hip fracture patients found good adherence and was effective as discussed earlier [32, 61]. With regard to exercise type, home exercise programs including balance exercises were associated with higher adherence [61]. Participants living alone, with higher socioeconomic status and better education, were more likely to adhere to exercise programs [62]. Further, adults with better health status (measured by fewer health conditions, better self-rated health, taking fewer medications) and lower-body mass index are more likely to adhere to exercise programs [62]. In contrast, participants affected by psychological challenges including depression, loneliness, psychoactive medication use, and a higher perceived risk of falling or with cognitive impairment (lower scores on the Mini-Mental Status Examination) showed poorer adherence [62]. Interventions focusing on physical activity and exercise as a fun, sociable, and achievable leisure-time activity with relevant short-term health benefits were reported to be more likely to lead to high adherence [63]. Finally, personal goal-setting is important for adherence to exercise and might differ greatly within younger and older age groups [64].

8.5 Guidelines and Recommendations

Physical exercise has been included in various official guidelines and recommendations and is a major topic in most prevention programs related to falls reduction across countries. Further, the importance of general practitioners (GPs) and health care professionals (HCP) to implement exercise programs for falls prevention successfully in the field of secondary prevention has been recognized.

In the United Kingdom (UK), the guideline of the National Institute for Health and Care Excellence (NICE) recommends muscle strength and balance exercises to prevent falls among community-dwelling older adults, especially for those who experienced repeated falls [65]. In their survey from 2019 (2019 surveillance of falls in older people: assessing risk and prevention, NICE guideline CG161), NICE found that according to the current evidence, an expansion of their guidance towards a broader set of physical exercise programs is needed [66]. The NICE guideline further states that exercise programs should be prescribed individually and delivered by trained HCP [65].

Following the NICE guideline, the British Geriatrics Society promotes the Falls Management Exercise (FaME) program. FaME includes a manual on how to implement the individually tailored and progressive exercise program in supervised groups, as well as on how to implement additional home exercises if appropriate [67]. The effects of the FaME program on the prevention of falls and physical function are currently studied in the "physical activity implementation study in community-dwelling adults" (PhISICAL) study at the University of Nottingham [68].

The United States Preventive Services Task Force (USPSTF) recommends exercise programs to prevent falls. Their recommendations are based on an analysis of 21 studies including 7297 participants aged 65 and older, whereas half of the studies reported effects among older adults at high risk for falls [69].

The US Centers for Disease Control and Prevention (CDC) promote comprehensive falls risk assessments through GPs and HCPs and provide prevention strategies via their STAEDI initiative (STEADI—Stopping Elderly Accidents, Deaths & Injuries) [70]. The STAEDI initiative recommends strength and balance exercises (including Tai Chi) and provides a comprehensive website focusing on the prevention of falls among community-dwelling older adults as well as for those living in institutions—offering screening tools, background information, and recommendations for health care providers, older adults, and their relatives [71].

The updated joint guidelines of the UK/US geriatric societies recommend physical exercise programs delivered in groups or as individual home exercise programs, specifically including balance, gait, and strength training (including Tai Chi and physical therapy) [72].

In Switzerland, stakeholders from community and health care services (Beratungsstelle für Unfallverhütung (bfu), ProSenectue, Gesundheitsförderung Schweiz, Rheumaliga Schweiz, PhysioSwiss) launched the campaign «sicher stehen, sicher gehen», which promotes simple evidence-based exercises performed in supervised groups or individually at home [73–75]. The campaign website provides easy-to-follow exercise examples on different levels [76]. Further, courses for HCPs on how to instruct the exercises to patients are offered by the professional associations of the Physio- and Ergotherapists [76].

8.6 Implication for Research and Practice

8.6.1 Research Gaps

Research gaps include the feasibility and effects of exercise programs in general among frail older adults at high risk of falling, as well as of novel types of exercise such as balance training on platforms, step training, and the use of virtual reality or real-time online interventions. It is recommended that more exercise studies should include falls and fall-related injury as outcomes using the standardized definition of falls published by ProFaNE [77, 78]. For broad implementation of complex and individualized exercise programs, future research needs to include cost-benefit analyses [77]. Further, evidence about the frequency, safety, and intensity, as well about the most appropriate components of physical exercise programs among frail older adults and older adults with cognitive impairment, is needed. Finally, there is lack of evidence considering the long-term effects and characteristics of required maintenance schemes for exercise interventions. Finnegan et al. (2019) reported in a meta-analysis summarizing that exercise interventions aimed to prevent falls among community-dwelling older adults were sustained for up to 2 years after randomization concerning rate of falls (20 RCTs including 5929 participants, RaR 0.79, 95% CI 0.71–0.88) and risk of falling (16 RCTs, 4442 participants, RR 0.83, 95% CI 0.75–0.93) [79]. However, in this meta-analysis, only three studies evaluated follow-ups longer than 24 months, and for those, no effect on rate of falls and risk of falling was reported [79].

8.6.2 Promotion of Physical Exercise for Falls Prevention Through The Medical System

Senior trauma centers include a comprehensive fall assessment and implement fall prevention strategies as part of the fracture liaison service with acute care of older adults with fragility frac-

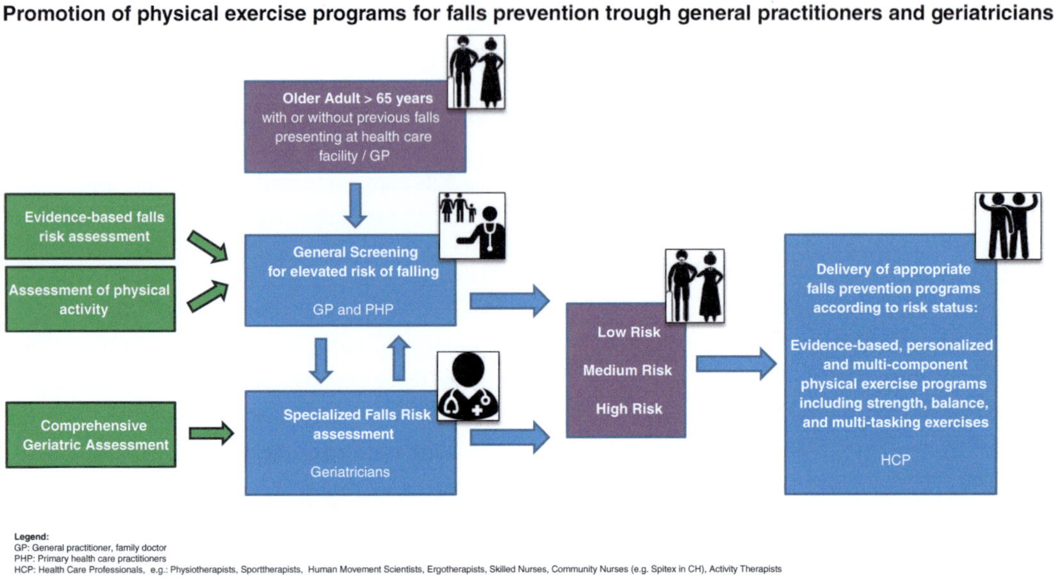

Fig. 8.1 Pathway of cooperation of different health care providers to implement fall prevention programs

tures or other fall-related injuries [80]. In such units, the comprehensive Geriatric assessment identifies key risk factors of falling (i.e., malnutrition, gait impairment, muscle weakness, sensory loss, impaired hearing and vision, fall-promoting medication use, comorbidities that increase fall risk and are not well-controlled, and cognitive impairment) and derives an individualized treatment plan implemented in the acute care early rehabilitation program. The early rehabilitation team consisting of physiotherapists and nurses monitors the patients regularly and adapts their exercise program to the current level of functionality and frailty. Once the patient is discharged to post-acute care or at home, the treating GPs and persons in charge of assisting living facilities or nursing homes are informed about the post-acute home exercise program instructed to the patient. Ideally, the patient is seen for a follow-up by the senior trauma center team, also to identify functional progress and possible challenges with the home exercise program. The GP has an important role as a gatekeeper and process-optimizer and builds the bridge not only to specialized care, but also to the community HPCs and therapists delivering evidence-based exercise programs. Telemedicine options could be introduced in the monitoring and supervision process. Figure 8.1 shows a proposed pathway of cooperation of GPs, primary health care practitioners (PHPs), Geriatricians, and HCPs to successfully implement fall prevention programs. The assessed level of risk of falling should be considered carefully when implementing the appropriate exercise program (see Fig. 8.2).

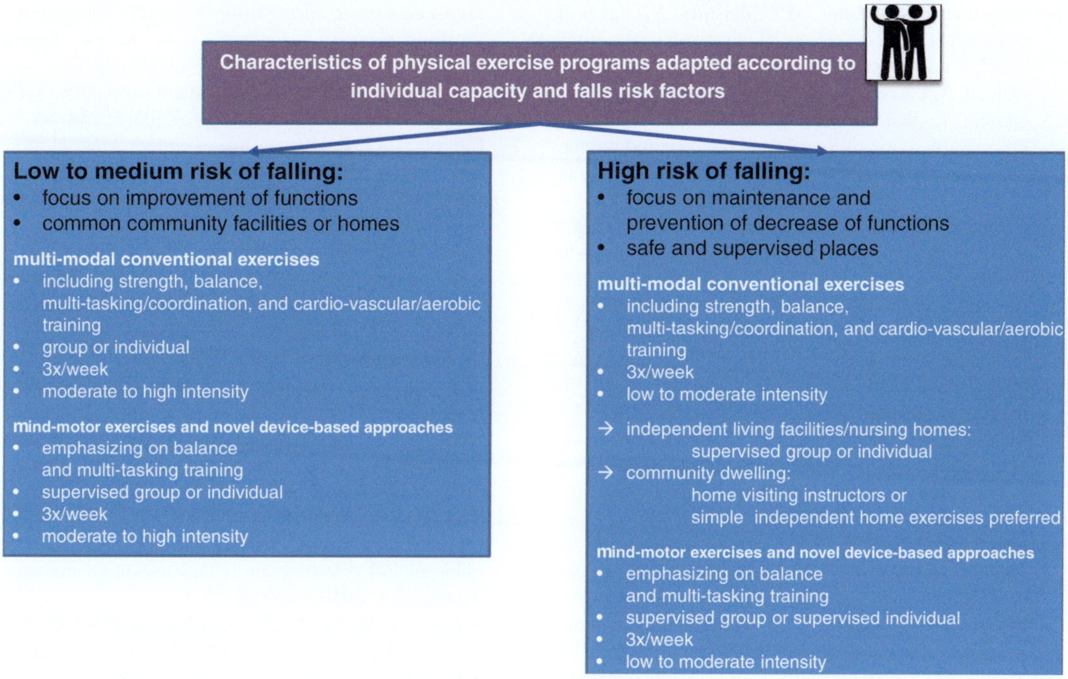

Fig. 8.2 Different types of fall prevention programs depending on fall risk

References

1. Bischoff-Ferrari HA. Chapter: fall prevention. In: ASBMR. 9th ed; 2018. p. 526–33.
2. Province MA, Hadley EC, Hornbrook MC, Lipsitz LA, Miller JP, Mulrow CD, et al. The effects of exercise on falls in elderly patients. A preplanned meta-analysis of the FICSIT Trials. Frailty and injuries: cooperative studies of intervention techniques. JAMA. 1995;273(17):1341–7.
3. Wolf SL, Barnhart HX, Kutner NG, McNeely E, Coogler C, Xu T. Reducing frailty and falls in older persons: an investigation of Tai Chi and computerized balance training. Atlanta FICSIT Group. Frailty and injuries: cooperative studies of intervention techniques. J Am Geriatr Soc. 1996;44(5):489–97.
4. Trombetti A, Hars M, Herrmann FR, Kressig RW, Ferrari S, Rizzoli R. Effect of music-based multitask training on gait, balance, and fall risk in elderly people: a randomized controlled trial. Arch Intern Med. 2011;171(6):525–33.
5. Gillespie LD, Robertson MC, Gillespie WJ, Sherrington C, Gates S, Clemson LM, et al. Interventions for preventing falls in older people living in the community. Cochrane Database Syst Rev. 2012;(9):CD007146.
6. Sherrington C, Fairhall NJ, Wallbank GK, Tiedemann A, Michaleff ZA, Howard K, et al. Exercise for preventing falls in older people living in the community. Cochrane Database Syst Rev. 2019;1:CD012424.
7. Peel NM, McClure RJ, Bartlett HP. Behavioral determinants of healthy aging1. Am J Prev Med. 2005;28(3):298–304.
8. Ekelund U, Tarp J, Steene-Johannessen J, Hansen BH, Jefferis B, Fagerland MW, et al. Dose-response associations between accelerometry measured physical activity and sedentary time and all cause mortality: systematic review and harmonised meta-analysis. BMJ. 2019;366:l4570.
9. Tricco AC, Thomas SM, Veroniki AA, Hamid JS, Cogo E, Strifler L, et al. Comparisons of interventions for preventing falls in older adults: a systematic review and meta-analysis. JAMA. 2017;318(17):1687–99.
10. Pichierri G, Wolf P, Murer K, de Bruin ED. Cognitive and cognitive-motor interventions affecting physical functioning: a systematic review. BMC Geriatr. 2011;11:29.
11. Segev-Jacubovski O, Herman T, Yogev-Seligmann G, Mirelman A, Giladi N, Hausdorff JM. The interplay between gait, falls and cognition: can cognitive therapy reduce fall risk? Expert Rev Neurother. 2011;11(7):1057–75.
12. Laatar R, Kachouri H, Borji R, Rebai H, Sahli S. Combined physical-cognitive training enhances postural performances during daily life tasks in older adults. Exp Gerontol. 2018;107:91–7.
13. Wolf SL, Sattin RW, Kutner M, O'Grady M, Greenspan AI, Gregor RJ. Intense tai chi exercise training and fall occurrences in older, transitionally frail adults: a randomized, controlled trial. J Am Geriatr Soc. 2003;51(12):1693–701.

14. Shigematsu R, Chang M, Yabushita N, Sakai T, Nakagaichi M, Nho H, et al. Dance-based aerobic exercise may improve indices of falling risk in older women. Age Ageing. 2002;31(4):261–6.
15. Okubo Y, Schoene D, Lord SR. Step training improves reaction time, gait and balance and reduces falls in older people: a systematic review and meta-analysis. Br J Sports Med. 2017;51(7):586–93.
16. Lamb SE, Becker C, Gillespie LD, Smith JL, Finnegan S, Potter R, et al. Reporting of complex interventions in clinical trials: development of a taxonomy to classify and describe fall-prevention interventions. Trials. 2011;12:125.
17. Huang ZG, Feng YH, Li YH, Lv CS. Systematic review and meta-analysis: Tai Chi for preventing falls in older adults. BMJ Open. 2017;7(2):e013661.
18. Merom D, Mathieu E, Cerin E, Morton RL, Simpson JM, Rissel C, et al. Social dancing and incidence of falls in older adults: a cluster randomised controlled trial. PLoS Med. 2016;13(8):e1002112.
19. Fernandez-Arguelles EL, Rodriguez-Mansilla J, Antunez LE, Garrido-Ardila EM, Munoz RP. Effects of dancing on the risk of falling related factors of healthy older adults: a systematic review. Arch Gerontol Geriatr. 2015;60(1):1–8.
20. Mattle M, Chocano-Bedoya PO, Fischbacher M, Meyer U, Abderhalden LA, Lang W, et al. Association of dance-based mind-motor activities with falls and physical function among healthy older adults: a systematic review and meta-analysis. JAMA Netw Open. 2020;3(9):e2017688.
21. Sivaramakrishnan D, Fitzsimons C, Kelly P, Ludwig K, Mutrie N, Saunders DH, et al. The effects of yoga compared to active and inactive controls on physical function and health related quality of life in older adults- systematic review and meta-analysis of randomised controlled trials. Int J Behav Nutr Phys Activity. 2019;16(1):33.
22. Youkhana S, Dean CM, Wolff M, Sherrington C, Tiedemann A. Yoga-based exercise improves balance and mobility in people aged 60 and over: a systematic review and meta-analysis. Age Ageing. 2016;45(1):21–9.
23. Gerards MHG, McCrum C, Mansfield A, Meijer K. Perturbation-based balance training for falls reduction among older adults: current evidence and implications for clinical practice. Geriatr Gerontol Int. 2017;17(12):2294–303.
24. Mansfield A, Wong JS, Bryce J, Knorr S, Patterson KK. Does perturbation-based balance training prevent falls? Systematic Review and meta-analysis of preliminary randomized controlled trials. Phys Ther. 2015;95(5):700–9.
25. Tripette J, Murakami H, Ryan KR, Ohta Y, Miyachi M. The contribution of Nintendo Wii Fit series in the field of health: a systematic review and meta-analysis. PeerJ. 2017;5:e3600.
26. Donath L, Rossler R, Faude O. Effects of virtual reality training (exergaming) compared to alternative exercise training and passive control on standing balance and functional mobility in healthy community-dwelling seniors: a meta-analytical review. Sports Med (Auckland, NZ). 2016;46(9):1293–309.
27. Tinetti ME, Kumar C. The patient who falls: "It's Always a Trade-off". JAMA. 2010;303(3):258–66.
28. Campbell AJ, Robertson MC, Gardner MM, Norton RN, Tilyard MW, Buchner DM. Randomised controlled trial of a general practice programme of home based exercise to prevent falls in elderly women. BMJ. 1997;315(7115):1065–9.
29. Liu-Ambrose T, Davis JC, Best JR, Dian L, Madden K, Cook W, et al. Effect of a home-based exercise program on subsequent falls among community-dwelling high-risk older adults after a fall: a randomized clinical trial effect of a home-based exercise program on subsequent falls among older adults after a falleffect of a home-based exercise program on subsequent falls among older adults after a fall. JAMA. 2019;321(21):2092–100.
30. Thomas S, Mackintosh S, Halbert J. Does the 'Otago exercise programme' reduce mortality and falls in older adults? A systematic review and meta-analysis. Age Ageing. 2010;39(6):681–7.
31. Stemmle J, Marzel A, Chocano-Bedoya PO, Orav EJ, Dawson-Hughes B, Freystaetter G, et al. Effect of 800 IU Versus 2000 IU Vitamin D3 with or without a simple home exercise program on functional recovery after hip fracture: a randomized controlled trial. J Am Med Direct Assoc. 2018;
32. Bischoff-Ferrari HA, Dawson-Hughes B, Platz A, Orav EJ, Stahelin HB, Willett WC, et al. Effect of high-dosage cholecalciferol and extended physiotherapy on complications after hip fracture: a randomized controlled trial. Arch Intern Med. 2010;170(9):813–20.
33. Theiler R, Freystätter G, Meyer U, Bischoff-Ferrari HA. Gezielte Trainingstherapie zur Sekundärprävention von Stürzen und Hüftfrakturen. Praxis. 2017;106(13):701–4.
34. Clemson L, Fiatarone Singh MA, Bundy A, Cumming RG, Manollaras K, O'Loughlin P, et al. Integration of balance and strength training into daily life activity to reduce rate of falls in older people (the LiFE study): randomised parallel trial. BMJ. 2012;345:e4547.
35. Weber M, Belala N, Clemson L, Boulton E, Hawley-Hague H, Becker C, et al. Feasibility and effectiveness of intervention programmes integrating functional exercise into daily life of older adults: a systematic review. Gerontology. 2018;64(2):172–87.
36. de Labra C, Guimaraes-Pinheiro C, Maseda A, Lorenzo T, Millan-Calenti JC. Effects of physical exercise interventions in frail older adults: a systematic review of randomized controlled trials. BMC Geriatr. 2015;15:154.
37. Voukelatos A, Cumming RG, Lord SR, Rissel C. A randomized, controlled trial of tai chi for the prevention of falls: the Central Sydney tai chi trial. J Am Geriatr Soc. 2007;55(8):1185–91.
38. Li F, Harmer P, Fisher KJ, McAuley E, Chaumeton N, Eckstrom E, et al. Tai Chi and fall reductions in

older adults: a randomized controlled trial. J Gerontol A Biol Sci Med Sci. 2005;60(2):187–94.
39. Tousignant M, Corriveau H, Roy PM, Desrosiers J, Dubuc N, Hebert R. Efficacy of supervised Tai Chi exercises versus conventional physical therapy exercises in fall prevention for frail older adults: a randomized controlled trial. Disabil Rehab. 2013;35(17):1429–35.
40. Berr C, Wancata J, Ritchie K. Prevalence of dementia in the elderly in Europe. Eur Neuropsychopharmacol. 2005;15(4):463–71.
41. Hendrie HC. Epidemiology of dementia and Alzheimer's disease. Am J Geriatr Psychiatry. 1998;6(2 Suppl. 1):S3–S18.
42. Prince M, Bryce R, Albanese E, Wimo A, Ribeiro W, Ferri CP. The global prevalence of dementia: a systematic review and metaanalysis. Alzheimer's Dement: J Alzheimer's Assoc 2013;9(1):63–75.e2
43. Feldman HH, Jacova C. Mild cognitive impairment. Am J Geriatr Psychiatry. 2005;13(8):645–55.
44. Roberts R, Knopman DS. Classification and epidemiology of MCI. Clin Geriatr Med. 2013;29(4):753–72.
45. Tinetti ME, Speechley M, Ginter SF. Risk factors for falls among elderly persons living in the community. N Engl J Med. 1988;319(26):1701–7.
46. Delbaere K, Kochan NA, Close JC, Menant JC, Sturnieks DL, Brodaty H, et al. Mild cognitive impairment as a predictor of falls in community-dwelling older people. Am J Geriatr Psychiatry. 2012;20(10):845–53.
47. Morris JC, Rubin EH, Morris EJ, Mandel SA. Senile dementia of the Alzheimer's type: an important risk factor for serious falls. J Gerontol. 1987;42(4):412–7.
48. Blondell SJ, Hammersley-Mather R, Veerman JL. Does physical activity prevent cognitive decline and dementia? A systematic review and meta-analysis of longitudinal studies. BMC Public Health. 2014;14:510.
49. Montero-Odasso M, Verghese J, Beauchet O, Hausdorff JM. Gait and cognition: a complementary approach to understanding brain function and the risk of falling. J Am Geriatr Soc. 2012;60(11):2127–36.
50. Boyle PA, Buchman AS, Wilson RS, Leurgans SE, Bennett DA. Association of muscle strength with the risk of Alzheimer disease and the rate of cognitive decline in community-dwelling older persons. Arch Neurol. 2009;66(11):1339–44.
51. Rolland Y, Pillard F, Klapouszczak A, Reynish E, Thomas D, Andrieu S, et al. Exercise program for nursing home residents with Alzheimer's disease: a 1-year randomized, controlled trial. J Am Geriatr Soc. 2007;55(2):158–65.
52. Verghese J, Lipton RB, Hall CB, Kuslansky G, Katz MJ, Buschke H. Abnormality of gait as a predictor of non-Alzheimer's dementia. N Engl J Med. 2002;347(22):1761–8.
53. Hauer K, Becker C, Lindemann U, Beyer N. Effectiveness of physical training on motor performance and fall prevention in cognitively impaired older persons: a systematic review. Am J Phys Med Rehab. 2006;85(10):847–57.
54. Burton E, Cavalheri V, Adams R, Browne CO, Bovery-Spencer P, Fenton AM, et al. Effectiveness of exercise programs to reduce falls in older people with dementia living in the community: a systematic review and meta-analysis. Clin Intervent Aging. 2015;10:421–34.
55. Chan WC, Fai Yeung JW, Man Wong CS, Wa Lam LC, Chung KF, Hay Luk JK, et al. Efficacy of physical exercise in preventing falls in older adults with cognitive impairment: a systematic review and meta-analysis. J Am Med Direct Assoc. 2015;16(2):149–54.
56. Lipardo DS, Aseron AMC, Kwan MM, Tsang WW. Effect of exercise and cognitive training on falls and fall-related factors in older adults with mild cognitive impairment: a systematic review. Arch Phys Med Rehab. 2017;98(10):2079–96.
57. Booth V, Hood V, Kearney F. Interventions incorporating physical and cognitive elements to reduce falls risk in cognitively impaired older adults: a systematic review. JBI Database Syst Rev Implement Rep. 2016;14(5):110–35.
58. Shier V, Trieu E, Ganz DA. Implementing exercise programs to prevent falls: systematic descriptive review. Injury Epidemiol. 2016;3(1):16.
59. Franco MR, Howard K, Sherrington C, Ferreira PH, Rose J, Gomes JL, et al. Eliciting older people's preferences for exercise programs: a best-worst scaling choice experiment. J Physiother. 2015;61(1):34–41.
60. Sherrington C. Prevention of fractures in older people: what does the evidence say? Physiother Canada Physiother Canada. 2011;63(2):146–51.
61. Picorelli AMA, Pereira LSM, Pereira DS, Felício D, Sherrington C. Adherence to exercise programs for older people is influenced by program characteristics and personal factors: a systematic review. J Physiother. 2014;60(3):151–6.
62. Simek EM, McPhate L, Haines TP. Adherence to and efficacy of home exercise programs to prevent falls: a systematic review and meta-analysis of the impact of exercise program characteristics. Prev Med. 2012;55(4):262–75.
63. Devereux-Fitzgerald A, Powell R, Dewhurst A, French DP. The acceptability of physical activity interventions to older adults: a systematic review and meta-synthesis. Social Sci Med. 2016;158:14–23.
64. Campbell PG, MacAuley D, McCrum E, Evans A. Age differences in the motivating factors for exercise. J Sport Exerc Psychol. 2001;23(3):191–9.
65. Excellence NIfHaC. Falls in older people: assessing risk and prevention United Kingdom: National Institute for Health and Care Excellence; 2019 [cited 2019 July 27]. Available from: https://www.nice.org.uk/guidance/cg161/chapter/1-Recommendations.
66. Excellence NIoHaC. 2019 surveillance of falls in older people: assessing risk and prevention (NICE guideline CG161) 2019 [Available from: https://www.nice.org.uk/guidance/cg161/resources/2019-surveillance-of-falls-in-older-people-assessing-risk-

and-prevention-nice-guideline-cg161-6784064895/chapter/Surveillance-decision?tab=evidence].
67. Society BG. Falls Management Exercise (FaME) Implementation Toolkit [cited 2019 July 27]. Available from: https://www.bgs.org.uk/resources/falls-management-exercise-fame-implementation-toolkit.
68. Research IEaP, Nottingham TUo. The physical activity implementation study in community-dwelling adults (PhISICAL) study: Investigating the implementation of the FaME falls prevention exercise programme [cited 2019 July 27]. Available from: https://www.nottingham.ac.uk/research/groups/injuryresearch/projects/phisical/index.aspx.
69. Grossman DC, Curry SJ, Owens DK, Barry MJ, Caughey AB, Davidson KW, et al. Interventions to prevent falls in community-dwelling older adults: US Preventive Services Task Force Recommendation Statement. JAMA. 2018;319(16):1696–704.
70. Prevention CfDCa. Older adult falls [cited 2019 July 27]. Available from: https://www.cdc.gov/homeandrecreationalsafety/falls/index.html.
71. Prevention CfDCa. STEADI—older adult fall prevention [cited 2019 July 27]. Available from: https://www.cdc.gov/steadi/index.html.
72. Summary of the Updated American Geriatrics Society/British Geriatrics Society clinical practice guideline for prevention of falls in older persons. J Am Geriatr Soc. 2011;59(1):148–57.
73. Unfallverhütung Bf. Für Fachpersonen – Sturzprävention [cited 2019 July 27]. Available from: https://www.bfu.ch/de/fuer-fachpersonen/sturzprävention/.
74. Lacroix A, Kressig RW, Muehlbauer T, Gschwind YJ, Pfenninger B, Bruegger O, et al. Effects of a supervised versus an unsupervised combined balance and strength training program on balance and muscle power in healthy older adults: a randomized controlled trial. Gerontology. 2016;62(3):275–88.
75. Lacroix A, Kressig RW, Mühlbauer T, Brügger O, Granacher U. Wirksamkeit eines Trainingsprogramms zur Sturzprävention. bfu-Report; 2016.
76. Unfallverhütung Bf. Die Kampagne "Sicher stehen – sicher gehen". [cited 2019 July 27]. Available from: http://www.sichergehen.ch/jetztstarten/.
77. Sherrington C, Fairhall N, Wallbank G, Tiedemann A, Michaleff ZA, Howard K, et al. Exercise for preventing falls in older people living in the community: an abridged Cochrane systematic review. Br J Sports Med. 2020;54(15):885–91.
78. Lamb SE, Jørstad-Stein EC, Hauer K, Becker C. Development of a common outcome data set for fall injury prevention trials: the Prevention of Falls Network Europe consensus. J Am Geriatr Soc. 2005;53(9):1618–22.
79. Finnegan S, Seers K, Bruce J. Long-term follow-up of exercise interventions aimed at preventing falls in older people living in the community: a systematic review and meta-analysis. Physiotherapy. 2019;105(2):187–99.
80. Andreasen C, Solberg LB, Basso T, Borgen TT, Dahl C, Wisloff T, et al. Effect of a fracture Liaison service on the rate of subsequent fracture among patients with a fragility fracture in the norwegian capture the fracture initiative (NoFRACT): a trial protocol. JAMA Netw Open. 2018;1(8):e185701.

Falls Risk Assessment

9

Jesse Zanker, Steven Phu, and Gustavo Duque

9.1 Introduction

Health care and socioeconomic advancement have led to aging of the global population. This is arguably one of the twenty-first century's greatest achievements. With this demographic shift comes an evolution of population health needs and a requirement for health care systems to be responsive to society's changing needs. An increase in age-related causes of morbidity and mortality (such as falls) has thus been observed and pose a significant public health challenge in the decades ahead [1]. Clinical interactions with older adults in the hospital and community setting present an important opportunity to undertake a falls risk assessment, which can be used to inform the multifactorial and interdisciplinary approach to interventions aimed at mitigating falls risk.

This chapter will examine the epidemiology falls, falls risk factors, the clinician's approach to falls assessment (history, examination, and investigations), and review the tools at the clinician's disposal when undertaking a falls risk assessment in both inpatient and community settings.

9.2 Epidemiology of Falls

A fall is defined as "an event which results in a person coming to rest inadvertently on the ground of floor, or other lower level" [2]. Approximately one third of adults over the age of 65 fall each year, and this proportion increases with each decade of life lived [3]. Falls are the second leading cause of accidental injury resulting in death after road traffic accidents [2]. However, nonfatal effects of falls are far more frequent. For every death due to a fall, there are approximately four people who experience disability, 13 people who require admission to hospital for greater than 10 days, and 690 people who will seek primary medical care [2].

The impacts of falls on older adults, carers, community, health care systems, economies, and governments are extensive and wide-ranging.

J. Zanker · G. Duque (✉)
Australian Institute for Musculoskeletal Science (AIMSS), The University of Melbourne and Western Health, St Albans, VIC, Australia

Department of Medicine—Western Health, Melbourne Medical School, The University of Melbourne, St Albans, VIC, Australia

Department of Subacute and Aged Care, Western Health, St Albans, VIC, Australia
e-mail: jesse.zanker@unimelb.edu.au; gustavo.duque@unimelb.edu.au

S. Phu
Australian Institute for Musculoskeletal Science (AIMSS), The University of Melbourne and Western Health, St Albans, VIC, Australia

Department of Medicine—Western Health, Melbourne Medical School, The University of Melbourne, St Albans, VIC, Australia

Falls, Balance and Injury Research Centre, Neuroscience Research Australia, Randwick, NSW, Australia
e-mail: steven.phu@unimelb.edu.au

H.-C. Pape et al. (eds.), *Senior Trauma Patients*, https://doi.org/10.1007/978-3-030-91483-7_9

Many of the injuries and impacts resulting from falls are obvious (such as fractures), yet other important impacts may be less obvious. At an individual level, falls can limit the ability of individuals to perform their activities of daily living (ADLs) and precipitate a cascade of adverse syndromes such as recurring fear of falling, social withdrawal, immobilization, depression, and dependence [4].

9.3 Falls Risk Factors

Over 400 risk factors for falls have been identified in older adults [5]. While it is not practical nor feasible to identify every falls risk factor, a targeted history, physical examination, and investigations focused on the risk factors most likely to contribute to falls risk should be undertaken. A single, major risk factor can be identified in approximately 20% of falls [6]. The greatest risk factor for a fall is a previous fall [7]. Therefore, any clinical encounter resulting from a fall or for which a fall is identified in the history should prompt exploration for falls risk factors. Falls risk factors have a cumulative effect on total falls risk [8]. A key component of the falls risk assessment is identifying risk factors that are modifiable, or reversible, which become the targets of interventions aimed at mitigating falls risk. Common potentially modifiable and non-modifiable falls risk factors are listed in Table 9.1.

Table 9.1 Risk factors for falls in older adults

Potentially modifiable	Non-modifiable
Cardiac	Age
Arrhythmias	Arthritis
Congestive cardiac failure	Dementia
Hypertension and hypotension	Female sex
Environmental	History of stroke
Carpets, rugs, crowding (people, objects), tripping hazards within the home	History of falling
Pets	History of fractures
Functional	Recent discharge from hospital
Use of a gait aid or assistive device	
Impairment in activities of daily living	
Medications	
Antidepressants, sedatives, hypnotics, narcotics, antipsychotics, and beta-blockers.	
Metabolic	
Diabetes Mellitus	
Low body mass index (BMI)	
Vitamin D deficiency	
Musculoskeletal	
Balance impairment	
Foot problems	
Gait impairment	
Limited activity	
Musculoskeletal pain	
Sarcopenia	
Neurological	
Delirium	
Dizziness or vertigo	
Movement disorder (Parkinson's disease)	
Peripheral neuropathy	
Psychological	
Depression	
Fear of falling	
Sensory impairment	
Visual impairment	
Auditory impairment	
Multifocal lens	
Other	
Acute illness	
Anemia	
Cancer	
Inappropriate footwear	
Nocturia	
Urinary or fecal incontinence	
Obstructive sleep apnea	
Postural hypotension	

Adapted from Moncada LVV, Mire LG. Preventing Falls in Older Persons. American family physician. 2017;96(4):240–7 [9]

9.4 Assessment

9.4.1 History

The falls risk assessment starts with clearly defining the fall and the history surrounding it. Among clinicians, there may be a consistent understanding of what constitutes a fall. However, lay people may understand a fall differently (i.e., an older adult might not consider a "trip" or a "slip" a fall). Individuals may tend to focus only on falls for which an injury was sustained [10]. The clinician should take care to ensure this understanding is established during the consultation. Furthermore, concomitant cognitive and sensory (hearing and visual) impairments are highly prevalent in older adults, particularly in those who experience falls. Clinicians may be required to use sensory assistive devices or obtain informant history from next of kin or carers to best establish an understanding of the fall(s) and associated risk factors. This is particularly important in older adults admitted to hospital, where the prevalence of delirium is high [11] and may impact upon the individual's ability to provide an accurate account of the fall.

An important element of the falls history is determining whether the fall was related to presyncope or syncope. Presyncope and syncope may reflect underlying cardiac or neurological pathology, and thus warrant targeted, specialist investigation. Other high-risk features that may prompt clinicians to refer to specialist clinics (such as falls clinic or a geriatrician-led clinic) include two or more falls in a year, unexplained falls, falls occurring in ADLs, recurrent falls occurring at home, fall with a long lie, or gait disturbance [12].

To complete the falls history, information should be obtained on medical comorbidities, medications (high-risk medications are listed in Table 9.1), continence, sensory impairments, cognition, and social and functional history.

9.4.2 Physical Examination

In both inpatient and community settings, the falls risk assessment must include a physical examination. The physical examination in a falls risk assessment is a head-to-toe examination of physical characteristics and performance/function focusing on identifying falls risk factors and modifiable characteristics.

The co-occurrence of cognitive impairment and falls risk is high in older adults [13]. The clinician should examine for both delirium and background cognitive impairment. Useful delirium assessment tools include the Cognitive Assessment Method (CAM) [14], which has been validated in multiple demographics and settings, and the 4AT [15]. If delirium is not present, background cognitive screening tests such as the standardized mini-mental status examination (MMSE) [16], Montreal Cognitive Assessment (MoCA) [17], or Rowland Universal Dementia Assessment Scale (RUDAS) [18] should accompany the collateral cognitive history. A neurological examination follows and includes assessment of visual acuity, hearing, and peripheral sensation. A review of the feet and footwear is important as abnormalities are readily reversible and referral to a podiatrist may be indicated.

Frailty is common among older adults at risk of falling and is an independent risk factor for falls and morbidity [19]. There are numerous useful definitions of frailty, each with variable clinical application and predictive ability for adverse outcomes. The Clinical Frailty Scale by Rockwood et al. is a useful, rapidly applied frailty assessment tool that describes individuals on the basis of their phenotype, comorbidities, and function [20]. Individuals are classified into categories from 1 (Very Fit) through to 9 (Terminally Ill) [20] and these classifications can be used in communicating with other care providers the individual's level of function and morbidity.

Sarcopenia, a progressive condition of generalized loss of muscle mass, strength, and function [21], is related to but clinically distinct from frailty [22]. Sarcopenia independently predicts falls risk in older adults [23]. When sarcopenia coexists with osteoporosis or osteopenia, this condition is known as osteosarcopenia [24]. Some of the authors have previously argued that osteosarcopenia should be considered in any comprehensive geriatric assessment [25]. Osteosarcopenia may predict risk of falls and fractures beyond sarcopenia and osteoporosis individually; however, studies have been conflicting [26]. An international consensus has recommended that clinicians considering the diagnosis of sarcopenia can use any of the currently validated definitions of sarcopenia [27]. A diagnosis of osteosarcopenia can guide person-centered treatment decisions to reduce falls and fracture risk.

Both frailty and sarcopenia are addressed in detail in Section A of this text.

9.4.3 Investigations

A range of metabolic and endocrine conditions increase the risk of falls and fractures. Investigations should target those conditions which may be suggested by the history and physical examination, in addition to those which may guide treatment. However, some common conditions may be asymptomatic (such as vitamin d deficiency and hyperparathyroidism) and therefore screening investigations are recommended for those at high risk of falls and fractures. These investigations include vitamin D, calcium, parathyroid hormone, thyroid-stimulating hormone, creatinine, and serum testosterone (men) [28].

9.5 Inpatient vs. Community Falls Risk Assessment

The approach taken to the comprehensive falls risk assessment is dependent upon a range of factors including setting, clinician capacity, breadth of the interdisciplinary team, and availability of resources. There are unique differences between a clinical encounter with an older adult at risk of falls consulted in the community and that with the hospital. Clinicians, therefore, need to be agile in their falls risk assessments based on circumstances and setting. The National Institute of Clinical Excellence (NICE) has developed guidelines which aim to guide an individualized approach to hospital-based falls assessment in the United Kingdom [5]. A summary of the key NICE Quality Statements includes:

- Practitioners should ask older people about falls during routine assessments and hospital admissions;
- Multifactorial falls assessments are offered to older adults at risk of falling;
- Multifactorial fall prevention interventions are provided to those at risk of falling or those who have had a fall;
- Assessments of older adults who experience an in-hospital fall are medically examined for injury (fracture or spinal) before movement and receive a full medical examination thereafter;
- Community-dwelling older adults with a history of falls should receive a referral for strength and balance training; and
- A home safety assessment and appropriate interventions should be offered to older adults admitted to hospital following a fall [5].

9.5.1 Falls Risk Assessment Tools

Based on understanding the risk factors for falls in older adults, several assessment tools have been developed to assist the clinician in predicting the risk of falls. This includes the use of specific physical performance measures and questionnaires. These tools are designed to accompany the history, physical examination, and investigations as described. Given the diversity of falls mechanisms, this section has been divided into falls assessment tools for inpatient and community-dwelling older adults. An overview of each assessment tool will be provided, in addition to the available data regarding sensitivity (ability to correctly identify falls risk) and specificity (ability to correctly rule out those with low falls risk) and area under receiver operating curve (AUC) where available. A summary of the commonly used tools can be found in Table 9.2. Assessment tools with high values in each of these measures indicate good predictive value. However, in many cases cut-points presented are the result of a balancing of risks for over- and underdiagnosis.

9.5.1.1 Falls Risk Assessment in Acute Care (Inpatient) Settings

St Thomas's Risk Assessment Tool in Falling Elderly Patients (STRATIFY)

The STRATIFY falls risk assessment is a 5-item questionnaire which can be used to easily classify older adults presenting as inpatients in hospital, containing questions regarding a patient's fall history, transfers and mobility, continence, visual impairment, and emotional state (agitation) [29]. In this tool, a score greater than 2 is indicative of

Table 9.2 Overview of commonly used falls risk assessment tools

Risk assessment tool	Population	Assessment items	Time to administer	Proposed cut-points	Sensitivity	Specificity
STRATIFY [29]	Acute – Inpatient	5	<5 min	2	93%	88%
Hendrich II Fall Risk Model [33]	Acute – Inpatient	8	<5 min	5	86%	43%
Berg Balance Scale [37]	Community-dwelling older adults	14	20 min	45	64%	90%
FROP-COM [39]	Community-dwelling older adults	28	15 min	19	71%	56%
FAB Scale [42]	Community-dwelling older adults	10	15 min	25	75%	53%
Timed Up and Go [45]	Community-dwelling older adults	1	<5 min	13.5 sec	87%	87%

STRATIFY—St Thomas's Risk Assessment Tool in Falling Elderly Patients
FROP-COM—Falls Risk for Older People – Community
FAB Scale—Fullerton Advanced Balance Scale

falls risk, with the initial study finding a sensitivity of 93% and specificity of 88% in the original, local setting (St Thomas's Hospital).

Several studies including systematic reviews and meta-analysis have been conducted since the original study, with mixed findings for use of the STRATIFY tool. A multicentre study including six hospitals in Belgium found high sensitivity (90%) and low specificity (59%) in the total sample, with interesting results for subgroups, including high predictive value in inpatients under 65 years of age (sensitivity 92% and specificity 81%) [30]. More recently, a systematic review and meta-analysis reported low sensitivity (67%) and specificity (57%) for the STRATIFY tool, with the authors suggesting that it should not be used in isolation for falls risk assessment [31].

Hendrich II Fall Risk Model

The Hendrich II Fall Risk Model is a tool which contains 8-items, with each item assigned a score, increasing with risk and a cut-point of 5 used to indicate a high risk for falls [32]. Risk factors were designed for acute care settings and include depression, disorientation, continence, dizziness/vertigo, gender, medications, and lower limb strength.

An assessment of the Hendrich II fall risk model in geriatric inpatients of an Italian hospital found the tool to be easily administered with high sensitivity (86%) and low specificity (43%) with the depression and confusion components being the most significant risk factors [33]. Higher specificity (69%) but lower sensitivity (72%) was found when using this tool in a Chinese population [34]; however, both studies suggested results supported use of the Hendrich II Fall Risk Model for screening older inpatients. A comparison of the STRATIFY and Hendrick II Fall Risk Model found a higher AUC and sensitivity for the Hendrick II Fall Risk Model [35].

9.5.1.2 Falls Risk Assessment for Community-Dwelling Older Adults

Berg Balance Scale

The Berg Balance Scale is an assessment tool consisting of 14 different tasks to assess the static and dynamic balance of older adults and can be completed within 20 min [36]. Each test is scored out of 4, with a maximum score of 56 achievable and a score of 45 originally used to indicate falls risk.

In a study assessing use of the cut-point of 45 as a marker for those at risk of falls, a sensitivity of 64% and specificity of 90% were evident, with the authors stating that this was low as one third of individuals could be misclassified [37]. More recently, in a study assessing the use of the Berg Balance Scale score of 45 in predicting those to have (1) any falls, (2) multiple falls, and (3) injurious falls, the Berg Balance Scale did not show good sensitivity [38]. In this study, sensitivity for all three categories of falls did not exceed 42%, while specificity was near 87%, with the authors suggesting the use of 45 as a cut-off score should not be recommended. Meanwhile, AUC was greatest for multiple falls (0.68), highlighting some value of use of the Berg Balance Scale to predict those at risk for multiple falls as opposed to any or injurious falls. This was somewhat in agreement with the findings of a more recent study into the Berg Balance Scale, which found moderate predictive value (pooled sensitivity 0.72, pooled specificity 0.73) with the greatest predictive value for those with 2 or more falls (AUC 0.83) which was similar to previously mentioned.

Falls Risk for Older People-Community Setting (FROP-COM)

The FROP-COM is an assessment tool which assesses 13 risk factors of falls using 28 criteria, most of which are rated on scale from 0 to 3, with the total score (out of 60) used to determine risk for falls and need of specific interventions [39]. The original FROP-COM can be performed within 15 min and individuals can be classified as having a mild (score 0–11), moderate (score 12–18), or high (score 19–60) falls risk. Additionally, a 3-question screening tool (total score out of 9) has been developed with a score of 0–3, indicating low risk of falls and 4 or more recommending performance of the full FROP-COM [40].

Using this tool, correlations have been found between balance and mobility (timed up and go and functional reach), physical activity, and falls risk assessment efficacy [39]. The reported cut-point of 19 to indicate a high risk of falls provided a sensitivity of 71% and specificity of 56%. AUC was 0.68, indicating a moderate capacity to predict falls, and higher than the timed up and go test (AUC 0.63) and functional reach (0.60). With regard to the FROP-COM screening tool, a score of 3 provides a sensitivity of 80% and specificity of 50% [40].

However, it is important to note that the validity and reliability of this tool were assessed in community-dwelling adults presenting to a hospital emergency department with a fall, and therefore, results cannot be extrapolated to individuals with no history of falls or those in residential aged care.

Fullerton Advanced Balance (FAB) Scale

The FAB scale has been described as a performance-based measure which consists of 10 items scored from 0 to 4 to assess multiple dimensions of balance in community-dwelling older adults [41]. Each of the 10 tasks assesses a range of sensory and motor systems, including the somatosensory, visual, vestibular, and musculoskeletal systems, with the test able to be completed within 15 min.

Studies evaluating the FAB scale have typically focused on its ability to discriminate between those with and without a history of recurrent (2 or more) falls. Given the maximum achievable score of 40 points, an assessment of the tool to predict falls status found a cut-point score of 25, provided a sensitivity of 75% and specificity of 53% in determining history of 2 or more falls [42]. This was in contrast with another study with fewer participants which reported greater sensitivity (85%) and specificity (65%) using a cut-point of 22 and AUC of 0.72, with results similar to that of the Berg Balance Scale [43].

Timed Up and Go test

The Timed Up and Go test is a simple measure of an individual's ability to transfer and change directions and mobility [44]. In this test, individuals begin in a seated position and are instructed to stand and walk to a marked area 3 m away, before turning and returning to the seated position. The time taken to complete this task is recorded, and several trials can be performed to ensure accuracy. Given its simplicity, testing can be completed efficiently.

As a screening tool for falls risk, this test has been commonly used in multiple studies to predict falls with the test itself showing high sensitivity and specificity (both 87%) and a cut-point of 13.5 s, providing a sensitivity and specificity of 80% and 100%, respectively [45]. Addition of a cognitive (subtraction task) and motor (carrying a cup of water) task was also found to be highly sensitive and specific for falls prediction. However, it is important to note that this study only provided a cross-sectional comparison of multiple fallers (2 or more) and non-fallers, and therefore, cannot provide predictive value.

In a recent systematic review and meta-analysis of use of the Timed Up and Go test in predicting falls in a period of 6 months up to 2 years, it was found that use of the Timed Up and Go test showed greater value (sensitivity of 73%) in identifying those with high risk of falls [46]. However, the ability to accurately rule out those with low risk of falls was reduced (specificity 32%). This resulted in poor predictive value, with an AUC of 0.57.

9.6 Fracture Risk Assessment

A falls risk assessment is a fundamental component in the comprehensive care of older adults. A falls risk assessment alone does not assist in guiding interventions to reduce the risk of injury related to falls. A significant and common outcome of falls are fractures. A marked proportion of fractures are avoidable with the appropriate primary and secondary prevention. The clinician should complete the falls risk assessment with a fracture risk assessment. Fracture risk assessment has been addressed in Chap. 12 of this book.

9.7 Conclusion

In summary, a wide range of assessment tools are available to the clinician for the assessment of falls risk in both inpatients and community-dwelling older adults. These tools should not be used in isolation, but accompany a comprehensive assessment including history, physical examination, and person-centered investigations. A large body of research has focused on the ability to diagnose a history of falls, with results used as a marker for future risk of falls given a history of falls is the primary risk factor for future falls. Currently, there is no single assessment which provides the highest sensitivity and specificity for assessing falls risk. As such, clinicians are recommended to employ a combination of tools to better classify falls risk and assist in the development of individualized falls prevention strategies.

References

1. Kannus P, Palvanen M, Niemi S, Parkkari J. Alarming rise in the number and incidence of fall-induced cervical spine injuries among older adults. J Gerontol Biol Sci Med Sci. 2007;62(2):180–3. https://doi.org/10.1093/gerona/62.2.180.
2. World Health Organisation (2018) Fact sheet: Falls. who.int/news-room/fact-sheets/detail/falls. Accessed 16 Sept 2019.
3. World Health Organization. Global report on falls prevention in older age. Geneva: World Health Organization; 2007.
4. Tinetti ME, Williams CS. The effect of falls and fall injuries on functioning in community dwelling older persons. J Gerontol Biol Sci Med Sci. 1998;53:112–M119.
5. National Institute of Clinical Excellence. Falls in older people. Quality standard: NICE, 2017. https://www.nice.org.uk/guidance/qs86/resources/falls-in-older-people-pdf-2098911933637. Accessed 30th August 2019
6. Campbell AJ, Borrie MJ, Spears GF. Risk factors for falls in a community-based prospective study of people 70 years and older. J Gerontol Biol Sci Med Sci. 1989;44:M112–7.
7. Deandrea S, Lucenteforte E, Bravi F, et al. Risk factors for falls in community-dwelling older people: a systematic review and meta-analysis. Epidemiology. 2010;215:658–68.
8. Zanker J, Duque G. Falls and fractures in older people: identifying patients at high risk. Endocrinol Today. 2017;6(2):12–8.
9. Moncada LVV, Mire LG. Preventing falls in older persons. Am Family Phys. 2017;96(4):240–7.
10. Zecevic AA, Salmoni AW, Speechley M, Vandervoort AA. Defining a fall and reasons for falling: comparisons among the views of seniors, health care

providers, and the research literature. Gerontologist. 2006;46:367–76.
11. Siddiqi N, House AO, Holmes JD. Occurrence and outcome of delirium in medical in-patients: a systematic literature review. Age Ageing. 2006;35:350–64.
12. Waldron N, Hill AM, Barker A. Falls prevention in older adults—assessment and management. Aust Fam Physician. 2012;41:930–5.
13. Muir SW, Gopaul K, Montero Odasso MM. The role of cognitive impairment in fall risk among older adults: a systematic review and meta-analysis. Age Ageing. 2012;41(3):299–308. https://doi.org/10.1093/ageing/afs012.
14. Inouye SK, VanDyck CH, Alessi CA, et al. Clarifying confusion: the Confusion Assessment Method. A new method for detecting delirium. Ann Intern Med. 1990;113:941–8.
15. Bellelli G, Morandi A, Davis DH, Mazzola P, et al. Validation of the 4AT, a new instrument for rapid delirium screening: a study in 234 hospitalised older people. Age Ageing. 2014;43:496–502.
16. Molloy M, Alemayehu E, Roberts R, et al. Reliability of a standardised MiniMental State Examination compared with the traditional Mini-Mental state Examination. Am J Psychiatry. 1991a;14:102–5.
17. Nasreddine ZS, Phillips NA, Bédirian V, Charbonneau S, et al. The Montreal cognitive assessment, MoCA: a brief screening tool for mild cognitive impairment. J Am Geriatr Soc. 2005;53:695–9. https://doi.org/10.1111/j.1532-5415.2005.53221.x.
18. Storey J, Rowland J, Conforti D, Dickson H. The Rowland Universal Dementia Assessment Scale (RUDAS): a multicultural cognitive assessment scale. Int Psychogeriatr. 2004;16(1):13–31. https://doi.org/10.1017/S1041610204000043.
19. Cheng M, Chang S. Frailty as a risk factor for falls among community dwelling people: evidence from a meta-analysis. J Nurs Scholar. 2017;49:529–36. https://doi.org/10.1111/jnu.12322.
20. Rockwood K, Song X, MacKnight C, et al. A global clinical measure of fitness and frailty in elderly people. Canadian Med Assoc J. 2005;73(5):489–95. https://doi.org/10.1503/cmaj.050051.
21. Cruz-Jentoft AJ, Bahat G, Bauer J, et al. Sarcopenia: revised European consensus on definition and diagnosis. Age Ageing. 2019;48(1):16–31. https://doi.org/10.1093/ageing/afy169.
22. Cesari M, Landi F, Vellas B, Bernabei R, Marzetti E. Sarcopenia and physical frailty: two sides of the same coin. Front Aging Neurosci. 2014;6:192. https://doi.org/10.3389/fnagi.2014.00192.
23. Yeung SSY, Reijnierse EM, Pham VK, et al. Sarcopenia and its association with falls and fractures in older adults: a systematic review and meta-analysis. J Cachexia Sarcopenia Muscle. 2019;10(3):485–500. https://doi.org/10.1002/jcsm.12411.
24. Hirschfeld HP, Kinsella R, Duque G. Osteosarcopenia: where bone, muscle, and fat collide. Osteoporos Int. 2017;28:2781. https://doi.org/10.1007/s00198-017-4151-8.
25. Zanker J, Duque G. Osteoporosis in older persons: old and new players. J Am Geriatr Soc. 2019;67:831–40. https://doi.org/10.1111/jgs.15716.
26. Nielsen BR, Abdulla J, Andersen HE, et al. Sarcopenia and osteoporosis in older people: a systematic review and meta-analysis. Eur Geriatr Med. 2018;9:419. https://doi.org/10.1007/s41999-018-0079-6.
27. Dent E, Morley JE, Cruz-Jentoft AJ, et al. International Clinical Practice Guidelines for Sarcopenia (ICFSR): screening, diagnosis and management. J Nutr Health Aging. 2018;22:1148. https://doi.org/10.1007/s12603-018-1139-9.
28. Johnson K, Suriyaarachchi P, Kakkat M, et al. Yield and cost-effectiveness of laboratory testing to identify metabolic contributors to falls and fractures in older persons. Archiv Osteopor. 2015;10:226.
29. Oliver D, Britton M, Seed P, Martin FC, Hopper AH. Development and evaluation of evidence based risk assessment tool (STRATIFY) to predict which elderly inpatients will fall: case-control and cohort studies. BMJ. 1997;315:1049–53.
30. Milisen K, Staelens N, Schwendimann R, et al. Fall prediction in inpatients by bedside nurses using the St. Thomas's Risk Assessment Tool in Falling Elderly Inpatients (STRATIFY) instrument: a multicenter study. J Am Geriatr Soc. 2007;55:725–33.
31. Billington J, Fahey T, Galvin R. Diagnostic accuracy of the STRATIFY clinical prediction rule for falls: a systematic review and meta-analysis. BMC Fam Pract. 2012;13:76.
32. Hendrich AL, Bender PS, Nyhuis A. Validation of the Hendrich II Fall Risk Model: a large concurrent case/control study of hospitalized patients. Appl Nurs Res. 2003;16:9–21.
33. Ivziku D, Matarese M, Pedone C. Predictive validity of the Hendrich fall risk model II in an acute geriatric unit. Int J Nurs Stud. 2011;48:468–74.
34. Zhang C, Wu X, Lin S, Jia Z, Cao J. Evaluation of reliability and validity of the Hendrich II fall risk model in a Chinese Hospital Population. PLoS One. 2015;10:e0142395.
35. Kim EA, Mordiffi SZ, Bee WH, Devi K, Evans D. Evaluation of three fall-risk assessment tools in an acute care setting. J Adv Nurs. 2007;60:427–35.
36. Berg KO, Wood-Dauphinee SL, Williams JI, Maki B. Measuring balance in the elderly: validation of an instrument. Can J Public Health. 1992;83(Suppl. 2):S7–11.
37. Riddle DL, Stratford PW. Interpreting validity indexes for diagnostic tests: an illustration using the Berg balance test. Phys Ther. 1999;79:939–48.
38. Muir SW, Berg K, Chesworth B, Speechley M. Use of the Berg Balance Scale for predicting multiple falls in community-dwelling elderly people: a prospective study. Phys Ther. 2008;88:449–59.
39. Russell MA, Hill KD, Blackberry I, Day LM, Dharmage SC. The reliability and predictive accuracy of the falls risk for older people in the community assessment (FROP-Com) tool. Age Ageing. 2008;37:634–9.

40. Russell MA, Hill KD, Day LM, Blackberry I, Gurrin LC, Dharmage SC. Development of the Falls Risk for Older People in the Community (FROP-Com) screening tool. Age Ageing. 2009;38:40–6.
41. Rose DJ, Lucchese N, Wiersma LD. Development of a multidimensional balance scale for use with functionally independent older adults. Arch Phys Med Rehabil. 2006;87:1478–85.
42. Hernandez D, Rose DJ. Predicting which older adults will or will not fall using the Fullerton Advanced Balance scale. Arch Phys Med Rehabil. 2008;89:2309–15.
43. Jeon YJ, Kim GM. Comparison of the Berg balance scale and fullerton advanced balance scale to predict falls in community-dwelling adults. J Phys Ther Sci. 2017;29:232–4.
44. Podsiadlo D, Richardson S. The timed "Up & Go": a test of basic functional mobility for frail elderly persons. J Am Geriatr Soc. 1991;39:142–8.
45. Shumway-Cook A, Brauer S, Woollacott M. Predicting the probability for falls in community-dwelling older adults using the Timed Up & Go Test. Phys Ther. 2000;80:896–903.
46. Barry E, Galvin R, Keogh C, Horgan F, Fahey T. Is the Timed Up and Go test a useful predictor of risk of falls in community dwelling older adults: a systematic review and meta-analysis. BMC Geriatr. 2014;14:14.

FRAX

10

John A. Kanis, Nicholas C. Harvey, Helena Johansson, Mattias Lorentzon, Enwu Liu, William D. Leslie, and Eugene V. McCloskey

10.1 Introduction

Osteoporosis is operationally defined on the basis of bone mineral density (BMD) assessment by dual-energy X-ray absorptiometry (DXA), with recent refinements of the description focusing on measurements at the femoral neck as a reference standard [1]. The WHO-defined T-score of −2.5 SD or lower, originally designed for classification in epidemiological studies, has since been widely adopted as both diagnostic and intervention thresholds. The principal difficulty for fracture risk assessment is that whereas this threshold has high specificity, it has low sensitivity, such that the majority of fragility fractures occur in individuals with BMD values above the osteoporosis threshold [2]. Many risk factors have been identified over the last two decades that contribute to fracture risk, at least partly if not wholly independently of DXA BMD. These include age, sex, a prior fracture, a family history of fracture, and lifestyle risk fac-

J. A. Kanis (✉)
Centre for Metabolic Bone Diseases, University of Sheffield Medical School, Broomhall, Sheffield, UK

Mary McKillop Institute for Health Research, Australian Catholic University, Melbourne, Australia
e-mail: w.j.pontefract@sheffield.ac.uk

N. C. Harvey
MRC Lifecourse Epidemiology Unit, University of Southampton, Southampton, UK

NIHR Southampton Biomedical Research Centre, University of Southampton and University Hospital Southampton NHS Foundation Trust, Southampton, UK
e-mail: nch@mrc.soton.ac.uk

H. Johansson
Centre for Metabolic Bone Diseases, University of Sheffield Medical School, Broomhall, Sheffield, UK

Mary McKillop Institute for Health Research, Australian Catholic University, Melbourne, Australia

Sahlgrenska Osteoporosis Centre, Institute of Medicine, University of Gothenburg, Gothenburg, Sweden
e-mail: helena@statiq.se

M. Lorentzon
Geriatric Medicine, Department of Internal Medicine and Clinical Nutrition, Institute of Medicine, University of Gothenburg, Gothenburg, Sweden

Region Västra Götaland, Geriatric Medicine Clinic, Sahlgrenska University Hospital, Mölndal, Sweden
e-mail: mattias.lorentzon@medic.gu.se

E. Liu
Mary McKillop Institute for Health Research, Australian Catholic University, Melbourne, Australia
e-mail: enwu.liu@acu.edu.au

W. D. Leslie
University of Manitoba, Winnipeg, Canada
e-mail: bleslie@sbgh.mb.ca

E. V. McCloskey
Centre for Metabolic Bone Diseases, University of Sheffield Medical School, Broomhall, Sheffield, UK

Centre for Integrated research in Musculoskeletal Ageing (CIMA), Mellanby Centre for Bone Research, University of Sheffield, Sheffield, UK
e-mail: e.v.mccloskey@sheffield.ac.uk

H.-C. Pape et al. (eds.), *Senior Trauma Patients*, https://doi.org/10.1007/978-3-030-91483-7_10

tors such as physical inactivity and smoking [3]. These and other factors have been combined in analyses of individual cohort studies to develop algorithms and scores to characterise future risk at the level of an individual. Such independent risk factors used with BMD can enhance fracture risk assessment; additionally, the incorporation of risk factors that correlate with BMD (e.g. age, fracture, body mass index (BMI)) can also facilitate fracture risk assessment in situations in which DXA is not available. These were the considerations underlying the development of the FRAX® tool, which was devised by the former WHO Collaborating Centre at the University of Sheffield.

10.2 Components of FRAX

The principal aim of treatments for osteoporosis is to decrease the risk of fragility fractures. Thus, the ability to assess fracture risk is critical in identifying patients who are eligible for therapeutic intervention. FRAX—a fracture risk assessment tool for estimating individualised 10-year probability of hip and major osteoporotic fracture (hip, clinical spine, distal forearm, or proximal humerus) [3, 4], integrates eight clinical risk factors (CRFs: prior fragility fracture, parental hip fracture, smoking, systemic glucocorticoid use, excess alcohol intake, BMI, rheumatoid arthritis, and other causes of secondary osteoporosis), which, in addition to age and sex, contribute to a 10-year fracture risk estimate independently of BMD [3, 4]. BMD at the femoral neck is an optional input variable.

FRAX computes fracture probability, accounting for both the risk of fracture and the risk of death. This is important because some of the risk factors affect both of these outcomes. Examples include increasing age, low BMI, low BMD, glucocorticoids, and smoking. Other risk engines calculate the risk of a clinical event without taking into account the possibility of death [5–7].

10.3 Models and Uptake of FRAX

Fracture probability differs markedly within and across regions of the world [8, 9], and thus FRAX models are calibrated to the epidemiology of fracture and mortality in individual countries. Models are currently available for 78 nations or territories covering more than 80% of the world population [10]. The FRAX web site (http://www.shef.ac.uk/FRAX) receives approximately three million visits annually, and the tool is available in 34 languages. Website usage markedly underestimates the uptake of FRAX since it is not the sole portal for the calculation of fracture probabilities using the FRAX tool. For example, FRAX is available in BMD equipment, on smartphones and, in some countries, through handheld calculators.

10.4 Performance Characteristics

The characteristic of major importance, for the purpose of risk assessment, is the ability of a tool to correctly predict the occurrence of new fractures, traditionally expressed as the increase in relative risk per standard deviation (SD) unit increase in risk score. This is termed the gradient of risk. The gradient of risk with the use of FRAX is shown in Table 10.1 for the use of the clinical risk factors alone, femoral neck BMD alone, and the combination [11]. Overall, the predictive value compares very favourably with other risk engines such as the Gail score for breast cancer [12].

Whereas both BMD and the CRFs alone provide significant gradients of risk, the best performance (highest gradients of risk) is observed when BMD is also entered into the FRAX model. Importantly, the impact of the CRFs and BMD is not purely multiplicative as there is some interdependence ($r = -0.25$). The importance of this observation is that the selection of patients with high FRAX probability, but without knowing their BMD, will preferentially select patients with low BMD and that the higher the fracture probability, the lower will be the BMD [13, 14].

Table 10.1 Gradients of risk (RR per SD change in with 95% confidence intervals) with the use of BMD at the femoral neck, clinical risk factors, or the combination [[11] with kind permission from Springer Science+Business Media B.V]

	Gradient of risk		
Age (years)	BMD only	Clinical risk factors alone	Clinical risk factors + BMD
(a) Hip fracture			
50	3.68 (2.61–5.19)	2.05 (1.58–2.65)	4.23 (3.12–5.73)
60	3.07 (2.42–3.89)	1.95 (1.63–2.33)	3.51 (2.85–4.33)
70	2.78 (2.39–3.23)	1.84 (1.65–2.05)	2.91 (2.56–3.31)
80	2.28 (2.09–2.50)	1.75 (1.62–1.90)	2.42 (2.18–2.69)
90	1.70 (1.50–1.93)	1.66 (1.47–1.87)	2.02 (1.71–2.38)
(b) Other osteoporotic fractures			
50	1.19 (1.05–1.34)	1.41 (1.28–1.56)	1.44 (1.30–1.59)
60	1.28 (1.18–1.39)	1.48 (1.39–1.58)	1.52 (1.42–1.62)
70	1.39 (1.30–1.48)	1.55 (1.48–1.62)	1.61 (1.54–1.68)
80	1.54 (1.44–1.65)	1.63 (1.54–1.72)	1.71 (1.62–1.80)
90	1.56 (1.40–1.75)	1.72 (1.58–1.88)	1.81 (1.67–1.97)

These findings consistently indicate that the categorisation of patients at high risk on the basis of FRAX without the use of DXA selects patients with low BMD, and the higher the probability, the lower the BMD. This has obvious significance for case finding in the absence of access to DXA scanning.

10.4.1 Validation

The performance characteristics of FRAX have been evaluated in eleven independent cohorts that did not participate in the model synthesis. In all the validation cohorts, the use of clinical risk factors alone or in combination with BMD gave gradients of fracture risk that differed significantly from unity and which were comparable to those in the original cohorts used for model building (see Table 10.1) [11].

10.4.2 Calibration

Since age-specific rates of fracture and death differ across the world, all FRAX models are calibrated with regard to the epidemiology of hip fracture (preferably from national sources) and mortality (usually UN source). Thus, where the population of each country is "FRAXed", the numbers of hip fractures and deaths estimated would match those indicated by the source data. It follows that the calibration of the FRAX algorithms is only as good as the epidemiology with which the tools are populated. Additionally, any validation exercise will be critically dependent on the representativeness of the population tested for the index country. There are several studies which have examined populations that are nationally representative. The first was based on a UK prospective open cohort study of over two million men and women aged 30–85 years using routinely collected data from 357 general practices [7]. The area under the ROC curve (AUC) for the FRAX algorithm in hip fracture prediction was 0.85 for women and 0.82 for men. Given the small differences in the incidence of hip fracture assumed by FRAX and that observed in the cohort, FRAX appears well-calibrated for the UK. Similar findings were reported from Norway: AUC for hip fracture was 0.81 (0.78–0.83) for women and 0.79 (0.76–0.83) for men [15]. In a study from Israel, the AUC for hip fracture was 0.82 (0.81–0.82) [16].

Fracture probabilities based on the Canadian FRAX tool (both without and with BMD) were compared with observed 10-year fracture incidence from men and women in the CaMos study in Canada (n = 1919 and 4778, respectively) [17]. FRAX-estimated 10-year probability for a major osteoporotic fracture did not differ from the incidence rates in men (5.4% vs. 6.4%, respectively) and was very similar in women (10.8% vs. 12.0%). Results for hip fracture risk were similar. Comparable findings were reported in a large Canadian BMD referral population from Manitoba [18] (Fig. 10.1). A strength of these studies is that fracture incidence was collected over 10 years and only the first major fracture taken into account. Note, however, that incidence is compared with probability so that, as expected from a comparison of incidence and probability, incidence values are higher than probability values as they do not account for the competing hazard of death. Nevertheless, FRAX appears well-calibrated for Canada.

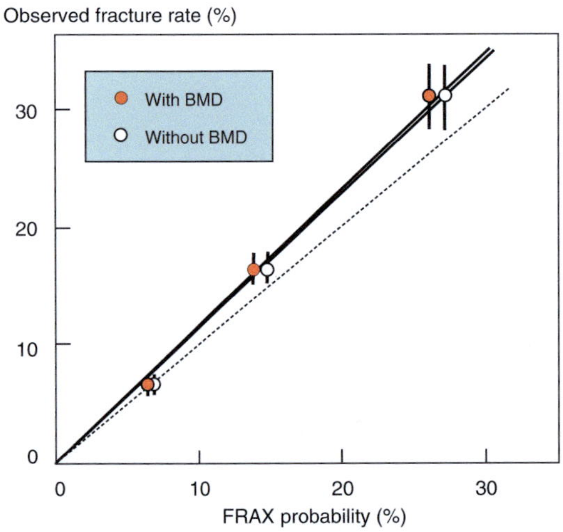

Fig. 10.1 10-year fracture probability for a major fracture derived from the Canadian FRAX tool with and without BMD versus observed 10-year fracture rates (95% confidence interval) by risk category (low, less than 10%; moderate, 10–20%; high, greater than 20%) with BMD (solid circles) and without BMD (open circles). The dashed line depicts the line of identity. Redrawn from [18]

10.5 The Use of FRAX in Assessment Guidelines

FRAX has been incorporated into more than 80 guidelines worldwide [19], although the nature of this application has been heterogeneous. Several guidelines have adopted FRAX into pre-existing guidelines. In the US, for example, the gateway to treatment includes either a prior fracture (hip or spine fracture) or a BMD T-score of <−2.5 SD [20] irrespective of FRAX probability. FRAX is reserved for individuals in whom the T-score is in the osteopenic range and treatment is recommended if the probability of a major fracture or hip fracture lies at 20% or more or 3% or more, respectively. Similarly in Japan, the use of FRAX is reserved for individuals without a prior fracture and a BMD that lies between a T-score of −1.8 to −2.7 SD and treatment is recommended if the probability of a major fracture is 15% or more (Fig. 10.2) [21].

Fig. 10.2 Algorithm for the assessment of patients in Japan [adapted from Orimo 2012]. YAM = young adult mean. A YAM of 70% and 80% is equivalent to a T-score of −2.7 SD and −1.8 SD, respectively, using the NHANES III reference for BMD at the femoral neck in Caucasian women aged 20–29 years (the international T-score referent used in FRAX)

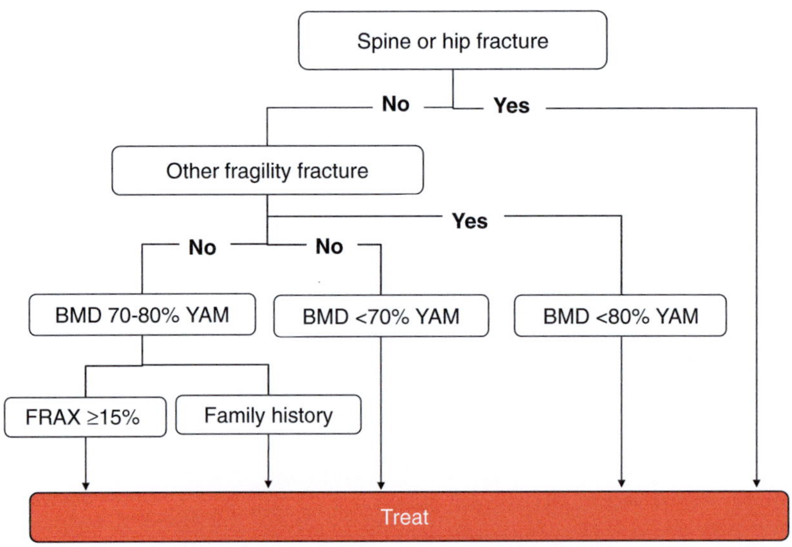

The intervention thresholds in the US, set at 20% for a major osteoporotic fracture and 3% for hip fracture probability, were based on an economic analysis [22]. While such analyses are appropriate for North America (at least at the time they were undertaken), they should not be indiscriminately applied elsewhere: there are many differences in fracture risks, cost of fracture, willingness to pay, and a myriad of other factors to be considered in health-economic evaluation. Notwithstanding such considerations, some countries have adopted these thresholds for no other reason that they were used in the National Osteoporosis Foundation guideline.

Other countries (e.g. China, Finland, Greece, Poland, Switzerland, Sri Lanka, and Sweden) have determined intervention thresholds more appropriate to the local health care setting [19].

Like the National Osteoporosis Foundation, the US Preventive Services Task Force recommends BMD testing in all women aged 65 years or older. For younger women aged 50-65 years, FRAX is recommended as a screening tool for BMD testing. A probability threshold of 8.4% for a major fracture is currently recommended for the following reason: A BMD test is recommended in younger women whose fracture probability is equal to or greater than that of a 65-year-old white woman who has no additional risk factors. With the US FRAX tool, a 65-year-old white woman of average BMI with no other risk factors has a 9.3% 10-year risk for a major osteoporotic fracture. In women aged 50–65 years who exceed this threshold, a BMD test is indicated and treatment recommended in those in whom BMD is in the range for osteoporosis [23, 24].

The probability threshold of 8.4% used by the USPSTF appears logical, but is actually inappropriate for the stated objective "to identify postmenopausal women with T-scores of −2.5 SD or lower" [25]. If detection of osteoporosis is the goal, it is clearly more appropriate to use algorithms that detect osteoporosis rather than a tool to assess fracture risk [26]. Appropriate tools include the Osteoporosis Self-Assessment Tool (OST) and Simple Calculated Osteoporosis Risk Estimation Tool (SCORE), which have higher sensitivity than FRAX for the detection of osteoporosis [27, 28]. A similar error of logic is made in the Scottish Intercollegiate Guidelines Network [29].

The use of BMD alone or BMD with prior fracture as a gateway to assessment is not without problems, as recently reviewed [26]. First, although reduced bone mass is easily quantifiable and strongly related to fracture risk, most fragility fractures occur in individuals with a BMD T-score above the operational threshold for osteoporosis [30]. Second, the significance of any given T-score threshold differs by age [31]. For example, at 65 years, a T-score of −2.5 SD confers a modest increase in the probability of fracture compared with women with no clinical risk factors and in whom BMD is not measured. With advancing age, the difference in the probability of fracture between the general population and those with a T-score of −2.5 SD reduces; indeed, from the age of 78 years in the US, fracture probability becomes progressively lower than that of the age and sex-matched general population (Fig. 10.3) [26]. Thus, a T-score of −2.5 SD becomes a protective factor from the age of 78 years in the US, relative to the general population. Third, fracture rates differ widely between countries, much more so than can be explained by variations in BMD [32]. Thus, the T-score at a given probability will vary from country to country. For example, when an intervention threshold is set at a 10-year probability of a major fracture of 20% (as used in Canada and the US) in women aged 65 years, the femoral neck T-score ranges from −4.6 SD in Venezuela to −2.0 SD in Iceland [26].

For the reasons above, many countries have used FRAX rather than BMD as the principal gateway for assessment. The approach is summarised in Fig. 10.4 [4]. The management process begins with the assessment of fracture probability and the categorisation of fracture risk on the basis of age, sex, BMI, and the clinical risk factors. Using this information alone, some patients at high fracture risk may be offered treatment without use of BMD testing (e.g. prior fracture). There will be other instances where the probability will be so low that a decision not to treat can be made without BMD. An example might be the well woman at

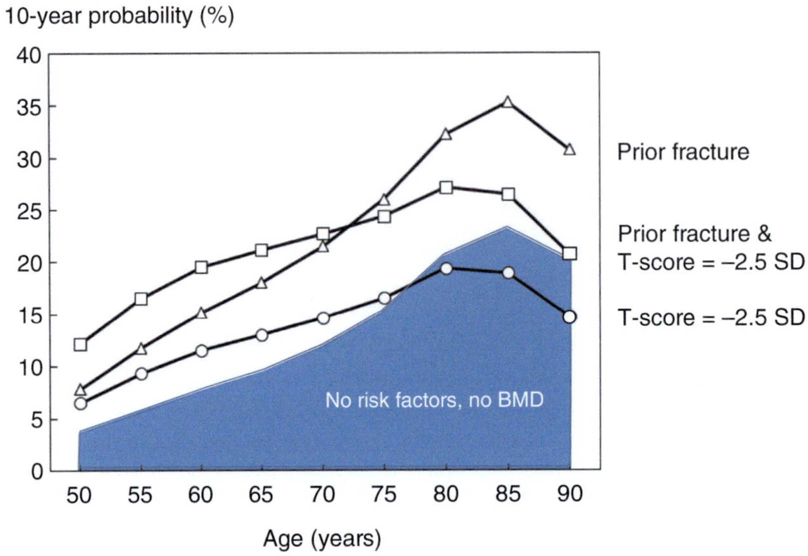

Fig. 10.3 Ten-year probabilities (%) of a major osteoporotic fracture for white women from the United States according to a T-score of −2.5 SD (circle), prior fracture (triangle), or the combination (square) (BMI is set to 24 kg/m^2) [http://www.shef.ac.uk/FRAX]. Note the decreased probability after the age of 85 years attributable to the competing effect of mortality. Redrawn from [6]

menopause with no clinical risk factors. Thus, not all individuals require a DXA scan and are thus excluded from the intermediate category in Fig. 10.4.

The size of the latter category will vary in different countries. In the US, this would be a large category, whereas in a large number of countries with limited or no access to DXA, the size of the intermediate group will necessarily be small. In other countries (e.g. the UK), where provision for BMD testing is suboptimal [33], the intermediate category will lie between the two extremes. It has been conservatively estimated that a minimum of 10 DXA units are required per million of the population and such provision is available for less than 20 countries worldwide [33].

The first step in defining the intermediate group is to establish an intervention threshold and target DXA scans to those lying at or around this threshold, in order to maximise the impact of the scan on decision making. Nearly all guidelines internationally recommend that women with a prior fragility fracture should be considered for intervention without the necessity for a DXA scan (other than to monitor treatment). Since a prior fracture is associated with sufficient risk that treatment can

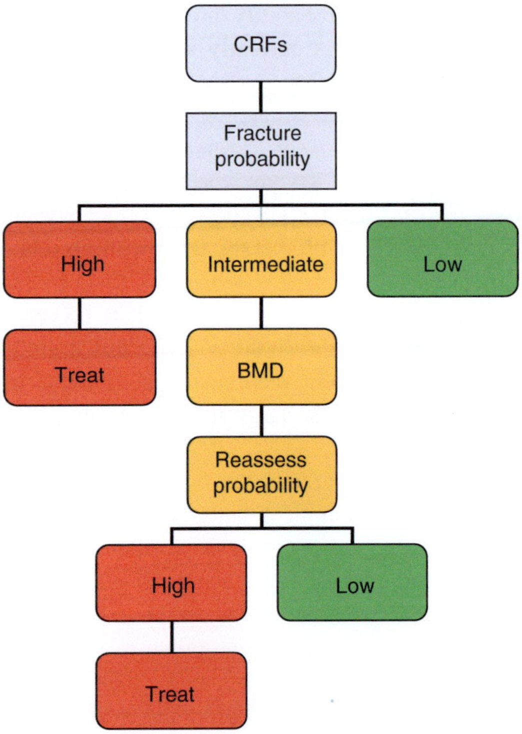

Fig. 10.4 Management algorithm for the assessment of individuals at risk of fracture. CRFs, clinical risk factors. Adapted from [4] with kind permission from Springer Science and Business Media

be recommended, the intervention threshold in women without a prior fracture can be set at the age-specific fracture probability equivalent to women with a prior fragility fracture [4] and therefore rises with age, for example from a 10-year probability of 8 to 33% in the UK. This may be termed the 'fracture threshold'. This is the approach to intervention thresholds first used by the UK National Osteoporosis Guideline Group (NOGG) [34] and has since been adopted into European guidelines [35, 36] and elsewhere [19, 37]. The same intervention threshold is applied to men, since the effectiveness and cost-effectiveness of interventions in men are broadly similar to those in women for equivalent risk [38].

10.6 FRAX and Efficacy of Intervention

European guidelines on the evaluation of medicinal products in the treatment of primary osteoporosis [39] place an emphasis on the study of patients at high fracture risk. As a consequence, FRAX has been applied to several phase 3 studies in order to determine the enrolment characteristics of patients. This information has also been used to determine whether treatment efficacy varies according to baseline fracture risk. Interventions studied include abaloparatide, raloxifene, bazedoxifene, clodronate, daily and weekly teriparatide, denosumab, alendronate, and strontium ranelate as well as a basket of interventions used by general practitioners in the UK [36]. Most of these were post hoc, but, in the case of denosumab, was a pre-planned analysis. In addition, the 'screening for prevention of fractures in older women' (SCOOP) study was a prospective randomised trial in which screening older women for treatment on the basis of FRAX hip fracture probability led to a 28% reduction in hip fracture occurrence over 5 years [40].

Greater efficacy against fracture in individuals at higher risk treated with clodronate, denosumab, and bazedoxifene (Fig. 10.5) [41] has been demonstrated. This FRAX-dependency has marked economic consequences, illustrated when comparing two hypothetical treatments with similar

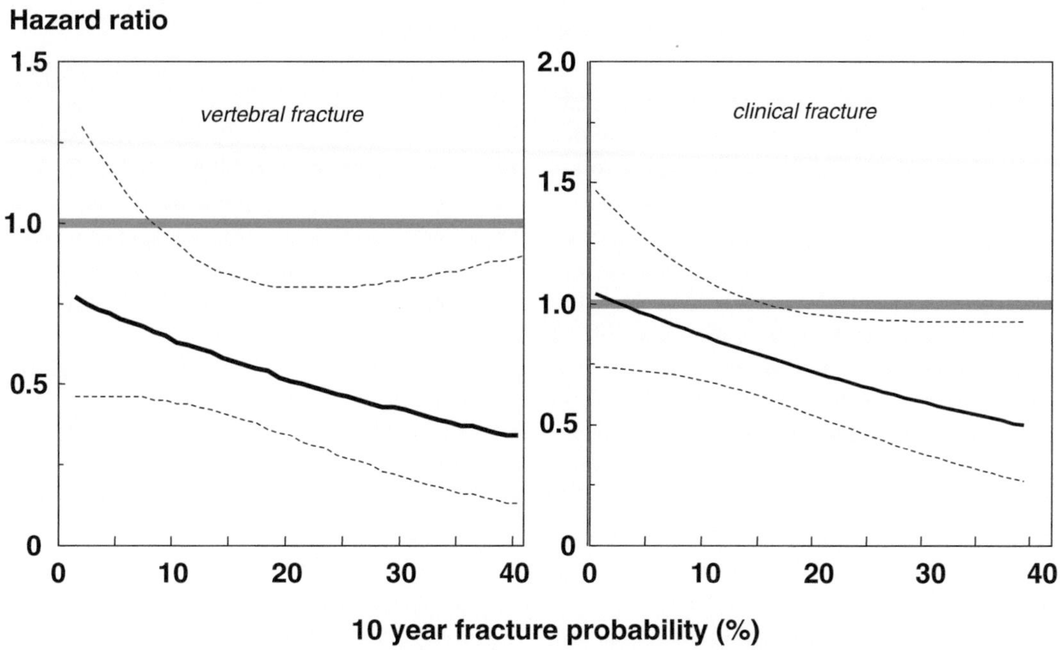

Fig. 10.5 Hazard ratio between treatments (bazedoxifene versus placebo) for vertebral fracture and all clinical fractures according to the 10-year probability of a major osteoporotic fracture calculated with BMD and other risk variables included in FRAX. Redrawn from [41]

Table 10.2 Contrasting effects on the number of fractures saved with an intervention, the efficacy of which is that the relative risk reduction (RRR) is independent or dependent on FRAX (average RRR set at 40%)

	A. FRAX independent		B. FRAX dependent	
Fracture probability (%)	RRR (%)	Fractures saved	RRR (%)	Fractures saved
0	40	0	0	0
5	40	2	14	1
10	40	4	27	3
15	40	6	40	6
20	40	8	54	11
25	40	10	68	17
30	40	12	80	24
Total		42		62

overall effectiveness on fracture risk, but the efficacy of one increases in women with higher baseline fracture probability (treatment B). In contrast, the relative risk reduction with the other is constant over the range of fracture probabilities studied (treatment A) (Table 10.2). As a consequence, treatment A has better cost-effectiveness in terms of fractures saved at low fracture probabilities, whereas treatment B has the better cost-effectiveness at high baseline fracture probabilities [36].

These results have a number of important implications. First, they remove any concern that patients identified on the basis of clinical risk factors with FRAX would not respond to pharmacologic interventions. Indeed, these studies showed that high FRAX probabilities are associated with efficacy, even when BMD is not used to characterise risk. Second, they support the views of the regulatory agencies that treatments should be targeted preferentially to men and women at high fracture risk. Third, the finding of greater efficacy at higher fracture probabilities with some interventions has important implications for health technology assessments and challenges the current meta-analytic approach. Finally, since treatments directed to high-risk patients improve the budget impact, greater efficacy in the higher risk groups will improve still further the budget impact and the cost-effectiveness of intervention.

10.7 Addressing the Limitations of FRAX

The limitations of FRAX have been extensively reviewed [19, 42] and are only briefly addressed here. The risk factors included in FRAX were carefully chosen to limit complexity, for ease of input, and to include only well-established, independent contributors to fracture risk. In addition, it was important that the factors used identified a risk that was amenable to an intervention [42]. The FRAX tool has been appreciated for its simplicity of use in primary care, but criticised for the same reason because it does not take account of exposure response. For example, the risk of fracture increases with exposure to glucocorticoids, but FRAX only accommodates a yes/no response to the relevant question. Other well-researched examples of 'dose–response' include the number of prior fractures and the consumption of alcohol. Other concerns are the lack of provision for lumbar spine BMD (which is commonly recommended in treatment guidelines) and the absence of measurements of the material or structural properties of bone. A concern that treatment might invalidate the interpretation of FRAX appears misplaced [43].

Relatively simple arithmetic procedures have been proposed, in order to address some of these limitations, which can be applied to conventional FRAX estimates of probabilities of hip fracture and a major osteoporotic fracture to adjust the probability assessment. Thus, adjustments have been devised to accommodate knowledge of the following:

- High, moderate, and low exposure to glucocorticoids [44].
- Concurrent data on lumbar spine BMD [45, 46].
- Information on trabecular bone score (TBS) [47, 48].
- Hip axis length [49].
- Falls history [50].
- Type 2 diabetes [51].
- Immigration status [52].
- Recency of prior fracture [53, 54].

With regard to glucocorticoids, for example, a woman aged 75 years from the UK taking glucocorticoids for rheumatoid arthritis (no other risk factors and BMI of 24 kg/m^2) has a 10-year probability for a major fracture of 29%. If she is on a higher than average dose of prednisolone (>7.5 mg daily), then the revised probability should be uplifted by 15% (29 × 1.15 = 33) [44]. Such analyses can inform the clinician how to temper clinical judgement on the existing output of the FRAX models. More precise adjustments are available through the FRAX website (FRAX$_{plus}$).

10.8 Summary

The FRAX fracture risk assessment tool provides country-specific algorithms for estimating individualised 10-year probability of hip and major osteoporotic fracture (hip, clinical spine, distal forearm, or proximal humerus). Following its release in 2008, 86 models are now available for 78 countries or territories covering more than 80% of the world population. The FRAX website receives approximately three million visits annually. Following independent validation, FRAX has been incorporated into more than 80 guidelines worldwide. However, the application of FRAX in guidelines has been heterogeneous with the adoption of several different approaches to setting intervention thresholds. The relationship between FRAX and efficacy of intervention has been explored and is expected to influence treatment guidelines in the future. A more unified approach to setting intervention thresholds with FRAX is a research priority.

Acknowledgements Some text is reproduced from Kanis JA, Cooper C, Rizzoli R, Reginster J-Y; Scientific Advisory Board of the European Society for Clinical and Economic Aspects of Osteoporosis (ESCEO); and the Committees of Scientific Advisors and National Societies of the International Osteoporosis Foundation (IOF) (2019) European guidance for the diagnosis and management of osteoporosis in postmenopausal women. Osteoporosis International 30: 3-44; Kanis JA, Harvey NC, Johansson H, Odén A, Leslie WD McCloskey EV (2017) FRAX update. Journal of Clinical Densitometry. 20: 360–367.

Competing interests Professor Kanis led the team that developed FRAX as director of the WHO Collaborating Centre for Metabolic Bone Diseases; he has no financial interest in FRAX. Professors McCloskey, Harvey, and Dr. Johansson are members of the FRAX team. Professors Kanis, Harvey, and McCloskey are members of the advisory body of the National Osteoporosis Guideline Group, UK. William D Leslie declares no competing interests.

References

1. Kanis JA, McCloskey EV, Johansson H, Oden A, Melton LJ 3rd, Khaltaev N. A reference standard for the description of osteoporosis. Bone. 2008;42(467-475):18180210.
2. WHO. Assessment of fracture risk and its application to screening for postmenopausal osteoporosis. Geneva: World Health Organization; 1994.
3. Kanis JA, on behalf of the World Health Organization Scientific Group (2008) Assessment of osteoporosis at the primary health-care level. Technical Report. WHO Collaborating Centre, University of Sheffield, UK. Available at http://www.shef.ac.uk/FRAX/index.htm
4. Kanis JA, McCloskey EV, Johansson H, Strom O, Borgstrom F, Oden A, the National Osteoporosis Guideline Group. Case finding for the management of osteoporosis with FRAX®—assessment and intervention thresholds for the UK. Osteoporos Int. 2008;19:1395–408.
5. Nguyen ND, Frost SA, Center JR, Eisman JA, Nguyen TV. Development of prognostic nomograms for individualizing 5-year and 10-year fracture risks. Osteoporos Int. 2008;19:1431–44.
6. Hippisley-Cox J, Coupland C. Derivation and validation of updated QFracture algorithm to predict risk of osteoporotic fracture in primary care in the United Kingdom: prospective open cohort study. BMJ. 2012:344. https://doi.org/10.1136/bmj.e3427.
7. Hippisley-Cox J, Coupland C. Predicting risk of osteoporotic fracture in men and women in England and Wales: prospective derivation and validation of QFractures Scores. Br Med J. 2009;339:b4229.
8. Kanis JA, Odén A, McCloskey EV, et al. A systematic review of hip fracture incidence and probability of fracture worldwide. Osteoporos Int. 2012;23:2239–56.
9. Cauley JA, Chalhoub D, Kassem AM, Fuleihan GEH. Geographic and ethnic disparities in osteoporotic fractures. Nat Rev Endocrinol. 2014;10:338–51.
10. Kanis JA, Johansson H, Oden A, Cooper C, McCloskey EV, the Epidemiology and Quality of Life Working Group of IOF. Worldwide uptake of FRAX. Arch Osteoporos. 2014;9:166.
11. Kanis JA, Oden A, Johnell O, et al. The use of clinical risk factors enhances the performance of BMD in the prediction of hip and osteoporotic fractures in men and women. Osteoporos Int. 2007;18:1033–46.
12. Chlebowski RT, Anderson GL, Lane DS, et al. Predicting risk of breast cancer in postmenopausal women by hormone receptor status. J Natl Cancer Inst. 2007;99:1695–705.

13. Johansson H, Oden A, Johnell O, et al. Optimisation of BMD measurements to identify high risk groups for treatment—a test analysis. J Bone Miner Res. 2004;19:906–13.
14. Leslie WD, Morin S, Lix LM, et al. Fracture risk assessment without bone density measurement in routine clinical practice. Osteoporos Int. 2012;23:75–85.
15. Hoff M, Meyer HE, Skurtveit S, Langhammer A, Søgaard AJ, Syversen U, Dhainaut A, Skovlund E, Abrahamsen B, Schei B. Validation of FRAX and the impact of self-reported falls among elderly in a general population: the HUNT study, Norway. Osteoporos Int. 2017;28:2935–44.
16. Goldshtein I, Gerber Y, Ish-Shalom S, Leshno M. Fracture risk assessment with FRAX using real-world data in a population-based cohort from Israel. Am J Epidemiol. 2018;187:94–102.
17. Fraser LA, Langsetmo L, Berger C, et al. Fracture prediction and calibration of a Canadian FRAX® tool: a population-based report from CaMos. Osteoporos Int. 2011;22:829–37.
18. Leslie WD, Lix LM, Johansson H, Oden A, McCloskey E, Kanis JA. Manitoba bone density program. Independent clinical validation of a Canadian FRAX((R)) tool: Fracture prediction and model calibration. J Bone Miner Res. 2010;25:2350–8.
19. Kanis JA, Harvey NC, Cooper C, Johansson H, Odén A, McCloskey EV, the Advisory Board of the National Osteoporosis Guideline Group. A systematic review of intervention thresholds based on FRAX. Arch Osteoporos. 2016;11:25. https://doi.org/10.1007/s11657-016-0278-z.
20. Cosman F, de Beur SJ, LeBoff MS, et al. Clinician's guide to prevention and treatment of osteoporosis. Osteoporos Int. 2014;25:2359–81.
21. Orimo H, Nakamura T, Hosoi T, et al. Japanese 2011 Guidelines for prevention and treatment of osteoporosis—Executive summary. A report of the committee for developing guidelines for prevention and treatment of osteoporosis: Japan Osteoporosis Society, Japanese Society for Bone and Mineral Research, and Japan Osteoporosis Foundation. Arch Osteoporos. 2012;7:3–20.
22. Tosteson AN, Melton LJ 3rd, Dawson-Hughes B, National Osteoporosis Foundation Guide Committee, et al. Cost-effective osteoporosis treatment thresholds: The United States perspective. Osteoporos Int. 2008;19:437–47.
23. US Preventive Services Task Force, Curry SJ, Krist AH, Owens DK, Barry MJ, Caughey AB, Davidson KW, Doubeni CA, Epling JW Jr, Kemper AR, Kubik M, Landefeld CS, Mangione CM, Phipps MG, Pignone M, Silverstein M, Simon MA, Tseng CW, Wong JB. Screening for osteoporosis to prevent fractures: US Preventive Services Task Force Recommendation Statement. JAMA. 2018;319:2521–31.
24. Nelson HD, Haney EM, Chou R, Dana T, Fu R, Bougatsos C (2010) Screening for osteoporosis: systematic review to update the 2002 US Preventive Services Task Force Recommendation. Evidence Syntheses No. 77. AHRQ Publication No. 10-05145-EF-1.
25. Crandall CJ, Larson J, Gourlay M, et al. Osteoporosis screening in postmenopausal women 50-64 years-old: Comparison of U.S. Preventive Services Task Force strategy and two traditional strategies in the Women's Health Initiative. J Bone Miner Res. 2014;29:1661–6.
26. Kanis JA, McCloskey EV, Harvey NC, Johansson H, Leslie WD. Intervention thresholds and the diagnosis of osteoporosis. J Bone Miner Res. 2015;30:1747–53.
27. Lydick E, Cook K, Turpin J, Melton M, Stine R, Byrnes C. Development and validation of a simple questionnaire to facilitate identification of women likely to have low bone density. Am J Manag Care. 1998;4:37–48.
28. Koh LK, Sedrine WB, Torralba TP, et al. A simple tool to identify Asian women at increased risk of osteoporosis. Osteoporos Int. 2001;12:699–705.
29. Scottish Intercollegiate Guidelines Network (SIGN) (2015) Management of osteoporosis and the prevention of fragility fractures. Edinburgh: SIGN publication no. 142. [March 2015]. Available from URL: http://www.sign.ac.uk accessed May 11th, 2018.
30. World Health Organisation (1994) Assessment of fracture risk and its application to screening for postmenopausal osteoporosis. WHO Technical Report Series 843. WHO, Geneva.
31. Kanis JA, Johnell O, Oden A, Jonsson B, De Laet C, Dawson A. Risk of hip fracture according to World Health Organization criteria for osteoporosis and osteopenia. Bone. 2000;27:585–90.
32. Kanis JA, Odén A, EV MC, Johansson H, Wahl D, Cyrus Cooper C on behalf of the IOF Working Group on Epidemiology and Quality of Life. A systematic review of hip fracture incidence and probability of fracture worldwide. Osteoporos Int. 2012;23:2239–56.
33. Kanis JA, Johnell O. Requirements for DXA for the management of osteoporosis in Europe. Osteoporosis Int. 2005;16:229–38.
34. Compston J, Cooper A, Cooper C, on behalf of the National Osteoporosis Guideline Group (NOGG), et al. Guidelines for the diagnosis and management of osteoporosis in postmenopausal women and men from the age of 50 years in the UK. Maturitas. 2009;62:105–8.
35. Lekawasam S, Adachi JD, Agnusdei D, et al. A framework for the development of guidelines for the management of glucocorticoid-induced osteoporosis. Osteoporos Int. 2012;23:2257–76.
36. Clark P, Denova-Gutiérrez E, et al. FRAX-based intervention and assessment thresholds in seven Latin American countries. Osteoporos Int. 2018;29:707–15.
37. Kanis JA, Cooper C, Rizzoli R, Reginster J-Y, Scientific Advisory Board of the European Society for Clinical and Economic Aspects of Osteoporosis (ESCEO), the Committees of Scientific Advisors and National Societies of the International Osteoporosis Foundation (IOF). European guidance for the diagnosis and management of osteoporosis in postmenopausal women. Osteoporos Int. 2019;30:3–44.

38. Kanis JA, Stevenson M, McCloskey EV, Davis S, Lloyd-Jones M. Glucocorticoid-induced osteoporosis: a systematic review and cost-utility analysis. Health Technol Assess. 2007;11:1–256.
39. Committee for Medicinal Products for Human Use (CHMP) (2006) Guideline on the evaluation of medicinal products in the treatment of primary osteoporosis. Ref CPMP/EWP/552/95Rev2 London, CHMP Nov 2006.
40. Shepstone L, Lenaghan E, Cooper C, et al. A randomized controlled trial of screening in the community to reduce fractures in older women—The SCOOP Study. Lancet. 2018;391:741–7.
41. Kanis JA, Johansson H, Oden A, McCloskey EV. Bazedoxifene reduces vertebral and clinical fractures in postmenopausal women at high risk assessed with FRAX®. Bone. 2009;44:49–54.
42. Kanis JA, McCloskey E, Johansson H, Oden A, Leslie WD. FRAX with and without BMD. Calcif Tissue Int. 2012;90:1–13.
43. Leslie WD, Lix LM, Johansson H, Oden A, McCloskey E, Kanis J. Does osteoporosis therapy invalidate FRAX for fracture prediction? J Bone Miner Res. 2012;27:1243–51.
44. Kanis JA, Johansson H, Oden A, McCloskey EV. Guidance for the adjustment of FRAX according to the dose of glucocorticoids. Osteoporos Int. 2011;22:809–16.
45. Leslie WD, Lix LM, Johansson H, Oden A, McCloskey EV, Kanis JA, for the Manitoba Bone Density Program. Spine-hip discordance and fracture risk assessment: A physician-friendly FRAX enhancement. Osteoporos Int. 2011;22:839–47.
46. Johansson H, Kanis JA, Odén A, et al. Impact of femoral neck and lumbar spine BMD discordances on FRAX probabilities in women: a meta-analysis of international cohorts. Calc Tiss Int. 2014;95:428–35.
47. Leslie WD, Johansson H, Kanis JA, et al. Lumbar spine texture enhances ten-year fracture probability assessment. Osteoporos Int. 2014;25:2271–7.
48. McCloskey EV, Odén A, Harvey NC, et al. A meta-analysis of trabecular bone score in fracture risk prediction and its dependence on FRAX. J Bone Miner Res. 2016;31:940–8.
49. Leslie WD, Lix LM, Morin SN, et al. Adjusting hip fracture probability in men and women using hip axis length: the Manitoba Bone Density Database. J Clin Densitom. 2015;19:326–31. https://doi.org/10.1016/j.jocd.2015.07.004.
50. Masud T, Binkley N, Boonen S, Hannan MT, on behalf of the FRAX Position Conference Members. Can falls and frailty be used in FRAX? J Clin Densitom. 2011;14:194–204.
51. Leslie WD, Johansson H, McCloskey EV, Harvey NC, Kanis JA, Hans D. Comparison of methods for improving fracture risk assessment in diabetes: The Manitoba BMD Registry. J Bone Miner Res. 2018;33:1923–30.
52. Johansson H, Odén A, Lorentzon M, et al. Is the Swedish FRAX model appropriate for immigrants to Sweden? Osteoporos Int. 2015;26:2617–22.
53. Kanis JA, Johansson H, Odén A, Harvey NC, Gudnason V, Sanders K, Sigurdsson G, Siggeirsdottir K, Borgström F, McCloskey EV. Characteristics of recurrent fractures. Osteoporos Int. 2018;29:1747–57.
54. Kanis JA, Harvey NC, McCloskey E, Bruyère O, Veronese N, Lorentzon M, Cooper C, Rizzoli R, Reginster J-Y. Algorithm for the management of patients at low/middle/high risk of osteoporotic fracture: a global perspective. Osteoporos Int. 2019;

11 Falls' Prevention by Self-Managed Scoring

Sascha Halvachizadeh, Christian Hierholzer, and Hans-Christoph Pape

11.1 Introduction

The demographic changes occur mostly in western societies. An increasing number of traumatic events are associated with these changes [1–6]. In general, falls are a major global public health problem and leading cause of accidental or unintentional injury and hospitalization. If occurring in hospitals, they are associated with a longer length of stay, need for readmissions, and adverse outcomes. Overall, they are accompanied by a dramatic increase in health care costs, both for in-hospital and outpatient treatments. In the elderly population, its influence is potentially underestimated, as even in the cognitively functioning patients, reconstructing the fall may not be possible [7]. Only few studies examined falls' risk and those were performed in health care facilities, e.g., hospitals or nursing homes [8]. According to home-based video analysis of falls, it became evident that only few falls happen during the day – most occur in the morning or in the evening [2].

Moreover, those falls leading to readmission to a hospital have been closely examined. In a large study [9], out of 358.581 initial fall-related readmissions (FRR) in geriatric adults, 21,713 experienced ≥1 fall-related readmission (6.06%). The authors describe independent predictors, such as age (OR 1.007, 95% CI 1.005–1.009), depression (OR 1.25, 95% CI 1.21–1.30), drug abuse (OR 1.37, 95% CI 1.15–1.63), liver disease (OR 1.25, 95% CI 1.15–1.43, $P < 0.001$), psychosis (OR 1.16, 95% CI 1.09–1.23), valvular heart disease (OR 1.07, 95% CI 1.02–1.12), chronic pulmonary disease (OR 1.10, 95% CI 1.06–1.13), and number of chronic conditions (OR 1.022, 95% CI 1.016–1.29). Patients in the FRR group were less likely to be discharged to their previous residence (5.9% versus 21.0%).

In addition, previous gait or balance disabilities seem to be strong and reliable predictors of future falls. Simple screening questions might therefore perform well enough in predicting falls. It has been discussed that little or no additional value may be gained by performing a complex screening test [10–12].

It has clearly been shown that a previous fall is a strong predictor [10], and further ones are impairments of strength, gait, and balance impairments. The causes of falls can be multifactorial and may derive from cardiac arrhythmias, cerebrovascular, neurologic causes, or are well-described to require the care of an ear, nose, and throat physician.

S. Halvachizadeh (✉) · C. Hierholzer · H.-C. Pape
Department of Trauma, University Hospital Zurich, Zürich, Switzerland
e-mail: Sascha.Halvachizadeh@usz.ch

H.-C. Pape et al. (eds.), *Senior Trauma Patients*, https://doi.org/10.1007/978-3-030-91483-7_11

11.2 The Role of Proprioception in The Prevention of Falls

Proprioception plays an important role in maintaining balance and controlling body posture. With aging, deterioration of the proprioceptive mechanisms occurs and involves changes in peripheral and central nervous system. Due to alterations in proprioception, the neuromuscular control of the limbs changes, resulting in the balance disturbances. The proprioceptive functions decline during the aging process, which has been associated with the balance deficits, thus resulting in an increase in the likelihood of falls [13, 14]. An associated decrease in the dynamic response of muscle spindles and the atrophy of axons reduces the speed of translation by nerve fibers. In geriatric patients, exercise programs have been shown to improve muscle function despite older age [15]. Most of the available falls' assessment scales use a variety of questions in order to demonstrate a well-rounded picture of the patient at risk [10, 16, 17].

The main purpose of a less complex first screening tool is the identification of a potential balance problem [11, 12, 17, 18]. Simple screening questions have been reported to perform as well as more complex screening tests in predicting who will fall [10]. The American Geriatric Society/ British Geriatric Society guidelines therefore suggest that all older individuals should be assessed regarding the incidence and number of falls within the year prior to the assessment. Furthermore, the evaluation should include a detailed physical examination and a timed performance test. Those found by this screen to be at higher risk should be given more intensive assessment and intervention [10, 11].

11.3 Self-Assessment Tool

In addition, it has been shown that the involvement of affected patients may be helpful in determining the risk analysis and effectively reduce the number of falls [19]. Our group has previously developed a self-assessment tool in order to minimize the risk of falls in the elderly population [20]. This was performed by using certain *A-priori assumptions, as summarized in* Table 11.1. *We* concluded that the compilation of questions covers the most important diseases known to contribute to ground level falls (Table 11.2).

Table 11.1 Prerequisites for the development of a self-assessment

• Each individual should be able to assess his/her own risk at defined time points.
• The assessment should be feasible by any layman. Assistance from a physician should not be required.
• Among the causes of falls, those caused by medical, neurologic, and orthopaedic reasons should be covered.
• The assessment should combine a questionnaire and a practical part.
• There should be no risk of a fall of the elderly while performing the practical part.
• The assessment should be reliable and repeatable to allow for longitudinal comparison.
• Feasibility represents a key factor, thus a 10-question limit was selected.

These screening algorithms usually have in common that the evaluation is undertaken by trained individuals in a hospital setting. This leads to the inclusion of a high proportion of low-risk people and a waste of resources, while at the same time the omission of a large proportion of people at high risk limits the potential reduction in falls achievable [10].

In this light, it would be advantageous to pretest the individuals at risk in their own environment using a simple self-assessment approach.

We thus searched to develop a scale that can be used by older citizen at higher risk of falling. The current manuscript summarizes the results of this review, consensus, and selection process. It was designed to allow for a prospective test of ease of use, validity, and specificity.

Runge et al. suggest five musculoskeletal tests. According to their study, self-selected gait velocity represented the most important predictive parameter, when frailty was used as determining factor [18]. However, all their assessments used an environment where helpers were close to the individual at risk. It is evident that these tests cannot be for self-assessment.

Table 11.2 Aachen falls prevention scale

Part I	
Self-questionnaire (10 questions, one point per question answered 'yes', 10 points max.):	
	Yes → no
1. Do you have problems with hearing or vision?	
2. Do you feel unsafe or have you been falling recently?	
3. Are you afraid of falling?	
4. Do you take medication for sleep, cardiac problems, diuretics, or sedatives?	
5. Do you loose urine or stool involuntarily?	
6. Do you have memory problems?	
7. Do you feel lonely at times and think that your life is without value?	
8. Do you use a walking aid on a regular basis?	
9. Do you suffer from Parkinson's, Arthritis, or Rheumatism?	
10. Are there many traps that might cause a fall in your home?	
Part II	
Self-Test with your partner	
Stand freely, do not lean or hold on anybody, measure the time until you have to do a corrective action with your arm, upper body, or lower extremity.	
Standing test	
Successfully completed:	10 s or more
Failed:	less than 10 s
	Yes → no

Assessment tools for gait and balance are straightforward, self-contained, fast to apply, and can apparently be used to predict the risk of falling [21]. However, there is a lack of evidence that any of the available screening tests is clearly useful for identifying fallers [10]. Evaluation of these tests has mostly been performed in single studies or in multiple but diverse and incomparable studies in terms of sample size or study design [10].

11.4 Screening for Mobility

Currently, the Timed Up and Go Test (TUG) is the most frequently recommended screening test for mobility. It is even used for assessment of certain fracture-associated scenarios, such as pelvic ring injuries [22]. It uses agreement in stop-watch durations instead of rating scales, thus probably making it the most reliable test [17, 23]. The most frequently evaluated tool is the Tinetti balance, gait, and mobility scales. However, different versions of the test were used by different studies [24]. Disadvantages of the scale include difficulty to assess many of the items on a 3-point scale and its poor specificity. Despite being widely used in gerontology, the gait section is seldom used [23]. The Berg Balance Scale (BBS) is easy to use and shows strong internal consistency and a high intra- and interrater reliability. On the other hand, the sensitivity is only poor to moderate [25]. In line with several other clinical tests, it is poor at identifying the affected subcomponents of gait and balance [17]. The Tandem Stance is reported to have poor discriminatory ability and sensitivity, but good specificity [26]. One-leg stance duration with eyes closed is often too difficult and variable to serve as a useful clinical test so that the eyes open version is generally used. Disadvantages include the difficult nature of the test and its lack of evaluating dynamic balance control [17].

In this light, we think the introduction of the combination of a simple questionnaire with a safe and quick balance tool, such as the 10 s standing test ('Aachen Falls Prevention Scale'), meets the criteria to identify whether or not a balance problem exists. An elderly patient who fails this quick balance screen should have a more complete balance or gait evaluation by a physician or occupational therapist. Balance disorders can have serious consequences for the social function. Fear of falls leads to activity restriction and social isolation. However, in the light of lacking evidence on the accuracy of screening tools for predicting falls risk [10], the 'Aachen Falls Prevention Scale' finally uses a self-assessment tool grading falls' risk on a scale of 1–10 by the individual itself after completion of Part I and Part II. This summarizes the felt falling risk resulting from the multidimensional evaluation of risk factors and the balance control.

11.5 Co-Managed Care in the Case of a Fall

If a fall requires hospitalization or even surgical intervention, the co-managed care concept foresees initial geriatric assessment. This implies a common treatment plan both for the fracture and the comorbidities. During the hospital stay, common ward rounds between geriatricians, orthopaedic trauma surgeons, social workers, and specialized nurses have become the rule, at least in geriatric fracture centers [4]. In some areas, even hospitals were built that focused on co-managed care [5]. Some studies document that the implementation of a standardized orthopaedic-geriatric care plan improves the outcome of proximal femur fractures [6, 27]. It appears, though, that the current literature about prospective studies regarding interdisciplinary treatment in hip fractures is difficult to prove and inconsistent results were shown. Furthermore, there is no consensus on efficacy of the different ways of cooperation between orthopaedic surgeons and geriatricians [28]. Using multidimensional assessment strategies, it is difficult to identify the specific patient cohorts who could potentially benefit from this complex cooperation [29]. In addition, attention should be paid to cost-value ratios [29]. Several countries in Europe have begun a process of certification in order to improve the issues of co-managed care. Among others, our group has contributed to the selection process and the standardization of criteria for geriatric trauma centers [30].

It has been discussed that multiple factors are important for rendering effective falls programs difficult. Among these, time constraints, competing demands, and inadequate reimbursement appear to be relevant factors [31, 32].

11.6 Conclusion

Certain medical comorbidities are associated with increased risk of falling. Especially, cardiac and neurologic disorders as well as the time of day increase susceptibility of the elderly to fall. It is of high importance to screen risk factors that are associated with falling and to control for these risk factors as early as possible in order to decrease the risk of falls and fall-associated injuries.

References

1. Moore L, Turgeon AF, Sirois M-J, Lavoie A. Trauma centre outcome performance: a comparison of young adults and geriatric patients in an inclusive trauma system. Injury. 2012;43(9):1580–5.
2. Vlaeyen E, Deschodt M, Debard G, Dejaeger E, Boonen S, Goedeme T, et al. Fall incidents unraveled: a series of 26 video-based real-life fall events in three frail older persons. BMC Geriatrics. 2013;13
3. Liem IS, Kammerlander C, Suhm N, Blauth M, Roth T, Gosch M, et al. Identifying a standard set of outcome parameters for the evaluation of orthogeriatric co-management for hip fractures. Injury. 2013;44(11):1403–12.
4. Kammerlander C, Gosch M, Blauth M, Lechleitner M, Luger TJ, Roth T. The Tyrolean geriatric fracture center an orthogeriatric co-management model. Zeitschrift Fur Gerontologie Und Geriatrie. 2011;44(6):363–7.
5. Bielza Galindo R, Ortiz Espada A, Arias Munana E, Guzman V, de Lazaro R, Mora Casado A, Moreno Martin R, et al. Opening of an acute orthogeriatric unit in a general hospital. Revista espanola de geriatria y. Gerontologia. 2013;48(1):26–9.
6. Patel NK, Sarraf KM, Joseph S, Lee C, Middleton FR. Implementing the National Hip Fracture Database: an audit of care. Injury. 2013;44(12):1934–9.
7. Ungar A, Rafanelli M, Iacomelli I, Brunetti MA, Ceccofiglio A, Tesi F, et al. Fall prevention in the elderly. Clin Cases Miner Bone Metab. 2013;10(2):91–5.
8. Nevitt MC, Cummings SR, Kidd S, Black D. Risk-factors for recurrent nonsyncopal falls—a prospective-study. J Am Med Assoc. 1989;261(18):2663–8.
9. Prabhakaran K, Gogna S, Pee S, Samson DJ, Con J, Latifi R. Falling again? Falls in geriatric adults-risk factors and outcomes associated with recidivism. J Surg Res, 2019.
10. Gates S, Smith LA, Fisher JD, Lamb SE. Systematic review of accuracy of screening instruments for predicting fall risk among independently living older adults. J Rehabil Res Dev. 2008;45(8):1105–16.
11. Lundebjerg N, Rubenstein LZ, Kenny RA, Koval KJ, Martin FC, Tinetti ME, et al. Guideline for the prevention of falls in older persons. J Am Geriatr Soc. 2001;49(5):664–72.
12. Ganz DA, Bao Y, Shekelle PG, Rubenstein LZ. Will my patient fall? JAMA. 2007;297(1):77–86.

13. Ribeiro F, Oliveira J. Aging effects on joint proprioception: the role of physical activity in proprioception preservation. Eur Rev Aging Phys Act. 2007;4(2):71–6.
14. Petrella RJ, Lattanzio PJ, Nelson MG. Effect of age and activity on knee joint proprioception. Am J Phys Med Rehabil. 1997;76(3):235–41.
15. Martinez-Amat A, Hita-Contreras F, Lomas-Vega R, Caballero-Martinez I, Alvarez PJ, Martinez-Lopez E. Effects of 12-week proprioception training program on postural stability, gait, and balance in older adults: a controlled clinical trial. J Strength Cond Res. 2013;27(8):2180–8.
16. Tinetti ME, Kumar C. The patient who falls "It's Always a Trade-off". J Am Med Assoc. 2010;303(3):258–66.
17. Mancini M, Horak FB. The relevance of clinical balance assessment tools to differentiate balance deficits. Eur J Phys Rehabil Med. 2010;46(2):239–48.
18. Runge M, Hunter G. Determinants of musculoskeletal frailty and the risk of falls in old age. J Musculoskelet Neuronal Interact. 2006;6(2):167–73.
19. Radecki B, Keen A, Miller J, McClure JK, Kara A. Innovating fall safety: engaging patients as experts. J Nurs Care Qual, 2019.
20. Pape HC, Schemmann U, Foerster J, Knobe M. The 'Aachen Falls Prevention Scale'—development of a tool for self-assessment of elderly patients at risk for ground level falls. Patient Saf Surg. 2015;9:6.
21. Berg K, Norman KE. Functional assessment of balance and gait. Clin Geriatr Med. 1996;12(4):705.
22. Pastor T, Tiziani S, Kasper CD, Pape H-C, Osterhoff G. Quality of reduction correlates with clinical outcome in pelvic ring fractures. Injury. 2019;50(6):1223–6.
23. Yelnik A, Bonan I. Clinical tools for assessing balance disorders. Neurophysiol Clin-Clin Neurophysiol. 2008;38(6):439–45.
24. Koepke S, Meyer G. The Tinetti test—Babylon in geriatric assessment. Zeitschrift Fur Gerontologie Und Geriatrie. 2006;39(4):288–91.
25. Berg K, Wooddauphinee S, Williams JI. The balance scale—reliability assessment with elderly residents and patients with an acute stroke. Scand J Rehabil Med. 1995;27(1):27–36.
26. Stel VS, Pluijm SMF, Deeg DJH, Smit JH, Bouter LM, Lips P. A classification tree for predicting recurrent falling in community-dwelling older persons. J Am Geriatr Soc. 2003;51(10):1356–64.
27. Bachmann S, Finger C, Huss A, Egger M, Stuck AE, Clough-Gorr KM. Inpatient rehabilitation specifically designed for geriatric patients: systematic review and meta-analysis of randomised controlled trials. Br Med J. 2010;340
28. Kammerlander C, Roth T, Friedman SM, Suhm N, Luger TJ, Kammerlander-Knauer U, et al. Ortho-geriatric service-a literature review comparing different models. Osteoporos Int. 2010;21:S637–S46.
29. Knobe M, Siebert CH. Hip fractures in the elderly: osteosynthesis versus joint replacement. Orthopade. 2014;43(4):314–24.
30. Pape HC, Friess T, Liener U, Ruchholtz S, Schmucker U, Sturm JA, et al. Development of geriatric trauma centers: an effort by the German Society for Trauma and Orthopaedics. Injury. 2014;45(10):1513–5.
31. Baker DI, King MB, Fortinsky RH, Graff LG, Gottschalk M, Acampora D, et al. Dissemination of an evidence-based multicomponent fall risk-assessment and -management strategy throughout a geographic area. J Am Geriatr Soc. 2005;53(4):675–80.
32. Tinetti ME, Gordon C, Sogolow E, Lapin P, Bradley EH. Fall-risk evaluation and management: challenges in adopting geriatric care practices. Gerontologist. 2006;46(6):717–25.

12 Pharmacological Treatment of Patients with Osteoporosis

René Rizzoli

12.1 Introduction

Osteoporosis is defined as a systemic skeletal disease characterized by low bone mass and microarchitectural deterioration of bone tissue, with a consequent increase in bone fragility and susceptibility to fracture risk [1]. At the age of 50, the lifetime risk of sustaining an osteoporotic fracture is close to 50% for women and more than 20% for men [1, 2]. Major osteoporotic fractures comprise spine, hip, distal forearm, and proximal humerus fractures.

Despite a rising number of old subjects and a forecasted increase of absolute number and incidence of hip fractures, a decrease in age-adjusted incidence has been observed in several regions, thus a reversal of a secular trend [3]. However, the incidence of other osteoporotic fractures is continuing to increase, as is the total number of days in orthopedic and rehabilitation wards, because of more frequent multiple fractures and higher number of co-morbidities [4]. This underlines the need for anti-osteoporosis treatment.

R. Rizzoli (✉)
Service of Bone Diseases, Geneva University Hospitals and Faculty of Medicine, Geneva 14, Switzerland
e-mail: rene.rizzoli@unige.ch

12.2 Whom to Treat

An osteoporosis diagnosis threshold as determined by DXA-provided areal bone mineral density (BMD) values should not be automatically translated into a therapeutic threshold. Other factors such as age, clinical risk factors (prevalent fracture, parental hip fracture, smoking, ≥3 alcoholic drinks/day, rheumatoid arthritis, current corticosteroid use, body mass index (BMI) <20 kg/m^2, or secondary osteoporosis), bone turnover level, or treatment cost/benefits should be included into the treatment decision [1]. In terms of fracture risk, the same T-score has different significances at different ages. For any BMD, fracture risk is much higher in the elderly than in younger individuals [1]. The objective of the risk assessment is to identify the individuals at higher fracture risk and to provide them with treatment [1].

Of the various fracture risk assessments developed in osteoporosis, the FRAX® tool is the most widely used. FRAX® is a computer-based algorithm (http://www.shef.ac.uk/FRAX) that calculates the 10-year probability of a major osteoporotic fracture (hip, clinical spine, humerus, or wrist fracture) and the 10-year probability of hip fracture. It has been updated to take into account glucocorticoid dose [5], large differences between femoral neck and lumbar spine BMD [6]. This tool adjusts the result in very old patients for the competing hazard of death and for country-specific fracture epidemiology. The

H.-C. Pape et al. (eds.), *Senior Trauma Patients*, https://doi.org/10.1007/978-3-030-91483-7_12

intervention thresholds for osteoporosis depend on regional guidances and country-specific reimbursement policies. These are increasingly guided by economic evaluations to determine cost-effective intervention thresholds. All treatments are cost-effective, and even cost-saving in the oldest old [1, 7].

There are two main approaches for determining an intervention threshold (Fig. 12.1). One approach suggests a fixed age-independent threshold. A treatment is recommended for *T*-score of ≤−2.5 at femoral neck; or, if the *T*-score is between −1.0 and −2.5, for a 10-year probability of fracture (based on FRAX) of ≥3% for hip or ≥20% for a major fragility fracture [8]. Another approach is to treat when the age-related fracture probability exceeds a threshold given by FRAX, equivalent to the fracture risk of a woman with a prior fragility fracture [1]. The argument for an age-dependent intervention threshold is to avoid under-prescription of treatment in eligible younger patients as well as the over-prescription in older age groups that could arise from a fixed threshold [9]. For instance, using an anti-osteoporosis treatment intervention threshold of 20% for major fractures, 10-year probability would concern 70% of a population older than 75 years [7]. Most guidelines recommend that women with a prior fragility fracture should be considered for intervention without the necessity for a BMD test (other than to monitor treatment). Therefore, a prior fragility fracture can be considered to carry a sufficient risk that treatment can be recommended. To identify these patients and ensure an optimal osteoporosis treatment for secondary fracture prevention, the Fracture Liaison Services are playing a major role [10, 11]. FRAX tool can also be applied in an osteoporosis screening approach, as shown in the SCOOP trial (SCreening of Older wOmen for the Prevention of fractures) [12]. The application of this screening algorithm resulted in an increase in the use of anti-osteoporosis medication, a greater compliance with therapy, and a lower hip fracture risk.

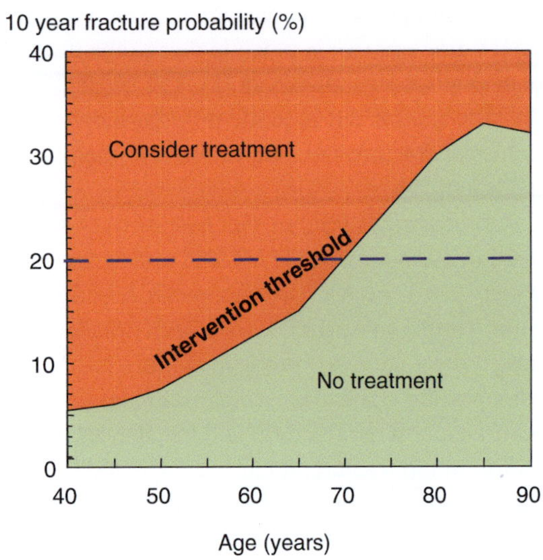

Fig. 12.1 Intervention threshold according to FRAX-determined 10-year fracture probability. The age-dependent threshold corresponds to the risk equivalent to that associated with a prevalent fragility fracture

12.3 General Management: Strategies to Prevent Bone Loss in Older Individuals (Fig. 12.2)

Physical activity: Weight bearing exercise forms an integral component of osteoporosis management [13]. At all times, increased muscle strength through resistance training contributes to reduce fracture risk by maintaining bone mass through a stimulation of bone formation and a decrease of bone resorption [14]. Mixed loading exercise appears to be effective to reduce bone loss in postmenopausal women [15, 16]. Some prevention of hip fracture by physical activity has been consistently reported [17].

Vitamin D supplementation: Vitamin D plays an essential role in the maintenance of bone strength and muscle function [18]. Many older people suffer from hypovitaminosis D. This is particularly true in patients with hip fracture [19]. A large number of clinical studies have tested the effects of vitamin D supplementation (often in combination with calcium) on fracture risk in older and/or osteoporotic population samples. Meta-analyses of these trials have provided inconsistent results. However, in a pooled analysis of 11 trials ($N = 31{,}000$), a lower fracture risk

Fig. 12.2 Management of patients with osteoporosis (adapted from Kanis et al Calcif Tissue Int 2019) [94]

Osteoporosis Management

Lifestyle
- Nutrition: calcium 800-1000 mg/day, protein ≥ 1g/kg BW/day
- Vitamin D: 800 IU/day
- Daily weight bearing physical activity
- Fall prevention measures

Pharmacological treatment

a. Intervention threshold
- FRAX® Score for major osteoporotic fractures or hip fracture ≥ risk equivalent to that associated with a prevalent fragility fracture
- Fragility spine or hip fracture (role of Fracture liaison service)

b. Intervention type (selection based on osteoporosis severity, patient preference and regional drug reimbursement policy)
- Oral bisphosphonates (gastro-resistant formulation may increase adherence)
- Intravenous bisphosphonates
- Denosumab
- Menopausal Hormone Therapy, raloxifene, bazedoxifene
- Teriparatide (if high fracture risk or imminent risk), or romosozumab followed by an anti-resorber
- Local osteo-enhancement procedure (if increased hip fracture risk)

was observed in patients having a plasma concentration of 25-hydroxyvitamin D (25-(OH)D) of at least 60 nmol/L at baseline as compared with those having levels below 30 nmol/L [20]. Vitamin D supplementation has beneficial effects beyond a direct effect on bone health. Raising the levels of 25-(OH)D decreased the incidence of falls in older persons by 19%.

Sufficient levels of vitamin D are a prerequisite for the efficacy of anti-osteoporosis medication, as all studies on these agents have been conducted in calcium and vitamin D-supplemented patients. The recommendation of a dose of 800 IU/day (20 μg/day) in older adults (>70 years) has been adopted by most European guidelines, as well as the International Osteoporosis Foundation (IOF) and the Institute of Medicine (IOM), and was also advised in a recent ESCEO consensus paper [18, 21, 22]. There is no strong necessity to systematically measure circulating levels of 25-(OH)D in older patients with suspected high fracture risk since the cost of testing far exceeds that of supplementation. Vitamin D supplementation should precede any anti-osteoporosis therapy. The adverse effects of hypercalcemia/hypercalciuria and nephrolithiasis are more frequently associated with high serum 25-(OH)D levels (>125 nmol/L), which has been set as the potential upper limit of adequacy. Studies with large annual doses of vitamin D have reported an increased risk of falls and hip fracture [23]. Thus, a yearly regimen of vitamin D high-dose supplementation should be avoided.

Calcium supplementation: Calcium and vitamin D supplements decrease secondary hyperparathyroidism and reduce the risk of proximal femur fracture, particularly in the elderly living in nursing homes [24]. Overall, the literature can be summarized as follows: (1) calcium and vitamin D supplementation may lead to a modest reduction in fracture risk; (2) supplementation with calcium alone does not reduce fracture risk; (3) side effects of calcium supplementation include renal stones (mostly driven by the WHI trials results) and gastrointestinal symptoms; (4) increased cardiovascular risk consequent to calcium supplementation is not convincingly supported by current evidence; (5) calcium and vitamin D supplementation is recommended for patients at high risk of calcium and vitamin D insufficiency and in those who are receiving treatment for osteoporosis [25]. Intakes of 800–1000 mg/day of calcium in addition to 800 IU of vitamin D can be recommended in the general management of patients with osteoporosis [1].

Dietary protein: Correction of protein insufficiency can lead to a rapid normalization of IGF-I levels in frail older adults and in patients with a recent hip fracture, together with a favourable outcome [26]. In view of the impaired protein assimilation of older individuals, the RDA (0.8 g/kg body weight) should be increased to 1.0 or 1.2 g/kg per day in the older age group without adverse event [27, 28]. Dairy products are a source of both protein and calcium, since one litre of milk provides 32 g of protein and 1200 mg of calcium. Dairy products, some being fortified with calcium or vitamin D, decrease circulating PTH, increase IGF-I, and decrease bone resorption markers [29]. Dairy products are associated with higher bone strength [30]. In older men and women, higher dairies consumption is associated with a lower hip fracture risk [31, 32].

12.4 Drugs Strategies (Fig. 12.3)

12.4.1 Efficacy of Anti-Osteoporotic Drugs

Anti-osteoporosis drugs are either inhibitors of bone resorption (anti-resorbers) or stimulators of bone formation. The efficacy of the available anti-osteoporotic agents in increasing bone strength and reducing osteoporotic fracture risk is well-established [1, 9]. For some of the anti-osteoporosis agents, the beneficial effect of treatment has also been demonstrated on hip fractures (Table 12.1). Agents that have been approved for the treatment of osteoporosis in postmenopausal women include selective bisphosphonates (alendronate, risedronate, zoledronic acid, and ibandronate), denosumab, oestrogen-receptor modulators, and teriparatide [1].

Osteoporosis Management Follow-up

Follow-up

- Assess compliance and/or side effects
- Bone turnover markers to verify compliance to bone resorption inhibitors (after 3-6 months)
- Consider continuing or changing treatment:
  - ➢ After 3 years for iv or 5 years for oral bisphosphonates
  - ➢ If incident fracture
  - ➢ Low risk patients: possible discontinuation for 2 years (reconsider yearly)
  - ➢ High risk patients: continue treatment
- Denosumab discontinuation may be associated with vertebral (multiple) fractures, consider then bisphosphonates for 1-2 years

Fig. 12.3 Follow-up of patients treated for osteoporosis (adapted from Kanis et al Calcif Tissue Int 2019) [94]

Table 12.1 Anti-fracture efficacy of the most frequently used treatments for postmenopausal osteoporosis when given with calcium and vitamin D, as derived from randomized controlled trials [updated from [1]]

	Effect on vertebral fracture risk		Effect on non-vertebral fracture risk	
	Osteoporosis	Established osteoporosis[a]	Osteoporosis	Established osteoporosis[a]
Alendronate	+	+	NA	+ (including hip)
Risedronate	+	+	NA	+ (including hip)
Ibandronate	NA	+	NA	+[b]
Zoledronic acid	+	+	NA	+[c]
HRT	+	+	+	+ (including hip)
Raloxifene	+	+	NA	NA
Teriparatide	NA	+	NA	+
Denosumab	+	+[c]	+ (including hip)	+[c]

NA No evidence available
+ Effective drug
[a]Women with a prior vertebral fracture
[b]In subsets of patients only (post-hoc analysis)
[c]Mixed group of patients with or without prevalent vertebral fractures

12.4.1.1 Bisphosphonates

Bisphosphonates are stable analogues of pyrophosphate characterized by a P-C-P bond. Their potency depends on the length and structure of the side chains [33]. Bisphosphonates have a strong affinity for bone hydroxyapatite and are potent inhibitors of bone resorption. They reduce the recruitment and activity of osteoclasts and increase their apoptosis. Aminobisphosphonates (alendronate, risedronate, ibandronate, zoledronic acid) inhibit the farnesyl pyrophosphate synthase step in the mevalonate pathway, thereby modifying the isoprenylation of guanosine triphosphate-binding proteins. Non-nitrogen containing bisphosphonates (clodronate, etidronate, tiludronate) act as ATP competitors. The potency and chemical affinity to bone of bisphosphonates determines their effect to inhibit bone resorption and varies greatly from compound to compound [33].

Oral bioavailability of bisphosphonates is around 1% of the dose ingested and is impaired by food, calcium, iron, coffee, tea, and orange juice. The oral formulation needs a 30- to 60-minute fast after ingestion and before any meal, without standing up, to ensure optimal intestinal absorption and prevent oesophageal damages. Bisphosphonates are quickly cleared from plasma, about 50% being deposited in bone and the remainder excreted in urine. Their half-life in bone is very prolonged.

12.4.1.2 Alendronate

Daily oral alendronate lowers the incidence of vertebral, wrist, and hip fractures by approximately 50% in women with prevalent vertebral fractures [34, 35]. In women without prevalent vertebral fractures, there is no significant decrease in clinical fractures in the overall population, but a reduction in those patients with baseline hip BMD *T*-score lower than −2.5 SD [36]. In a case-control study performed in more than 90,000 men and women aged 80 years and older and with a prevalent fracture, alendronate use is associated with a 34% decrease in hip fracture risk and a 12% lower mortality risk, but with a 58% increase in the risk of mild upper gastrointestinal symptoms [37]. Pivotal trials have been conducted with a daily dose. The efficacy of the weekly 70 mg regimen has been shown in bridging studies with BMD and bone turnover markers as outcome [38].

12.4.1.3 Risedronate

Daily oral risedronate reduces the risk of vertebral and non-vertebral fractures by 40–50% and 30–36%, respectively, in women with prevalent vertebral fractures [39, 40]. In a large population of elderly women, risedronate decreases the risk of hip fractures by 30%. This effect is greater in osteoporotic women aged 70–79 years (–40%), but not significant in women over the age of 80 years without evidence of osteoporosis [41]. A delayed-release formulation of 35 mg risedronate weekly allows osteoporotic patients to take their risedronate dose immediately after breakfast, offering thereby a potentially improved adherence to treatment [42].

12.4.1.4 Ibandronate

Daily oral ibandronate (2.5 mg) reduces the risk of vertebral fractures by 50–60%, whereas a lower non-vertebral fracture risk was only demonstrated in a post-hoc analysis of women with a baseline BMD *T*-score below −3 SD [43–45]. In bridging studies, oral ibandronate 150 mg once monthly or intravenous ibandronate 3 mg every 3 months are equivalent or superior to daily regimen in increasing BMD and decreasing biochemical markers of bone turnover [46, 47]. In post-hoc analyses, ibandronate regimens with annual cumulative exposure ≥10.8 g increase time-to-fracture for all clinical fractures versus placebo [48].

12.4.1.5 Zoledronic Acid

In a large phase III trial comprising 7700 postmenopausal osteoporotic patients, the yearly perfusion of zoledronic acid 5 mg over 3 years reduces the incidence of vertebral, non-vertebral, and hip fractures by 70%, 25%, and 40%, respectively [49]. Intravenous zoledronic acid decreases fracture risk and mortality when given shortly after a first hip fracture [50]. From an extension study to 6 [51] and 9 [52] years, it appears that prolonging treatment beyond 6 years does not provide additional benefits. In a 6-year randomized placebo-controlled trial conducted in osteopenic non-osteoporotic women, zoledronic acid given at 18-month interval instead of yearly reduces non-vertebral and symptomatic vertebral fracture risk, as well as height loss [53].

Bisphosphonates Safety [54]*:* Upper GI events with oral bisphosphonates include irritation of the oesophagus, dysphagia, and heartburn. Generic versions of bisphosphonates may be associated with higher rates of GI events and greater risk of treatment discontinuation [55]. Weekly or monthly dosing formulations are associated with lower rates of upper GI effects than daily dosing. Of potential interest for the oldest old is the development of an alendronate formulation in effervescent forms that are easier to swallow.

Bone pain, as well as joint and muscle pain, has been frequently associated with bisphosphonates use, both oral and IV (about 5–10% of patients), and also to some extent with raloxifene and teriparatide [54].

Intravenous bisphosphonates are associated with transient flu-like symptoms (myalgia, arthralgia, headache, and fever), collectively called an acute phase reaction (APR) [54]. Rates of fever of about 30% have been reported post-dosing with zoledronic acid. The symptoms of APR seem to be evoked by the release of pro-inflammatory cytokines from circulating T cells, generally appear 24–48 h after administration and resolve within 48 h. The likelihood of having an APR after an IV bisphosphonate may be reduced by administration of acetaminophen (paracetamol) prior to dosing.

Rare cases of oesophageal cancer have been reported in patients exposed to oral bisphosphonates. But the results from epidemiological studies on prescription databases have been conflicting. In the most recent analysis performed on the UK GPRD, 95 out of the 4442 annually reported cases of upper gastrointestinal cancer could be linked to bisphosphonate use (Odds Ratio of 1.34 for bisphosphonates) [56].

An increased risk of atrial fibrillation (AF) reported as a severe adverse event was observed in the pivotal HORIZON study with zoledronic acid. Post-hoc analyses of other bisphosphonate trials and several large population-based studies have not confirmed this suspicion. No increase in risk of cardiovascular mortality with use of bisphosphonates is reported and indeed a decrease in myocardial infarction has been associated with bisphosphonate use in patients with rheumatoid arthritis [57]. In patients with hip fracture, alendronate was associated with a lower risk of 1-year cardiovascular mortality (HR 0.33) and incident myocardial infarction (HR 0.55), whereas marginally significant reduction in risk of stroke was observed at 5 and 10 years [58].

There is no evidence for impaired fracture healing. Cases of osteonecrosis of the jaw (ONJ) have been reported [59]. They are defined as exposed bone in the maxillofacial region that shows negligible healing over a period of 8 weeks. They are mostly reported in cancer patients receiving high-dose IV bisphosphonates for the prevention or treatment of cancer-related bone disease.

Atypical subtrochanteric, low-trauma, and femur fractures in bisphosphonate-treated patients have been reported, some with prodromal thigh pain in the preceding period. Although there is an association with duration of BP use, atypical fractures can also be observed in untreated patients [60, 61].

Impaired renal function is common in older patients causing concern for various drug treatments, including bisphosphonates, since these are excreted via the kidney [33]. Therefore, these products (both oral and IV forms) are not recommended in patients with creatinine clearance <30–35 mL/min.

12.4.1.6 Denosumab

Receptor activator of nuclear factor NFkB (RANK), its ligand RANKL, a member of the tumour necrosis factor (TNF) superfamily, and osteoprotegerin (OPG), which acts as a decoy receptor for RANKL, are critical molecules for differentiation and action of osteoclast and hence for bone resorption. The fully human antibody against RANKL denosumab prevents the interaction of RANKL with the receptor RANK.

Over a 3-year placebo-controlled pivotal trial, there is a 68% reduction in the incidence of new vertebral fractures with denosumab given subcutaneously every 6 months at a dose of 60 mg. Non-vertebral fracture risk is reduced by 20% and hip fractures by 40% [62]. In an extension study, women from the denosumab group had seven more years of treatment (long-term group) and those in the placebo group received seven years of denosumab (cross-over group) [63]. The yearly incidence of new vertebral fractures remained low during the extension, whereas non-vertebral fractures further decreased to reach a stable level [63].

Discontinuation of denosumab is associated with a rapid increase in bone turnover, even above pretreatment levels, a BMD decrease, and a marked increase in vertebral fracture rate [64]. Multiple vertebral fracture risk was even higher than in the placebo group. A short duration of bisphosphonate could be considered when discontinuing denosumab to prevent the rebound turnover [65].

Denosumab is not excreted by the kidney and could therefore be used in patients with impaired renal function. However, the administration of such a potent bone resorption inhibitor in patients with terminal renal failure and possibly adynamic bone disease may further inhibit bone turnover. Regarding adverse events, seven cases of ONJ were reported in the long-term group and six cases in the cross-over group [63]. Their incidence rates seem to be similar to those of zoledronic acid [66]. In a meta-analysis of four trials, a non-statistically significant relative risk of serious adverse events for the denosumab group compared with the placebo group was 1.33, of serious adverse events related to infection 2.10, of neoplasm 1.11, of study discontinuation due to adverse events 1.10, and of death 0.78 [67].

12.4.1.7 Selective Oestrogen-Receptor Modulators

Selective oestrogen-receptor modulators are non-steroidal agents that bind to the oestrogen-receptor and act as oestrogen agonists or antagonists, depending on the target tissue. Raloxifene is available for the prevention and treatment of postmenopausal osteoporosis. Raloxifene prevents bone loss and reduces the risk of vertebral fractures by 30–50% in postmenopausal women with low bone mass, with or without prior vertebral fractures as shown in the MORE trial [68]. There is no significant reduction of non-vertebral fractures, except in women with severe vertebral fractures at baseline [69].

As adverse events, there is an increase of deep venous thrombo-embolism, of hot flushes, and of lower limb cramps. The risk of invasive breast cancer is reduced by about 60% [70]. Raloxifene is approved for the prevention and treatment of postmenopausal osteoporosis.

Though approved in Europe, bazedoxifene is only available in Spain and Germany. It reduces the risk of new vertebral fracture, with favourable effects on BMD, bone turnover markers, and lipid profile [71, 72]. In a subgroup of women at increased risk of fracture, bazedoxifene decreases non-vertebral fracture risk. Like with raloxifene, venous thromboembolic events, deep vein thromboses, leg cramps, and hot flushes are reported adverse events [73]. Bazedoxifene is also combined with conjugated equine estrogen to create a tissue selective estrogen complex for the management of vasomotor symptoms and the prevention of osteoporosis associated with menopause (bazedoxifene 20 mg/conjugated equine estrogen 0.45 mg) [74]. This association improves vasomotor symptoms, while opposing breast and endometrial proliferation, preventing bone resorption, increasing BMD, and improving lipid profile [74].

12.4.1.8 Menopausal Hormone Therapy (MHT)

MHT decreases the risk of vertebral and non-vertebral fractures (including hip fracture) by about 30%, regardless of baseline BMD [75, 76]. In a recent re-assessment of the long-term outcomes of WHI trials, MHT with conjugated oestrogen and medroxyprogesterone acetate for a median of 5.6 years or with conjugated oestrogen alone for a median of 7.2 years was not associated with an increased risk of all-cause, cardiovascular, or cancer mortality during a cumulative follow-up of 18 years [77].

12.4.1.9 Teriparatide

While a continuous increase of endogenous production of parathyroid hormone (PTH) is deleterious for the skeleton, intermittent administration of PTH (e.g. daily subcutaneous injections) leads to an increase in bone mass and an improvement in skeletal microstructure at both cancellous and cortical skeletal sites [78]. At a daily subcutaneous dose of 20 μg, the 1-34 N-terminal fragment (teriparatide) reduces the risk of vertebral fractures (−65%) and non-vertebral fractures (−53%) [79]. Treatment with PTH is registered for 18–24 months, and beneficial effects on non-vertebral fracture with teriparatide persist for up to 30 months after stopping teriparatide [80].

Adverse events with teriparatide are nausea, pain in the limbs, headache, and dizziness. Slight and transient elevations of serum calcium concentrations have been observed following the injection of teriparatide. The use of peptides of the PTH family is contraindicated in conditions such as hypercalcemia, metabolic bone diseases other than osteoporosis, Paget's disease, prior radiation therapy to the skeleton, in malignancies, or bone metastasis or severe renal impairment. In rats, very high doses of teriparatide since weaning increase the risk of osteosarcoma [81]. There is no confirmation of these findings in human.

12.5 Perspectives

Abaloparatide is a 34-amino-acid peptide with 76% homology to parathyroid-related protein (PTHrP) (1–34) and 41% homology to PTH (1–34) [82]. Abaloparatide is a potent and selective activator of the PTH receptor type 1 (PTHR1) signaling pathway.

At a daily subcutaneous dose of 80 μg, abaloparatide increases BMD more than teriparatide and reduces major osteoporotic fractures to a greater extent than teriparatide, with a possible more rapid onset of action [83, 84]. Use of abaloparatide for 18 months followed by alendronate for 24 months improves spine, total hip, and femoral neck BMD and reduces vertebral, non-vertebral, major, and clinical fractures compared to that observed after 18 months of placebo followed by 24 months of alendronate [85]. Adverse events are nausea, dizziness, headaches, and palpitations, which are generally mild to moderate in severity [86]. Presently, abaloparatide is approved in the US.

Romosozumab is an anti-sclerostin monoclonal antibody, which transiently stimulates bone formation and more persistently inhibits bone resorption [87]. In a one-year placebo-controlled study, followed by one year of denosumab in both groups, romosozumab given subcutaneously monthly reduced vertebral fracture risk by 73%, while the −25% observed for non-vertebral fracture was not statistically significant [88]. In another trial, romosozumab was compared to weekly alendronate during the first year and then both groups received the bisphosphonate for one year. By 2 years, vertebral, non-vertebral, and hip fracture risk was decreased by 48, 19, and 38%, respectively [89]. In the latter trial, a higher number of adjudicated severe cardiovascular events were recorded in the romosozumab-treated patients. These results open the way to sequential regimens for the treatment of osteoporotic patients. Romosozumab has just been registered in the US.

12.6 Early Onset of Anti-Fracture Efficacy

Anti-osteoporosis treatments are frequently under-prescribed, even in women who have sustained an osteoporotic fracture and are at increased risk of a subsequent fracture [90]. Clinicians may be reluctant to prescribe treatment because of doubts they might have over the effectiveness of treatment in a short period of time in patients with a limited life expectancy. Clinically significant benefits in terms of fracture reduction have been demonstrated within the first year of treatment [9]. Thus, even in an oldest old patient population, treatment with an anti-osteoporosis agent is worth to be introduced, because of an early onset of fracture risk reduction. Over the long-term, anti-osteoporosis treatments seem to maintain effectiveness and remain safe [91]. Various guidelines recommend bisphosphonate treatment re-evaluation after 3 years for parenteral administration and 5 years for oral formulations [92].

12.7 Treatment Adherence in Osteoporosis

Yearly persistence rates in osteoporosis are from 26% to 56% for daily anti-osteoporosis regimens and from 36% to 70% for weekly regimens. Estimates of compliance (medication possession ratio) range from 46% to 64% and 58% to 76%, respectively. Compliance tends to diminish with increasing follow-up duration and the drop is particularly rapid over the first 2 years of treatment. In a meta-analysis of six studies (171,063 patients), the increase in fracture risk for non-compliant patients was 28% for hip fractures and 43% for clinical vertebral fractures [93].

The main reasons underlying non-adherence are the financial limitation of paying for the treatment, the fear or experience of side effects, concerns about pharmacological treatments in general, and lack of perceived need for an anti-osteoporosis treatment. Given the rather wide range of side effects outlined earlier, many patients are likely to believe that the negative effects of anti-osteoporosis medication outweigh any possible benefits. Patients with fragility fractures may deny that their facture is related to bone health, attributing all causality to the fall [10].

12.8 Conclusions

The risk of osteoporotic fractures is a major healthcare concern. The impact of a major fracture on patients' quality of life is immense, often heralding the transition to frailty and dependence. The costs borne by society are also significant, both in terms of immediate care and rehabilitation, and over the longer term if dependence begins to take hold. Many people at high risk of fracture receive no treatment or highly inadequate treatment [1]. There is now sufficient evidence of the short-term benefits of treatment and of the long-term safety profile of anti-osteoporosis treatments. Many older people are undernourished and vitamin D-deficient. These are situations that should be easily improved. In order to promote awareness and encourage proactive treatment in high-risk patients, the *Capture the Fracture Campaign* of the IOF and a wide implementation of fracture liaison services [10, 11] to strengthen secondary fracture prevention should be strongly advocated.

References

1. Kanis JA, Cooper C, Rizzoli R, Reginster JY. European guidance for the diagnosis and management of osteoporosis in postmenopausal women. Osteoporos Int. 2019;30:3–44.
2. Lippuner K, Johansson H, Kanis JA, Rizzoli R. Remaining lifetime and absolute 10-year probabilities of osteoporotic fracture in Swiss men and women. Osteoporos Int. 2009;20:1131–40.
3. Chevalley T, Guilley E, Herrmann FR, Hoffmeyer P, Rapin CH, Rizzoli R. Incidence of hip fracture over a 10-year period (1991-2000): reversal of a secular trend. Bone. 2007;40:1284–9.
4. Lippuner K, Popp AW, Schwab P, Gitlin M, Schaufler T, Senn C, Perrelet R. Fracture hospitalizations between years 2000 and 2007 in Switzerland: a trend analysis. Osteoporos Int. 2011;22:2487–97.
5. Kanis JA, Johansson H, Oden A, McCloskey EV. Guidance for the adjustment of FRAX according to the dose of glucocorticoids. Osteoporos Int. 2011;22:809–16.
6. Johansson H, Kanis JA, Oden A, et al. Impact of femoral neck and lumbar spine BMD discordances on FRAX probabilities in women: a meta-analysis of international cohorts. Calcif Tissue Int. 2014;95:428–35.
7. Lippuner K, Johansson H, Borgstrom F, Kanis JA, Rizzoli R. Cost-effective intervention thresholds against osteoporotic fractures based on FRAX(R) in Switzerland. Osteoporos Int. 2012;23:2579–89.
8. Cosman F, de Beur SJ, LeBoff MS, Lewiecki EM, Tanner B, Randall S, Lindsay R. Clinician's guide to prevention and treatment of osteoporosis. Osteoporos Int. 2014;25:2359–81.
9. Rizzoli R, Branco J, Brandi ML, et al. Management of osteoporosis of the oldest old. Osteoporos Int. 2014;25:2507–29.
10. Chevalley T, Hoffmeyer P, Bonjour JP, Rizzoli R. An osteoporosis clinical pathway for the medical management of patients with low-trauma fracture. Osteoporos Int. 2002;13:450–5.
11. Wu CH, Tu ST, Chang YF, Chan DC, Chien JT, Lin CH, Singh S, Dasari M, Chen JF, Tsai KS. Fracture

liaison services improve outcomes of patients with osteoporosis-related fractures: a systematic literature review and meta-analysis. Bone. 2018;111:92–100.
12. Shepstone L, Lenaghan E, Cooper C, et al. Screening in the community to reduce fractures in older women (SCOOP): a randomised controlled trial. Lancet. 2018;391:741–7.
13. Howe TE, Shea B, Dawson LJ, Downie F, Murray A, Ross C, Harbour RT, Caldwell LM, Creed G. Exercise for preventing and treating osteoporosis in postmenopausal women. Cochrane Database Syst Rev. 2011:Cd000333.
14. Girgis CM. Integrated therapies for osteoporosis and sarcopenia: from signaling pathways to clinical trials. Calcif Tissue Int. 2015;96:243–55.
15. Martyn-St James M, Carroll S. A meta-analysis of impact exercise on postmenopausal bone loss: the case for mixed loading exercise programmes. Br J Sports Med. 2009;43:898–908.
16. Kelley GA, Kelley KS, Kohrt WM. Effects of ground and joint reaction force exercise on lumbar spine and femoral neck bone mineral density in postmenopausal women: a meta-analysis of randomized controlled trials. BMC Musculoskelet Disord. 2012;13:177.
17. Karlsson MK, Nordqvist A, Karlsson C. Physical activity, muscle function, falls and fractures. Food Nutr Res. 2008;52
18. Rizzoli R, Boonen S, Brandi ML, Bruyere O, Cooper C, Kanis JA, Kaufman JM, Ringe JD, Weryha G, Reginster JY. Vitamin D supplementation in elderly or postmenopausal women: a 2013 update of the 2008 recommendations from the European Society for Clinical and Economic Aspects of Osteoporosis and Osteoarthritis (ESCEO). Curr Med Res Opin. 2013;29:305–13.
19. Bischoff-Ferrari HA, Can U, Staehelin HB, Platz A, Henschkowski J, Michel BA, Dawson-Hughes B, Theiler R. Severe vitamin D deficiency in Swiss hip fracture patients. Bone. 2008;42:597–602.
20. Bischoff-Ferrari HA, Willett WC, Orav EJ, et al. A pooled analysis of vitamin D dose requirements for fracture prevention. N Engl J Med. 2012;367:40–9.
21. Dawson-Hughes B, Mithal A, Bonjour JP, Boonen S, Burckhardt P, Fuleihan GE, Josse RG, Lips P, Morales-Torres J, Yoshimura N. IOF position statement: vitamin D recommendations for older adults. Osteoporos Int. 2010;21:1151–4.
22. Ross AC, Manson JE, Abrams SA, et al. The 2011 report on dietary reference intakes for calcium and vitamin D from the Institute of Medicine: what clinicians need to know. J Clin Endocrinol Metab. 2011;96:53–8.
23. Sanders KM, Stuart AL, Williamson EJ, Simpson JA, Kotowicz MA, Young D, Nicholson GC. Annual high-dose oral vitamin D and falls and fractures in older women: a randomized controlled trial. Jama. 2010;303:1815–22.
24. Tang BM, Eslick GD, Nowson C, Smith C, Bensoussan A. Use of calcium or calcium in combination with vitamin D supplementation to prevent fractures and bone loss in people aged 50 years and older: a meta-analysis. Lancet. 2007;370:657–66.
25. Harvey NC, Biver E, Kaufman JM, et al. The role of calcium supplementation in healthy musculoskeletal ageing: an expert consensus meeting of the European Society for Clinical and Economic Aspects of Osteoporosis, Osteoarthritis and Musculoskeletal Diseases (ESCEO) and the International Foundation for Osteoporosis (IOF). Osteoporos Int. 2017;28:447–62.
26. Rizzoli R. Nutritional aspects of bone health. Best Pract Res Clin Endocrinol Metab. 2014;28:795–808.
27. Bauer J, Biolo G, Cederholm T, et al. Evidence-based recommendations for optimal dietary protein intake in older people: a position paper from the PROT-AGE Study Group. J Am Med Dir Assoc. 2013;14:542–59.
28. Rizzoli R, Biver E, Bonjour JP, et al. Benefits and safety of dietary protein for bone health-an expert consensus paper endorsed by the European Society for Clinical and Economical Aspects of Osteopororosis, Osteoarthritis, and Musculoskeletal Diseases and by the International Osteoporosis Foundation. Osteoporos Int. 2018;
29. Rizzoli R. Dairy products, yogurts, and bone health. Am J Clin Nutr. 2014;99:1256s–62s.
30. Durosier-Izart C, Biver E, Merminod F, van Rietbergen B, Chevalley T, Herrmann FR, Ferrari SL, Rizzoli R. Peripheral skeleton bone strength is positively correlated with total and dairy protein intakes in healthy postmenopausal women. Am J Clin Nutr. 2017;105:513–25.
31. Feskanich D, Meyer HE, Fung TT, Bischoff-Ferrari HA, Willett WC. Milk and other dairy foods and risk of hip fracture in men and women. Osteoporos Int. 2018;29:385–96.
32. Bian S, Hu J, Zhang K, Wang Y, Yu M, Ma J. Dairy product consumption and risk of hip fracture: a systematic review and meta-analysis. BMC Public Health. 2018;18:165.
33. Rizzoli R. Bisphosphonates for post-menopausal osteoporosis: are they all the same? Qjm. 2011;104:281–300.
34. Black DM, Cummings SR, Karpf DB, et al. Randomised trial of effect of alendronate on risk of fracture in women with existing vertebral fractures. Fracture Intervention Trial Research Group. Lancet. 1996;348:1535–41.
35. Cranney A, Guyatt G, Griffith L, Wells G, Tugwell P, Rosen C. Meta-analyses of therapies for postmenopausal osteoporosis. IX: Summary of meta-analyses of therapies for postmenopausal osteoporosis. Endocr Rev. 2002;23:570–8.
36. Cummings SR, Black DM, Thompson DE, et al. Effect of alendronate on risk of fracture in women with low bone density but without vertebral fractures: results from the Fracture Intervention Trial. JAMA. 1998;280:2077–82.
37. Axelsson KF, Wallander M, Johansson H, Lundh D, Lorentzon M. Hip fracture risk and safety with alen-

dronate treatment in the oldest-old. J Intern Med. 2017;282:546–59.
38. Rizzoli R, Greenspan SL, Bone G 3rd, et al. Two-year results of once-weekly administration of alendronate 70 mg for the treatment of postmenopausal osteoporosis. J Bone Miner Res. 2002;17:1988–96.
39. Harris ST, Watts NB, Genant HK, et al. Effects of risedronate treatment on vertebral and nonvertebral fractures in women with postmenopausal osteoporosis: a randomized controlled trial. Vertebral Efficacy With Risedronate Therapy (VERT) Study Group. JAMA. 1999;282:1344–52.
40. Reginster J, Minne HW, Sorensen OH, et al. Randomized trial of the effects of risedronate on vertebral fractures in women with established postmenopausal osteoporosis. Vertebral Efficacy with Risedronate Therapy (VERT) Study Group. Osteoporos Int. 2000;11:83–91.
41. McClung MR, Geusens P, Miller PD, et al. Effect of risedronate on the risk of hip fracture in elderly women. Hip Intervention Program Study Group. N Engl J Med. 2001;344:333–40.
42. McClung MR, Balske A, Burgio DE, Wenderoth D, Recker RR. Treatment of postmenopausal osteoporosis with delayed-release risedronate 35 mg weekly for 2 years. Osteoporos Int. 2013;24:301–10.
43. Chesnut CH 3rd, Skag A, Christiansen C, et al. Effects of oral ibandronate administered daily or intermittently on fracture risk in postmenopausal osteoporosis. J Bone Miner Res. 2004;19:1241–9.
44. Delmas PD, Recker RR, Chesnut CH 3rd, Skag A, Stakkestad JA, Emkey R, Gilbride J, Schimmer RC, Christiansen C. Daily and intermittent oral ibandronate normalize bone turnover and provide significant reduction in vertebral fracture risk: results from the BONE study. Osteoporos Int. 2004;15:792–8.
45. Harris ST, Blumentals WA, Miller PD. Ibandronate and the risk of non-vertebral and clinical fractures in women with postmenopausal osteoporosis: results of a meta-analysis of phase III studies. Curr Med Res Opin. 2008;24:237–45.
46. Reginster JY, Adami S, Lakatos P, et al. Efficacy and tolerability of once-monthly oral ibandronate in postmenopausal osteoporosis: 2 year results from the MOBILE study. Ann Rheum Dis. 2006;65:654–61.
47. Delmas PD, Adami S, Strugala C, et al. Intravenous ibandronate injections in postmenopausal women with osteoporosis: one-year results from the dosing intravenous administration study. Arthritis Rheum. 2006;54:1838–46.
48. Miller PD, Recker RR, Harris S, Silverman S, Felsenberg D, Reginster J, Day BM, Barr C, Masanauskaite D. Long-term fracture rates seen with continued ibandronate treatment: pooled analysis of DIVA and MOBILE long-term extension studies. Osteoporos Int. 2014;25:349–57.
49. Black DM, Delmas PD, Eastell R, et al. Once-yearly zoledronic acid for treatment of postmenopausal osteoporosis. N Engl J Med. 2007;356:1809–22.
50. Lyles KW, Colon-Emeric CS, Magaziner JS, et al. Zoledronic acid and clinical fractures and mortality after hip fracture. N Engl J Med. 2007;357:1799–809.
51. Black DM, Reid IR, Boonen S, et al. The effect of 3 versus 6 years of zoledronic acid treatment of osteoporosis: a randomized extension to the HORIZON-Pivotal Fracture Trial (PFT). J Bone Miner Res. 2012;27:243–54.
52. Black DM, Reid IR, Cauley JA, et al. The effect of 6 versus 9 years of zoledronic acid treatment in osteoporosis: a randomized second extension to the HORIZON-Pivotal Fracture Trial (PFT). J Bone Miner Res. 2015;30:934–44.
53. Reid IR, Horne AM, Mihov B, Stewart A, Garratt E, Wong S, Wiessing KR, Bolland MJ, Bastin S, Gamble GD. Fracture prevention with zoledronate in older women with osteopenia. N Engl J Med. 2018;379:2407–16.
54. Rizzoli R, Reginster JY, Boonen S, Breart G, Diez-Perez A, Felsenberg D, Kaufman JM, Kanis JA, Cooper C. Adverse reactions and drug-drug interactions in the management of women with postmenopausal osteoporosis. Calcif Tissue Int. 2011;89:91–104.
55. Kanis JA, Reginster JY, Kaufman JM, Ringe JD, Adachi JD, Hiligsmann M, Rizzoli R, Cooper C. A reappraisal of generic bisphosphonates in osteoporosis. Osteoporos Int. 2012;23:213–21.
56. Wright E, Schofield PT, Seed P, Molokhia M. Bisphosphonates and risk of upper gastrointestinal cancer—a case control study using the General Practice Research Database (GPRD). PLoS One. 2012;7:e47616.
57. Wolfe F, Bolster MB, O'Connor CM, Michaud K, Lyles KW, Colon-Emeric CS. Bisphosphonate use is associated with reduced risk of myocardial infarction in patients with rheumatoid arthritis. J Bone Miner Res. 2013;28:984–91.
58. Sing CW, Wong AY, Kiel DP, Cheung EY, Lam JK, Cheung TT, Chan EW, Kung AW, Wong IC, Cheung CL. Association of alendronate and risk of cardiovascular events in patients with hip fracture. J Bone Miner Res. 2018;33:1422–34.
59. Rizzoli R, Burlet N, Cahall D, et al. Osteonecrosis of the jaw and bisphosphonate treatment for osteoporosis. Bone. 2008;42:841–7.
60. Rizzoli R, Akesson K, Bouxsein M, Kanis JA, Napoli N, Papapoulos S, Reginster JY, Cooper C. Subtrochanteric fractures after long-term treatment with bisphosphonates: a European Society on Clinical and Economic Aspects of Osteoporosis and Osteoarthritis, and International Osteoporosis Foundation Working Group Report. Osteoporos Int. 2011;22:373–90.
61. Meier RP, Perneger TV, Stern R, Rizzoli R, Peter RE. Increasing occurrence of atypical femoral fractures associated with bisphosphonate use. Arch Intern Med. 2012;172:930–6.
62. Cummings SR, San Martin J, McClung MR, et al. Denosumab for prevention of fractures in postmeno-

pausal women with osteoporosis. N Engl J Med. 2009;361:756–65.
63. Bone HG, Wagman RB, Brandi ML, et al. 10 years of denosumab treatment in postmenopausal women with osteoporosis: results from the phase 3 randomised FREEDOM trial and open-label extension. Lancet Diabetes Endocrinol. 2017;5:513–23.
64. Cummings SR, Ferrari S, Eastell R, et al. Vertebral fractures after discontinuation of denosumab: a post hoc analysis of the randomized placebo-controlled FREEDOM trial and its extension. J Bone Miner Res. 2018;33:190–8.
65. Meier C, Uebelhart B, Aubry-Rozier B, et al. Osteoporosis drug treatment: duration and management after discontinuation. A position statement from the SVGO/ASCO. Swiss Med Wkly. 2017;147:w14484.
66. Saad F, Brown JE, Van Poznak C, et al. Incidence, risk factors, and outcomes of osteonecrosis of the jaw: integrated analysis from three blinded active-controlled phase III trials in cancer patients with bone metastases. Ann Oncol. 2012;23:1341–7.
67. von Keyserlingk C, Hopkins R, Anastasilakis A, Toulis K, Goeree R, Tarride JE, Xie F. Clinical efficacy and safety of denosumab in postmenopausal women with low bone mineral density and osteoporosis: a meta-analysis. Semin Arthritis Rheum. 2011;41:178–86.
68. Ettinger B, Black DM, Mitlak BH, et al. Reduction of vertebral fracture risk in postmenopausal women with osteoporosis treated with raloxifene: results from a 3-year randomized clinical trial. Multiple Outcomes of Raloxifene Evaluation (MORE) investigators. JAMA. 1999;282:637–45.
69. Delmas PD, Genant HK, Crans GG, Stock JL, Wong M, Siris E, Adachi JD. Severity of prevalent vertebral fractures and the risk of subsequent vertebral and nonvertebral fractures: results from the MORE trial. Bone. 2003;33:522–32.
70. Cummings SR, Eckert S, Krueger KA, et al. The effect of raloxifene on risk of breast cancer in postmenopausal women: results from the MORE randomized trial. Multiple outcomes of raloxifene evaluation. JAMA. 1999;281:2189–97.
71. Silverman SL, Christiansen C, Genant HK, Vukicevic S, Zanchetta JR, de Villiers TJ, Constantine GD, Chines AA. Efficacy of bazedoxifene in reducing new vertebral fracture risk in postmenopausal women with osteoporosis: results from a 3-year, randomized, placebo-, and active-controlled clinical trial. J Bone Miner Res. 2008;23:1923–34.
72. Silverman SL, Chines AA, Kendler DL, Kung AW, Teglbjaerg CS, Felsenberg D, Mairon N, Constantine GD, Adachi JD. Sustained efficacy and safety of bazedoxifene in preventing fractures in postmenopausal women with osteoporosis: results of a 5-year, randomized, placebo-controlled study. Osteoporos Int. 2012;23:351–63.
73. de Villiers TJ, Chines AA, Palacios S, Lips P, Sawicki AZ, Levine AB, Codreanu C, Kelepouris N, Brown JP. Safety and tolerability of bazedoxifene in postmenopausal women with osteoporosis: results of a 5-year, randomized, placebo-controlled phase 3 trial. Osteoporos Int. 2011;22:567–76.
74. Umland EM, Karel L, Santoro N. Bazedoxifene and conjugated equine estrogen: a combination product for the management of vasomotor symptoms and osteoporosis prevention associated with menopause. Pharmacotherapy. 2016;36:548–61.
75. Torgerson DJ, Bell-Syer SE. Hormone replacement therapy and prevention of nonvertebral fractures: a meta-analysis of randomized trials. JAMA. 2001;285:2891–7.
76. Cauley JA, Robbins J, Chen Z, et al. Effects of estrogen plus progestin on risk of fracture and bone mineral density: the Women's Health Initiative randomized trial. Jama. 2003;290:1729–38.
77. Manson JE, Aragaki AK, Rossouw JE, et al. Menopausal hormone therapy and long-term all-cause and cause-specific mortality: the women's health initiative randomized trials. JAMA. 2017;318:927–38.
78. Kraenzlin ME, Meier C. Parathyroid hormone analogues in the treatment of osteoporosis. Nat Rev Endocrinol. 2011;7:647–56.
79. Neer RM, Arnaud CD, Zanchetta JR, et al. Effect of parathyroid hormone (1-34) on fractures and bone mineral density in postmenopausal women with osteoporosis. N Engl J Med. 2001;344:1434–41.
80. Prince R, Sipos A, Hossain A, Syversen U, Ish-Shalom S, Marcinowska E, Halse J, Lindsay R, Dalsky GP, Mitlak BH. Sustained nonvertebral fragility fracture risk reduction after discontinuation of teriparatide treatment. J Bone Miner Res. 2005;20:1507–13.
81. Vahle JL, Sato M, Long GG, Young JK, Francis PC, Engelhardt JA, Westmore MS, Linda Y, Nold JB. Skeletal changes in rats given daily subcutaneous injections of recombinant human parathyroid hormone (1-34) for 2 years and relevance to human safety. Toxicol Pathol. 2002;30:312–21.
82. Hattersley G, Dean T, Corbin BA, Bahar H, Gardella TJ. Binding selectivity of abaloparatide for PTH-type-1-receptor conformations and effects on downstream signaling. Endocrinology. 2016;157:141–9.
83. Reginster JY, Al Daghri NM, Bruyere O. Abaloparatide Comparator Trial In Vertebral Endpoints (ACTIVE) confirms that abaloparatide is a valuable addition to the armamentarium against osteoporosis. Expert Opin Pharmacother. 2017;18:1811–3.
84. Miller PD, Hattersley G, Lau E, Fitzpatrick LA, Harris AG, Williams GC, Hu MY, Riis BJ, Russo L, Christiansen C. Bone mineral density response rates are greater in patients treated with abaloparatide compared with those treated with placebo or teriparatide: results from the ACTIVE phase 3 trial. Bone. 2019;120:137–40.
85. Bone HG, Cosman F, Miller PD, et al. ACTIVExtend: 24 months of alendronate after 18 months of abaloparatide or placebo for postmenopausal osteoporosis. J Clin Endocrinol Metab. 2018;
86. Miller PD, Hattersley G, Riis BJ, et al. Effect of abaloparatide vs placebo on new vertebral fractures in

postmenopausal women with osteoporosis: a randomized clinical trial. JAMA. 2016;316:722–33.
87. Appelman-Dijkstra NM, Papapoulos SE. Sclerostin inhibition in the management of osteoporosis. Calcif Tissue Int. 2016;98:370–80.
88. Cosman F, Crittenden DB, Adachi JD, et al. Romosozumab treatment in postmenopausal women with osteoporosis. N Engl J Med. 2016;375:1532–43.
89. Saag KG, Petersen J, Brandi ML, Karaplis AC, Lorentzon M, Thomas T, Maddox J, Fan M, Meisner PD, Grauer A. Romosozumab or alendronate for fracture prevention in women with osteoporosis. N Engl J Med. 2017;377:1417–27.
90. Kanis JA, Borgstrom F, Compston J, Dreinhofer K, Nolte E, Jonsson L, Lems WF, McCloskey EV, Rizzoli R, Stenmark J. SCOPE: a scorecard for osteoporosis in Europe. Arch Osteoporos. 2013;8:144.
91. Cooper C, Reginster JY, Cortet B, Diaz-Curiel M, Lorenc RS, Kanis JA, Rizzoli R. Long-term treatment of osteoporosis in postmenopausal women: a review from the European Society for Clinical and Economic Aspects of Osteoporosis and Osteoarthritis (ESCEO) and the International Osteoporosis Foundation (IOF). Curr Med Res Opin. 2012;28:475–91.
92. Adler RA, El-Hajj Fuleihan G, Bauer DC, et al. Managing osteoporosis in patients on long-term bisphosphonate treatment: report of a task force of the American Society for Bone and Mineral Research. J Bone Miner Res. 2016;31:16–35.
93. Imaz I, Zegarra P, Gonzalez-Enriquez J, Rubio B, Alcazar R, Amate JM. Poor bisphosphonate adherence for treatment of osteoporosis increases fracture risk: systematic review and meta-analysis. Osteoporos Int. 2010;21:1943–51.
94. Kanis JA, Cooper C, Rizzoli R, Reginster JY. Executive summary of the European guidance for the diagnosis and management of osteoporosis in postmenopausal women. Calcif Tissue Int. 2019;104:235–8.

Part III

Geriatric Care Concepts in Acute Care

Prevention of Delirium in The Elderly

13

Egemen Savaskan

Delirium or acute confusional state is a clinical syndrome that manifests as fluctuations in mental status. It is characterized by disturbed consciousness, cognitive function, and perception. The Diagnostic and Statistical Manual of Mental Disorders, DSM-5, of the American Psychiatric Association describes delirium as a disturbance in attention and awareness which develops over a short period of time and tends to fluctuate in severity during the course of the day [1]. Additional disturbances in cognition (e.g., memory deficit, disorientation, language, visuospatial ability, or perception) can be part of the acute syndrome. These disturbances are not better explained by a preexisting, established, or evolving neurocognitive disorder and do not occur in the context of a severely reduced level or arousal such as coma. There is evidence from the history, physical examination, or laboratory findings that the disturbance is a direct physiological consequence of a medical condition.

Several international guidelines focus on prevention, diagnostic, and therapy of delirium representing clinical evidence and expertise of the professionals and practitioners [2–24]. Some of them are developed for delirium in the elderly [2, 7, 10–17, 20, 21, 23, 24]. The "Recommendations for the Prevention, Diagnostic and Therapy of Delirium in the Elderly" of the Swiss Society for Gerontopsychiatry are the most recently published guidelines for delirium in the elderly [23, 24].

The prevalence of delirium in the population among the elderly aged 65+ years is 1–2% and rises up to 10% among a general population aged 85+ and up to 22% in a population with dementia [25]. In long-term care, prevalence ranges between 1.4 and 70%, depending on diagnostic criteria and the prevalence of dementia. Delirium is highly prevalent among persons with Alzheimer's disease who are hospitalized: 56% developed a delirium during hospitalization [26]. These patients experienced greater cognitive deterioration in the year following the hospitalization relative to patients who had not developed delirium. Therefore, strategies to prevent delirium in patients with dementia may help to slow cognitive deterioration.

13.1 Clinical Subtypes of Delirium

Delirium is not a homogenous syndrome and three subtypes have been described in the literature: hyperactive, hypoactive, and mixed [23, 24, 27, 28]. Although the hyperactive subtype with the prominent psychomotor disturbance may be recognized more readily, hypoactive and mixed subtypes are more common. Verbal and physical agitations are the core symptoms of the hyperactive subtype. Hallucinations, delusions,

E. Savaskan (✉)
Department of Geriatric Psychiatry, University Hospital of Psychiatry, Zürich, Switzerland
e-mail: egemen.savaskan@puk.zh.ch

H.-C. Pape et al. (eds.), *Senior Trauma Patients*, https://doi.org/10.1007/978-3-030-91483-7_13

sleep-wake cycle disturbances, disorientation, and cognitive deficits are other clinical symptoms of the hyperactive subtype. These patients may be hyperalert and have vegetative symptoms. In the hypoactive variant, reduced motor activity and apathy are the prominent features. The patients are lethargic and quiet and easily overlooked on an acute clinical setting. Psychotic symptoms are present in more than half of the patients with hypoactive type of delirium, but often underdiagnosed. Finally, in the mixed subtype, the patients can alternate unpredictably between hyperactive and hypoactive subtypes within a single day or over the course of a few days. While the mixed subtype has the worst prognosis, the hyperactive subtype shows the best.

13.2 Risk Factors of Delirium

Delirium is a complex syndrome, mostly of multifactorial origin. While in some cases delirium may be caused by a single factor, in the majority of cases delirium is a result of combined action of predisposing and precipitating factors in the elderly [29].

The most common predisposing risk factors for delirium are as follows [23, 24, 29]:

- Older Age
- Preexisting cognitive impairment or dementia
- Sex (male)
- Severe underlying illness
- Multiple comorbidities (more than 3)
- Polypharmacy (more than 3 drugs)
- Renal impairment
- Hepatic impairment
- Drug/Alcohol withdrawal
- Sensory impairment (deafness, vision impairment)
- Post-general anesthesia
- (Postfracture) surgery

The most common precipitating factors for delirium are as follows [23, 24, 27]:

- Infection
- Dehydration
- Malnutrition
- Use of physical restraints
- Use of urinary catheter
- More than 3 medications added
- Drugs (particularly psychoactive drugs and drugs with anticholinergic properties)
- Any iatrogenic event
- Electrolyte disturbance
- Immobility
- Constipation
- Pain
- Urinary retention
- Metabolic disturbances
- Environmental change (ward transfer, lack of orientation cues)
- Sensory deprivation (hearing or visual aid not available)
- Sleep deprivation

13.3 Diagnosis and Assessment of Delirium

Identification of risk factors and underlying causes of delirium is essential for the prevention and therapy. A detailed clinical history (including preexisting diseases and drugs/medication) followed by physical examination (including neurological examination) is the basis of diagnostic procedure. Since the delirium is an acute syndrome laboratory testing of electrolytes, signs of infection, etc. should be performed urgently. Additional diagnostic procedures (ECG, EEG, imaging, lumbar puncture, chest X-ray, etc.) may be necessary depending on the findings from history and examination [23, 24].

The following assessment instruments have been recommended for the screening of delirium in the elderly depending on setting [23, 24]:

- Delirium Observation Screening Scale (DOS) [30]
- Confusion Assessment Method (CAM) [31]
- Confusion Assessment Method for Intensive Care Unit (CAM-ICU) [32]

- Modified Confusion Assessment Method for the Emergency Department (mCAM-ED) [33]
- Delirium Rating Scale Revision 1998 (DRS-R-98) [34]
- Intensive Care Delirium Screening Checklist (ICDSC) [35]

The "Delirium Risk Assessment Tool" detects patients with high risk of delirium [18]. When people first present to hospital or long-term care, the person is at risk of delirium if any of the following risk factors is present:

- Age 65 years or older
- Cognitive impairment (past or present) and/or dementia
- Current hip fracture
- Severe illness

Two new assessment scales, I-AgeD (Informant Assessment of Geriatric Delirium Scale) for caregivers and 4AT (4 A's Test for Delirium Screening), are in development as useful instruments in delirium screening.

13.4 Non-Pharmacological Interventions for The Prevention of Delirium

Multicomponent intervention strategies have been recommended for the prevention of delirium in hospitalized (postoperative, post-trauma) patients [7, 10, 11, 18, 20, 23, 24, 29, 36, 37] as follows:

1. Collect information: Age, indication for hospitalization, medication, substance dependency, cognitive impairment, severe illness.
2. Orientation aids for patients with cognitive impairment (regular and repeated cues, at least three times daily), cognitively stimulating activities. Appropriate environmental stimuli. Use of clocks and calendars.
3. Eyeglasses and hearing aids for vision and hearing impairment.
4. Regulation of sleep-wake-cycle disturbances and minimization of sleep deprivation.
5. Appropriate lighting levels during daytime.
6. Elimination of unexpected and irritating noise.
7. Early mobilization (postoperative) and rehabilitation. Physiotherapeutical interventions for mobilization and to avoid falls.
8. Adequate CNS oxygen delivery (assessing for pain, looking for nonverbal signs, appropriate pain management).
9. Monitoring/restoring fluid/electrolyte balance.
10. Treatment of pain.
11. Monitoring medication (interactions), elimination of unnecessary medication (especially benzodiazepines, anticholinergics, antihistaminergics).
12. Regulation of bowel, bladder function.
13. Adequate nutritional intake.
14. Address constipation.
15. Avoid fixation and physical restraints.
16. Avoid catheterization if possible.
17. Prevention and treatment of infections (urinary tract infection, pneumonia).
18. Early detection and treatment of major postoperative complications (myocardial infarction, arrhythmias, pneumonia, embolus).
19. Treatment of agitated delirium.
20. Educate and train the multidisciplinary team.
21. Continuity of care from nursing staff.
22. Ensure/improve communication (patient and caregiver)
23. Involve and inform caregivers, family members. Explain the cause of delirium. Encourage family members to help calm the patient.

13.5 Pharmacological Prophylaxis of Delirium

Several drugs have been investigated as prophylactic intervention strategy for delirium [23, 24, 38–44]. However, since the results of the medical intervention studies are conflicting, no recommendation can be made for the moment for a medical prophylactic intervention. Pharmacological therapies should be restricted to patients with delirium; when the non-pharmacological interventions are not effective, the patients or staff are out in danger by symptoms such as agitation and aggression, and the symptoms of delirium severely impair the patient's capacity to cooperate with diagnostic and therapeutic procedures.

Antipsychotics are the best investigated drugs as prophylactic therapy strategy [38]. Perioperative prophylactic haloperidol administration reduced delirium duration and total hospital days when compared to placebo, but not the incidence of delirium in patients presenting for hip surgery [39]. There are also some studies demonstrating that prophylactic haloperidol [40] or olanzapine [41] administration after noncardiac surgery decreases the incidence of delirium. However, antipsychotics are highly associated with side effects and increased mortality in elderly multimorbid patients. Therefore, the use of antipsychotics in the prevention of postoperative delirium may be restricted to certain high-risk subgroups of the surgical population.

Since cholinergic depletion is a causative factor for delirium development, acetylcholinesterase inhibitors have been investigated as prophylactic therapy strategy. But both perioperative rivastigmine [42] and donepezil [43, 44] administration have failed to show any impact on delirium development.

Other substances such as dexmedetomidine, ketamine, statins, and steroids have been investigated as prophylactic agents [38]. However, the results do not allow a recommendation for these drugs as a medical prevention strategy for delirium at this point.

References

1. American Psychiatric Association. Diagnostic and Statistical Manual of Mental Disorders, 5th ed (DSM-5). Washington, DC: APA; 2013.
2. Young L, George J. Guidelines for the diagnosis and management of delirium in the elderly. London: Royal College of Physicians; 1997. www.bgs.org.uk
3. American Psychiatric Association. Practice guideline for the treatment of patients with delirium. Am J Psychiatry. 1999;156(5 Suppl):1–20.
4. Leentjens AF, Diefenbacher A. A survey of delirium guidelines in Europe. J Psychosom Res. 2006;61:123–8.
5. Van der Mast RC, Huyse FJ, Droogleever Fortuijn HA, Heeren TJ, Izaks GJ, Kalisvaart CJ, Klijn FAM, Leentjens AFG, Sno HN, Schuurmans MJ, Wilterdink J. Richtlijn delirium. Amsterdam: Nederlandse Vereniging voor Psychiatrie; 2004.
6. Van der Mast RC, Huyse FJ, Rosier PFWM. Richtlijn "Delirium". Nederlands Tijdschrift voor Geneeskunde. 2005;149(19):1027–32.
7. British Geriatrics Society. Guidelines for the prevention, diagnosis and management of delirium in older people in hospital. London: BGS; 2005.
8. Deutsche Gesellschaft für Neurologie (DGN): Alkoholdelir und Verwirrtheitszustände. DGN Leitlinien für Diagnostik und Therapie in der Neurologie. DGN, 2002. www.dgn.org
9. Leentjens AFG, Rundell J, Rummans T, Shim JJ, Oldham R, Peterson L, Philbrick K, Soellner W, Wolcott D, Freudenreich O. Delirium: an evidence-based medicine (EBM) monograph for psychosomatic medicine practice, commissioned by the Academy of Psychosomatic Medicine (APM) and the European Association of Consultation Liaison Psychiatry and Psychosomatics (EACLPP). J Psychosom Res. 2012;73:149–52.
10. British Geriatrics Society (BGS) and Royal College of Physicians (RCP). Guidelines for the prevention, diagnosis and management of delirium in older people: National Guidelines. Concise guidance to good practice series, No 6. London: RCP; 2006.
11. Potter J, George J. Guideline Development Group. The prevention, diagnosis and management of delirium in older people: concise guidelines. Clin Med. 2006;6(3):303–8.
12. Clinical Epidemiology and Health Services Evaluation. Clinical Practice Guidelines for the Management of Delirium in Older People, Melbourne: Victorian Government Department of Human Services; 2006. https://www2.health.vic.gov.au
13. Tropea J, Slee JA, Brand CA, Gray L, Snell T. Clinical practice guidelines for the management of delirium in older people in Australia. Australas J Ageing. 2008;27(3):150–6.
14. Hogan D, Gage L, Bruto V, et al. National guidelines for seniors' mental health: the assessment and treatment of delirium. Can Geriatr J. 2006;9:42–51.
15. Canadian Coalition for Seniors' Mental Health (CCSMH). National Guidelines for Senior's Mental Health—The Assessment and Treatment of Delirium. Toronto: CCSMH; 2006. www.ccsmh.ca
16. Sendelbach S, Finch GP. Acute confusion/delirium. In: Titler MG, editor. Series on evidence-based practice for older adults. Iowa City, IA: The University of Iowa College of Nursing Gerontological Nursing

Interventions Research Center, Research Translation and Dissemination Core; 2009.
17. Canadian Coalition for Seniors' Mental Health (CCSMH). Guideline on the assessment and treatment of delirium in older adults at the end of life. Adapted from the CCSMH National guidelines for seniors' mental health. The assessment and treatment of delirium. Toronto: CCSMH; 2010.
18. National Clinical Guideline Centre. Delirium: diagnosis, prevention and management. London: National Clinical Guideline Centre—Acute and Chronic Conditions; 2010. http://www.nice.org.uk/guidance
19. Barr J, Fraser GL, Puntillo K, Ely EW, Gélinas C, Dasta JF, Davidson JE, Devlin JW, Kress JP, Joffe AM, Coursin DB, Herr DL, Tung A, Robinson BR, Fontaine DK, Ramsay MA, Riker RR, Sessler CN, Pun B, Skrobik Y, Jaeschke R, American College of Critical Care Medicine. Clinical practice guidelines for the management of pain, agitation, and delirium in adult patients in the intensive care unit. Crit Care Med. 2013;41(1):263–306.
20. American Geriatrics Society (AGS) Expert Panel on Postoperative Delirium in Older Adults. Clinical practice guideline for postoperative delirium in older adults. New York: AGS; 2014. http://geriatricscareonline.org
21. American Geriatrics Society Expert Panel on Postoperative Delirium in Older Adults. American Geriatrics Society abstracted clinical practice guideline for postoperative delirium in older adults. J Am Geriatr Soc. 2015;63(1):142–50.
22. Michaud L, Büla C, Berney A, Camus V, Voellinger R, Stiefel F, Burnand B, Delirium Guidelines Development Group. Delirium: guidelines for general hospitals. J Psychosom Res. 2007;62(3):371–83.
23. Savaskan E, Baumgartner M, Georgescu D, Hafner M, Hasemann W, Kressig RW, Popp J, Rohrbach E, Schmid R, Verloo H. Recommendations for the prevention, diagnostic and therapy of delirium in the elderly (in German). Praxis. 2016;105(16):941–52.
24. Savaskan E, Hasemann W, editors. Guidelines for delirium: recommendations for the prevention, diagnostic and therapy of delirium in the elderly (in german). Bern: Hogrefe; 2017.
25. de Lange E, Verhaak PF, van der Meer K. Prevalence, presentation and prognosis of delirium in older people in the population, at home and in long term care: a review. Int J Geriatr Psychiatry. 2013;28(2):127–34.
26. Gross AL, Jones RN, Habtemariam DA, Fong TG, Tommet D, Quach L, Schmitt E, Yap L, Inouye SK. Delirium and long-term cognitive trajectory among persons with dementia. Arch Intern Med. 2012;172(17):1324–31.
27. Stagno D, Gibson C, Breitbart W. The delirium subtypes: a review of prevalence, phenomenology, pathophysiology, and treatment response. Palliat Support Care. 2004;2(2):171–9.
28. O'Keeffe ST. Clinical subtypes of delirium in the elderly. Dement Geriatr Cogn Disord. 1999;10:380–5.
29. Inouye SK. Prevention of delirium in hospitalized older patients: risk factors and targeted intervention strategies. Ann Med. 2000;32(4):257–63.
30. Schuurmans MJ, Shortridge-Baggett LM, Duursma SA. The delirium observation screening scale: a screening instrument for delirium. Res Theory Nurs Pract. 2003;17(1):31–50.
31. Inouye SK, van Dyck CH, Alessi CA, Balkin S, Siegal AP, Horwitz R. Clarifying confusion: the confusion assessment method. A new method for detection of delirium. Ann Intern Med. 1990;113(12):941–8.
32. Guenther U, Popp J, Koecher L, Muders T, Wrigge H, Ely EW, Putensen C. Validity and reliability of the CAM-ICU Flowsheet to diagnose delirium in surgical ICU patients. J Crit Care. 2010;25(1):144–51.
33. Grossmann FF, Hasemann W, Graber A, Bingisser R, Kressig RW, Nickel CH. Screening, detection and management of delirium in the emergency department—a pilot study on the feasibility of a new algorithm for use in older emergency department patients: the modified Confusion Assessment Method for the Emergency Department (mCAM-ED). Scand J Trauma Resusc Emerg Med. 2014;22:19.
34. Trzepacz PT, Mittal D, Torres R, Kanary K, Norton J, Jimerson N. Validation of the Delirium Rating Scale-revised-98: comparison with the delirium rating scale and the cognitive test for delirium. J Neuropsychiatry Clin Neurosci. 2001;13(2):229–42.
35. Radtke FM, Franck M, Oppermann S, Lütz A, Seeling M, Heymann A, Kleinwächter R, Kork F, Skrobik Y, Spies CD. The Intensive Care Delirium Screening Checklist (ICDSC)—translation and validation of intensive care delirium checklist in accordance with guidelines. Anasthesiol Intensivmed Notfallmed Schmerzther. 2009;44(2):80–6.
36. Marcantonio ER, Flacker JM, Wright RJ, Resnick NM. Reducing delirium after hip fracture: a randomized trial. J Am Geriatr Soc. 2001;49(5):516–22.
37. Inouye SK, Bogardus ST Jr, Charpentier PA, Leo-Summers L, Acampora D, Holford TR, Cooney LM Jr. A multicomponent intervention to prevent delirium in hospitalized older patients. N Engl J Med. 1999;340(9):669–76.
38. Rengel KF, Pandharipande PP, Hughes C. Postoperative delirium. Presse Med. 2018;47:e53–64.
39. Kalisvaart KJ, de Jonghe JF, Bogaards MJ, Vreeswijk R, Egberts TC, Burger BJ, Eikelenboom P, van Gool WA. Haloperidol prophylaxis for elderly hip-surgery patients at risk for delirium: a randomized placebo-controlled study. J Am Geriatr Soc. 2005;53(10):1658–66.
40. Wang W, Li HL, Wang DX, Zhu X, Li SL, Yao GQ, Chen KS, Gu XE, Zhu SN. Haloperidol prophylaxis decreases delirium incidence in elderly patients after noncardiac surgery: a randomized controlled trial. Crit Care Med. 2012;40(3):731–9.
41. Larsen KA, Kelly SE, Stern TA, Bode RH Jr, Price LL, Hunter DJ, Gulczynski D, Bierbaum BE, Sweeney GA, Hoikala KA, Cotter JJ, Potter

AW. Administration of olanzapine to prevent postoperative delirium in elderly joint-replacement patients: a randomized, controlled trial. Psychosomatics. 2010;51(5):409–18.
42. Gamberini M, Bolliger D, Lurati Buse GA, Burkhart CS, Grapow M, Gagneux A, Filipovic M, Seeberger MD, Pargger H, Siegemund M, Carrel T, Seiler WO, Berres M, Strebel SP, Monsch AU, Steiner LA. Rivastigmine for the prevention of postoperative delirium in elderly patients undergoing elective cardiac surgery—a randomized controlled trial. Crit Care Med. 2009;37(5):1762–8.
43. Liptzin B, Laki A, Garb JL, Fingeroth R, Krushell R. Donepezil in the prevention and treatment of post-surgical delirium. Am J Geriatr Psychiatry. 2005;13(12):1100–6.
44. Marcantonio ER, Palihnich K, Appleton P, Davis RB. Pilot randomized trial of donepezil hydrochloride for delirium after hip fracture. J Am Geriatr Soc. 2011;59(Suppl 2):S282–8.

14 Frailty Assessment and Treatment

Michael Gagesch and Olga Theou

14.1 Integrated Approach to the Frail Older Adult

The complex care of older adults warrants a holistic approach beyond the disease-centered perspective of today's highly specialized and fragmented medical care tailored to younger patients [1]. Geriatric medical care should focus on being appropriate, timely, and identifying reduced functional capacities and abilities (e.g., mobility and activities of daily living) [2]. This is especially important for the care of frail older patients. Frailty (described in detail in Sect. 14.5) is a state associated with an increased risk of adverse outcomes due to age-related multidimensional decline. Frailty is linked to accelerated functional decline and diminished resistance to even minor external stressors [3]. Over the past 20 years, the literature on frailty has increased exponentially and various frailty operationalizations and screening tools have been published [4]. However, no single screening tool has emerged to be of superior feasibility, validity, and reliability across care settings and therefore no undisputed gold standard exists [5].

As clinical experts in the field, geriatricians use a patient-centered treatment and management plan based on a comprehensive geriatric assessment (CGA); the diagnostic instrument of choice in primary and acute care settings. Performing a CGA identifies deficits and resources in aging body systems such as cognition, musculoskeletal strength and function, nutrition, and environment in order to determine individual patient care needs [6]. The efficacy of a structured geriatric evaluation and management plan based on CGA has already been investigated by multiple randomized controlled trials and meta-analyses, including for orthogeriatric patients with fragility fractures [7–11].

While CGA can be considered the gold standard for the evaluation and management of older patients [12], its application is often considered time-consuming for the first step of evaluation (screening) [13], especially for the acute care of older trauma patients. Including a validated screening tool for frailty in the CGA framework has been recommended by the 2017 Asia-Pacific guidelines for frailty management [14].

M. Gagesch (✉)
Department of Aging Medicine, University Hospital Zurich and University of Zurich, Zurich, Switzerland
e-mail: michael.gagesch@usz.ch

O. Theou
Physiotherapy and Geriatric Medicine, Dalhousie University, Halifax, Nova Scotia, Canada
e-mail: olga.theou@dal.ca

H.-C. Pape et al. (eds.), *Senior Trauma Patients*, https://doi.org/10.1007/978-3-030-91483-7_14

14.2 Frailty in The Acute Care Setting

Important factors that inform about the acute care of older adults include physiological changes that occur with aging, such as musculoskeletal, cardiopulmonary and neuropsychological decline, nutritional impairments, multimorbidity, and polypharmacy [15]. These factors (described in detail in other sections of this textbook), in addition to the often atypical disease presentation—which can be considered "typical" for frail patients [16], can explain the substantially higher risk for adverse outcomes that older patients experience in the face of external stressors [12, 17]. These stressors range from minor infections (e.g., upper respiratory or lower urinary tract infections) to acute organ decompensation (e.g., decompensated heart failure), medical interventions (e.g., invasive diagnostic procedures or percutaneous coronary interventions), or environmental challenges (e.g., enduring heat waves) and can lead to accelerated or acute functional deterioration, increased morbidity, and premature mortality. Due to this, early detection and treatment of frailty is a priority for public health [18]. Frailty could be integrated in a comprehensive geriatric care framework with the aim of countering the risk of functional decline and the adverse outcomes associated with increased health care costs (e.g., permanent care dependency, institutionalization).

Experts in the field of acute care see frailty as an emerging "geriatric giant" [2, 3, 19]. Consequently, whether the assessment of frailty is done using case finding screening or embedded within a CGA, it is a timely window of opportunity to support the early identification of risk for adverse outcomes from acute to long-term care settings.

The two most widely used frailty concepts are the syndromic frailty phenotype (with its five components of fatigue, low physical activity level, slowness, weakness, and unintentional weight loss) and the deficit accumulation approach, operationalized in a Frailty Index (i.e., the ratio of deficits by the total number of items assessed) [4]. Although there is no agreement on a universal frailty screening tool, a frailty consensus in 2013 recommended frailty screening in all adults aged 70 years or older using tools such as the Fried Phenotype, the FRAIL scale, or the Clinical Frailty Scale [20]. Similarly, the British Geriatric Society recommended in their 2014 best practice guidelines on frailty that all formal health care encounters with community-dwelling older adults include frailty screening, using tools such as the PRISMA-7 or mobility assessments (standardized gait speed test or the Timed Up and Go test) [21].

A recent scoping review identified 204 studies that measured frailty in an acute care setting [22]. They concluded that most frailty studies were conducted in non-geriatric settings and the most commonly used tools were the Clinical Frailty Scale, the Frailty Index, and the Frailty Phenotype. Even though there was great variability in the tools used, frailty was a good predictor of acute care outcomes including mortality, length of stay, complications, and rehospitalization. They recommended that a validated frailty assessment should be used in acute care to assist with formulating the care plan and improving informed and shared decision making [16].

14.3 Frailty in The Geriatric Trauma Setting

Frail older adults have a high risk of falls and fractures [23], and older trauma patients generally experience worse outcomes than their younger counterparts [24]. Therefore, optimizing care of older trauma patients is of growing importance. Frailty is now among the nine core components of the geriatric assessment (together with cognitive/behavioral disorders, cardiac evaluation, pulmonary evaluation, functional/performance status, nutritional status, medication management, patient counseling, and preoperative testing) as defined by the 2015 Best Practices Guideline from ACS NSQIP®/American Geriatrics Society for optimal perioperative management of geriatric patients [25]. In a joint statement, the American College of Surgeons and the American Geriatric Society recommended frailty assessment in geriatric surgical patients, including in traumatology settings [26].

Postsurgical complications in older patients often arise from nonsurgical factors (e.g., postoperative pneumonia, heart failure, or gastrointestinal bleeding), as demonstrated in hip fracture patients [27]. Frailty tools used to assess orthogeriatric patients must consider functional limitations due to acute illness and should not be too time-consuming or invasive [24]. A multidisciplinary team made up of surgeons, geriatricians, and other health care professionals may be useful. Furthermore, using physical and occupational therapy soon after admission has proven beneficial compared to geriatric liaison services [28]. More evidence is needed from large randomized controlled trials with standardized measures for the widespread implementation of geriatric comanagement programs.

14.4 Frailty Tools

Frailty assessment in the acute care of older trauma patients requires the selection of a suitable screening tool for the individual care environment. This depends largely on the local structural and personal resources, the availability of geriatric expertise, and the characteristics of the targeted patient population. A frailty screening tool used in the orthogeriatric setting should be validated for geriatric trauma patients and should be reliable, feasible, and easy to administer.

The phenotypic frailty approach focuses more on physical frailty and can add a structured measurement to the "eyeball-exam" of clinical experts. It also allows for follow-up after care transitions when patient clinical data might not be as easily available as in the acute care setting. Our group demonstrated in 2017 the feasibility of frailty screening based on the frailty phenotype in an investigation of the association of impaired nutritional status and frailty in older trauma patients [29].

The Frailty Index approach, utilizing patient-related data without a physical examination, has been validated for the prediction of institutionalization and mortality in the orthogeriatric setting [30, 31]. Strengths of the Frailty Index approach are that it can be constructed using existing data (not every index need includes the same items to achieve closely comparable estimates in frailty levels), it is a comprehensive assessment of health, and it provides a continuous score from fitness to frailty. Joseph and colleagues demonstrated in 2014 the superiority of a Frailty Index for predicting adverse outcomes in geriatric trauma patients beyond chronological age alone [32]. A national initiative is currently ongoing in Switzerland (Swiss Frailty Network and Repository) to investigate a harmonized Frailty Index in older acute care inpatients at all five Swiss university hospitals using data from electronic health records.

Both frailty approaches can trigger a CGA and management plan for patients classified as frail or at risk for frailty. This two-step case finding concept could be applied in clinical settings to deal with the influx of frail older patients.

In summary, the frailty screening tool of choice should be reliable and validated in the desired setting. Table 14.1 provides a brief summary of validated frailty tools for older adult trauma patients; a complete overview of available instruments is beyond the scope of this chapter. Additionally, the cited literature contains key papers for implementing frailty assessment in the orthogeriatric setting.

14.5 Comprehensive Treatment Approach

Targeting frailty requires a multisystem treatment approach. Like other progressive conditions affecting older adults, early identification and intervention is a key to success. Interventions should consider the characteristic deficits of frail older adults and focus on improving physical function and activity and counteracting malnutrition and polypharmacy [33–37].

So far, evidence for frailty interventions comes mainly from observational studies in community-dwelling older adults. However, a small number of clinical trials have investigated

Table 14.1 Commonly used frailty tools in the acute care setting

Description	Operationalization/Components	Score	Type of assessment	Approximate duration	
Fried Phenotype[a]	Fatigue (self-report) Low Physical Activity Level (self-report) Slowness (Walking Speed) Weakness (Grip Strength) Weight Loss (unintentional)	0–5 points (0/1 for each item) 0 = robust 1–2 = pre-frail (at-risk) ≥3 = frail	Patient-based	10–20 min	Fried LP, et al. Gerontology 2001 [42]
Frailty Index	30+ items. Not every frailty index includes the same number and type of items. Commonly used items: Activities of Daily Living, Musculoskeletal Function, Cognitive Function and Mood, Cardiovascular Function, Comorbidities, Medication, (+/– Laboratory abnormalities)	Continuous 0–1	Varies; it could be chart-based	Varies	Mitnitski AB, et al. Scientific World Journal 2001 [43]
Trauma-Specific Frailty Index	15 items: Comorbidities, Daily Activities, Health Attitude, Nutrition, Sexual Function	Continuous 0–1	(Mainly) chart-based	10–20 min	Joseph B, et al. J Am Coll Surg 2014 [44]
Modified Frailty Index	11 items based on NSQIP data: (1) history of diabetes; (2) impaired functional status; (3) history of chronic obstructive pulmonary disease or pneumonia; (4) history of congestive heart failure; (5) history of myocardial infarction within 6 months of surgery; (6) history of percutaneous coronary intervention cardiac surgery or angina; (7) receipt of hypertensive medications; (8) peripheral vascular disease, rest pain, or gangrene; (9) impaired sensorium; (10) transient ischemic attack or cerebrovascular accident (CVA) defined as focal neurological deficits of sudden onset and brief duration; and (11) CVA with deficit defined by history of CVA with persistent residual dysfunction.	Stepwise increase from 0-1 through 0.09, 0.18, 0.27, 0.36, 0.45, 0.54, 0.63, 0.72, 0.81, and 1.0.	(Strictly) chart based	10–20 min	Velanovich V, et al. J Surg Research 2013 [45]
Clinical Frail Scale	Overall impression of clinician after the evaluation of comorbidity, function, and cognition.	(1) Very Fit (2) Well (3) Managing Well (4) Vulnerable (5) Mildly Frail (6) Moderately Frail (7) Severely Frail (8) Very Severely Frail (9) Terminally Ill	Clinical judgment-based	2–5 min	Rockwood K, et al. CMAJ, 2005 [46]

FRAIL scale	Fatigue (self-report) Resistance (self-report) Ambulation (self-report) Illnesses (self-report) Weight loss (unintentional)	0–5 points (0/1 for each item) 0 = robust 1–2 = pre frail (at-risk) ≥3 = frail	Patient-based	5–10 min	Abellan van Kan G, et al., J Am Med Dir Assoc, 2008 [47] Morley JE, et al. J Nutr Health Aging 2012 [48]
Edmonton Frail Scale	Cognition (Clock Drawing Test) General Health (self-report) Functional Status (self-report) Functional performance (Timed Up and Go Test) Social Support (self-report) Polypharmacy (self-report) Nutrition (self-report) Mood (self-report) Continence (self-report)	Scoring from 0 to 17 points 0–5 points = robust 6–7 points = vulnerable 8–9 points = mildly frail 10–11 points = moderately frail 12–17 points = severely frail	Patient-based	20–30 min	Rolfson DB, et al. Age Ageing, 2006 [49]

[a]Various operationalizations of the five phenotypic criteria exist in the literature

the efficacy of nutritional or exercise-based interventions in the acute care setting.

A 2011 systematic review by Theou and colleagues examined 47 randomized controlled trials on exercise interventions for the management of frailty [37]. They included participants aged 60 years or older recruited from community and hospital settings and found that multicomponent exercise programs of 30–45 min duration, performed 3 or more times a week for ≥5 months, generally resulted in better outcomes compared to other exercise programs. Of note, in this systematic review, the heterogeneity of studies was large and only a minority used a validated frailty measure.

Among older trauma patients, malnutrition is associated with the development of frailty yet remains underdiagnosed [38]. In an orthogeriatric unit at a tertiary medical center in Switzerland, 50% of patients were at risk of malnutrition, 7% were malnourished, and 33% of frail patients had impaired nutritional status (vs. 8% for non-frail) [29]. The authors recommended screening for malnutrition in all older trauma patients. For community-dwelling frail older adults, there is evidence for improving nutrition using protein [39] and vitamin D3 [40, 41] supplementation. A promising but challenging approach might be to prevent frailty and its long-term detrimental outcomes at mid-life while reducing falls as the main cause of trauma for older adults.

14.6 Summary

Frailty assessment in the orthogeriatric setting seems promising to further improve patient-centered care and promote beneficial outcomes in this vulnerable population. However, there is currently no universally recommended frailty instrument for this setting. A Frailty Index based on the deficit accumulation approach is useful for the assessment of frailty and perioperative risk and does not require additional examinations since it can be constructed using existing patient data. On the other hand, a frailty assessment which includes performance-based measures of health such as the frailty phenotype might provide more in-depth information about the patients' functional impairments. In summary, assessing frailty using a validated tool independent of the selected approach provides a timely window of opportunity to further improve outcomes for older adults in the acute trauma setting.

References

1. Tinetti ME, Fried T. The end of the disease era. Am J Med. 2004;116(3):179–85.
2. Cesari M, Marzetti E, Thiem U, Perez-Zepeda MU, Abellan Van Kan G, Landi F, et al. The geriatric management of frailty as paradigm of "The end of the disease era". Eur J Intern Med. 2016;31:11–4.
3. Rodriguez-Manas L, Feart C, Mann G, Vina J, Chatterji S, Chodzko-Zajko W, et al. Searching for an operational definition of frailty: a Delphi method based consensus statement: the frailty operative definition-consensus conference project. J Gerontol A Biol Sci Med Sci. 2013;68(1):62–7.
4. Buta BJ, Walston JD, Godino JG, Park M, Kalyani RR, Xue QL, et al. Frailty assessment instruments: Systematic characterization of the uses and contexts of highly-cited instruments. Ageing Res Rev. 2016;26:53–61.
5. Warnier RM, van Rossum E, van Velthuijsen E, Mulder WJ, Schols JM, Kempen GI. Validity, reliability and feasibility of tools to identify frail older patients in inpatient hospital care: a systematic review. J Nutr Health Aging. 2016;20(2):218–30.
6. Bandeen-Roche K, Seplaki CL, Huang J, Buta B, Kalyani RR, Varadhan R, et al. Frailty in older adults: a nationally representative profile in the United States. J Gerontol A Biol Sci Med Sci. 2015;70(11):1427–34.
7. Stuck AE, Siu AL, Wieland GD, Adams J, Rubenstein LZ. Comprehensive geriatric assessment: a meta-analysis of controlled trials. Lancet. 1993;342(8878):1032–6.
8. Ellis G, Whitehead MA, Robinson D, O'Neill D, Langhorne P. Comprehensive geriatric assessment for older adults admitted to hospital: meta-analysis of randomised controlled trials. BMJ. 2011;343:d6553.
9. Talevski J, Sanders KM, Duque G, Connaughton C, Beauchamp A, Green D, et al. Effect of clinical care pathways on quality of life and physical function after fragility fracture: a meta-analysis. J Am Med Dir Assoc. 2019;20(7):926.e1–926.e11.
10. Van Craen K, Braes T, Wellens N, Denhaerynck K, Flamaing J, Moons P, et al. The effectiveness of inpatient geriatric evaluation and management units: a systematic review and meta-analysis. J Am Geriatr Soc. 2010;58(1):83–92.
11. Prestmo A, Hagen G, Sletvold O, Helbostad JL, Thingstad P, Taraldsen K, et al. Comprehensive geriatric care for patients with hip fractures: a pro-

spective, randomised, controlled trial. Lancet. 2015;385(9978):1623–33.
12. Clegg A, Young J, Iliffe S, Rikkert MO, Rockwood K. Frailty in elderly people. Lancet. 2013;381(9868):752–62.
13. Seematter-Bagnoud L, Bula C. Brief assessments and screening for geriatric conditions in older primary care patients: a pragmatic approach. Public Health Rev. 2018;39:8.
14. Dent E, Lien C, Lim WS, Wong WC, Wong CH, Ng TP, et al. The Asia-Pacific clinical practice guidelines for the management of frailty. J Am Med Dir Assoc. 2017;18(7):564–75.
15. Fulop T, Larbi A, Witkowski JM, McElhaney J, Loeb M, Mitnitski A, et al. Aging, frailty and age-related diseases. Biogerontology. 2010;11(5):547–63.
16. Theou O, Rockwood K. Frailty in aging. In: Fulop T, editor. Basel. New York: Karger; 2015. 200 p.
17. Dent E, Kowal P, Hoogendijk EO. Frailty measurement in research and clinical practice: A review. Eur J Intern Med. 2016;31:3–10.
18. Beard JR, Bloom DE. Towards a comprehensive public health response to population ageing. Lancet. 2015;385(9968):658–61.
19. Morley JE, Vellas B, van Kan GA, Anker SD, Bauer JM, Bernabei R, et al. Frailty consensus: a call to action. J Am Med Dir Assoc. 2013;14(6):392–7.
20. Vanpottelbergh G, Vaes B, Adriaensen W, Mathei C, Legrand D, Wallemacq P, Degryse JM. The glomerular filtration rate estimated by new and old equations as a predictor of important oucomes in elderly patients. BMC Med. 2014;12(27) https://doi.org/10.11186/11741.
21. Turner G, Clegg A. Best practice guidelines for the management of frailty: a British Geriatrics Society, Age UK and Royal College of General Practitioners report. Age Ageing. 2014;43(6):744–7.
22. Theou O, Squires E, Mallery K, Lee JS, Fay S, Goldstein J, et al. What do we know about frailty in the acute care setting? A scoping review. BMC Geriatrics. 2018;18(1):139.
23. Ensrud KE, Ewing SK, Taylor BC, Fink HA, Stone KL, Cauley JA, et al. Frailty and risk of falls, fracture, and mortality in older women: the study of osteoporotic fractures. J Gerontol A Biol Sci Med Sci. 2007;62(7):744–51.
24. McDonald VS, Thompson KA, Lewis PR, Sise CB, Sise MJ, Shackford SR. Frailty in trauma: a systematic review of the surgical literature for clinical assessment tools. J Trauma Acute Care Surg. 2016;80(5):824–34.
25. Mohanty S, Rosenthal RA, Russell MM, Neuman MD, Ko CY, Esnaola NF. Optimal perioperative management of the geriatric patient: a best practices guideline from the American College of Surgeons NSQIP and the American Geriatrics Society. J Am Coll Surg. 2016;222(5):930–47.
26. Chow WB, Rosenthal RA, Merkow RP, Ko CY, Esnaola NF. Optimal preoperative assessment of the geriatric surgical patient: a best practices guideline from the American College of Surgeons National Surgical Quality Improvement Program and the American Geriatrics Society. J Am Coll Surg. 2012;215(4):453–66.
27. Roche JJ, Wenn RT, Sahota O, Moran CG. Effect of comorbidities and postoperative complications on mortality after hip fracture in elderly people: prospective observational cohort study. BMJ. 2005;331(7529):1374.
28. Van Grootven B, Flamaing J, Dierckx de Casterle B, Dubois C, Fagard K, Herregods MC, et al. Effectiveness of in-hospital geriatric co-management: a systematic review and meta-analysis. Age Ageing. 2017:1–8.
29. Muller FS, Meyer OW, Chocano-Bedoya P, Schietzel S, Gagesch M, Freystaetter G, et al. Impaired nutritional status in geriatric trauma patients. Eur J Clin Nutr. 2017;71(5):602–6.
30. Maxwell CA, Patel MB, Suarez-Rodriguez LC, Miller RS. Frailty and prognostication in geriatric surgery and trauma. Clin Geriatr Med. 2019;35(1):13–26.
31. Joseph B, Pandit V, Zangbar B, Kulvatunyou N, Tang A, O'Keeffe T, et al. Validating trauma-specific frailty index for geriatric trauma patients: a prospective analysis. J Am Coll Surg. 2014;219(1):10-7.e1.
32. Joseph B, Pandit V, Zangbar B, Kulvatunyou N, Hashmi A, Green DJ, et al. Superiority of frailty over age in predicting outcomes among geriatric trauma patients: a prospective analysis. JAMA Surg. 2014;149(8):766–72.
33. Cruz-Jentoft AJ, Kiesswetter E, Drey M, Sieber CC. Nutrition, frailty, and sarcopenia. Aging Clin Exp Res. 2017;29(1):43–8.
34. Ng TP, Feng L, Nyunt MSZ, Feng L, Niti M, Tan BY, et al. Nutritional, physical, cognitive, and combination interventions and frailty reversal among older adults: a randomized controlled trial. Am J Med. 2015;128(11):1225–1236.e1.
35. Tarazona-Santabalbina FJ, Gomez-Cabrera MC, Perez-Ros P, Martinez-Arnau FM, Cabo H, Tsaparas K, et al. A multicomponent exercise intervention that reverses frailty and improves cognition, emotion, and social networking in the community-dwelling frail elderly: a randomized clinical trial. J Am Med Dir Assoc. 2016;17(5):426–33.
36. Puts MT, Toubasi S, Andrew MK, Ashe MC, Ploeg J, Atkinson E, et al. Interventions to prevent or reduce the level of frailty in community-dwelling older adults: a scoping review of the literature and international policies. Age Ageing. 2017;
37. Theou O, Stathokostas L, Roland KP, Jakobi JM, Patterson C, Vandervoort AA, et al. The effectiveness of exercise interventions for the management of frailty: a systematic review. J Aging Res. 2011;2011:569194.
38. Bischoff HA, Staehelin HB, Willett WC. The effect of undernutrition in the development of frailty in older persons. J Gerontol A Biol Sci Med Sci. 2006;61(6):585–9.
39. Tieland M, Borgonjen-Van den Berg KJ, van Loon LJC, de Groot LCPGM. Dietary protein intake in community-dwelling, frail, and institutionalized

elderly people: scope for improvement. Eur J Nutr. 2012;51(2):173–9.

40. Pabst G, Zimmermann AK, Huth C, Koenig W, Ludwig T, Zierer A, et al. Association of low 25-hydroxyvitamin D levels with the frailty syndrome in an aged population: results from the KORA-age Augsburg study. J Nutr Health Aging. 2015;19(3):258–64.
41. Halfon M, Phan O, Teta D. Vitamin D: a review on its effects on muscle strength, the risk of fall, and frailty. BioMed Res Int. 2015;2015:953241.
42. Fried LP, Tangen CM, Walston J, Newman AB, Hirsch C, Gottdiener J, Seeman T, Tracy R, Kop WJ, Burke G, McBurnie MA. Frailty in Older Adults: Evidence for a Phenotype. The Journals of Gerontology Series A: Biological Sciences and Medical Sciences 2001;56(3):M146–M157 https://doi.org/10.1093/gerona/56.3.M146.
43. Arnold B, Mitnitski Alexander J, Mogilner KR. Accumulation of Deficits as a Proxy Measure of Aging. The Scientific World JOURNAL 2001;1323–336. https://doi.org/10.1100/tsw.2001.58.
44. Joseph Viraj B, Bardiya P, Narong Z, Andrew K, Terence T, O'Keeffe Donald J, Gary G, Vercruysse Mindy J, Fain Randall S, Rhee FP. Validating trauma-specific frailty index for geriatric trauma patients: a prospective analysis. Journal of the American College of Surgeons. 2014;219(1):10-17.e1. https://doi.org/10.1016/j.jamcollsurg.2014.03.020.
45. Velanovich Heath V, Andrew A, David S, Rubinfeld PI. Accumulating deficits model of frailty and post-operative mortality and morbidity: its application to a national database. Journal of Surgical Research 2013;183(1):104–10. https://doi.org/10.1016/j.jss.2013.01.02.
46. Rockwood K. A global clinical measure of fitness and frailty in elderly people. Canadian Medical Association Journal. 2005;173(5):489–95. https://doi.org/10.1503/cmaj.050051.
47. Abellan G, van Kan Yves M, Rolland John E, Morley Bruno V. Frailty: Toward a Clinical Definition. Journal of the American Medical Directors Association 2008;9(2):71–72:10. https://doi.org/1016/j.jamda.2007.11.005.
48. John E, Morley TK, Malmstrom DK, Miller. A simple frailty questionnaire (FRAIL) predicts outcomes in middle aged African Americans. The journal of nutrition health & aging 2012;16(7):601–8. https://doi.org/10.1007/s12603-012-0084-2.
49. Darryl B, Rolfson Sumit R, Majumdar Ross T, Adeel T, Kenneth T. Rockwood validity and reliability of the edmonton frail scale. Age and Ageing. 2006;35(5):526–9. https://doi.org/10.1093/ageing/afl041.

15 Pain Management

Markus Gosch

Uncontrolled pain is a common contributor to poor outcomes. In contrast, adequate pain management enhances early mobilization, lowers delirium rates, and may shorten the length of hospital stay. It may also lead to a reduced cardiovascular, renal, respiratory, and gastrointestinal morbidity [1]. Early onset of sufficient pain control—ideally at the scene of trauma or at least in the emergency room—is of importance, and more than that, has been shown to reduce the rate of delirium. However, pain treatment in older adults is difficult, complicated in patients with comorbidities and impaired cognition, and may be harmful because of the vulnerability of these patients. In light of the many factors necessary to achieve safe and adequate pain control, a thoughtful and thorough approach is required to manage pain appropriately.

15.1 Types of Pain

For clinical work, it is useful to distinguish between different types of pain. From the timeline, pain can be characterized as acute or chronic pain. Acute pain is defined by an abrupt onset, caused by a specific trauma, and only lasts for a relatively short period of time. Chronic pain persists for more than 3–6 months and is not linked to special event or trauma. Prevalence of chronic pain ranges from 20% to 46% in community-dwelling older adults and from 28% to 73% in older adults in long-term care [2]. Older women have higher prevalence rates of pain than older men [2]. The reported effect of age on pain prevalence in older people is inconsistent, with some studies reporting an increase in prevalence with age and others reporting a decrease in prevalence with age. The effect also varies by sites of pain. The three most common sites of pain in older adults are the back, leg/knee, or hip and other joints [2].

There are three different pathophysiological subtypes of pain [3]: nociceptive, neuropathic, and mixed. Pain related to a hip fracture is typically a nociceptive, somatic type of pain. It is due to the activation of sensory receptors by noxious stimuli. This kind of pain tends to originate in the skin, muscle, or bone and it is easily localized. Another form of nociceptive pain is visceral pain. In contrast to somatic type, visceral pain is caused by internal organs such as the heart, lung, or gastrointestinal tract. Usually visceral pain is difficult to localize and it is described as aching, dull, or vague. Neuropathic pain is caused by irritation or inflammation of nerve fibres and/or neurons. It is described as burning, tingling, or numbness. It is localized easily, but may have a radiating component that follows path of the nerves itself. Neuropathic pain may have an insufficient

M. Gosch (✉)
Department for Geriatric Medicine, Paracelsus Private Medical University, General Hospital Nuremberg, Nuremberg, Germany
e-mail: markus.gosch@pmu.ac.at

H.-C. Pape et al. (eds.), *Senior Trauma Patients*, https://doi.org/10.1007/978-3-030-91483-7_15

response to typical pain medication, including non-steroidal-anti-inflammatory drugs (NSAID) or opioids. In that case, anticonvulsants or antidepressants may be more effective. In mixed pain, we find a combination of nociceptive and neuropathic pain. Mixed pain can be seen in patients with vertebral fractures, as well as in patients with hip fractures, if nerve fibres are disturbed by the fracture itself, a hematoma, oedema, or inflammation.

15.2 Pain Assessment

Pain has to be assessed as the fifth vital sign. Its assessment is quite difficult in younger age groups, but it is really challenging in older fragility fracture patients, especially in patients with multiple comorbidities, polypharmacy, cognitive impairment, or pre-existing pain medication. Each treatment has to be based on an appropriate assessment.

Different pain assessment tools are available. The most frequent used tools are the Visual Analog Scale (VAS) and the Numeric or Verbal Rating Scale (NRS, VRS). These scores are based on patient's self-reporting. Therefore, it is obvious that their value is extremely dependent on the cognitive function of patients. In our daily clinical work, we have to distinguish between older patients with preserved cognition and those with an impaired cognition.

Cognitive function should be assessed as soon as possible. The point is to evaluate the patient if he/she is able to use a VAS or VRS or not. The goal is not to screen or to diagnose dementia. There are many reasons for an impaired cognition after sustaining a trauma like a hip fracture. It is not indicated to use complex assessment tools like a Mini-Mental-State-Examination (MMSE). Cognition should be checked by an experienced physician, ideally a geriatrician. If emergency physicians or orthopaedic surgeons are not familiar to diagnose a cognitive impairment, they may use simple assessment tools like the Clock Drawing Test or a short memory test.

15.2.1 Assessment of Patients with Preserved Cognition

The NRS is a verbally obtained pain scale from 0 to 10 (0 is considered no pain and 10 the most severe pain imaginable). The NRS is the most common valid pain scale in older adults capable of self-report [4]. The VAS is a related tool that asks a patient to rate their pain on a printed line between 0 (no pain) to 10 (maximum pain). This tool has limitations, not only in patients with cognitive impairment, but also in other older adults and it is seen as less effective and has a high rate of errors [5]. The VRS has also been validated in older adults and assesses pain by using verbal indicators, like mild, moderate, or severe, to quantify the intensity of pain. The VRS is preferred for older adults and can also be used in patients with mild to moderate dementia [4]. Pain intensity varies a lot during day and different situations, like mobilization or toileting. Therefore, it is an obligation to assess pain on different time during a day and during different activities.

15.2.2 Assessment of Patients with Impaired Cognition

In this group of patients, pain assessment has to be focused on observation of nonverbal indicators of pain. The American Geriatric Society (AGS) recommends the evaluation of six behavioural domains: facial expression, verbalization/vocalization, body movements, changes in interpersonal interactions, changes in activity patterns, and changes in mental status [5].

Fractures are associated with pain. Therefore, older fragility fracture patients usually receive any kind of pain medication, mostly according to a local guideline or standard operating procedure (SOP). Even under treatment in many patients, a complete pain relief is not realistic. Overtreatment can be as harmful as undertreatment. For a sufficient and safe pain treatment, we have to take into account the individual tolerability to pain of our patients. A trigger to increase the dose of pain killers is not the question "Do you have pain?", but "Do you need more pain medication?". From a personal clinical experience, this is a simple, but very valuable question, even in patients with moderate and sometimes also severe dementia, to find the adequate dose of pain medication.

15.3 Treatment of Pain

Physiological changes in older adults increase the sensitivity to some analgesic drugs, resulting in them sometimes requiring lower doses and with a higher risk for adverse drug events (ADR). Analgesics should always be titrated to response. To minimize the risk of side effects, usually we start with low dose, particularly regarding strong opioids. Although the risk of ADRs is high in older patient, sufficient pain treatment is essential for good outcome and reluctance could be harmful. Considering existing comorbidities and polypharmacy, analgesics can still be safe and effective. Besides pharmacological treatment, non-pharmacological strategies such as counselling, bedding of patients, or physiotherapy and mobilization should be considered. For sure, these measures alone are not sufficient, but may help to reduce the doses of analgesics.

NSAIDs are one of the most widely prescribed pain killers. However, in older adults with relevant comorbidities and polypharmacy, NSAIDs should no longer play a major role in pain management. Despite good efficacy, NSAIDs have a high risk of potentially serious and life-threatening side effects. The gastrointestinal bleeding risk of the upper gastrointestinal tract can be minimized by the additional prescription of proton pump inhibitors. Remaining risks of bleeding of the lower gastrointestinal tract, renal, and cardiovascular side effects exclude NSAIDs as an option for pain treatment in older fragility fracture patients.

15.3.1 Preoperative Phase

Pain treatment should start as soon as possible. Transportation, transfers, or x-rays can be very painful. Usually, medical pain treatment of fragility fracture patients starts with intravenous opioids. In some patients, who report only few pain or present with minor injuries, acetaminophen or metamizol is sufficient. If pharmacological pain treatment is not sufficient or there is a need for optimization of the patient that leads to a significant delay of surgery, local nerve blocks should be considered as an additional option. There is evidence for adequate pain relief by regional anaesthesia using femoral nerve blocks preoperatively. Apart from that, nerve blocks reduce the need for opioids and significantly reduce the incidence of pulmonary complications [6]. Nerve blocks are also a good option in the first hours or days after surgery.

Hydromorphone is the preferred opiate for older adults, particularly in patients with renal impairment. Starting dose is 0.2 mg intravenous. Application can be repeated every 30 min until pain relief is achieved, followed by an application every 2–4 h. Morphine is another option. However, ADRs increase in patients with renal failure (eGFR < 35 mL/min). Starting dose is 1 mg intravenous; it should be repeated every 30 min until sufficient pain relief, followed by an application every 2–4 h. Fentanyl is an option for patients who are already on transdermal pain treatment with fentanyl. Starting dose is 10 mcg, every 15 min until pain relief, afterwards every 30 min.

Weak opioids do not play a role in the preoperative setting. They are less effective but the risk of ADRs is similar to strong opioids. Acetaminophen and metamizol are an option as mentioned above. For both, the dose is 1 g intravenous. In contrast to metamizol, acetaminophen should be infused over a very short time. Intravenous metamizol has the risk of acute hypotension, especially if the infusion rate is too fast. Therefore, application rate should be below 0.5 g per minute. The application of both can be repeated in 4–6 h. If pain relief is insufficient after the first applications, strong opioids should be used.

15.3.2 Postoperative Phase

Postoperative pain management should be standardized using a SOP or a guideline. The whole team should be familiar with the recommended drugs, doses, and possible side effects. Complete pain relief could not be a realistic goal in patients after fragility fracture. However, treatment has to be sufficient to allow early mobilization and physiotherapy.

15.3.3 Pharmacological Treatment

Acetaminophen is widely used. It can be prescribed as oral or intravenous application. Pain relief and efficacy have been shown especially for intravenous application [7]. Although acetaminophen is generally well-tolerated, we have to be aware of some side effects. Gastrointestinal bleeding increases by the factor 3.6, if doses more than 2 g are prescribed [8]. In combination with Vitamin K antagonists, acetaminophen leads to a significant increase of the INR resulting in a higher bleeding risk [9]. Apart from that, the use of acetaminophen results in a higher risk for mortality, hypertension, and cardiovascular complications [10]. A dose of more than 7 g per day could lead to acute liver failure. A dose of 4 g per day is usually safe, but oral prescription should be limited to 2 g per day to avoid a potential lethal overdose.

Metamizol is not available in every country. It is the most relevant pyrazolon. It has high analgesic, good antipyretic, but no antiphlogistic effects. Usually, metamizol is well-tolerated and side effects are rare. But, there are also ongoing discussion about severe side effects, like agranulocytosis or hypotension caused by intravenous application. The risk of agranulocytosis varies from doses as well as from countries. The incidence ranges from 1.1 per million in Spain to 1 per 1439 persons in Sweden. In literature, we find two different kinds of agranulocytosis. One is dose-independent, caused by an allergic reaction that leads to a toxic effect on granulocytes. The other one is only toxic and dose-dependant [11]. The mortality of metamizol-induced agranulocytosis is low (9%), and leucopenia is reversible after withdrawal of metamizol. More hazardous is the intravenous application. Hypotension can be caused by the high osmolarity and the relaxing effect on smooth muscles. Mortality can be up to 25% [12].

In many fragility fracture patients, opioids are required for sufficient pain relief, at least for some days. On one hand, starting dose should be low, on the other hand sufficient pain treatment from the beginning is crucial for the outcome. So it is reasonable to start with a single low dose and adapt the dose immediately, if pain relief is not sufficient. Especially for starting opioids, nausea, vomiting, and obstipation are frequent side effects. To minimize these side effects, opioids should be prescribed in combination with antiemetics, like metoclopramide, and laxatives. The risk of interactions with other drugs is small. Hydromorphone is recommended as first choice. It can also be used in patients with impaired renal function. In patients with a combination of nociceptive and neuropathic pain, tapendatol (starting does 50 mg twice) is a good option. Oral application is always first choice. Intravenous is an alternative way, if swallowing is impossible or not safe. Transdermal application is not useful.

Adjuvant drugs, like antidepressants, do not play any role in this indication. Antiepileptics may help in some patients with mixed pain. However, possible side effects are more relevant than the benefit of pain treatment.

15.3.4 Non-Pharmacological Treatment

Besides drug treatment, non-pharmacological interventions should be integrated in pain management. Benefit to risk ratio is excellent. Early mobilization, physical therapy, positioning, ice, massage therapy, acupuncture/acupressure, and the use of transcutaneous electrical nerve stimulation (TENS) help to save drugs and their doses, and for some intervention, there is evidence in terms of reduction of mortality, reduced length of stay, and physical disability [13].

Key Messages

Pain has to be seen as the fifth vital sign.

Pain assessment in older fragility patients is difficult and needs special consideration.

Sufficient pain relief is essential for good outcome.

NSAIDs are more or less contraindicated.

Non-opioids: use Acetaminophen and Metamizol (be aware of local situation)

Opioids: first choice Hydromorphone or Tapentadol

Create an own SOP, in accordance to your local situation.

Do not forget non-pharmacological treatment of pain!

References

1. Liu SS, Wu CL. The effect of analgesic technique on postoperative patient-reported outcomes including analgesia: a systematic review. Anesth Analg. 2007;105(3):789–808.
2. Abdulla A, Adams N, Bone M, Elliott AM, Gaffin J, Jones D, et al. Guidance on the management of pain in older people. Age Ageing. 2013;42(Suppl 1):i1–57.
3. Fillit HM, Rockwood K, Woodhouse K, editors. B B. Pain in older adults. 7th ed. Philadelphia: Saunders/ Elsevier Health Science; 2010.
4. Lukas A, Niederecker T, Gunther I, Mayer B, Nikolaus T. Self- and proxy report for the assessment of pain in patients with and without cognitive impairment: experiences gained in a geriatric hospital. Z Gerontol Geriatr. 2013;46(3):214–21.
5. Hadjistavropoulos T, Herr K, Prkachin KM, Craig KD, Gibson SJ, Lukas A, et al. Pain assessment in elderly adults with dementia. Lancet Neurol. 2014;13(12):1216–27.
6. Guay J, Parker MJ, Griffiths R, Kopp S. Peripheral nerve blocks for hip fractures. Cochrane Database Syst Rev. 2017;5:CD001159.
7. Sinatra RS, Jahr JS, Reynolds L, Groudine SB, Royal MA, Breitmeyer JB, et al. Intravenous acetaminophen for pain after major orthopedic surgery: an expanded analysis. Pain Pract. 2012;12(5):357–65.
8. Gonzalez-Perez A, Rodriguez LA. Upper gastrointestinal complications among users of paracetamol. Basic Clin Pharmacol Toxicol. 2006;98(3):297–303.
9. Mahe I, Bertrand N, Drouet L, Bal Dit Sollier C, Simoneau G, Mazoyer E, et al. Interaction between paracetamol and warfarin in patients: a double-blind, placebo-controlled, randomized study. Haematologica. 2006;91(12):1621–7.
10. Roberts E, Delgado Nunes V, Buckner S, Latchem S, Constanti M, Miller P, et al. Paracetamol: not as safe as we thought? A systematic literature review of observational studies. Ann Rheum Dis. 2016;75(3):552–9.
11. Gosch M, Bohmdorfer B, Benvenuti-Falger U, Dovjak P, Iglseder B, Lechleitner M, et al. Polypharmacy and pain treatment. Wien Med Wochenschr. 2010;160(11–12):286–92.
12. Lampl C, Likar R. Metamizole (dipyrone): mode of action, drug-drug interactions, and risk of agranulocytosis. Schmerz. 2014;28(6):584–90.
13. Siu AL, Penrod JD, Boockvar KS, Koval K, Strauss E, Morrison RS. Early ambulation after hip fracture: effects on function and mortality. Arch Intern Med. 2006;166(7):766–71.

Polypharmacy: Less is More

16

Thomas Münzer

16.1 Introduction

Older trauma patients often present with chronic disease that may interfere or even complicate perioperative management. As with the number of diseases, the number of medical treatments is rising significantly. Especially frail older persons take more medications than non-frail persons [1]. While the primary focus of care should be trauma surgery, geriatric medical expertise may help to improve outcome [2, 3]. Pharmacological treatment of geriatric trauma patients is complex because of several services and disciplines are involved. This includes emergency room staff, anesthesiologists, surgeons, and geriatricians. To provide a structured approach to the complex management of polypharmacy in geriatric trauma patients, the following chapter is divided into six periods that aim to follow a typical patient pathway with focus on pharmacological treatment of geriatric trauma patients. During the clinical course, these periods normally overlap (Fig. 16.1). Given that polypharmacy is associated with higher mortality in geriatric patients, all measures to reduce medication load may improve outcome [4].

T. Münzer (✉)
Geriatric Medicine, University of Zurich Medical School, Zurich, Switzerland

Geriatrische Klinik St. Gallen, St. Gallen, Switzerland
e-mail: thomasmuenzer@geriatrie-sg.ch

16.2 Pre-Trauma Period

At a first glance, it does not seem important to collect a medication history of drugs older people took before a trauma event. Nevertheless, such information might help to avoid serious perioperative adverse events. This is especially true, when information is not transferred adequately or even missing. For example: knowing the type and the dose of a sleeping pill in an old person suffering from chronic insomnia and reinstalling this drug immediately after surgery may help to avoid severe postoperative withdrawal delirium [5]. Similarly, alcohol or drug abuse information is very helpful for the estimation of the perioperative delirium risk. Furthermore, information on chronic pain as well as type and dose and pain medication might help to give guidance for postoperative pain management. Finally, functional and cognitive capacities during the time preceding the trauma are important elements for the management of polypharmacy. Information on both factors may help to determine the degree of preoperative medication adherence. A patient who was not able to take the medication because of functional problems or did not take the medication as prescribed because of cognitive problems might be at extremely high risk for postoperative complications [6]. The initial trauma is a risk factor for following trauma events in an older person.

H.-C. Pape et al. (eds.), *Senior Trauma Patients*, https://doi.org/10.1007/978-3-030-91483-7_16

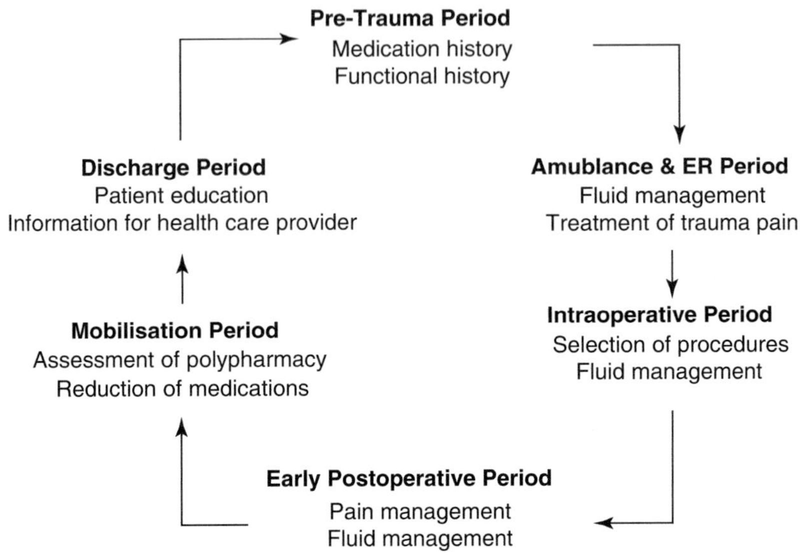

Fig. 16.1 Geriatric trauma treatment periods and key tasks

16.3 Ambulance and Emergency Room Period

Several key elements characterize geriatric acute trauma patients during transportation and their stay in an emergency room. In this early phase, most older trauma patients receive an intravenous line and crystalloid fluids or plasma extenders. After an acute trauma, patients are often not able to take their regular oral medication. Usually pain management involves intravenous opioids or other anesthetics. Thus, medication is rather *added* than reduced. From a geriatric point of view, preoperative fluid management in old trauma patients should be monitored very carefully. The goal of fluid therapy should be to compensate for potential blood loss and to provide a physiological circulating volume. Older persons usually have a low thirst and drink less [7]. It is clinically very difficult to estimate hydration status in geriatric patients [8, 9]. Thus in this early phase, volume management should be the main pharmacological intervention. The goal should be to avoid postoperative fluid overload which is associated with higher mortality [10]. Due to the several consequences of preoperative volume overload, all disciplines involved in the management of the geriatric trauma patients should receive appropriate training.

16.4 Intraoperative Period

The time interval between trauma and surgery, the type of the surgical approach as well as the selection of prosthetic materials that allow immediate postoperative full weight bearing are key elements of a successful geriatric trauma management [11]. In addition, the selection of the anesthesia method in geriatric trauma patients is as important as using an operation procedure that induces minimal surgical trauma. Regional anesthesia is the preferred method in geriatric patients since they have lesser delirium risks [12]. Combined methods using low doses of analgetic and anesthetic drugs may be beneficial for geriatric trauma patients [12]. Older persons tend to be very sensitive to anesthetics and might suffer from severe drops in blood pressure during general anesthesia. Normally, such a situation triggers an increase in crystalloid infusion rate. Thus, intraoperatively fluid management should be tailored to the minimal amount of volume possible.

16.5 Early Postoperative Period

In this early phase, geriatric trauma patients suffer from immobilization and pain and have a high risk of venous thromboembolism which leads to increased mortality [13, 14]. Usually they have indwelling catheters and still receive intravenous fluids. Due to several factors, geriatric patients are prone to edema that may impact upon wound healing [15]. Given that geriatric trauma patients should be mobilized as early as possible, this phase should preferably concentrate on optimal pain management. Usually WHO step 1 medication such as paracetamol (acetaminophen) is well-tolerated and can be given intravenously [16]. Although there is no clear recommendation for geriatric patients, dose should be reduced in frail persons with low body weight [17]. If opioids are needed, short acting drugs are recommended in order to avoid overdoses [18]. Due to age-associated changes in body composition such as decreased muscle mass and increased fat mass, older patients are at higher risk for opioid accumulation and should be frequently assessed for incidental delirium and opioid toxicity [19]. A structured pain assessment in geriatric trauma patients helps to apply the lowest possible dose and serves as a basis for the adaptation of pain medication during early mobilization (see also Chap. 15).

16.6 Mobilization and Discharge Period

This period is characterized by therapeutic interventions aiming at "getting the persons back on their feet". The analgetic drugs should now be tailored to the patient's therapy schedule allowing additional on-demand drug doses prior to a given therapeutic session. Again, a structured pain assessment helps to adjust the patient's analgetic needs and to determine the minimally effective dose. Removal of indwelling bladder catheters and unnecessary intravenous lines is a simple measure to decrease the incidence perioperative delirium [20]. Postoperative early mobilization might be accompanied with orthostatic dysregulation which is associated with a high risk of falls [21]. To approach this problem, fast acting antihypertensive drugs such as calcium channel blockers should be used with caution.

Several studies have examined the use of proton pump inhibitors (PPI) in geriatric patients in the perioperative setting. Due to low evidence and the number of adverse events, PPI should be tapered as soon as possible in all patients without a medical indication for the long-term use [22]. Insomnia is a common perioperative problem. In patients complaining about sleep problems, all avoidable factors causing sleeplessness should be identified. Non-pharmacological interventions should be tried first. A good alternative to benzodiazepines and z-drugs are low dose antidepressants with sleep-inducing properties such as mirtazapine.

Geriatricians systematically assess and manage comorbidities and over- or undertreatment in old patients [23]. The goal of such an intervention is to reduce medication-associated adverse events. Potentially inappropriate medications (PIMS) can cause significant medical problems and are associated with increased mortality [24] or delayed recovery [25]. Indeed, many prescribed drugs may lead to falls [26, 27] or induce delirium [28]. Thus, polypharmacy poses a high risk for older persons. This is especially true for drugs that act centrally such as benzodiazepines, z-drugs (e.g., zolpidem), antidepressants, or neuroleptic drugs. However, other commonly used medications such as opioids, GABA receptor agonists, or dopaminergic substances do have significant central activities and are frequently associated with falls and fractures.

To manage polypharmacy, several positive and negative lists provide evidenced-based recommendations on which medication should be prescribed, avoided, or replaced [29]. Other lists have used a Delphi method approach having experts in the field decide on which drugs may help or harm older patients [30]. Finally, geriatric societies from different countries have made recommendations on the use of pharmaceutical drugs in older persons [31].

All these recommendations have been developed for a *non-trauma* setting and do not necessarily reflect the needs of a geriatric trauma patient. In this special situation, the decision on which medication can be tapered, stopped, or replaced is far more difficult [32]. In preparation for discharge, regular medication lists should be screened based on a benefit to risk ratio approach. Drugs with high risks of adverse events and low long-term benefit to the patients (see Fig. 16.2) should be replaced or avoided at all. This is especially important in frail person with limited life expectancy [33]. The major goal of perioperative medication management should be to tailor all pharmacological interventions to the patients' individual needs and always aim to the lowest effective dose [23]. A simple categorization of drugs ranging from A to D has been shown to induce a deprescribing process in a nonsurgical setting [31]. A few services have managed to decrease the number of PIMS during a hospital stay using a comanagement approach in trauma patients [34].

During ward rounds, geriatric trauma patients should be regularly informed about modifications of their drug regimen. Important additional measures to improve adherence to reductions or adaptations is to involve family members and caregivers [35]. The explanation of a change in a new regimen can, however, be time-consuming and sometimes needs several attempts. In preparation for discharge, a medication plan that explains the dosage and reason to take any given drug improves adherence significantly [35]. Relevant modifications in the medication plan should be also communicated to the primary care providers [36]. This will help to reduce barriers and implement such recommendations effectively.

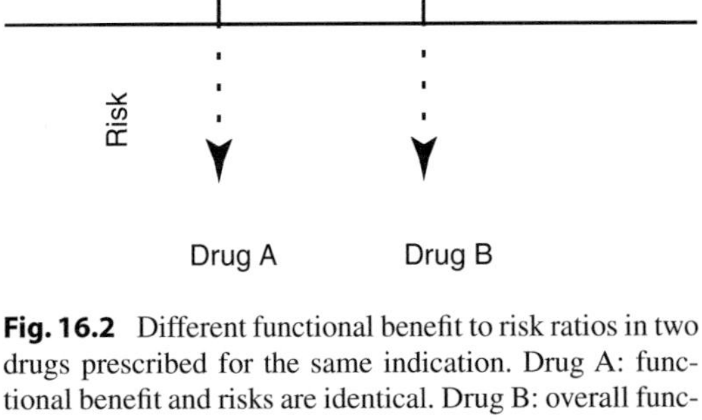

Fig. 16.2 Different functional benefit to risk ratios in two drugs prescribed for the same indication. Drug A: functional benefit and risks are identical. Drug B: overall functional benefit exceeds functional risk

In summary, managing medical treatment in geriatric trauma patients can be divided into several periods. Each period has a specific treatment focus that may increase the total medication load. As soon as older trauma patients are stable and during early mobilization, a sound assessment of current drugs and pre-trauma polypharmacy should trigger interventions that aim to reduce potentially dangerous drugs. Several tables and list may provide information on medications that should be avoided. These are currently not different from those used in a non-trauma setting.

References

1. Bennett A, Gnjidic D, Gillett M, Carroll P, Matthews S, Johnell K, et al. Prevalence and impact of fall-risk-increasing drugs, polypharmacy, and drug-drug interactions in robust versus frail hospitalised falls patients: a prospective cohort study. Drugs Aging. 2014;31(3):225–32.
2. Knobe M, Pape H-C. Focus on co-management in geriatric fracture care. Eur J Trauma Emerg Surg. 2016;42(5):533–5.
3. Gosch M, Hoffmann-Weltin Y, Roth T, Blauth M, Nicholas JA, Kammerlander C. Orthogeriatric co-management improves the outcome of long-term care residents with fragility fractures. Arch Orthop Trauma Surg. 2016;136(10):1403–9.
4. Nossaman VE, Larsen BE, DiGiacomo JC, Manuelyan Z, Afram R, Shukry S, et al. Mortality is predicted by Comorbidity Polypharmacy score but not Charlson Comorbidity Index in geriatric trauma patients. Am J Surg. 2018;216(1):42–5.
5. Ng BJ, Le Couteur DG, Hilmer SN. Deprescribing benzodiazepines in older patients: impact of interventions targeting physicians, pharmacists, and patients. Drugs Aging. 2018;35(6):493–521.
6. Yang Y, Zhao X, Dong T, Yang Z, Zhang Q, Zhang Y. Risk factors for postoperative delirium following hip fracture repair in elderly patients: a systematic review and meta-analysis. Aging Clin Exp Res. 2017;29(2):115–26.
7. Volkert D, Kreuel K, Stehle P. Fluid intake of community-living, independent elderly in Germany--a nationwide, representative study. J Nutr Health Aging. 2005;9(5):305–9.
8. Johnson P, Hahn RG. Signs of dehydration in nursing home residents. J Am Med Dir Assoc. 2018;19(12):1124–8.

9. Hooper L, Abdelhamid A, Attreed NJ, Campbell WW, Channell AM, Chassagne P, et al. Clinical symptoms, signs and tests for identification of impending and current water-loss dehydration in older people. Cochrane Database Syst Rev. 2015;(4):Cd009647.
10. Malbrain ML, Marik PE, Witters I, Cordemans C, Kirkpatrick AW, Roberts DJ, et al. Fluid overload, de-resuscitation, and outcomes in critically ill or injured patients: a systematic review with suggestions for clinical practice. Anaesthesiol Intensive Ther. 2014;46(5):361–80.
11. Neuerburg C, Gosch M, Bocker W, Blauth M, Kammerlander C. Proximal femoral fractures in the elderly. Z Gerontol Geriatr. 2015;48(7):647–59; quiz 60-1
12. Luger MF, Luger TJ. Anesthesiological care of trauma patients in orthogeriatric co-management. Anaesthesist. 2017;66(5):375–92.
13. Kim DY, Kobayashi L, Barmparas G, Fortlage D, Curry T, Coimbra R. Venous thromboembolism in the elderly: the result of comorbid conditions or a consequence of injury? J Trauma Acute Care Surg. 2012;72(5):1286–91.
14. Siu CW, Sun NC, Lau TW, Yiu KH, Leung F, Tse HF. Preoperative cardiac risk assessment in geriatric patients with hip fractures: an orthopedic surgeons' perspective. Osteoporos Int. 2010;21(Suppl 4):S587–91.
15. Myles PS, Andrews S, Nicholson J, Lobo DN, Mythen M. Contemporary approaches to perioperative IV fluid therapy. World J Surg. 2017;41(10):2457–63.
16. McNicol ED, Ferguson MC, Haroutounian S, Carr DB, Schumann R. Single dose intravenous paracetamol or intravenous propacetamol for postoperative pain. Cochrane Database Syst Rev. 2016;(5):Cd007126.
17. What dose of paracetamol for older people? Drug Ther Bull. 2018;56(6):69–72.
18. Miller M, Barber CW, Leatherman S, Fonda J, Hermos JA, Cho K, et al. Prescription opioid duration of action and the risk of unintentional overdose among patients receiving opioid therapy. JAMA Intern Med. 2015;175(4):608–15.
19. Swart LM, van der Zanden V, Spies PE, de Rooij SE, van Munster BC. The comparative risk of delirium with different opioids: a systematic review. Drugs Aging. 2017;34(6):437–43.
20. Inouye SK, Bogardus ST Jr, Charpentier PA, Leo-Summers L, Acampora D, Holford TR, et al. A multicomponent intervention to prevent delirium in hospitalized older patients. N Engl J Med. 1999;340(9):669–76.
21. Jans O, Bundgaard-Nielsen M, Solgaard S, Johansson PI, Kehlet H. Orthostatic intolerance during early mobilization after fast-track hip arthroplasty. Br J Anaesth. 2012;108(3):436–43.
22. Alhazzani W, Alshamsi F, Belley-Cote E, Heels-Ansdell D, Brignardello-Petersen R, Alquraini M, et al. Efficacy and safety of stress ulcer prophylaxis in critically ill patients: a network meta-analysis of randomized trials. Intensive Care Med. 2018;44(1):1–11.
23. Colburn JL, Mohanty S, Burton JR. Surgical guidelines for perioperative management of older adults: what geriatricians need to know. J Am Geriatr Soc. 2017;65(6):1339–46.
24. Muhlack DC, Hoppe LK, Weberpals J, Brenner H, Schottker B. The association of potentially inappropriate medication at older age with cardiovascular events and overall mortality: a systematic review and meta-analysis of cohort studies. J Am Med Dir Assoc. 2017;18(3):211–20.
25. Iaboni A, Rawson K, Burkett C, Lenze EJ, Flint AJ. Potentially inappropriate medications and the time to full functional recovery after hip fracture. Drugs Aging. 2017;34(9):723–8.
26. Kragh Ekstam A, Elmstahl S. Do fall-risk-increasing drugs have an impact on mortality in older hip fracture patients? A population-based cohort study. Clin Interv Aging. 2016;11:489–96.
27. Rubenstein LZ. Falls in older people: epidemiology, risk factors and strategies for prevention. Age Ageing. 2006;35(Suppl 2):ii37–41.
28. Marcantonio ER. Delirium in hospitalized older adults. N Engl J Med. 2017;377(15):1456–66.
29. American Geriatrics Society 2015 updated beers criteria for potentially inappropriate medication use in older adults. J Am Geriatr Soc. 2015;63(11):2227–46.
30. Wehling M, Burkhardt H, Kuhn-Thiel A, Pazan F, Throm C, Weiss C, et al. VALFORTA: a randomised trial to validate the FORTA (Fit fOR The Aged) classification. Age Ageing. 2016;45(2):262–7.
31. American Geriatrics Society identifies another five things that healthcare providers and patients should question. J Am Geriatr Soc. 2014;62(5):950–60.
32. Lester E, Dykstra M, Grant C, Fawcett V, Tsang B, Widder S. High-risk medications in older patients with trauma: a cross-sectional study of risk mitigation. Can J Surg. 2019;62(2):100–4.
33. Lavan AH, Gallagher P, Parsons C, O'Mahony D. STOPPFrail (Screening Tool of Older Persons Prescriptions in Frail adults with limited life expectancy): consensus validation. Age Ageing. 2017;46(4):600–7.
34. Gleich J, Pfeufer D, Zeckey C, Bocker W, Gosch M, Kammerlander C, et al. Orthogeriatric treatment reduces potential inappropriate medication in older trauma patients: a retrospective, dual-center study comparing conventional trauma care and co-managed treatment. Eur J Med Res. 2019;24(1):4.
35. Reeve E, Thompson W, Farrell B. Deprescribing: A narrative review of the evidence and practical recommendations for recognizing opportunities and taking action. Eur J Intern Med. 2017;38:3–11.
36. Gillespie RJ, Harrison L, Mullan J. Deprescribing medications for older adults in the primary care context: A mixed studies review. Health Sci Reports. 2018;1(7):e45.

17 Perioperative Care Program: Zurich-POPS Zurich-PeriOperative-care-for-older-PatientS

Heike A. Bischoff-Ferrari

17.1 Introduction

Perioperative care of patients aged 70 and older who suffered a fall-related injury such as a fragility fracture poses many challenges such as delirium and multi-morbidity plus polypharmacy as well as malnutrition and frailty [1–3]. The need for new care concepts and research to overcome these challenges is enormous.

While fracture liaison services (FLS) have been successfully implemented in many acute care settings worldwide [4, 5], senior trauma centers that follow a next level shared-care concept are being established and evaluated [6]. In this chapter, we describe Zurich-POPS, as a model for an integrated care concept developed at the University Hospital in Zurich (Zurich-POPS). Next to its clinical concept of shared and integrated care described below, Zurich-POPS defined a complete research agenda to further improve care of older adults with fall-related injuries and fragility fractures.

17.2 Evidence for Shared-Care Models

Zurich-POPS builds on prior evidence that shared care between traumatologists and geriatricians reduces length-of-stay and post-surgery complications most effectively compared to consultation models [7]. A recent meta-analysis compared 18 studies with 9094 patients for three subgroups of orthogeriatric care after hip fracture: routine geriatric consultation, geriatric ward with orthopedic consultation, and shared care [7]. The overall results suggested that ortho-geriatric collaboration was associated with a significant reduction of in-hospital mortality (RR 0.60, 95%CI 0.43, 0.84) and long-term mortality (RR 0.83, 95%CI 0.74, 0.94). Also, length of stay (SMD −0.25, 95%CI −0.44, −0.05) was significantly reduced, and this was most pronounced in the shared-care model (SMD −0.61, 95%CI −0.95, −0.28) [7].

With regard to health economic considerations, based on data from 11 acute hospitals in a region of England [8], both nurse-led FLS models and shared-care models between orthopedic surgery and geriatrics were cost-effective, while the shared-care model was the most cost-effective [8].

H. A. Bischoff-Ferrari (✉)
Department of Aging Medicine and Aging Research, City Hospital Zurich-Waid, Zurich University, Zürich, Switzerland
e-mail: heike.bischoff@usz.ch

H.-C. Pape et al. (eds.), *Senior Trauma Patients*, https://doi.org/10.1007/978-3-030-91483-7_17

17.3 Zurich-POPS Shared and Integrated Care Model

At a clinical level, Zurich-POPS follows a shared-care concept between traumatologists and geriatrics. Every patient aged 70 and older admitted to the traumatology unit for fall-related injuries is seen by a geriatrician within 24 h including pre-surgery recommendations on delirium prevention, medication use, and post-surgery care. Once a patient is enrolled in the shared-care concept, a geriatrician sees the patient regularly together with the traumatologist. Two to 8 weeks after discharge, the patient is seen by both the traumatologist and the geriatrician to define secondary prevention concepts based on the repeat comprehensive geriatric assessment, including fall risk and bone density measurement.

17.3.1 Specific Clinical Care Components of Zurich-POPS

Zurich-POPs developed a comprehensive geriatric assessment from which individualized recommendations are derived and implemented by an interprofessional team of doctors, physiotherapists, expert nurses, dieticians, and social workers—see Zurich-POPS communication tool in Fig. 17.1.

Further, Zurich-POPs includes an **early rehabilitation program** implemented by an interprofessional team of geriatricians, physiotherapist, dieticians, and nursing experts in parallel to acute medical care. Early rehabilitation includes two therapy sessions per day, protein supplementation, and weekly interprofessional team meetings to define goals and progress of the patient. In addition to acute care and rehabilitation treatment recommendations, the Zurich-POPS assessment supports post-hospital care need planning of post-hospital care needs, involving family and other proxies, as well as the general practitioner of the patient.

17.4 Zurich POPS 3-Step Research Agenda

- *Step 1:* To assess the risk of frailty, comorbidity, polypharmacy, functional impairment, malnutrition, delirium risk, cognitive impairment, and quality of life among consecutive patients admitted to the senior trauma center at the University Hospital Zurich [1–3].
- *Step 2:* To test new treatment strategies for both muscle and bone health in high-quality randomized controlled trials for their effect on the outcome after a fall or after a fragility fracture among older adults.

  - The Zurich Disability Prevention trial [9–11] and the Zurich Hip Fracture trial [1, 12–14]) focused on vitamin D supplementation and a simple home exercise program.
  - The ongoing trials focus on whey protein with or without exercise (STRONG ClinicalTrials.gov Identifier: NCT03417531) among pre-frail older adults with a fall-related injury and a home-based rehabilitation program among patients after acute hip fracture (STARK ClinicalTrials.gov Identifier: NCT03154684).
  - The largest European healthy aging trial focuses on vitamin D, omega-3, and a simple home exercise program for the prevention of falls, injurious falls, and fractures (DO-HEALTHClinicalTrials.gov Identifier: NCT01745263).

- *Step 3:* Collaboration within international guidelines on fragility fracture care [15–17], sarcopenia [16, 18–21], and frailty [21, 22].

In summary, the Zurich-POPS's shared- and integrated care concept may help to further advance shared- and integrated care concepts for older patients with fragility fractures.

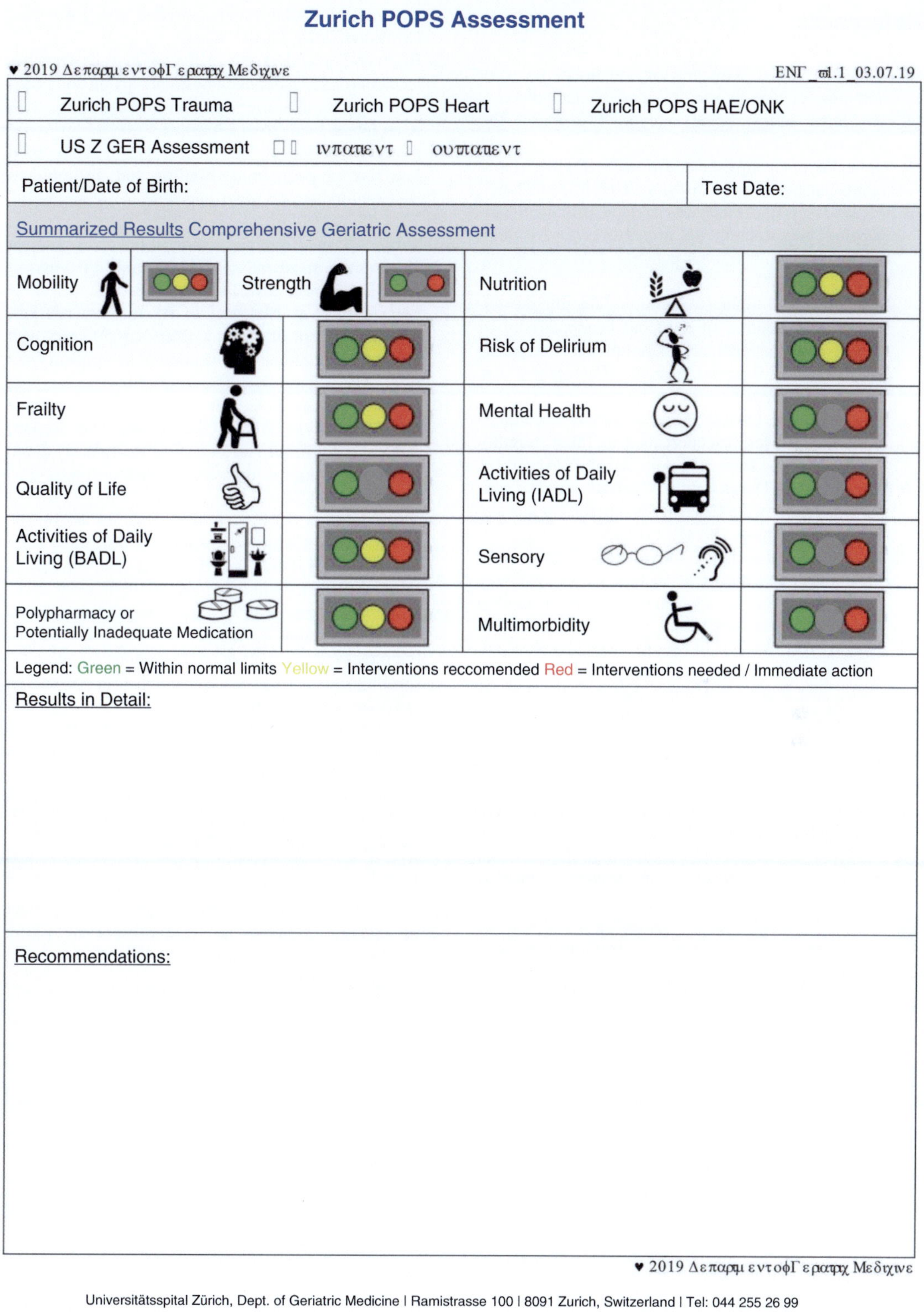

Zurich POPS Assessment

♥ 2019 Δεπαρτμεντοφ Γεριατριχ Μεδιχινε ENΓ_ϖl.1_03.07.19

☐ Zurich POPS Trauma	☐ Zurich POPS Heart	☐ Zurich POPS HAE/ONK
☐ US Z GER Assessment ☐ ☐ ινπατιεντ ☐ ουτπατιεντ		
Patient/Date of Birth:		Test Date:

Summarized Results Comprehensive Geriatric Assessment

Mobility		Nutrition	
Strength			
Cognition		Risk of Delirium	
Frailty		Mental Health	
Quality of Life		Activities of Daily Living (IADL)	
Activities of Daily Living (BADL)		Sensory	
Polypharmacy or Potentially Inadequate Medication		Multimorbidity	

Legend: Green = Within normal limits Yellow = Interventions reccomended Red = Interventions needed / Immediate action

Results in Detail:

Recommendations:

♥ 2019 Δεπαρτμεντ οφ Γεριατριχ Μεδιχινε

Universitätsspital Zürich, Dept. of Geriatric Medicine I Ramistrasse 100 I 8091 Zurich, Switzerland I Tel: 044 255 26 99

Fig. 17.1 Zurich-POPS assessment

References

1. Fischer K, et al. Timeline of functional recovery after hip fracture in seniors aged 65 and older: a prospective observational analysis. Osteoporos Int. 2019;30(7):1371–81.
2. Muller FS, et al. Impaired nutritional status in geriatric trauma patients. Eur J Clin Nutr. 2017;71(5):602–6.
3. Wiegand A, et al. Association of depression with malnutrition, grip strength and impaired cognitive function among senior trauma patients. J Affect Disord. 2019;247:175–82.
4. Javaid MK, et al. Effective secondary fracture prevention: implementation of a global benchmarking of clinical quality using the IOF Capture the Fracture(R) Best Practice Framework tool. Osteoporos Int. 2015;26(11):2573–8.
5. Bunta AD, et al. Own the bone, a system-based intervention, improves osteoporosis care after fragility fractures. J Bone Joint Surg Am. 2016;98(24):e109.
6. Pape HC, et al. Development of geriatric trauma centers—an effort by the German Society for Trauma and Orthopaedics. Injury. 2014;45(10):1513–5.
7. Grigoryan KV, Javedan H, Rudolph JL. Orthogeriatric care models and outcomes in hip fracture patients: a systematic review and meta-analysis. J Orthop Trauma. 2014;28(3):e49–55.
8. Judge A, et al.. Models of care for the delivery of secondary fracture prevention after hip fracture: a health service cost, clinical outcomes and cost-effectiveness study within a region of England. Southampton (UK); 2016.
9. Bischoff-Ferrari HA, et al. Monthly high-dose vitamin D treatment for the prevention of functional decline: a randomized clinical trial. JAMA Intern Med. 2016;176(2):175–83.
10. Gugger A, et al. Effect of monthly high-dose vitamin D on mental health in older adults: secondary analysis of a RCT. J Am Geriatr Soc. 2019;67(6):1211–7.
11. Schlogl M, et al. Effect of monthly vitamin D on chronic pain among community-dwelling seniors: a randomized, double-blind controlled trial. J Am Med Dir Assoc. 2019;20(3):356–61.
12. Bischoff-Ferrari HA, et al. Effect of high-dosage cholecalciferol and extended physiotherapy on complications after hip fracture: a randomized controlled trial. Arch Intern Med. 2010;170(9):813–20.
13. Finsterwald M, et al. Gender-specific hip fracture risk in community-dwelling and institutionalized seniors age 65 years and older. Osteoporos Int. 2014;25(1):167–76.
14. Teister CJ, et al. Which method of fall ascertainment captures the most falls in prefrail and frail seniors? Am J Epidemiol. 2018;187(10):2243–51.
15. Lems WF, et al. EULAR/EFORT recommendations for management of patients older than 50 years with a fragility fracture and prevention of subsequent fractures. Ann Rheum Dis. 2017;76(5):802–10.
16. Bischoff-Ferrari HA. Three steps to unbreakable bones: the 2011 World Osteoporosis Day Report; 2011. https://www.iofbonehealth.org/news/three-steps-unbreakable-bones-world-osteoporosis-day. Accessed 6/11/2016.
17. Vellas B, et al. Designing drug trials for sarcopenia in older adults with hip fracture—a task force from the international conference onfrailty and sarcopenia research (Icfsr). J Frailty Aging. 2014;3(4):199–204.
18. Bischoff-Ferrari HA, et al. Comparative performance of current definitions of sarcopenia against the prospective incidence of falls among community-dwelling seniors age 65 and older. Osteoporos Int. 2015;26(12):2793–802.
19. Abellan van Kan G, et al. Carla task force on sarcopenia: propositions for clinical trials. J Nutr Health Aging. 2009;13(8):700–7.
20. Reginster JY, et al. Recommendations for the conduct of clinical trials for drugs to treat or prevent sarcopenia. Aging Clin Exp Res. 2016;28(1):47–58.
21. Rizzoli R, et al. Quality of life in sarcopenia and frailty. Calcif Tissue Int. 2013;93(2):101–20.
22. Bischoff HA, Staehelin HB, Willett WC. The effect of undernutrition in the development of frailty in older persons. J Gerontol A Biol Sci Med Sci. 2006;61(6):585–9.

18 Palliative Care Concepts

Mathias Schlögl

18.1 The Need for Palliative Care

Palliative care is an approach that improves the quality of life of patients and their families who are facing problems associated with life-threatening illness [1]. It prevents and relieves suffering through the early identification, correct assessment, and treatment of pain and other problems. Palliative care is the prevention and relief of suffering of any kind—physical, psychological, social, or spiritual—experienced by patients living with life-limiting health problems. It promotes dignity, quality of life, and adjustment to progressive illnesses, using best available evidence. It already begins when the illness is diagnosed—and continues regardless of whether or not a patient receives treatment directed at the disease [2].

Several trends in healthcare suggest that there is an urgent need for integrating palliative care into trauma care [3]. First, despite all efforts, 10–15% of trauma patients who make it to the hospital will die from their injuries. Second, as the geriatric population in the United States increases, trauma centers across the country are seeing older trauma patients. Patients aged 65 years or older account for 20% of all hospital trauma-related admissions [3]. Of trauma patients admitted to the intensive care unit (ICU) in this age group, 10–20% die of their injuries [4, 5]. Finally, in recent years, a greater focus on quality of life and functional outcomes as endpoints along with survival became important in trauma care. Several studies, for example, suggest that if greater attention is paid to interventions in the acute hospital setting to improve parameters such as psychosocial support and symptom management, long-term functional outcomes and quality of life may be improved [6, 7].

18.2 Palliative Care Interventions and Concepts for Surgical Patients

In 2003, the American College of Surgeons Palliative Care Workgroup [8] identified the following seven domains as potential research targets for studying the applications of palliative care in surgical settings: (a) surgical decision-making, (b) patient decision-making, (c) end-of-life (EOL) decision-making, (d) symptom management, (e) communication, (f) processes of care, and (g) surgical education about palliative care [9].

18.2.1 Surgical Decision-Making

Although innovations to improve preoperative communication and decision-making have been

M. Schlögl (✉)
Department of Acute Geriatric Care, University Clinic for Acute Geriatric Care, City Hospital Waid, Zurich, Switzerland
e-mail: mathias.schloegl@waid.zuerich.ch

H.-C. Pape et al. (eds.), *Senior Trauma Patients*, https://doi.org/10.1007/978-3-030-91483-7_18

described, whether these strategies improve the quality of surgical decisions (i.e., better patient understanding of their disease and procedure, realistic expectations of recovery, reduced decisional regret) or other patient-oriented outcomes is unknown because assessment of these interventions is fraught with multiple serious methodological challenges [9, 10].

For example, Miner and colleagues used a communication technique, the palliative triangle, to guide decisions about palliative surgery for patients with advanced cancer [11]. This model incorporated patients' symptoms, values, and treatment goals to create a context for decisions about surgery or medical treatments. In total, 227 patients symptomatic from advanced incurable cancer receiving a procedure to palliate symptoms of advanced cancer were identified prospectively from all surgical palliative care consultations and observed for at least 90 days or until death. Patients selected for palliative operations using the palliative triangle approach had higher rates of symptom resolution (90.7% vs 80.0%), longer overall survival (median, 528 vs 194 days), and lower associated 30-day morbidity (20.1% vs 40%) and mortality (3.9% vs 11.0%) [11].

In another study, Tan and colleagues tailored perioperative care to older patients who underwent major colorectal surgery with emphasis on preoperative evaluation, pre-rehabilitation, psychosocial needs, and functional recovery [12]. The broad input from a transdisciplinary team informed surgical decision-making. Compared with patients receiving usual care, patients whose treatment was managed by this team demonstrated lower rates of 30-day mortality (6.9%vs 9.6%) and major complications (17.2%vs 30.8%) [12].

Finally, other cohort studies by Moorhouse and colleagues suggested that preoperative interventions to better clarify patients' disease understanding and treatment preferences are associated with a decrease in surgical procedures among frail older adults [13].

18.2.2 Patient Decision-Making

Because patients who have surgery are at risk of losing decision-making capacity for prolonged periods, it is important to clarify—before surgery—the desired outcome from the patient's perspective, treatments patients are willing to endure to achieve those outcomes, and postoperative outcomes patients find unacceptable (i.e., prolonged ventilator dependence) [10]. Patients who have major surgical procedures may also have desires to limit burdensome life-supporting treatments after surgery, and those with preexisting directives restricting specific treatments may want to suspend these restrictions during the acute, perioperative period to achieve specific goals [10]. Despite the importance of clarifying treatment preferences before surgery, some surgeons are resistant or reluctant to pursue preoperative advance care planning and data suggest that such conversations are often incomplete, or altogether absent, which can lead to unwanted postoperative treatment and conflict between surgeons and patients. Unless preferences are clarified beforehand, surgeons and surrogates may presume that permission for surgery implies permission for all postoperative treatments necessary to avoid postoperative death [10].

Legal standards for decision-making capacity for consent to treatment vary somewhat across jurisdictions, but generally they embody the following [14]:

- Cognitive ability: the ability to grasp at least the fundamental elements of the information relevant for the decision
- Evaluative ability: the ability to assign a personal meaning to the decision situation, in the light of the various options available
- Decisional ability: the ability to make a decision based on the information available and one's own experience, motives, and values
- Expressive ability: the ability to communicate and defend this decision. The more complex the decision, the greater the demands placed on the mental abilities. Appropriate assessment of these abilities calls for a holistic view of the person concerned.

18.2.3 End-of-Life Decision-Making

Early psychosocial and bereavement support, as well as communication with physicians and nurses, has clearly been shown to improve later

EOL decision-making and reduce conflict. Again, in the trauma setting, this support should be offered to all patients and families, regardless of prognosis; data suggest it not only facilitates EOL care, but may improve overall quality of care in the ICU [15, 16].

For example, a study by Swetz and colleagues found that palliative care consultation for preparedness planning did not increase documentation of advance directives; however, the small sample size was inadequately powered to detect statistically significant differences [17]. In another study, Grimaldo and colleagues found that a brief, anesthesiologist-led information session was associated with a 32% increase in preoperative EOL conversations between patients and their proxies and with a 170% increase in documentation of durable power of attorney compared with the control group [18].

18.2.4 Symptom Management

Several studies examined the role of palliative care in providing symptom management for patients after surgery. In 1997, Axelsson and colleagues [19] studied a home-based palliative support service for postoperative care of patients with symptomatic incurable cancer. Compared with controls, patients receiving the intervention had a shorter median duration of terminal hospitalization (3 vs 10 days), more days at home in the last 2 months of life (44vs 38.5 days), and a mean cost savings of $2500 per patient [19].

Studies by McCorkle and colleagues [20, 21] used home nursing care for postoperative treatment of patients with cancer that involved tailored, specialized care by an advanced practice nurse specializing in oncology, including symptom management, emotional support, and care coordination [20, 21]. Overall, they found increased survival [21], less uncertainty [21], and less symptom distress [20].

18.2.5 Communication

There is an urgent need for an improved communication as a central element in providing goal-concordant care and reducing health care utilization and costs among seriously ill older patients. Given high rates of surgery in the last weeks of life, high risk of poor outcomes after emergency operations in these patients, and barriers to quality communication in the acute setting, it is necessary to support surgeons in communicating with seriously ill, older patients with surgical emergencies [22]

In 1995, a landmark study [23] (The Study to Understand Prognoses and Preferences for Outcomes and Risks of Treatments, SUPPORT) aimed to improve EOL decision-making and reduce the frequency of a mechanically supported, painful, and prolonged process of dying. Overall, this 2-year prospective observational study (phase I) with 4301 patients was followed by a 2-year controlled clinical trial (phase II) with 4804 patients and their physicians randomized by specialty group to the intervention group ($n = 2652$) or control group ($n = 2152$). Physicians in the intervention group received estimates of the likelihood of 6-month survival for every day up to 6 months, outcomes of cardiopulmonary resuscitation (CPR), and functional disability at 2 months. A specifically trained nurse had multiple contacts with the patient, family, physician, and hospital staff to elicit preferences, improve understanding of outcomes, encourage attention to pain control, and facilitate advance care planning and patient-physician communication [23].

In detail, the phase I observation documented shortcomings in communication, frequency of aggressive treatment, and the characteristics of hospital death: only 47% of physicians knew when their patients preferred to avoid CPR; 46% of do-not-resuscitate (DNR) orders were written within 2 days of death; 38% of patients who died spent at least 10 days in an ICU; and for 50% of conscious patients who died in the hospital, family members reported moderate to severe pain at least half the time [23].

During the phase II intervention, patients experienced no improvement in patient-physician communication (e.g., 37% of control patients and 40% of intervention patients discussed CPR preferences) or in the five targeted outcomes, i.e., incidence or timing of written DNR orders (adjusted ratio, 1.02; 95% confidence interval [CI], 0.90 to 1.15), physicians' knowledge of their patients' preferences not to be resuscitated (adjusted ratio, 1.22; 95% CI, 0.99 to 1.49), number of days spent in an ICU, receiving mechanical ventilation, or comatose before death (adjusted ratio, 0.97; 95% CI, 0.87–1.07), or level of reported pain (adjusted ratio, 1.15; 95% CI, 1.00–1.33). The intervention also did not reduce use of hospital resources (adjusted ratio, 1.05; 95% CI, 0.99–1.12) [23].

In 2003, Schneidermann and colleagues investigated whether ethics consultations in the intensive care setting reduce the use of life-sustaining treatments delivered to patients who ultimately did not survive to hospital discharge, as well as the reactions to the consultations of physicians, nurses, and patients/surrogates. This prospective, multicenter, randomized controlled trial in adult ICUs of seven US hospitals representing a spectrum of institutional characteristics enrolled 551 patients who were randomly assigned either to an intervention (ethics consultation offered) ($n = 278$) or to usual care ($n = 273$). Overall, the intervention and usual-care groups showed no difference in mortality. However, ethics consultations were associated with reductions in hospital (−2.95 days, $P = 0.01$) and ICU (−1.44 days, $P = 0.03$) days and life-sustaining treatments (−1.7 days with ventilation, $P = 0.03$) in those patients who ultimately did not survive to discharge. The majority (87%) of physicians, nurses, and patients/surrogates agreed that ethics consultations in the ICU were helpful in addressing treatment conflicts [24].

In 2014, an interdisciplinary panel of 23 national leaders in surgery, palliative medicine, critical care, emergency medicine, geriatrics, anesthesiology, and health care innovation provided a communication framework to help surgeons (1) contextualize how an acute surgical condition relates to the patient's underlying illness; (2) elucidate the patient's goals and priorities with respect to prolonging life, achieving cure, maintaining function and quality of life, and achieving life goals24; (3) understand how to describe treatments, including palliative approaches, that are most closely aligned with patient goals; (4) direct treatment to achieve these outcomes and allow opportunities to reconsider if necessary; and (5) affirm continued commitment to the patient's goals of care no matter their treatment decisions (Table 18.1) [25].

Table 18.1 Key elements of a communication framework [25]

Guide	Clinician steps	Clinician prompts
Prognosis	Gather data about illness trajectory and formulate prognosis. Review prior advance directives.	
Connect and elicit	Address symptoms, express concern for patient's well-being, elicit patient illness understanding	"How would you describe your overall health/functioning lately?
Inform	Disclose information about the acute problem in context of illness trajectory	"It seems that we've hit something today that changes the course of things …"
Summarize	Establish shared understanding of patient's overall condition	"The way I am seeing things is that you have both a serious ongoing medical issue, and a new acute surgical crisis. I think what this means is that …"
Pause	Allow the patient to process the information; respond to patient's emotion	"I can see how upsetting this is …"
Options	Describe the benefits, burdens, and likely outcomes of surgical and nonsurgical options, including palliative treatments, in context of patient's goals	"In your situation, here is what we expect this could look like …"

Table 18.1 (continued)

Guide	Clinician steps	Clinician prompts
Goals	Understand patient's goals, priorities, and tradeoffs. Discuss existing advance directives with the patient or designated surrogate.	"Have you thought about the kind of medical care you would want if you became very sick?" "Are there any treatments or health states that are intolerable to you?" "How much are you willing to go through to try to get you over this crisis?"
Recommend	Recommend a course of treatment in the context of the patient's goals. Consider time-limited trials.	"Based on your priorities, I would recommend we do x. We can meet again in x time and see whether things are getting better or worse and reconsider the options then."
Support	Affirm relationship, describe next steps to patient, document the conversation in the medical record, and communicate with clinical team	"We are all committed to taking great care of you, and respecting your goals."

18.2.6 Process of Care

Several studies aimed to identify surgical patients who could benefit from palliative care consultation that is critical to improving access to these services. In 1991, Fisher and colleagues instituted weekly joint palliative care and surgical ward rounds with a hospital palliative care physician and a general surgeon who specialized in oncologic surgery. Overall, they found a 140% increase in palliative care team referrals after initiation of joint ward rounds and an increase in consultations for symptom management [26]. In 2010, Bradley and colleagues performed a retrospective, pre- and post-intervention study examining the effect of an initiative involving palliative care consultation in a 21-bed ICU at an urban, tertiary referral center [27]. The initiative identified patients meeting a set of consultation triggers suggested by a group of physicians with expertise in surgical palliative care. The charts of 300 patients were reviewed retrospectively before the initiative (Group I), and 344 charts were reviewed after the initiative (Group II) for the presence of a trigger and/or subsequent palliative care consultation.

Less than 30% of patients who met at least one trigger criterion were referred for palliative care consultation, indicating a lack of investment among treating surgeons and intensivists and among patients and their families about the benefits of palliative care in this setting. The triggers, including futility considered or declared by the medical team, death expected during the same surgical ICU stay, and multiple-organ system failure involving more than three systems, identified patients with acute critical illness who were not expected to survive and only approximately 6% of patients met a single trigger [27].

In two studies [28, 29], the authors found an increased rate of palliative care consultation with the use of screening criteria that also identified patients with serious chronic illness who may benefit from palliative care. Furthermore, Ernst and colleagues found preoperative screening and palliative care consultation were associated with an increased rate of cancellations (19.3% vs 5.6%; $P < 0.05$) and decreased mortality among frail older patients at 30, 180, and 360 days [28]

18.2.7 Surgical Education

The need for surgical palliative care education has in part been spurred by the documentation of the shortcomings of the seriously ill, e.g., in the Study to Understand Prognoses and Preferences for Outcomes and Risks of Treatments (SUPPORT) [23, 30]. However, only one measured patient-oriented outcomes. Holloran and colleagues found that a case-based educational intervention for surgical residents improved communication and reduced the surgical ICU length of stay without increasing mortality [31]. Multiple-modality strategies for education, recognizing three different audiences (a) to the practicing surgeon, (b) to surgical educators, and (c) to those who were still in training, are urgently needed [30].

18.2.8 Quality Measures in Surgical Palliative Care

In 2017, the American College of Surgeons conceptualized the surgical episode over five phases of surgical care, including preoperative evaluation, immediate preoperative readiness, intraoperative, postoperative, and post discharge phases. Examples of overlapping and potentially adaptable quality measures are summarized in Table 18.2 [32].

Table 18.2 Existing quality measures relevant for palliative care delivery to surgical patients [32]

Phase of surgical episode	Example quality measures that overlap between surgery and palliative care (*N* = 18)	Examples of palliative care quality measures potentially applicable to surgical patients (*N* = 71)
Preoperative Evaluation and Preparation	Percentage of elderly patients with preoperative discussions of goals and treatment preferences (ACOVE/QIESP)	Percentage of seriously ill patients who received a physical symptom assessment during an inpatient palliative care encounter (NQF/MWM) Percentage of patients with a documented surrogate decision-maker (ACOVE/ASSIST/CCB)
Immediate Preoperative Readiness	None	Proportion of vulnerable elders with continuity of advance directive or care preference documentation between health care settings (ACOVE)
Intraoperative	None	None
Postoperative	Patient's experience with postoperative communication or communication after cancer surgery (CAHPS) Percentage of elderly patients whose documented treatment preferences were followed postoperatively (QIESP)	Percentage of ICU patients with documentation of an interdisciplinary meeting with patient/family (CCB) Percentage of seriously ill patients with documentation of life-sustaining treatment preferences (NQF/ACOVE/MWM)
Postdischarge	Percentage of adult patients with improved ability to self-manage (measured by the Patient Activation Measures questionnaire) in the year after orthopedic surgery (NQF)	Percentage of cancer patients with screening for pain during a cancer-related outpatient visit (ASSIST)
End-of-Life	None	Proportion of older patients with documentation of end of life discussion if diagnosed with incurable cancer (ACOVE) Proportion of patients who died from cancer not admitted to hospice (NQF)

Abbreviations: *ACOVE* Assessing Care of Vulnerable Elders, *CAHPS* Consumer Assessment of Healthcare Providers and Systems, *Cancer-Quality ASSIST* Addressing Symptoms, Side Effects, and Indicators of Supportive Treatment, *CCB* Care and Communication Bundle, *ICU* Intensive care unit, *MWM* Measuring What Matters, *NQF* National Quality Forum, *QIES* Quality Indicators for Elderly Surgical Patients

Importantly, measures unique to surgery, such as documenting preoperative life-sustaining treatment preferences or preoperative palliative symptom assessment for palliative operations, are not captured among current measures. There is an urgent need to adapt and create palliative care quality measures relevant to seriously ill surgical patients. For this, these measures should be tested to establish baseline performance and set goals for improvement, then ultimately integrated into quality improvement programs to improve the value of surgical care for complex seriously ill patients [32].

18.2.9 Evidence-Based Outcomes in Surgical Palliative Care for Frail Elderly Patients

Despite the increasing availability of palliative care, elderly trauma patients continue to have unmet palliative care needs. This is especially true for those who survive their hospital stay but have diminished functional outcomes. It is increasingly clear that frailty and preinjury function are more important predictors of outcome than severity of injury in this population [10].

In 2016, McGreevy, Mosenthal, and colleagues performed a retrospective study of trauma patients aged 55 years or older admitted to the surgical ICU [33]. Using logistic regression, the Palliative Performance Scale (PPS) was assessed as a predictor of mortality, Glasgow Outcome Scale, and discharge destination. Out of 153 patients, 28 died; 28% of the survivors had a Glasgow Outcome Scale 3 or less, and 13% were discharged to dependent care. PPS score of 80 or less was an independent predictor of mortality (odds ratio [OR]: 2.97 [1.08–8.66]), poor functional outcome (OR: 12.59 [4.81–37.07]), and discharge to dependent care (OR: 8.13 [2.64–30.09]), yet only 52% of the patients with PPS of 80 or less received palliative care [33]. Although the same size is relatively small, this study clearly demonstrated that a prognostic tool capable of predicting poor functional outcomes on admission to the trauma center is valuable as a trigger for delivery of palliative care services in this vulnerable population.

In another study, Hwang, Mosenthal, and colleagues performed a prospective observational study of 516 trauma patients aged ≥55 years (mean age 70 years) with preinjury PPS assessed at admission [34]. Primary outcomes were mortality and functional outcomes, measured by Extended Glasgow Outcome Scale (GOSE), at discharge and 6 months. Poor functional outcomes were defined as GOSE score of four or less. Secondary outcomes were patient-reported outcomes at 6 months: EuroQol-5D and 36-ItemShort Form Survey. In summary, older trauma patients with decreased performance status prior to injury are more likely to die in hospital and have poor functional outcomes at discharge and 6 months. Although the overall cohort of survivors improved their functional outcomes over 6 months, those with low PPS had much less improvement, which further highlights the importance of long-term evaluations in multiple domains to assess outcomes and recovery [34].

18.2.10 Defining The Research Priorities

In 2018, the National Institutes of Health and the National Palliative Care Research Center convened researchers from several medical subspecialties to develop a national agenda for palliative care research. The surgeon work group reviewed the existing surgical literature to identify critical knowledge gaps [10]. Priorities for future research on palliative care in surgery include: (1) aligning surgical quality with outcomes that matter to patients [10, 35], (2) communication and decision-making, and (3) delivery of palliative care to surgical patients.

For example, one of the current major pitfalls is the assessment of 30-day mortality, which may motivate surgeons and hospitals to improve outcomes, and theoretically empower patients to make informed choices [35]. However, use of this single metric unintentionally fails to accommodate patients who might benefit from palliative surgery, or patients who would prefer death to prolonged postoperative treatment in the ICU or long-term chronic care after a major complication [10, 35]. Furthermore, defining surgical quality and value based solely on survival duration incentivizes surgeons to prolong life, not improve it, and can impede integration of palliative care. Alternatively, measures of functional independence [36], disability-free survival [37], days spent at home [38], or freedom from pain after surgery provide information on outcomes that are both clinically meaningful and important to patients [10]. Valuable palliative care outcomes should include the alignment between patients' goals and the likely outcomes of surgery, reduction of burdensome, unwanted or non-beneficial postoperative interventions, and improvement in physical and psychological outcomes after surgery [10].

In this context, currently little is known about the palliative care utilization among patients with dementia in possible need of surgical intervention [39]. In 2017, Berlin, Mosenthal, and colleagues retrospectively queried the National Inpatient Sample for patients aged >50 years with dementia and acute abdominal emergency who were admitted nonelectively 2009–2013, utilizing ICD-9-CM codes for dementia and surgical indication and identified predictors of palliative care utilization. Among 15,209 patients, in-hospital mortality was 10.2%, the nonroutine discharge rate was 67.2%, and 7.5% received palliative care. Patients treated operatively were less likely to receive palliative care than those who did not undergo operation (adjusted OR = 0.50; 95% CI 0.41–0.62). Only 6.4% of patients discharged nonroutinely received palliative care. This study clearly demonstrated that patients with dementia and acute abdominal emergency have considerable in-hospital mortality, a high frequency of nonroutine discharge, and low palliative care utilization [39].

In another study, Baker and colleagues performed a qualitative analysis of in-depth elite interviews conducted with a clinical care team involved in management of patients with dementia after hospitalization for hip fractures. Hip fractures in older individuals, even without the presence of dementia, increase the risk of mortality (20%–30% within a year), secondary osteoporotic fractures, and multiple medical complications [40]. These fractures decrease the patient's quality of life due to impaired mobility and the need for increased level of care and supervision [41]. Among survivors, 25% of previously independent patients end up in nursing homes and 60% cannot perform at least one activity of daily living a year after a hip fracture [42]. Patients with dementia are at increased risk for hip fractures, and outcomes after hip fractures are worse [41]. Baker and colleagues showed that the three main themes that most interviewees discussed were pain control, functional status, and medical comorbidities [41]. The emphasis on dementia, advanced directives, and involving family or caregivers by the geriatricians indicated the importance of including geriatricians in the decision-making team for these patients.

In conclusion, as the population ages and technical innovation advances, surgical patients will become increasingly complex. Building the science around palliative care in surgery will require the engagement and support of stakeholders, interdisciplinary collaboration, and development of new, well-trained researchers with interest in this field. The proposed research priorities will provide evidence to support lasting improvements and establish palliative care as a core tenet of high-quality surgical car [10].

References

1. Knaul F, Bhadelia A, Atun R, De Lima L, Radbruch L. Palliative care: an essential facet of universal health coverage. Lancet Glob Health. 2019;7(11):e1488.
2. Powell RA, Mwangi-Powell FN, Radbruch L, Yamey G, Krakauer EL, Spence D, et al. Putting palliative care on the global health agenda. Lancet Oncol. 2015;16(2):131–3.
3. Mosenthal AC, Murphy PA. Trauma care and palliative care: time to integrate the two? J Am Coll Surg. 2003;197(3):509–16.
4. Khandelwal N, Benkeser D, Coe NB, Engelberg RA, Teno JM, Curtis JR. Patterns of cost for patients dying in the intensive care unit and implications for cost savings of palliative care interventions. J Palliat Med. 2016;19(11):1171–8.
5. Zafar SN, Obirieze A, Schneider EB, Hashmi ZG, Scott VK, Greene WR, et al. Outcomes of trauma care at centers treating a higher proportion of older

patients: the case for geriatric trauma centers. J Trauma Acute Care Surg. 2015;78(4):852–9.
6. Michaels AJ, Michaels CE, Smith JS, Moon CH, Peterson C, Long WB. Outcome from injury: general health, work status, and satisfaction 12 months after trauma. J Trauma. 2000;48(5):841–8; discussion 848-850.
7. Schelling G, Stoll C, Haller M, Briegel J, Manert W, Hummel T, et al. Health-related quality of life and posttraumatic stress disorder in survivors of the acute respiratory distress syndrome. Crit Care Med. 1998;26(4):651–9.
8. Office of Promoting Excellence in End-of-Life Care: Surgeon's Palliative Care Workgroup report from the field. J Am Coll Surg. 2003;197(4):661–86.
9. Lilley EJ, Khan KT, Johnston FM, Berlin A, Bader AM, Mosenthal AC, et al. Palliative care interventions for surgical patients: a systematic review. JAMA Surg. 2016;151(2):172–83.
10. Lilley EJ, Cooper Z, Schwarze ML, Mosenthal AC. Palliative care in surgery: defining the research priorities. Ann Surg. 2018;267(1):66–72.
11. Miner TJ, Cohen J, Charpentier K, McPhillips J, Marvell L, Cioffi WG. The palliative triangle: improved patient selection and outcomes associated with palliative operations. Arch Surg Chic Ill 1960. 2011;146(5):517–22.
12. Tan K-Y, Tan P, Tan L. A collaborative transdisciplinary "geriatric surgery service" ensures consistent successful outcomes in elderly colorectal surgery patients. World J Surg. 2011;35(7):1608–14.
13. Moorhouse P, Mallery LH. Palliative and therapeutic harmonization: a model for appropriate decision-making in frail older adults. J Am Geriatr Soc. 2012;60(12):2326–32.
14. Appelbaum PS. Clinical practice. Assessment of patients' competence to consent to treatment. N Engl J Med. 2007;357(18):1834–40.
15. Berlin A, Kunac A, Mosenthal AC. Perioperative goal-setting consultations by surgical colleagues: a new model for supporting patients, families, and surgeons in shared decision making. Ann Palliat Med. 2017;6(2):178–82.
16. McCahill LE, Dunn GP, Mosenthal AC, Milch RA, Krouse RS. Palliation as a core surgical principle: part 1. J Am Coll Surg. 2004;199(1):149–60.
17. Swetz KM, Freeman MR, Abou Ezzeddine OF, Carter KA, Boilson BA, Ottenberg AL, et al. Palliative medicine consultation for preparedness planning in patients receiving left ventricular assist devices as destination therapy. Mayo Clin Proc. 2011;86(6):493–500.
18. Grimaldo DA, Wiener-Kronish JP, Jurson T, Shaughnessy TE, Curtis JR, Liu LL. A randomized, controlled trial of advanced care planning discussions during preoperative evaluations. Anesthesiology. 2001;95(1):43–50; discussion 5A.
19. Axelsson B, Christensen SB. Evaluation of a hospital-based palliative support service with particular regard to financial outcome measures. Palliat Med. 1998;12(1):41–9.
20. McCorkle R, Dowd M, Ercolano E, Schulman-Green D, Williams A, Siefert ML, et al. Effects of a nursing intervention on quality of life outcomes in post-surgical women with gynecological cancers. Psychooncology. 2009;18(1):62–70.
21. McCorkle R, Strumpf NE, Nuamah IF, Adler DC, Cooley ME, Jepson C, et al. A specialized home care intervention improves survival among older post-surgical cancer patients. J Am Geriatr Soc. 2000;48(12):1707–13.
22. Fiorentino M, Hwang F, Pentakota SR, Livingston DH, Mosenthal AC. Palliative care in trauma: not just for the dying. J Trauma Acute Care Surg. 2019;87(5):1156–63.
23. A controlled trial to improve care for seriously ill hospitalized patients. The study to understand prognoses and preferences for outcomes and risks of treatments (SUPPORT), The SUPPORT Principal Investigators. JAMA. 1995;274(20):1591–8.
24. Schneiderman LJ, Gilmer T, Teetzel HD, Dugan DO, Blustein J, Cranford R, et al. Effect of ethics consultations on nonbeneficial life-sustaining treatments in the intensive care setting: a randomized controlled trial. JAMA. 2003;290(9):1166–72.
25. Cooper Z, Koritsanszky LA, Cauley CE, Frydman JL, Bernacki RE, Mosenthal AC, et al. Recommendations for best communication practices to facilitate goal-concordant care for seriously ill older patients with emergency surgical conditions. Ann Surg. 2016;263(1):1–6.
26. Fisher JA, Parker MC. Joint surgical/palliative care ward round in a district general hospital. Palliat Med. 1999;13(3):249–50.
27. Bradley C, Weaver J, Brasel K. Addressing access to palliative care services in the surgical intensive care unit. Surgery. 2010;147(6):871–7.
28. Ernst KF, Hall DE, Schmid KK, Seever G, Lavedan P, Lynch TG, et al. Surgical palliative care consultations over time in relationship to systemwide frailty screening. JAMA Surg. 2014;149(11):1121–6.
29. Sihra L, Harris M, O'Reardon C. Using the improving palliative care in the intensive care unit (IPAL-ICU) project to promote palliative care consultation. J Pain Symptom Manage. 2011;42(5):672–5.
30. Palliation as a core surgical principle: part 2. J Am Coll Surg. 2004;199(2):321–34.
31. Holloran SD, Starkey GW, Burke PA, Steele GJ, Forse RA. An educational intervention in the surgical intensive care unit to improve ethical decisions. Surgery. 1995;118(2):294–8; discussion 298-299.
32. Lee KC, Senglaub SS, Walling AM, Mosenthal AC, Cooper Z. Quality measures in surgical palliative care: adapting existing palliative care measures to improve care for seriously ill surgical patients. Ann Surg. 2019;269(4):607–9.
33. McGreevy CM, Bryczkowski S, Pentakota SR, Berlin A, Lamba S, Mosenthal AC. Unmet palliative care needs in elderly trauma patients: can the Palliative Performance Scale help close the gap? Am J Surg. 2017;213(4):778–84.

34. Hwang F, Pentakota SR, McGreevy CM, Glass NE, Livingston DH, Mosenthal AC. Preinjury Palliative Performance Scale predicts functional outcomes at 6 months in older trauma patients. J Trauma Acute Care Surg. 2019;87(3):541–51.
35. Schwarze ML, Brasel KJ, Mosenthal AC. Beyond 30-day mortality: aligning surgical quality with outcomes that patients value. JAMA Surg. 2014;149(7):631–2.
36. Berian JR, Mohanty S, Ko CY, Rosenthal RA, Robinson TN. Association of loss of independence with readmission and death after discharge in older patients after surgical procedures. JAMA Surg. 2016;151(9):e161689.
37. Shulman MA, Myles PS, Chan MTV, McIlroy DR, Wallace S, Ponsford J. Measurement of disability-free survival after surgery. Anesthesiology. 2015;122(3):524–36.
38. Groff AC, Colla CH, Lee TH. Days spent at home—a patient-centered goal and outcome. N Engl J Med. 2016;375(17):1610–2.
39. Berlin A, Hwang F, Singh R, Pentakota SR, Singh R, Chernock B, et al. Outcomes and palliative care utilization in patients with dementia and acute abdominal emergency: opportunities for surgical quality improvement. Surgery. 2018;163(2):444–9.
40. Bischoff-Ferrari HA, Willett WC, Orav EJ, Lips P, Meunier PJ, Lyons RA, et al. A pooled analysis of vitamin D dose requirements for fracture prevention. N Engl J Med. 2012;367(1):40–9.
41. Baker AC, Ambrose CG, Knudson PL, Saraykar SS, Piller LB, McCurdy SA, et al. Factors considered by interprofessional team for treatment decision in hip fracture with dementia. J Am Geriatr Soc. 2019;67(6):1132–7.
42. Grigoryan KV, Javedan H, Rudolph JL. Orthogeriatric care models and outcomes in hip fracture patients: a systematic review and meta-analysis. J Orthop Trauma. 2014;28(3):e49–55.

Part IV

Fracture Care Service Models

19 Fracture Liaison Service (FLS)—Intersectoral Treatment of the Disease After Osteoporosis-Associated Fractures

Wolfgang Böcker, Eric Hesse, and Christian Kammerlander

19.1 Current Situation

There is an increase in the life expectancy in western societies. Thus, the prevalence of age-related osteoporosis rises as well, leading to an increase in fractures after ground level falls. These patients frequently require in-house treatment and surgeries. The prevalence of osteoporosis in females >75 years is currently around 59.1% [1]. In Germany, about 6.3 million people are dealing with osteoporosis and about 885,000 new diagnoses are found per year [1]. In 2010, the incidence of osteoporosis-induced fractures was 725,000 and an increase up to 2025 might be as high as 928,000 per year [2]. The associated costs are estimated to be 4.5 Mrd. € per year [3].

Numerous studies confirmed that a specific treatment for osteoporosis is effective and can block up to 70% of subsequent fractures. Currently, there is a lack of preventive measures, especially for the prevention of secondary fractures. This appears to be a particular problem in the German-speaking countries [1, 4]. Due to this, subsequent fractures appear to be a particular issue. The risk of a secondary fracture appears to be most sustained within the first year after an osteoporotic fracture. Nevertheless, about 90% of females and 97% of males do not receive further treatment within 1 year after the first osteoporotic fracture [5, 6].

Even after adequate diagnostics and initiation of therapy, frequently there is a lack of adherence of medication, and in less than 30% of cases, there is continuation of the medical treatment [7]. One of the reasons may be the strict separation between the in- and outpatient treatment and reimbursement. There is a lack of structured care management for patients between in- and outpatient status [8]. To address these issues, the so-called fracture liaison service (FLS) has been developed, as described below.

19.2 Effects of a Fracture Liaison Service

It has been shown that the development of a FLS leads to a more frequent application of a standardized and guideline-adapted osteoporotic therapy. A meta-analysis of 74 controlled studies has shown to improve diagnostics. When com-

W. Böcker (✉)
Muskuloskeltal University Center Munich, Department of Orthopaedic and Trauma Surgery, University Hospital LMU, Munich, Germany
e-mail: Wolfgang.Boecker@med.uni-muenchen.de

E. Hesse
Muskuloskeltal University Center Munich, Institut for Muskuloskeltal Medicine, University Hospital LMU, Munich, Germany
e-mail: eric.hesse@med-uni-muenchen.de

C. Kammerlander
Muskuloskeltal University Center Munich, Department of Orthopaedic and Trauma Surgery, University Hospital LMU, Munich, Germany

AUVA-Trauma Hospital Styria, Graz, Austria
e-mail: christian.kammerlander@med.uni-muenchen.de

H.-C. Pape et al. (eds.), *Senior Trauma Patients*, https://doi.org/10.1007/978-3-030-91483-7_19

pared with standard treatment, there was a more frequent use of bone density measurements (48.0% vs. 23.5%) [9]. Also, the initiation of treatment began significantly more rapidly (38.0% vs. 17.2%), associated with better adherence to medical treatment (57.0% vs. 34.1%) [9]. This leads to a reduction in secondary fractures (33% over 2 years) and mortality rates (35%/2 years) [10, 11].

19.3 Practical Implications of a FLS

The main goal of a FLS program is to reduce the gap between in- and outpatient service by developing a so-called intersectoral care. To achieve this goal, a clinically active person is required to guide all treatment steps and connects the in-house care with outpatient follow-up. This is named an "*FLS-nurse*", whose primary location is usually the hospital. It is not important to be located in a level I trauma center, as the coordination can occur in multiple locations. Among the outpatient care physicians, multiple subspecialities can be effective, such as orthopedic surgeons, rheumatologists, gynecologists, or general practitioners.

Likewise, the qualification of a "*FLS-Nurse*" can vary, in some instances even a person without medical background can take care of this task. However, continuous education in falls' prevention and networking is crucial.

References

1. Hadji P, Klein S, Gothe H, et al. The epidemiology of osteoporosis—Bone Evaluation Study (BEST): an analysis of routine health insurance data. Dtsch Arztebl Int. 2013;110:52–7.
2. Linder R. Epidemiologie der Osteoporose in Deutschland, Frakturen und Kosten. 5 Jahrestagung der DGGÖ. Essen; 2013.
3. Klein S, Jessel S, Linder R, Verheyen F, Häussler B. Frakturen und Versorgungskosten bei Osteoporose: Analyse von Krankenkassen-Routinedaten im Rahmen der Bone Evaluation Study (BEST). Journal für Mineralstoffwechsel & Muskuloskelettale Erkrankungen. 2014;21:121–5.
4. Strom O, Borgstrom F, Kanis JA, et al. Osteoporosis: burden, health care provision and opportunities in the EU: a report prepared in collaboration with the International Osteoporosis Foundation (IOF) and the European Federation of Pharmaceutical Industry Associations (EFPIA). Arch Osteoporos. 2011;6:59–155.
5. Svedbom A, Hernlund E, Ivergard M, et al. Osteoporosis in the European Union: a compendium of country-specific reports. Arch Osteoporos. 2013;8:137.
6. Smektala R, Endres HG, Dasch B, Bonnaire F, Trampisch HJ, Pientka L. Quality of care after distal radius fracture in Germany. Results of a fracture register of 1,201 elderly patients. Unfallchirurg. 2009;112:46–54.
7. Hadji P, Claus V, Ziller V, Intorcia M, Kostev K, Steinle T. GRAND: the German retrospective cohort analysis on compliance and persistence and the associated risk of fractures in osteoporotic women treated with oral bisphosphonates. Osteoporos Int. 2012;23:223–31.
8. Schray D, Neuerburg C, Stein J, et al. Value of a coordinated management of osteoporosis via Fracture Liaison Service for the treatment of orthogeriatric patients. Eur J Trauma Emerg Surg. 2016;42:559–64.
9. Wu CH, Tu ST, Chang YF, Chan DC, Chien JT, Lin CH, Singh S, Dasari M, Chen JF, Tsai KS. Fracture liaison services improve outcomes of patients with osteoporosis-related fractures: a systematic literature review and meta-analysis. Bone. 2018;111:92–100.
10. Huntjens KM, van Geel TA, van den Bergh JP, et al. Fracture liaison service: impact on subsequent nonvertebral fracture incidence and mortality. J Bone Joint Surg Am. 2014;96:e29.
11. Nakayama A, Major G, Holliday E, Attia J, Bogduk N. Evidence of effectiveness of a fracture liaison service to reduce the re-fracture rate. Osteoporos Int. 2016;27:873–9.

Building A Senior Trauma Centre 20

Carl Neuerburg, Alexander Martin Keppler, Evi Fleischhacker, Johannes Gleich, and Christian Kammerlander

20.1 Early Identification of Seniors at Risk/Elements of Care

The development of a successful senior trauma centre is particularly dependent on an early identification of seniors at risk and their management in an effective, interdisciplinary team approach within the patient's journey. Within the course of treatment, some key elements have to be considered as summarized by Lisk et al. [1] and shown in Fig. 20.1 as follows:

- Prompt admission to orthopaedic care
- Rapid and comprehensive medical, surgical, and anaesthesiologic assessment
- Minimal delay to surgery
- Accurate and well-performed surgery (single-shot surgery)
- Prompt mobilization and rehabilitation
- Early supported discharge and ongoing community rehabilitation
- Secondary prevention, addressing bone protection and falls' assessment

C. Neuerburg (✉) · A. M. Keppler · E. Fleischhacker
J. Gleich
Department of Orthopaedics and Trauma Surgery, Musculoskeletal University Center Munich (MUM), University Hospital, LMU Munich, Munich, Germany
e-mail: carl.neuerburg@med.uni-muenchen.de

C. Kammerlander
AUVA Traumahospital Styria, Graz, Austria

There is growing emphasis on minimizing surgical delay for ortho-geriatric hip fracture patients [2]. It has been shown that a prolonged time to surgery is a risk factor for delirium, whereas delirium was found to be associated with a poor functional outcome and increased mortality [3, 4]. Therefore, a standardized involvement of the emergency department is a first-line requirement for an early identification of seniors at risk. The development of patient care pathways such as the ones presented in a publication from Murphy et al. can contribute to improved patient outcomes [5].

20.2 Treatment Pathways and Goal Setting

The implementation of standard operating procedures is a crucial part in the treatment of elderly trauma patients to ensure routine use of best practice in the areas of osteoporotic fracture repair, anticoagulant management, treatment of comorbidities, and early mobilization. Numerous guidelines for various indications have been published so far, such as the NICE guidelines (National Institute for Health and Care Excellence) in which standardized pathways for the individual surgical and medical management have been proposed. In order to gain the official certification for an ortho-geriatric centre, i.e. by the German Trauma Society (DGU), the guidelines are a prerequisite that are intensively studied within an audit. In a prospective study of ortho-geriatric patients who

H.-C. Pape et al. (eds.), *Senior Trauma Patients*, https://doi.org/10.1007/978-3-030-91483-7_20

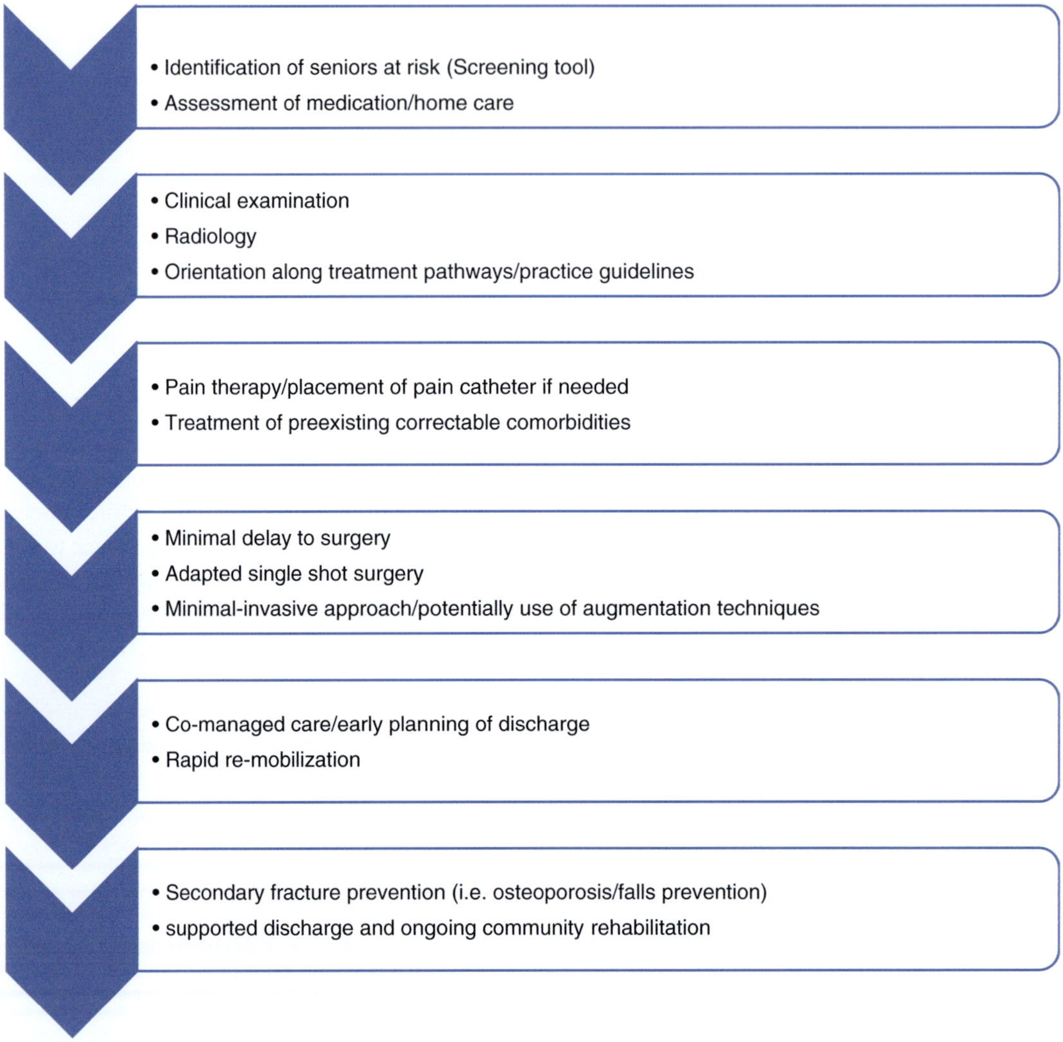
• Identification of seniors at risk (Screening tool)
• Assessment of medication/home care
• Clinical examination
• Radiology
• Orientation along treatment pathways/practice guidelines
• Pain therapy/placement of pain catheter if needed
• Treatment of preexisting correctable comorbidities
• Minimal delay to surgery
• Adapted single shot surgery
• Minimal-invasive approach/potentially use of augmentation techniques
• Co-managed care/early planning of discharge
• Rapid re-mobilization
• Secondary fracture prevention (i.e. osteoporosis/falls prevention)
• supported discharge and ongoing community rehabilitation

Fig. 20.1 Illustration of the treatment of care of elderly trauma patients and the key elements that have to be considered

suffered from a hip fracture, Ogilvie-Harris et al. [6] observed significantly improved outcomes for those patients treated with standardized medical and nursing protocols.

Another important issue of ortho-geriatric care is an early interdisciplinary goal setting for the individual patient. Based on protocols and guidelines, patient-specific short-term and medium-term treatment goals must be set and revised according to the dynamic status and functional potential of each patient. Diagnostic and therapeutic interventions must be aligned with those goals. Goal setting is an excellent technique to get all clinicians and family members on the same page and to ease interprofessional and interdisciplinary communication.

20.3 Organization Chart and Staff Structure

Ortho-geriatric patients can be challenging for the entire team and a structured approach and collaboration of all team members as illustrated in Fig. 20.2 are of major importance. Some countries have already included the interdisci-

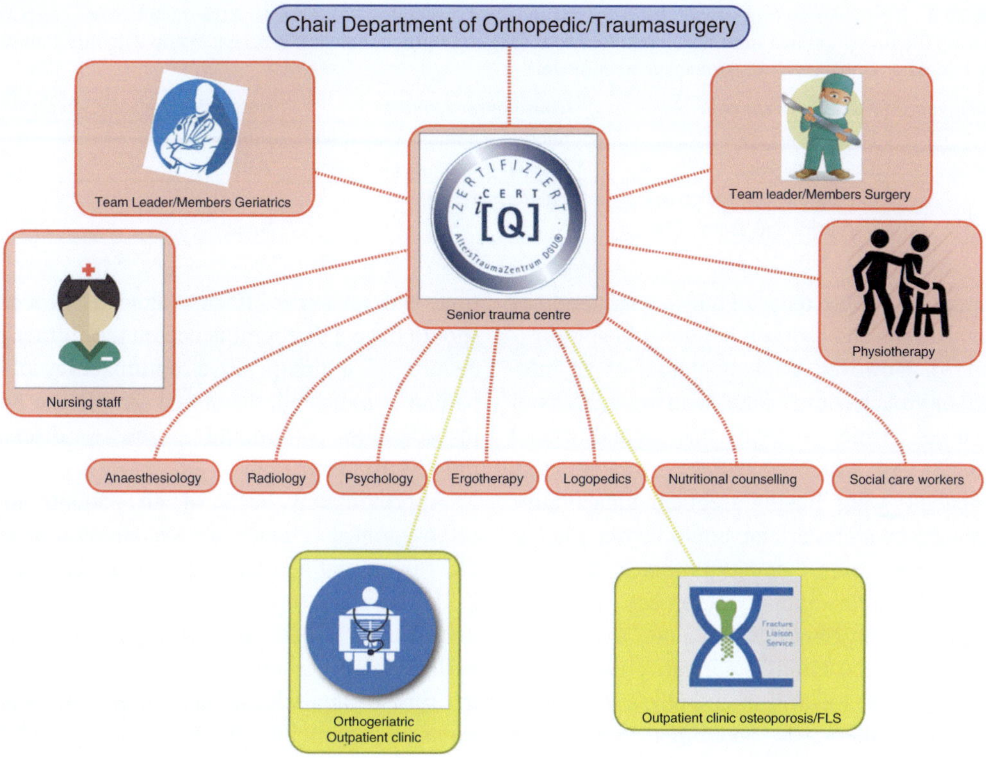

Fig. 20.2 Exemplary organization chart of a senior trauma centre illustrating the interaction of team members as implemented within the department of the authors. Each position has to be assigned to a specific team member

plinary approach in their guidelines, i.e. for the treatment of elderly hip fracture patients, thus the "Best Practice Tariff" in the UK and the decision of the German Joint Government Committee (G-BA) [7, 8].

20.4 Collaboration of Geriatricians and Surgeons

The standardized collaboration of orthopaedic surgeons and geriatricians (ortho-geriatric co-management) was developed in the UK. Originally, patients with frailty fractures were treated by an orthopaedic surgeon in charge, whereas specialists from other subject areas (in particular internists) were requested for a consultative service [9]. In this setting, neither the patients' comorbidities nor additional factors of influence for the patient are addressed adequately. As an attempt to reduce the mortality of these ortho-geriatric fracture patients, different models have been reported to reduce complications. Broadly speaking, four models of ortho-geriatric services have to be differentiated according to Pioli et al. (Table 20.1) [10].

According to the literature, the interdisciplinary model with an integrated approach appears to be the most effective symbiosis which is associated with a reduction of perioperative complications, reduced length of hospitalization, improved functional outcome, and reduction of costs in the treatment of aged patients with a hip fracture [11–13]. The relatively extensive ortho-geriatric co-management model was primarily reported by a group from Rochester (NY, USA) [14, 15], whereas reports from Asia [16] and Europe [17, 18] supported the investigations on an interdisciplinary approach. Treatment in an interdisciplinary team requires extended resources, yet Kates et al. showed that the overall costs in an interdis-

Table 20.1 It provides an overview of the different models of ortho-geriatric services in the treatment of aged patients with a hip fracture (modified from Kammerlander et al. [9]). *1* Traditional model; *2*, *3* Leadership with different bases; and *4* Integrated ortho-geriatric co-management model

Model type	Admitting care unit	Consultation service	Automated consultation service
1	Trauma surgery	Internal medicine /Geriatrics	No
2	Trauma surgery	Internal medicine /Geriatrics	Yes
3	Internal medicine/Geriatrics	Trauma surgery	Yes
4	Geriatrics and Trauma surgery	None	None

ciplinary team were reduced due to a reduction of complications and reduced length of hospitalization [19]. However, implementation of an integrated approach is associated with organizational difficulties, which is why the second model (Table 20.1) in which the patient is treated on an orthopaedic ward having frequent consultative treatments by a geriatrician could be regarded as a first step approach that could be extended.

In this interdisciplinary approach including orthopaedic surgeons, geriatricians, anaesthesiologists, etc., the multidisciplinarity of medical doctors, nurses, social workers, physiotherapists, occupational therapists, and others remains of primary importance, whereas decisions are made in a team with equal responsibilities [20].

20.5 Collaboration with Anaesthesiologists

Present comorbidities not only have a potential influence on the process of the underlying disease, the comorbidities could also have a relevant impact on the aetiology of the trauma. Thus, the trauma can be associated with an acute event such as a syncope, an apoplexy, or it can be the cause of a progressive deterioration of a chronic underlying disease. The immediate examination of the patient in the emergency department remains a major contribution of the ortho-geriatric co-management model.

Many of the aged patients take anticoagulants due to their underlying disease. Present treatment with anti-platelet agents, vitamin K antagonists such as warfarin, or treatment with an oral anticoagulant should not preclude surgery within an optimal time slot [21]. Given rationale preoperative diagnostic procedures, one could also save time and resources. Each diagnostic procedure should have a direct influence on the further procedure. If a preoperative optimization of the patient is indicated, the aimed time frame of the investigations should be discussed interdisciplinary.

Approximately, 60% of all patients in an ortho-geriatric fracture care system require a surgical treatment and have to undergo anaesthesia [17]. There is a higher anaesthesiological risk in ortho-geriatric patients with regard to intra- or perioperative complications. Thus, selection of the type of anaesthesia has a high significance. Local or regional anaesthesia is associated with reduced mortality and morbidity such as reduced peripheral thrombosis; lower rate of post-operative delirium tends to have fewer rates of myocardial infarction and lethal pulmonary embolisms [21]. General anaesthesia has the advantage of a decreased risk in drop of blood pressure such as reduced time of surgery. For those patients with a hip fracture, local or regional anaesthesia is the method of choice, while the choice of best anaesthesia in senior hip fracture patients is still a matter of current studies as investigated in the multicentre iHOPE study at present [22]. Given the variety of individual factors in elderly multi-morbid patients, the choice of anaesthesia should currently remain an individual decision [21].

Delirium remains a special challenge as it belongs to the most frequent complications and occurs in up to 60% of all bigger surgical interventions [23]. Thus, delirium increases the risk for further complications and leads to a direct and indirect impairment of the medical, functional, and cognitive outcome [23]. Given the limited scientific knowledge, treatment of this condition relies on preventive measures. Due to technical problems in the implementation of a non-pharmacological prevention, various substances have been analysed in the past regarding their potential to reduce a delirium. There are indications showing that haloperidol and other new atypical neuroleptics such as risperidone and olanzapine, or melatonin are able to reduce the incidence of a post-operative delirium [24]. However, general therapy recommendations cannot be provided. Pharmacological prophylaxis of delirium should therefore be reserved for patients with a high risk of suffering a delirium, taking the individual risk-benefit assessment into consideration [24]. Despite the advanced age and the remaining comorbidities, the immediate mortality risk associated with delirium is limited. Given a 30-day mortality risk, the delirium-associated risk has been shown to be 3.6%, whereas the majority was associated with a cardiovascular cause (41%) [25]. Apart from delirium, urinary infections remain the most frequent complication. Catheter and continence managements are still paid little attention in ortho-geriatric trauma surgery. An early removal of the catheter is known to significantly reduce the risk of urinary infections [20].

Apart from an ortho-geriatric co-management model, patients' multiple-medication remains another almost insurmountable challenge. Multiple drug usage leads to undesired pharmaceutical effects and interactions. Age-related physiological changes such as renal failure increase the risk of undesired pharmaceutical effects in ortho-geriatric patients. Especially, the implementation of an adapted analgesia has a crucial role in these patients. Non-steroidal anti-inflammatory drugs (NSAIDs) belong to the group of drugs with an increased risk and should be avoided in ortho-geriatric patients.

20.6 Collaboration with Nurses, Physiotherapists, and Social Workers

The interdisciplinary approach of ancillary personnel including physiotherapists, nurses, mid-level providers, and social workers is crucial to regain patient's autonomy and maintain best recovery of the patient. Thus, early mobilization, activation of the patient, nutritional management, and discharge management are of high relevance, which should be coordinated in regular team meetings as an integral part of the ortho-geriatric co-management model.

A first step towards early mobilization of the patient is a therapeutically active care accompanied by the nursing staff [26]. Thus, the patient has to be guided to carry out as many activities as possible on his own. However, it has to be considered that this approach to guide the patients is generally more time-consuming for the nursing staff compared to the treatment of the patient themselves. Persuasion of the patients to take the meal in a common room has been shown to be another beneficial way of activation [26]. Thus, patients also experience a daily routine which could also be beneficial for the prevention of delirium.

In ortho-geriatric patients, physiotherapy has the objective of early re-mobilization, prevention of load, and adjacent fractures. Thus, programs of back and spine exercise courses are a relevant part of a postural and behavioural training. Strengthening of muscles increases the patients' standing and walking ability, whereas on the other hand this leads to a stimulation of bone formation of the skeletal system [27, 28]. With these exercises, also, the coordinative abilities can be trained, whereas falls can be reduced [29]. Mobilization in the early post-operative phase is of superior importance, as a delay is associated with diminished physical function at 2 months, and a worse survival rate at 6 months [30, 31]. Further, additional physiotherapy during acute care reduces falls in the first 12 months after hip fracture [32]. These patients generally struggle to comply with partial weight-bearing, yet post-operative weight-bearing restrictions are still recommended by nearly 25% of surgeons [33]. Thus, post-operative recommendations should clearly support the physiotherapeutical approach to encourage early re-mobilization in senior trauma patients. Also, the home environment should be adjusted with regard to an age-based conversion to prevent falls.

A balanced nutrition including a sufficient intake of calcium and vitamin D, the reduction of risk factors such as smoking, and the intake of phosphate-rich food also play a relevant role in bone metabolism [34].

Besides these therapy approaches, depending on the patient's health condition and autonomy prior to fracture, an intensive follow-up rehabilitation is needed. Thus, the cooperation with rehabilitation facilities, geriatric facilities, and nursing homes could be beneficial for reduction of the length of hospitalization.

20.7 Adapting Facilities in a Senior Trauma Centre

Besides interdisciplinary care pathways, the ward/ICU facilities also have a major impact in a senior trauma centre. Thus, elderly trauma patients are at a high risk to suffer a post-operative delirium and the nonpharmacological treatment is also well-known to be very effective. Nowadays, nonpharmacologic approaches focus on risk factors such as immobility, functional decline, visual or hearing impairment, dehydration, and sleep deprivation that can be addressed by the inpatient infrastructure [35]. Many structural factors can be modified with regard to the geriatric requirements. These are, i.e. walls/colours, implementation of common rooms, adaptation of patient rooms/beds, and adjustment of washrooms and bathroom facilities such as implementation of nearby therapy rooms [36]. With these approaches, the special needs for elderly trauma patients can be influenced in many ways according to Mayr et al. Thus, a suitable equipment on the ward should consider a sufficient amount of handlebars and handrails. Also, the installation of large clocks can help to maintain orientation, while room changes throughout the course should be avoided. The rooms should also be spacious to store assistive devices for patients with difficult mobilization, while height-adjustable low-floor beds are beneficial. In common rooms, patients can have lunch together and chat with each other, while older posters may help to improve the recognition value.

Throughout the inpatient journey, many factors can have a beneficial impact on the outcome of geriatric trauma patients as reported recently in a comparative study with two different treatment structures for elderly hip fracture patients (Table 20.2).

Table 20.2 Modified comparison of two different treatment structures as published by our group recently in which the outcome of hip fracture patients in a hospital with conventional trauma care (CTC) and interdisciplinary ortho-geriatric care (OGC) was assessed [37]

	CTC	OTC
Department	• Department of Trauma Surgery • Other departments on consultation basis	• Department of Trauma Surgery with geriatricians working within the team
Facilities	• Trauma ward: Single-triple bed rooms on different trauma wards with up to 30 beds	• Specific designed ortho-geriatric ward: Single-double-bedrooms on one ward with up to 44 beds
Treatment	• Early mobilization after surgery • Physiotherapy 1×/day (30 min) • Social care workers on call	• Early mobilization after surgery • Physiotherapy 2×/day (30 min) • "activating care": help for body care with greatest possible participation of the patient, shared meals with other patients in a common room with independent transfer (as possible) • Interdisciplinary treatment with focus on: Somatic health, mental health, function, and social situation

20.8 Rehabilitation and Secondary Fracture Prevention

In ortho-geriatric patients, it is of particular importance to start rehabilitation straight after surgery and to continue in the inpatient as in the outpatient setting to prevent a loss of selfcare and autonomy. Especially in patients with various comorbidities, a multidisciplinary rehabilitation process is an important factor, besides the surgical procedure and the medical management of an aged person with complex diseases and polypharmacy [38]. Therefore, registration of the patients has to be ensured as early as possible, preferably starting on the day of admission to the hospital. To find out the best way of rehabilitation program, the individual's health status has to be assessed. Therefore, analysis of mobility, cognition, depression, the risk to suffer falls, nutritional status, continence, and visual function are of importance to rule out the right rehabilitation program [39]. To improve the physical outcome and the quality of life, such as daily activities, and reduce readmission rates, depression, and falls, an interdisciplinary rehabilitation program is known to have the best outcome [40].

Cooperation with rehabilitation facilities for elderly people, including departments for acute geriatrics, is a proven approach to ensure early discharge of the patient while connection of the patient with the hospital can be secured. Treatment of ortho-geriatric patients would be at its best if as much hospital-based care is guaranteed as necessary and as much home care provided as possible. Therefore, another new approach is the establishment of an Outreach Geriatric Re-mobilization which takes place in an environment that is familiar to patients and in which patients are mobilized in a place where they spend their everyday lives [38]. According to Pils et al., these projects have shown to contribute to a reduction of time spent as an inpatient, accelerate and encourage the reintegration of the patient in their familiar environment, and help maintain the patient's social network.

Regarding secondary fracture prevention and treatment of an underlying osteoporosis, fracture liason services (FLS), which coordinate diagnostics, treatment initiation, and therapy adherence, have shown encouraging results. Patients who suffer a fragility fracture and present with special risk factors for an osteoporosis are included and guideline-adapted treatment can be recommended [41].

The importance of secondary fracture prevention is also highlighted by a study of Ryg et al., who could show recurrent fractures following primary hip fracture [42]. Besides the FLS approach to improve bone quality and prevent fragility fractures, this includes adjustment of medication to decrease induced symptoms like dizziness, which is often followed by falls and removal of fall risk-increasing drugs.

20.9 Outcome and Quality Control

There are different outcome parameters to assess the effectiveness of an ortho-geriatric service (Table 20.3). Specific parameters of time including the time to surgery, length of hospitalization, and one year mortality are comparable measures to monitor a system's effectiveness. As stated above in patients with a hip fracture, longer preoperative waiting times increase the risk of medical complications due to immobility [9]. Similarly, the length of hospitalization is an important parameter as it can be associated with the formation of complications and there is a direct correlation with costs [25]. It has to be the goal to achieve an improvement or at least a restoring of the patients' function, whereas mortality should be lowered.

A new approach to monitor mobility, i.e. the cardiovascular system of elderly trauma patients, can be facilitated by the use of wearables. Various mobile systems including fitness/activity trackers such as specific pressure sensors have been introduced and proven to be feasible in elderly trauma patients [43, 44].

Table 20.3 Overview of the relevant outcome parameters, assessment tools, and their follow-up to monitor system's effectiveness adopted and modified from Liem et al. [25]

Outcome parameter	Assessment tool	Admission*	Discharge†	30 days	90 days	1 year
Mortality	Mortality rate (%)			X		X
Length of stay	Midnight census method		X			
Time to surgery	Time from admission until arrival in operating room (h)		X			
Complications:	Complication rate (%) using the complication list					
• Medical			X	X		
• Surgical			X	X		X
Readmission:	Readmission rate (%) using the complication list					
• Medical				X	X	
• Surgical				X	X	X
Mobility	• Parker Mobility Score	X			X	X
	• Timed Up and Go test				X	X
Quality of life	EQ-5D	X			X	X
Pain	Verbal rating scale	X‡			X	X
Satisfaction	No appropriate tool available					
Activities of daily living	Barthel Index	X	X		X	X
Falls	No appropriate tool available					
Medication use:						
• Inappropriate	• Adverse drug reaction with complications		X	X		
• Osteoporosis	• Medication list	X	X		X	X
Place of residence	Living situation list	X			X	X
Costs	Percentage of expected national costs		X			

Additionally, appropriate geriatric scores can be useful. Functional outcome and activities of daily living can be assessed, i.e. by the Barthel index which is used to measure performance in basic activities of daily living by scaling the presence or absence of faecal or urinary incontinence and the help needed with grooming, toilet use, feeding, transfers (e.g. from chair to bed), walking, dressing, climbing stairs, and bathing. For each question, there are 2–4 ordinal responses with a fixed count, which are summed up. The maximum of 100 points imply that the patient is independent in his basic activities of daily living. This score was found to be a reliable outcome parameter for hip fracture patients [45, 46].

Another frequently used index to assess activities of daily living is the Katz Score which analyses the patient's performance in six functions. Thus, the Katz Score uses yes or no questions to evaluate the functions of bathing, dressing, toileting, transferring, continence, and feeding, a score of 6 indicates full function, 4 moderate impairment, and 2 or less describes a relevant impairment of the patient's ADL. Also, the Functional Independence Measure (FIM) which uses similar items to evaluate motoric and cognitive performance is frequently used to describe the ADLs of the patient at discharge. Another simple tool to evaluate mobility is the Parker mobility scale. The Timed Up and Go (TUG) test is another commonly used mobility score which is known to be a valid and reliable tool to assess the patients' mobility [47].

Also, peri- and post-operative complications have to be evaluated. Thus, common complications of patients having suffered an ortho-geriatric fracture are cardiac, cerebral, thrombo-embolic, and pulmonary complications, such as, renal failure, urinary tract infection, delirium, pressure-ulcers, gastrointestinal (GI) complications, adverse drug reactions (ADR), and subsequent fractures. Further surgical problems are surgical site infection and other surgical complications [25].

Further parameters to assess quality improvement are the readmission rate, analysis of the quality of life, pain, and patients' satisfaction (i.e. with questionnaires such as the EQ-5D and the Visual analogue Scale).

Inadequate medication use remains another relevant issue which has to be assessed ideally within the time of hospitalization. Thus, specific screening tools have been described, such as the Screening Tool of Older Person's Prescriptions (STOPP) criteria, which consists of 65 clinically significant criteria for potentially inappropriate medications, and the Screening Tool to Alert doctors to Right Treatment (START) criteria, which consists of 22 evidence-based prescribing indicators for commonly encountered diseases in older adults [25]. Thus, the diagnosis of osteoporosis should also be assessed ideally within the time of hospitalization and appropriate medication should be initiated or mentioned in the discharge report.

Given the high financial burden of osteoporosis associated with osteoporotic fractures and estimated annual costs of 31.7 billion € in Europe [48], cost effectiveness remains another tool to evaluate a programme's effectiveness.

References

1. Lisk R, Yeong K. Reducing mortality from hip fractures: a systematic quality improvement programme. BMJ Qual Improv Rep. 2014;3
2. Khan SK, Jameson SS, Avery PJ, et al. Does the timing of presentation of neck of femur fractures affect the outcome of surgical intervention. Eur J Emerg Med. 2013;20:178–81.
3. Juliebo V, Bjoro K, Krogseth M, et al. Risk factors for preoperative and postoperative delirium in elderly patients with hip fracture. J Am Geriatrics Soc. 2009;57:1354–61.
4. Lee KH, Ha YC, Lee YK, et al. Frequency, risk factors, and prognosis of prolonged delirium in elderly patients after hip fracture surgery. Clin Orthop Relat Res. 2011;469:2612–20.
5. Murphy C, Mullen E, Hogan K, et al. Streamlining an existing hip fracture patient pathway in an acute tertiary adult Irish hospital to improve patient experience and outcomes. Int J Qual Health Care. 2019;31:45–51.
6. Ogilvie-Harris DJ, Botsford DJ, Hawker RW. Elderly patients with hip fractures: improved outcome with the use of care maps with high-quality medical and nursing protocols. J Orthop Trauma. 1993;7:428–37.
7. (G-Ba) GB. Beschluss des Gemeinsamen Bundesausschusses über eine Richtlinie zur Versorgung der hüftgelenknahen Femurfraktur; 2019.
8. Khan SK, Weusten A, Bonczek S, et al. The Best Practice Tariff helps improve management of neck of femur fractures: a completed audit loop. Br J Hosp Med (Lond). 2013;74:644–7.
9. Kammerlander C, Roth T, Friedman SM, et al. Ortho-geriatric service--a literature review comparing different models. Osteoporos Int. 2010;21:S637–46.
10. Pioli G, Giusti A, A B (2008) Orthogeriatric care for the elderly with hip fractures: where are we? Aging Clin Exp Res 20:113–122
11. Buecking B, Struewer J, Waldermann A, et al. What determines health-related quality of life in hip fracture patients at the end of acute care?—A prospective observational study. Osteoporos Int. 2014;25:475–84.
12. Prestmo A, Hagen G, Sletvold O, et al. Comprehensive geriatric care for patients with hip fractures: a prospective, randomised, controlled trial. Lancet. 2015;385:1623–33.
13. Rapp K, Becker C, Todd C, et al. The association between orthogeriatric co-management and mortality following hip fracture. Dtsch Arztebl Int. 2020;117:53–9.
14. Friedman S, Mendelson D, Kates S, et al. Geriatric co-management of proximal femur fractures: total quality management and protocol-driven care result in better outcomes for a frail patient population. J Am Geriatrics Soc. 2008;56:1349–56.
15. Kates SL, Mendelson DA, Friedman SM. Co-managed care for fragility hip fractures (Rochester model). Osteoporos Int. 2010;21:S621–5.

16. Shyu Y-IL, Liang J, Wu C-C, et al. Interdisciplinary intervention for hip fracture in older Taiwanese: benefits last for 1 year. J Gerontol A Biol Sci Med Sci. 2008;63:92–7.
17. Kammerlander C, Gosch M, Blauth M, et al. The Tyrolean Geriatric Fracture Center: an orthogeriatric co-management model. Zeitschrift fur Gerontologie und Geriatrie. 2011;44:363–7.
18. Singler K, Biber R, Wicklein S, et al. "N-active": a new comanaged, orthogeriatric ward: observations and prospects. Zeitschrift fur Gerontologie und Geriatrie. 2011;44:368–74.
19. Kates SL, Mendelson DA, Friedman SM. The value of an organized fracture program for the elderly: early results. J Orthop Trauma. 2011;25:233–7.
20. Mendelson DA, Friedman SM. Principles of comanagement and the geriatric fracture center. Clin Geriatr Med. 2014;30:183–9.
21. Luger TJ, Kammerlander C, Luger MF, et al. Mode of anesthesia, mortality and outcome in geriatric patients. Zeitschrift fur Gerontologie und Geriatrie. 2014;47:110–24.
22. Kowark A, Adam C, Ahrens J, et al. Improve hip fracture outcome in the elderly patient (iHOPE): a study protocol for a pragmatic, multicentre randomised controlled trial to test the efficacy of spinal versus general anaesthesia. BMJ Open. 2018;8:e023609.
23. Inouye SK. Delirium in older persons. N Engl J Med. 2006;354:1157–65.
24. Gosch M, Nicholas JA. Pharmacologic prevention of postoperative delirium. Zeitschrift fur Gerontologie und Geriatrie. 2014;47:105–9.
25. Liem IS, Kammerlander C, Suhm N, et al. Identifying a standard set of outcome parameters for the evaluation of orthogeriatric co-management for hip fractures. Injury. 2013;44:1403–12.
26. Werther SFJ, Mayr E. Interdisziplinäres Management im Zentrum für geriatrische Traumatologie. Orthopädie und Unfallchirurgie up2date. 2014;5:387–406.
27. Bonaiuti D, Shea B, Iovine R, et al. Exercise for preventing and treating osteoporosis in postmenopausal women. Cochrane Database Syst Rev. 2002:CD000333.
28. Huuskonen J, Vaisanen SB, Kroger H, et al. Regular physical exercise and bone mineral density: a four-year controlled randomized trial in middle-aged men. The DNASCO study. Osteoporos Int. 2001;12:349–55.
29. Willburger RE, Knorth H. Osteoporose der Wirbelsäule: Therapieoption und Präventionsstrategien. Dtsch Arztebl Int. 2003;100:1120.
30. Kammerlander C, Pfeufer D, Lisitano LA, et al. Inability of older adult patients with hip fracture to maintain postoperative weight-bearing restrictions. J Bone Joint Surg Am. 2018;100:936–41.
31. Siu AL, Penrod JD, Boockvar KS, et al. Early ambulation after hip fracture: effects on function and mortality. Arch Intern Med. 2006;166:766–71.
32. Hill K. Additional physiotherapy during acute care reduces falls in the first 12 months after hip fracture. J Physiother. 2010;56:201.
33. Ottesen TD, Mclynn RP, Galivanche AR, et al. Increased complications in geriatric patients with a fracture of the hip whose postoperative weight-bearing is restricted: an analysis of 4918 patients. Bone Joint J. 2018;100-B:1377–84.
34. Lunt M, Masaryk P, Scheidt-Nave C, et al. The effects of lifestyle, dietary dairy intake and diabetes on bone density and vertebral deformity prevalence: the EVOS study. Osteoporos Int. 2001;12:688–98.
35. Oh ES, Fong TG, Hshieh TT, et al. Delirium in older persons: advances in diagnosis and treatment. JAMA. 2017;318:1161–74.
36. Mayr E, Blauth M, Kates S, et al. 2.5 Adapting facilities to fragility fracture patients. In: Osteoporotic fracture care. Georg Thieme Verlag; 2019.
37. Neuerburg C, Forch S, Gleich J, et al. Improved outcome in hip fracture patients in the aging population following co-managed care compared to conventional surgical treatment: a retrospective, dual-center cohort study. BMC Geriatr. 2019;19:330.
38. Pils K, Muller W, Likar R, et al. Rehabilitation after hip fracture. Wiener medizinische Wochenschrift. 2013;163:462–7.
39. Givens JL, Sanft TB, Marcantonio ER. Functional recovery after hip fracture: the combined effects of depressive symptoms, cognitive impairment, and delirium. J Am Geriatrics Soc. 2008;56:1075–9.
40. Huusko TM, Karppi P, Avikainen V, et al. Intensive geriatric rehabilitation of hip fracture patients: a randomized, controlled trial. Acta Ortho Scand. 2002;73:425–31.
41. Schray D, Neuerburg C, Stein J, et al. Value of a coordinated management of osteoporosis via Fracture Liaison Service for the treatment of orthogeriatric patients. Eur J Trauma Emerg Surg. 2016;42:559–64.
42. Ryg J, Rejnmark L, Overgaard S, et al. Hip fracture patients at risk of second hip fracture: a nationwide population-based cohort study of 169,145 cases during 1977-2001. J Bone Miner Res. 2009;24:1299–307.
43. Keppler AM, Holzschuh J, Pfeufer D, et al. Postoperative physical activity in orthogeriatric patients—new insights with continuous monitoring. Injury. 2020;51:628–32.
44. Pfeufer D, Zeller A, Mehaffey S, et al. Weight-bearing restrictions reduce postoperative mobility in elderly hip fracture patients. Arch Orthop Trauma Surg. 2019;139:1253–9.
45. Bryant DM, Sanders DW, Coles CP, et al. Selection of outcome measures for patients with hip fracture. J Orthop Trauma. 2009;23:434–41.
46. Kammerlander C, Riedmuller P, Gosch M, et al. Functional outcome and mortality in geriatric distal femoral fractures. Injury. 2012;43:1096–101.
47. Hutchings L, Fox R, Chesser T. Proximal femoral fractures in the elderly: how are we measuring outcome? Injury. 2011;42:1205–13.
48. Kanis JA, Johnell O. Requirements for DXA for the management of osteoporosis in Europe. Osteoporos Int. 2005;16:229–38.

Part V

Specific Treatments in Acute Care

21 Specifics of Fracture Stabilization in Geriatric Bone

Richard Stange and Michael J. Raschke

21.1 Introduction

Fractures in the elderly patient represent a challenge to orthopaedic surgeons since osteoporosis does not only increase the risk of fracture but also represents a problem in fracture stabilization in the geriatric bone. The soft tissue envelope around the fracture often is compromised due to pre-existing diseases such as diabetes, chronic venous insufficiency or peripheral vascular disease. Therefore, the successful treatment of the fracture with fast recovery of the mobility is essential for the patient's survival and well-being. The goals of treatment differ from those, which are valid for younger adults. Primary goal is preserving independency of the elderly patient in his activities of daily life. Advantages and drawbacks of surgical procedures have to be balanced with those of conservative treatment.

When operative treatment is chosen, restoring stability with full weight-bearing has the highest priority, second priority is less invasive surgery, whereas restoring anatomy or optimal function becomes less important. The aim of surgical treatment mainly is to obtain a stable fixation that reduces pain and permits early mobilization. In some fracture types, restoration of stability has higher priority than preservation of blood supply. This shift is justified in the light of the different characteristics and functional requirements of geriatric patients. Optimal function of a shoulder, knee or hip joint was often not present prior to the injury; therefore, better function than before the accident cannot be expected. Being independent in activities of daily life such as personal hygiene, cooking, short walking or shopping is much more important than optimal function of a joint [1].

Geriatric, often osteoporosis-related, fractures are especially located meta-epiphyseal, in skeletal sites with particular morphological and biomechanical characteristic, complex and with more fragments, with slow healing process and co-morbidities. Typical osteoporotic fractures are vertebral compression fractures, hip fractures, proximal humerus and distal radius fractures. They are considered as "indicator-fractures" for osteoporosis. Bone mineral density has decreased, which enhances the risk of implant loosening. The major technical problem that surgeons face is the difficulty to obtain a stable fixation of an implant due to osteoporotic bone. Different biological, technical and surgical aspects have to be taken into account for fracture stabilization in geriatric bone. The treatment of osteoporotic

R. Stange (✉)
Department of Regenerative Musculoskeletal Medicine, Institute of Musculoskeletal Medicine (IMM), University Hospital Münster, Albert-Schweitzer-Campus 1, Gebäude W1, Münster, Germany
e-mail: richard.stange@ukmuenster.de

M. J. Raschke
Department of Trauma, Hand and Reconstructive Surgery, University Hospital Münster, Albert-Schweitzer-Campus 1, Gebäude W1, Münster, Germany
e-mail: michael.raschke@ukmuenster.de

H.-C. Pape et al. (eds.), *Senior Trauma Patients*, https://doi.org/10.1007/978-3-030-91483-7_21

fractures therefore can be demanding, despite optimal surgical techniques. Sometimes, replacement of fractured joints is superior to reconstruction to allow immediate bearing.

Remarkably the overall complication rate and mechanical implant failure following surgical treatment of geriatric fractures are significantly higher compared with non-fragility fractures [2]. Geriatric bone is the main cause of failure of fracture fixation rather than implant failure itself. Complication rates after surgical therapy of osteoporosis-related fractures are twice as high as after treatment of healthy bone. The implant-related failure rate in osteoporosis-related fractures is estimated to be about 10–25% [3]. Surgical treatment of these fragility fractures is also associated with a higher rate of complications as mal- or non-union [4]. Surgical success is based on the correct indication as well as on the correct surgical technique ("surgeon factor"), biological factors (e.g. perfusion of fracture fragments) and biomechanical factors (e.g. bone quality, fracture configuration and anatomical reduction). Over the last years, implant design in orthopaedic and trauma surgery continuously developed towards devices, which are optimized in size, shape and screw orientation in certain anatomic regions. Implant scale and (bio) mechanical properties have been progressively adapted to the biological surroundings and forces expected adapted to the technical surroundings discussed above.

A comprehensive strategy for improved treatment of geriatric fractures therefore should address biological and mechanical issues, and include the stimulation of fracture repair, removal of inhibitors to bone healing, improvements in surgical implants and application of augmentation.

21.2 Biological Aspects

The general ability of bone to resist fracture and withstand loads depends on the amount of bone (bone mass), its distribution in space and the intrinsic material properties of the bone tissue [5]. Age-related degradation of bone and the additional bone weakening through age-related diseases such as osteoporosis reduce the ability of bone to withstand increased loading. The biological situation of osteoporotic bone in geriatric patients is characterized by poor bone quality, loss of bone mass and microarchitectural deterioration of bone tissue [6] (Fig. 21.1). The reduction in bone mass mainly results from increased bone resorption and inadequate bone formation leading to a negative remodelling balance. Osteoporosis is further characterized by thinner cross-linking connections within trabecular bone [7]. At a tissue level, there is a decrease in the cancellous bone mineral density. There is also a decrease in the density of cortical bone, because of an increase in porosity, which can affect the holding capacity of screws. Intrinsic material properties of bone tissue are affected by ageing and osteoporosis [8] and include compositional factors such as mineralization distribution, content of collagen and cross-linking profiles of inter- and intrafibrillar collagen connections [9]. Bone fragility therefore results from typical modifications of mechanical and structural properties of the osteoporotic bone [10]:

- Reduction of mineral content (provides strength and stiffness) and protein content (limits the damage consequent to an impact and influences bone mechanical properties);
- Reduction of the ability to oppose to deformations (rigidity), to absorb energy (resistance), to adapt to repetitive loads (fatigue resistance) and to inhibit the progression of a lesion (resistance to fracture);
- Increase of anisotropy (major number of trabeculae with an orientation on the principal load axis) and therefore increase of fracture risk for abnormal loads (falls);
- Increase of microdamages (manifestation related to repetitive micro-stress on bony tissue, age-related).

Age-related endosteal diaphyseal resorption and medullary expansion are common in both men and women. The changes in diameter of the inner and outer cortices affect the bending and torsional characteristics of the entire bone

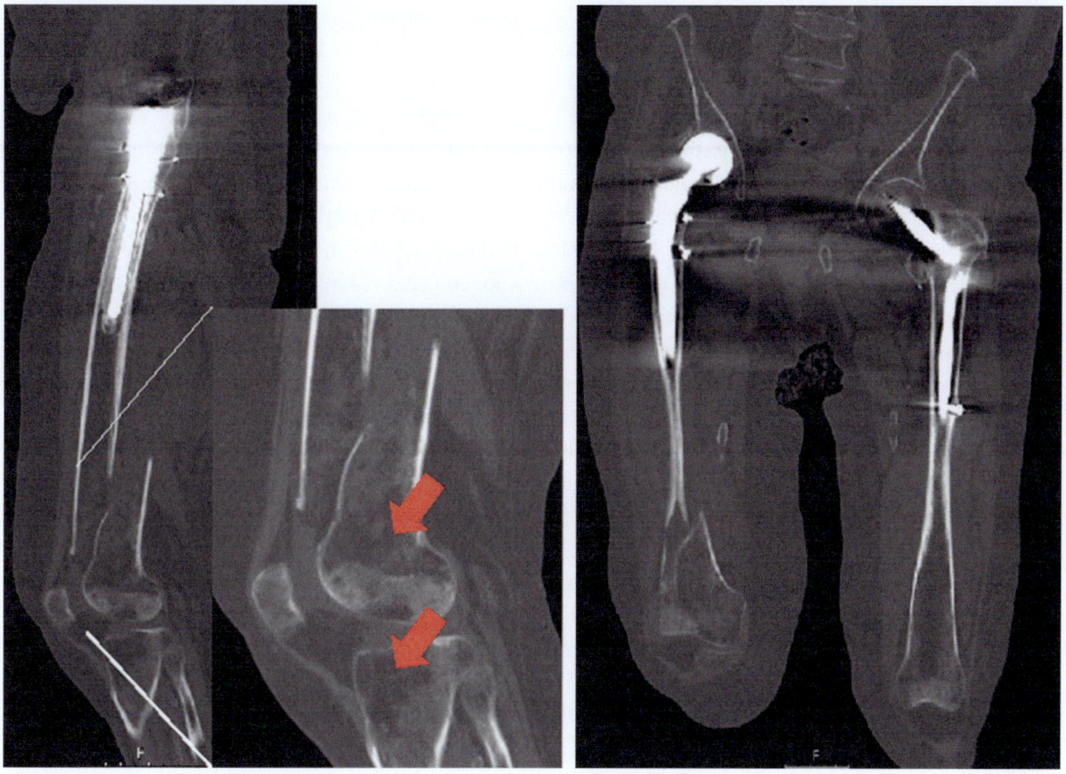

Fig. 21.1 85-year old female: Distal femoral periprosthetic fracture with severe osteoprosis: Reduction of bone mass and mineral content, disappearance of diaphyseal and metaphyseal trabecular bone structure (arrows). Thinning 1 of cortical diameter and widening of the intramedullary canal

and predispose to low-energy fractures, which often have a complex pattern. The load transmitted at the bone–implant interface can often exceed the reduced strain tolerance of osteoporotic bone [11].

Loss of bone mineral reflects the loss of bone mass in osteoporosis. Non-invasive evaluation of bone mineral has mainly been used to assess metabolic changes of bone. Non-invasive assessment of bone mineral is, today, mainly obtained by Dual X-ray Absorptiometry (DXA) and Quantitative Computed Tomography (QCT). The bone mineral content of cortical and cancellous bone is not distributed to meet similar demands in any one individual. Strong cortical bone does not imply strong cancellous bone, and vice versa. Although bone fragility in the elderly is a metabolic problem, it does not develop similarly in all bones. It seems, for example, that the distal radius and the spine differ from the proximal femur. This indicates that the use of non-invasive bone mineral assessment in defining mechanical strength of bone has to address the individual bone [12]. To estimate local geriatric bone quality and expected implant anchorage, mechanical methods may be promising to measure bone strength intraoperatively. Although not in regular clinical application, it has been shown that the mechanical peak torque correlates with the local bone mineral density and screw failure load in hip, hindfoot, humerus and spine in vitro [13].

With ageing it is possible to observe an increase of microdamages that the physiological mechanisms of repair are not able to contrast. The healing of fractures in osteoporotic bone passes through the normal stages and concludes with union of the fracture although the healing process is prolonged [14]. The biological activity of the osteoblast, as for other mesenchymal cells, is influenced negatively by ageing. Clinically, although delay in fracture healing is not always obvious, the decreased healing capacity in osteoporosis is reflected in a dramatic increase in the rate of failure of implant fixation [15].

There are several possible explanations for this effect. There might be fewer mesenchymal stem cells in osteoporotic individuals, which have a lower proliferative response [16]. This may explain the age-related decrease in the number of osteoblasts. Mesenchymal stem cells in post-menopausal women differ from those in the premenopausal by having a lower rate of growth and a deficiency in their ability to differentiate along the osteogenic lineage [17]. Finally, bone cells from osteoporotic patients may have an impaired long-term response to mechanical stress [18].

Biological support which enhances the healing potential of osteoporotic fractures should therefore also be considered as an adjunct to surgery, e.g. bone tissue-engineering using a suitable scaffold material, growth factors, bone grafts or adult mesenchymal stem cells [19].

21.3 Technical Aspects

The major problem facing the surgeon is the difficulty in obtaining secure fixation of an implant to geriatric bone. Osteoporotic bone structure provides less cortical and cancellous bone for the screw threads to gain purchase, so that the pull-out strength of implants is significantly reduced. Bone mineral density correlates linearly with the holding power of screws [20]. The load transmitted at the bone–implant interface can often exceed the reduced strain tolerance of osteoporotic bone. This may result in microfracture, resorption of the bone and loosening of the implant, with secondary failure of fixation [21]. Consequently, the common mode of failure of internal fixation in osteoporotic bone is bone failure rather than implant breakage (Fig. 21.2).

This high rate of complications in geriatric bone has encouraged extensive research into the development of implants, which can improve the bone–implant interface by preventing high stress and distributing the forces transmitted to bone in a load-sharing, rather than load-bearing way. The general principles of fracture management in osteoporotic bone require some changes in surgical technique in order to decrease the risk of failure at the bone–implant interface. These include the use of relative stability techniques such as intramedullary nails, bone impaction, buttress fixation, fixed-angle devices, bone augmentation and joint replacement [1, 11, 22]. Open reduction and internal fixation (ORIF) have been commonly developed for normal healthy bone but especially in geriatric bone it is paramount to apply these techniques subsequently. Techniques of internal fixation which aim to provide absolute stability with lag screws, however, are usually inappropriate in osteoporotic bone [3]. A biomechanical construct, which is adequate in younger adults, may fail in elderly persons with osteoporosis [13]. Relative stability techniques are the most efficient at reducing strain at the bone–implant interface, as the implant is within the load-bearing axis of the bone.

Several biomechanical principles can be employed to achieve sufficient primary stability in osteoporotic bone. Implants for osteosynthesis in osteoporosis must use the longest possible corridors, be angular stable and be inserted in regions with the highest bone mineral density [23–25]. Of uttermost importance in fracture fixation of geriatric bone is the interface between implant and bone. Internal fixation devices that allow load sharing with host bone should be chosen to minimize stress at the bone–implant interface. This can be achieved by employing fixation devices which have a maximum of contact area between implant and bone. Examples are long plates and nails with many locking options or plates with a larger surface area providing more possibilities for screw placement. Plates with a larger contact area effectively reduce the local compressional strain on the bone. Similarly, thinner screws generate smaller local strain in cortical as well as trabecular bone compared to thicker screws [26]. Thinner screws have the additional advantage of providing more flexibility and thus the ability to distribute the load within a larger volume of bone. External fixation devices may be difficult to apply to geriatric patients for a longer period since pin anchorage is hard to achieve in osteoporotic bone.

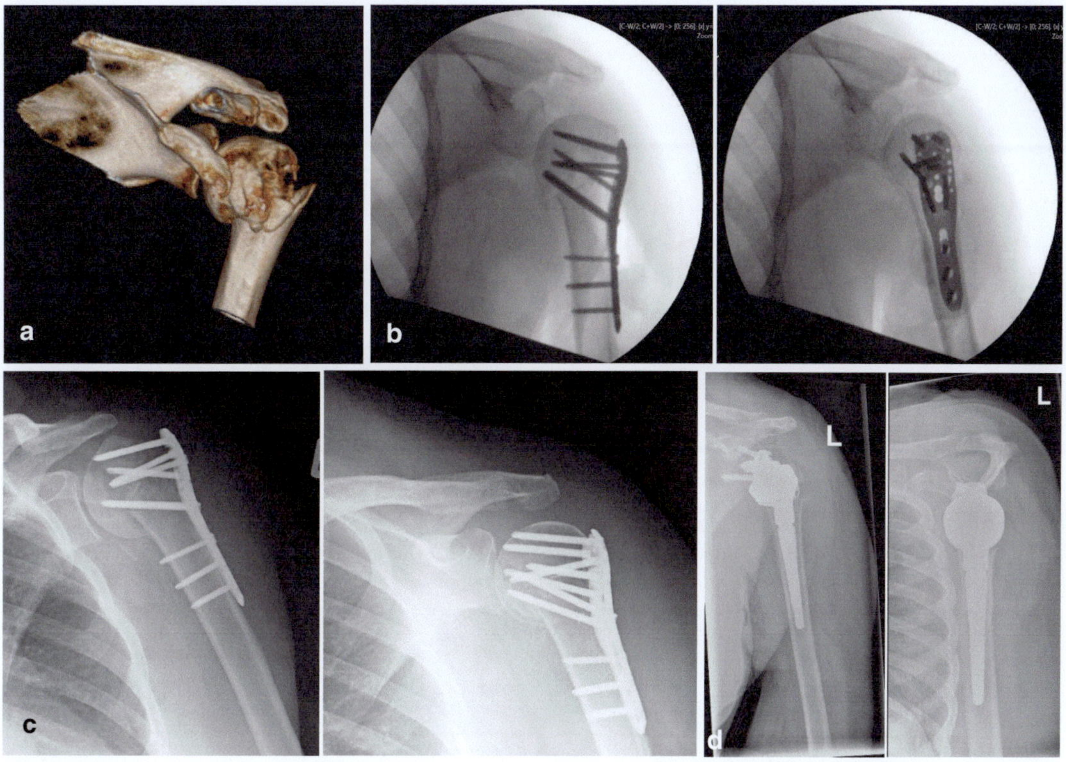

Fig. 21.2 73-year old female: Proximal humeral fracture (**a**): Initial osteosynthesis with angular stable proximal humerus plate (PHILOS, Synthes) (**b**). Secondary failure of fixation and loosening of the implant in osteoporotic bone (**c**). Revision and reverse total shoulder arthroplasty (**d**)

Secondary stability can only be achieved if sufficient primary stability is provided and bone fatigue by brittle failure, creep or trabecular crushing is prevented. The limiting factor for secondary stability is the limited fatigue strength of osteoporotic bone. Since bone fatigues at locations of high strain the primary principle of secondary stability is the prevention of excessive strain and strain concentrations. As mentioned above, implants which distribute the strain over a larger area by large surfaces or by more screws or bolts may prevent bone from early fatigue. Loading which generates excessive strains locally has to be avoided, e.g. by implants with additional features such as anti-rotation or anti-gliding mechanisms which can potentially prevent excessive shear or tensile loads (Fig. 21.3) [27]. In certain situations, additional augmentation of screws with bone cement is very effective in distributing the load from the metallic implant to the bone [28, 29].

Significant developments have taken place in order to address the difficulties which surgeons encounter in the stabilization of osteoporotic fractures. These can be summarized as being implant-related (fixed-angle devices, locking plates, coating of implants and joint replacement implants) or technique-related (bone impaction, buttress fixation, bone augmentation and lever-arm modification).

The specific demands involved in the treatment of osteoporotic fractures calls for specific solutions. Various treatment methods and innovations have been attempted in order to improve the past poor results. In general, researchers and developers have worked on three different approaches:

1. adapted design and anchoring of implants;
2. improved load distribution;
3. augmentation techniques using bone autograft or allograft, bone cement or bone substitute.

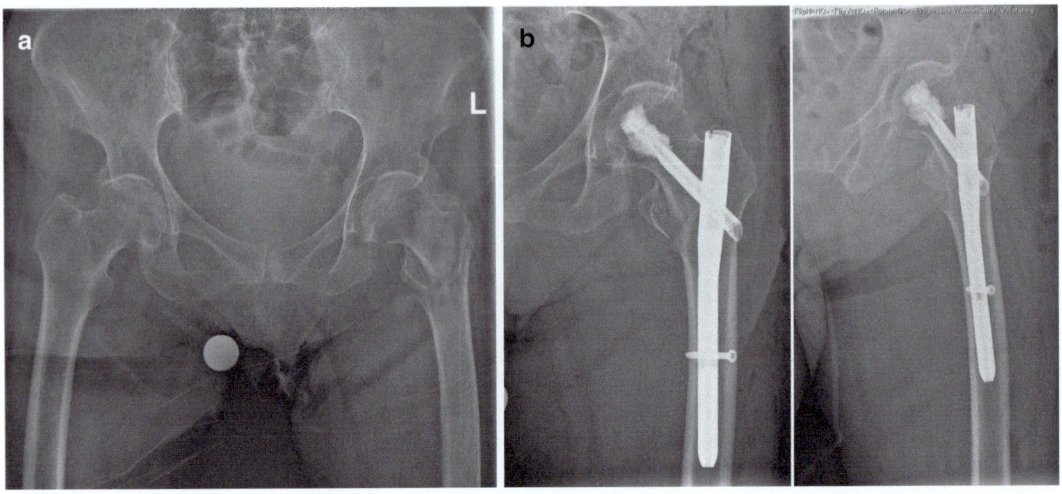

Fig. 21.3 95-year old female: Proximal femur fracture (**a**): Intramedullary nail with helical screw and augmentation (TFN, Synthes) (**b**), superior in resisting vertical or rotational displacement in comparison to conventional screws

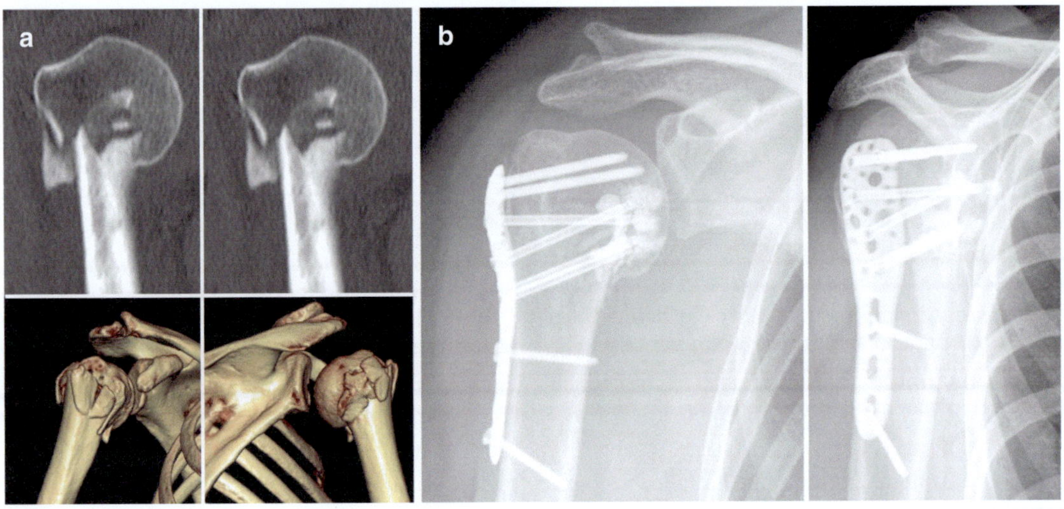

Fig. 21.4 64-year old female: proximal humeral fracture (**a**): angular stable plate osteosynthesis, augmentation (PHILOS, Synthes) (**b**)

21.3.1 Implant Design and Anchorage

21.3.1.1 Implant Design

Over the last years, implant design in orthopaedic and trauma surgery continuously developed towards devices, which are optimized in size, shape and screw orientation in certain anatomic regions. Implant scale and (bio)mechanical properties have been progressively adapted to the biological surroundings and forces expected adapted to the technical surroundings discussed above. Especially for geriatric bone and its "indicator fracture" regions huge progress has been made in terms of implant design and specialization. Implant devices, e.g. for the proximal humerus (Figs. 21.2 and 21.4) or periprosthetic fractures (Fig. 21.5), help to meet special demands of stabilization in geriatric bone through certain combinations of implant shape and screw arrangement that support fracture stabilization in geriatric bone in vulnerable anatomical regions. Double plating in 90–90° positioning of the implants further can increase torsional stability (Fig. 21.6).

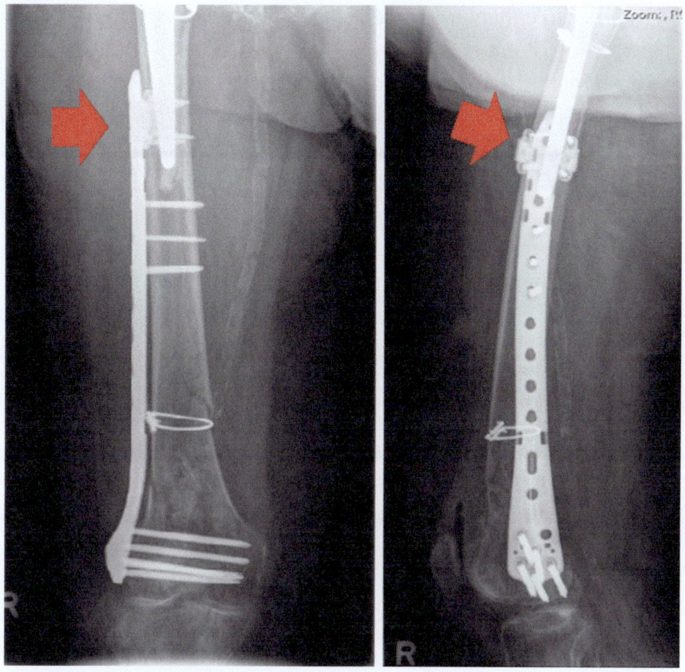

Fig. 21.5 Periprosthetic distal femur plate (Loqteq, aap) with hinges (arrows) attached laterally to a plate, adjusted as required and anchored in the bone around the prosthesis

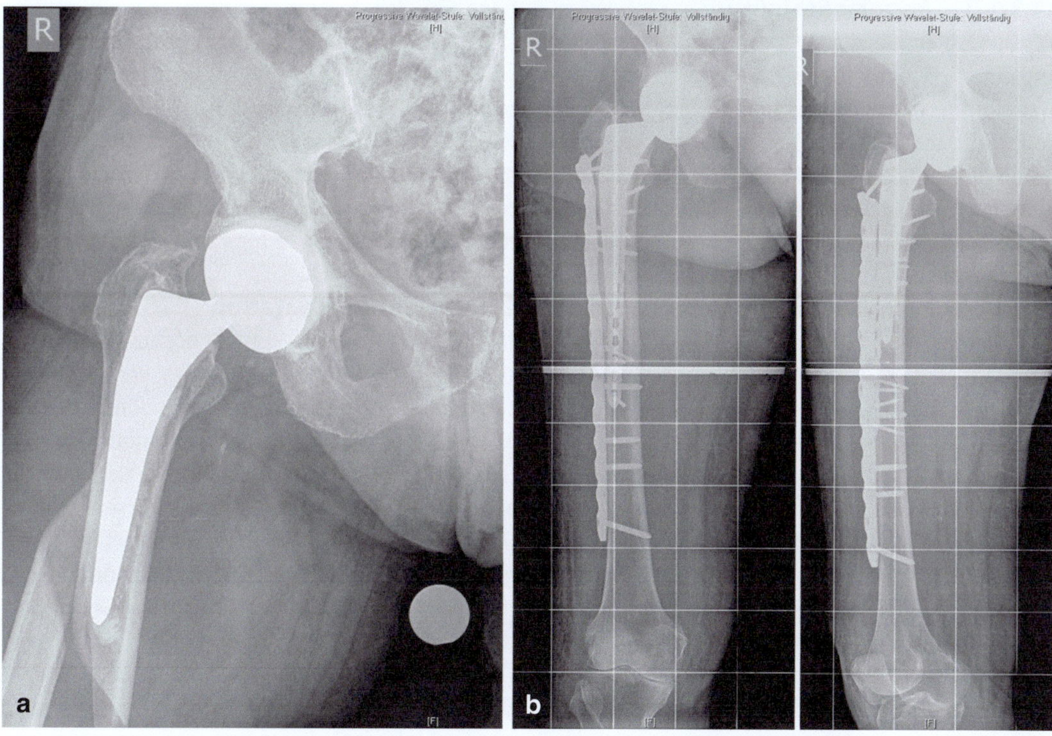

Fig. 21.6 85-year old female: Periprosthetic femoral fracture (**a**): double plating in 90–90° positioning (**b**)

In order to enhance the anchorage of screws in osteoporotic bone, efforts have been made to increase load distribution and to avoid stress risers at the implant interface by creating specialized fixation devices like helical screws (Fig. 21.3). The principle here is to compress the cancellous bone during insertion and hence increasing primary fixation.

On the other hand, this progress leads to an enormous increase of implants and devices that have to be stored and provided in each hospital treating geriatric patients. This affects not only storage but also economic capacities and may contribute to reserved treatment of geriatric fractures in specialized centres. Current developments of customized implants by individual 3D printing might help to overcome these developments and may help to provide appropriate implants for geriatric fracture stabilization in the future.

21.3.1.2 Angular Stability

Various techniques and implants have been implemented to improve initial fixation and minimize failure of open reduction and internal fixation, but the introduction of locking plates resulted in substantial increases in construct stiffness even in osteoporotic bone [30]. Numerous biomechanical studies have demonstrated that in osteoporotic bone locking plates create increased fatigue strength and improve ultimate failure loads compared to conventional plates [31, 32]. It is today generally accepted that locking plate constructs have mechanical advantages compared to conventional plate constructs and that these advantages are of particular benefit in osteoporotic bone [33].

The major difference between locking and conventional constructs is the load transfer between fracture fragments. Conventional plates rely on frictional load transfer between the plate and the bone. Thus loads are transferred from the bone to the plate across the fracture area and back to the bone again. The main advantage of the locking-plate device is the mechanical couple between the screw head and the plate (fixed-angle device) so that even if the screw–bone interface fails, the screw–plate interface remains intact (Fig. 21.2). In locked plating the plate is not compressed to the bone surface. This preserves periosteal perfusion and prevents delayed fracture healing. Therefore load transfer from the bone to the plate is achieved through the head of the locking screw. The load transfer from the bone to the screw is distributed along the length of the screw wherever the screw is in contact with bone. It has been shown that in osteoporotic bone locking plates indeed demonstrate clinical benefit by producing considerably lower tensile strains in the bone around the bone screws. This provides a mechanical explanation for the improved performance of locking plates in poorer bone quality and explains previously reported higher incidence of screw loosening using the conventional plates. Complete failure of fixation is still possible and can be seen in severe osteoporosis. Therefore, implants such as the locking compression plate and the less invasive stabilization system have significant advantages in osteoporotic bone [34, 35]. In intramedullary nailing, angular stable locking screws can also provide enhanced stability in geriatric bone by limiting the movement of the constructed. A balance must be achieved between construct stiffness and efficient load transfer because rigid constructs might result in stress shielding and thus cause a delay in tissue organization and mineralization.

21.3.1.3 Augmentation

In addition to altering implant design characteristics and screw fixation techniques, enhancing the surrounding bony environment is another method to enhance construct stability and minimize fixation failure in geriatric bone. This may be achieved at the fracture site or the screw–bone interface. Use of cancellous or structural bone grafts or synthetic bone graft substitutes can improve immediate screw purchase and even promote favourable bony remodelling.

Biological

Many biological adjuvants are available and widely utilized for general skeletal restoration. Their use for the specific task of osteoporotic fracture augmentation is less well recognized. Besides the autograft gold standard, allograft bone represents an attractive alternative for the treatment of fractures, non-unions and fusion augmentation for the osteoporotic population where autogenous harvest would be less than a satisfying experience, with low bone yields expected and all the attendant risks associated with the second surgical site. Therefore, non-biological augmentation for augmentation of osseous voids and fracture fixation has become a promising treatment option to improve fracture stability and ultimate healing.

Non-biological

Different biomaterials have been developed for reconstruction of osseous defects and enhance fixation in fragility fractures in different anatomic locations. Screw augmentation methods using polymethyl methacrylate (PMMA) or hydroxyapatite coatings have been used in an attempt to increase screw purchase in osteoporotic bone [36, 37]. PMMA is effective because it interdigitates with surrounding cancellous bone and screw threads to distribute holding force. Hydroxyapatite-coated screws directly stimulate bone remodelling to increase screw holding strength.

Cannulated screws with side openings in order to inject PMMA around the screws and thereby enhance their purchase in fractures of the humerus, femur and tibia are already in clinical practice (Figs. 21.3 and 21.4). A similar principle can be applied to a hip screw of the proximal femur nail and could show to improve fixation, although local cement application through the implant was limited [28]. Fragility fractures of the pelvis are a cumulative index fracture of osteoporosis, which can be addressed by PMMA augmented screw fixation (Fig. 21.7) [38, 39]. However, these methods are limited in that PMMA-induced thermal necrosis may result in local necrosis and might induce screw loosening.

Therefore calcium phosphate–based cements have been proposed for screw augmentation because the curing process is not exothermic and the material composition supports bone formation, which may promote fracture healing and long-term biologic fixation. Stadelmann et al. demonstrated that calcium phosphate–based bone cement substantially enhanced screw pullout force and reduced the dependence of screw pullout strength on cortical fixation [40]. Resorbable polymers could also be used to provide the additional stability needed in osteoporotic fractures until healing has occurred.

Strengthening implant fixation through the use of augmentation materials has shown promising mechanical and clinical results, with a majority of these materials showing remarkable biocompatibility. Given the demographic changes of our ageing population, the need for early weight-bearing and mobilization to avoid complications and the loss of function and independence in older patients is of great impor-

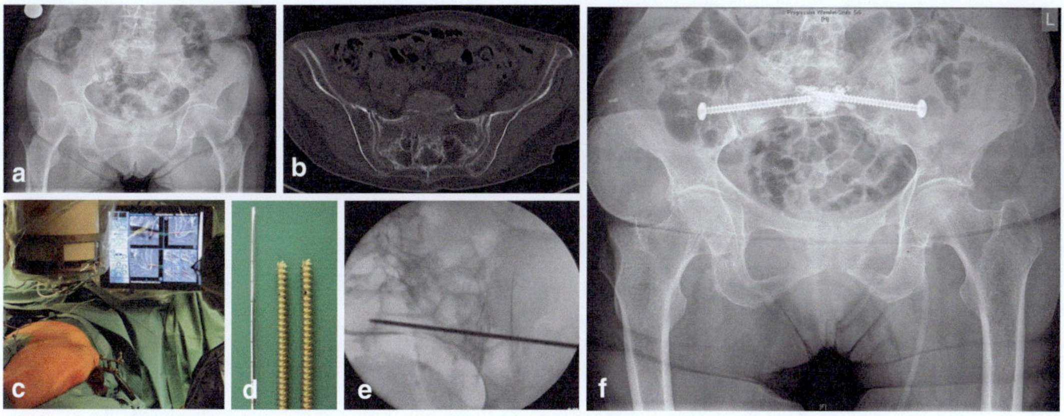

Fig. 21.7 89-year old female (**a**, **b**): bilateral fragility fracture of the sacrum: Bilateral navigated (**c**) and augmented screw osteosynthesis. Guided K-wire (**e**) and cannulated screws (**d**): Post op x-rays (**f**)

tance. Therefore, the need to develop biomaterials and composites that improve fixation in osteoporotic bone is of great importance.

First Line Arthroplasty

In case of severe joint comminution with osteoporotic bone and osteoarthritis, the benefit of internal fixation followed by prolonged non-weight-bearing is highly questionable. The indications for first-line arthroplasty in complex epiphyseal shoulder and elbow joint fractures are well established with the same rationale as for displaced femoral neck fracture in the elderly [41–43]. Primary arthroplasty is commonly used to treat acute fractures of the proximal femur, complex proximal humerus or elbow fractures, but is less common in other locations [44] (Fig. 21.8). However, there are good reasons for treating certain acute complex articular and metaphyseal fractures using primary replacement, such as: significant symptomatic osteoarthritis prior to the fracture, fracture complexity, especially of its articular part, bone fragility making fixation hazardous, and the need for early mobilization and the earliest possible resumption of walking in elderly patients, to avoid the decubitus complications and the risk of becoming bed-ridden [45].

Reconstruction using primary arthroplasty in case of complex geriatric articular fractures therefore might be an interesting and promising surgical option, limiting the number of revision surgeries while addressing several main objectives:

1. saving the patient's life by allowing early resumption of function and/or weight-bearing,
2. limiting the decubitus complications and preserving function, thanks to immediate unrestricted joint mobilization and limited loss of autonomy.

21.4 Surgical Aspects

Besides fracture configuration and bone quality, fracture stabilization in geriatric bone is determined by two other factors: The soft tissues and the patients' status. Besides bone aspects, these factors may present particular problems as thin soft tissues and skin due to atrophy or malnutrition, ischemic changes and poor healing, oedema, ulcers and chronic skin lesions. Even patient factors are often complex in the elderly, because the majority of patients also have medical comorbidities, which require careful treatment. The soft tissues surrounding geriatric fractures are fre-

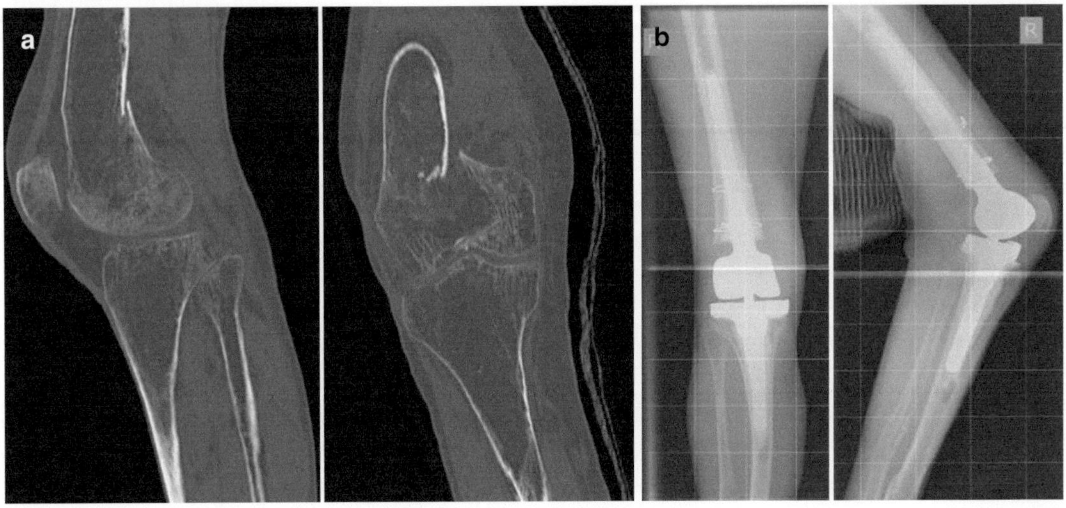

Fig. 21.8 80-year old female: Distal femoral fracture severe osteoporosis (**a**): primary arthroplasty (MUTARS distal femur, Implantcast) (**b**)

quently altered due to other concomitant diseases such as venous insufficiency, peripheral arterial disease, due to long-term cortisone intake or to pre-existing infections or decubitus. In these circumstances, there is a much higher risk of local complications when large incisions are made through compromised soft tissues or when long-lasting surgeries with aggressive manipulations are performed. Therefore, soft tissue management becomes even more important than in younger patients. The aim of surgical care after geriatric fracture in the elderly therefore is a single stop fracture management with stable fracture fixation facilitating early full weight-bearing. Techniques of osteosynthesis and approaches have to be as less invasive as possible. Minimal invasive plate osteosynthesis (MIPO), intramedullary nails, implants using long anatomical corridors and intra-osseous implants, using small incisions for insertion, are safe and prevent wound healing problems. An individual analysis of the specific benefits and drawbacks of conventional techniques and their alternatives is needed [1].

21.5 Summary

Fracture stabilization in geriatric bone remains to be challenging due to bone quality, fracture patterns and patients' general status. The goal of returning the patient to prefracture level of function is ambitious and often difficult to achieve. Significant developments have taken place in order to address the difficulties which surgeons have encountered over the years in the stabilization of osteoporotic fractures. These can be summarized as being technique-related (bone impaction, double plating and bone augmentation), implant-related (fixed-angle devices, locking plates, coating of implants and joint replacement implants) or surgery-related (less invasive).

However, since osteoporosis is a disease that is nearly always subclinical until a patient sustains a fragility fracture, and geriatric fractures are hard to treat, current management paradigms should continue to focus on prevention and on the concomitant treatment of the systemic disease.

References

1. Rommens PM. Paradigm shift in geriatric fracture treatment. Eur J Trauma Emerg Surg. 2019;45(2):181–9.
2. Barrios C, et al. Healing complications after internal fixation of trochanteric hip fractures: the prognostic value of osteoporosis. J Orthop Trauma. 1993;7(5):438–42.
3. Augat P, et al. Mechanics and mechano-biology of fracture healing in normal and osteoporotic bone. Osteoporos Int. 2005;16(Suppl 2):S36–43.
4. Marongiu G, Mastio M, Capone A. Current options to surgical treatment in osteoporotic fractures. Aging Clin Exp Res. 2013;25(Suppl 1):S15–7.
5. Bouxsein ML, Seeman E. Quantifying the material and structural determinants of bone strength. Best Pract Res Clin Rheumatol. 2009;23(6):741–53.
6. Silva MJ. Biomechanics of osteoporotic fractures. Injury. 2007;38(Suppl 3):S69–76.
7. Fuggle NR, et al. Fracture prediction, imaging and screening in osteoporosis. Nat Rev Endocrinol. 2019;15(9):535–47.
8. Zimmermann EA, Busse B, Ritchie RO. The fracture mechanics of human bone: influence of disease and treatment. Bonekey Rep. 2015;4:743.
9. Nyman JS, et al. Age-related effect on the concentration of collagen crosslinks in human osteonal and interstitial bone tissue. Bone. 2006;39(6):1210–7.
10. Pesce V, et al. Surgical approach to bone healing in osteoporosis. Clin Cases Miner Bone Metab. 2009;6(2):131–5.
11. Giannoudis PV, Schneider E. Principles of fixation of osteoporotic fractures. J Bone Joint Surg Br. 2006;88(10):1272–8.
12. Stromsoe K. Fracture fixation problems in osteoporosis. Injury. 2004;35(2):107–13.
13. Hoppe S, et al. Intraoperative mechanical measurement of bone quality with the DensiProbe. J Clin Densitom. 2015;18(1):109–16.
14. Nikolaou VS, et al. The influence of osteoporosis in femoral fracture healing time. Injury. 2009;40(6):663–8.
15. von Ruden C, Augat P. Failure of fracture fixation in osteoporotic bone. Injury. 2016;47(Suppl 2):S3–S10.
16. Bergman RJ, et al. Age-related changes in osteogenic stem cells in mice. J Bone Miner Res. 1996;11(5):568–77.
17. Rodriguez JP, et al. Abnormal osteogenesis in osteoporotic patients is reflected by altered mesenchymal stem cells dynamics. J Cell Biochem. 1999;75(3):414–23.
18. Sterck JG, et al. Response of normal and osteoporotic human bone cells to mechanical stress in vitro. Am J Physiol. 1998;274(6):E1113–20.
19. Everding J, et al. Stimulation of fracture healing by growth factors and cell-based technologies. Unfallchirurg. 2019;122(7):534–43.
20. Chapman JR, et al. Factors affecting the pullout strength of cancellous bone screws. J Biomech Eng. 1996;118(3):391–8.

21. Koval KJ, et al. An AOA critical issue. Geriatric trauma: young ideas. J Bone Joint Surg Am. 2003;85(7):1380–8.
22. Kammerlander C, et al. The use of augmentation techniques in osteoporotic fracture fixation. Injury. 2016;47(Suppl 2):S36–43.
23. Augat P, Goldhahn J. Osteoporotic fracture fixation—a biomechanical perspective. Injury. 2016;47(Suppl 2):S1–2.
24. Hepp P, et al. Where should implants be anchored in the humeral head? Clin Orthop Relat Res. 2003;415:139–47.
25. Kamer L, et al. Bone mass distribution of the distal tibia in normal, osteopenic, and osteoporotic conditions: an ex vivo assessment using HR-pQCT, DXA, and computational modelling. Calcif Tissue Int. 2016;99(6):588–97.
26. Hungerer S, et al. Biomechanical evaluation of subtalar fusion: the influence of screw configuration and placement. J Foot Ankle Surg. 2013;52(2):177–83.
27. Born CT, et al. Hip screw migration testing: first results for hip screws and helical blades utilizing a new oscillating test method. J Orthop Res. 2011;29(5):760–6.
28. Kammerlander C, et al. Standardised cement augmentation of the PFNA using a perforated blade: a new technique and preliminary clinical results. A prospective multicentre trial. Injury. 2011;42(12):1484–90.
29. Schliemann B, et al. How to enhance the stability of locking plate fixation of proximal humerus fractures? An overview of current biomechanical and clinical data. Injury. 2015;46(7):1207–14.
30. Cornell CN, Ayalon O. Evidence for success with locking plates for fragility fractures. HSS J. 2011;7(2):164–9.
31. Seide K, et al. Locked vs. unlocked plate osteosynthesis of the proximal humerus—a biomechanical study. Clin Biomech (Bristol, Avon). 2007;22(2):176–82.
32. Zehnder S, Bledsoe JG, Puryear A. The effects of screw orientation in severely osteoporotic bone: a comparison with locked plating. Clin Biomech (Bristol, Avon). 2009;24(7):589–94.
33. Miranda MA. Locking plate technology and its role in osteoporotic fractures. Injury. 2007;38(Suppl 3):S35–9.
34. Perren SM. Evolution of the internal fixation of long bone fractures. The scientific basis of biological internal fixation: choosing a new balance between stability and biology. J Bone Joint Surg Br. 2002;84(8):1093–110.
35. Schutz M, Sudkamp NP. Revolution in plate osteosynthesis: new internal fixator systems. J Orthop Sci. 2003;8(2):252–8.
36. Kammerlander C, et al. Cement augmentation of the Proximal Femoral Nail Antirotation (PFNA)—a multicentre randomized controlled trial. Injury. 2018;49(8):1436–44.
37. Rothberg DL, Lee MA. Internal fixation of osteoporotic fractures. Curr Osteoporos Rep. 2015;13(1):16–21.
38. Gruneweller N, et al. Biomechanical comparison of augmented versus non-augmented sacroiliac screws in a novel hemi-pelvis test model. J Orthop Res. 2017;35(7):1485–93.
39. Wahnert D, Raschke MJ, Fuchs T. Cement augmentation of the navigated iliosacral screw in the treatment of insufficiency fractures of the sacrum: a new method using modified implants. Int Orthop. 2013;37(6):1147–50.
40. Stadelmann VA, et al. Calcium phosphate cement augmentation of cancellous bone screws can compensate for the absence of cortical fixation. J Biomech. 2010;43(15):2869–74.
41. Parratte S, et al. Primary total knee arthroplasty in the management of epiphyseal fracture around the knee. Orthop Traumatol Surg Res. 2011;97(6 Suppl):S87–94.
42. Obert L, et al. Four-part fractures treated with a reversed total shoulder prosthesis: Prospective and retrospective multicenter study. Results and complications. Orthop Traumatol Surg Res. 2016;102(3):279–85.
43. Bohm ER, Tufescu TV, Marsh JP. The operative management of osteoporotic fractures of the knee: to fix or replace? J Bone Joint Surg Br. 2012;94(9):1160–9.
44. Ries MD. Primary arthroplasty for management of osteoporotic fractures about the knee. Curr Osteoporos Rep. 2012;10(4):322–7.
45. Boureau F, et al. Does primary total knee arthroplasty for acute knee joint fracture maintain autonomy in the elderly? A retrospective study of 21 cases. Orthop Traumatol Surg Res. 2015;101(8):947–51.

22 Orthogeriatric Inpatient Management

Zachary A. Kons, Sarah E. Hobgood, and Stephen L. Kates

22.1 Introduction

Fragility fractures represent a rapidly growing major medical problem in terms of patient outcome and cost. It is estimated that due to an aging population, the annual worldwide incidence of hip fractures will reach 6.26 million by the year 2050 [1]. There is a 5–8 times greater risk of all-cause mortality within the first 3 months following a hip fracture in older adults [2]. Independence also decreases sharply after fragility fracture, especially for patients whose fractures result in decreased mobility [3]. In a study following 733 subjects greater than 65 years of age after a hip fracture, only 36% of those who were independent in Activities of Daily Living (ADLs) prior to fracture returned to that level of independence [4]. The cost of treating hip fractures alone is estimated to increase to 62 billion dollars annually in the United States by the year 2040 [5]. The personal and economic impact of fragility fractures, especially those of the hip, clearly warrants a thorough examination of the process of inpatient management.

As the "Baby Boomer" (born between 1946 and 1964) generation ages, the incidence of fragility fractures is expected to increase. For each decade reached after the age of 50, the risk of hip fracture doubles [6]. As of 2011, the Baby Boomer generation started turning 65 years old. It is estimated that 74 million people in the United States will be 65 or older by 2030, a number that represents roughly 21% of the population [7]. With continued advances in medicine, the percentage of the population at increased risk for fragility fractures will also continue to rise due to longer life expectancy.

Poor bone health, often secondary to osteoporosis, contributes to fragility fractures [8]. Osteoporosis is the most common bone disease worldwide, causing an estimated 8.9 million fractures annually, a statistic that amounts to a fragility fracture approximately every 3 s [9]. One in three women over the age of 50 will sustain an osteoporotic fracture in their lifetime [10]. Osteoporosis is estimated to increase in incidence by 87% for those aged 65–74. Unfortunately osteoporosis is often clinically silent, going untreated and resulting in a major burden in cost to the healthcare system due to complications such as fragility fracture [11].

Z. A. Kons
Virginia Commonwealth University School of Medicine, Richmond, VA, USA
e-mail: konsza@mymail.vcu.edu

S. E. Hobgood
Department of Internal Medicine, Division of Geriatric Medicine, Virginia Commonwealth University, Richmond, VA, USA
e-mail: Sarah.hobgood@vcuhealth.org

S. L. Kates (✉)
Department of Orthopaedic Surgery, Virginia Commonwealth University, Richmond, VA, USA
e-mail: Stephen.Kates@vcuhealth.org

H.-C. Pape et al. (eds.), *Senior Trauma Patients*, https://doi.org/10.1007/978-3-030-91483-7_22

Fragility fractures and an aging population pose a threat to patients and the healthcare system. However, by understanding and optimizing the process of fragility fracture management, physicians have an opportunity to lessen these threats. Strong leadership and careful interdisciplinary teamwork can help improve patient outcomes and decrease the cost for the health system [12]. Orthopedic surgeons and geriatricians can improve how a health system approaches these patients by ensuring each member of the care team understands, accepts, and fulfills their role in the inpatient management of a fragility fracture. This chapter will discuss the role of different specialties in treating a fragility fracture optimizing patient safety and outcomes, and clearly defines the position orthopedic surgeons and geriatricians should assume in this process.

22.2 Establishing Goals of Orthogeriatric Inpatient Management

22.2.1 Surgery Within 24–48 h of Fracture

Surgical treatment of fragility fractures, especially those of the hip, within 24 h of the original fracture is ideal and is associated with better outcomes for patients including decreased length of stay and complications, including lower mortality rates, lower rates of postoperative pneumonia, and fewer pressure sores [13–16]. Although 24 h is ideal, given some variability among studies, surgery should certainly be performed within 48 h [17]. Patient safety is of utmost importance in the process of optimizing a patient for surgery; however, each test ordered should support the ultimate goal of early surgery. For example, although most institutions perform a full-body CT scan for high energy trauma patients, this "pan-scan" is typically not a necessary test for patients with a ground-level fall or fragility fracture of the hip and should therefore be avoided.

Reducing unnecessary testing is one method to decrease the time to surgery for patients with fragility fractures. Once the patient is determined to be stable, tests not needed for the surgical decision and that do not provide obvious and immediate benefit to the patient should be avoided. Every specialty involved with the care of a fragility fracture patient should share a common goal for early surgical care within 24–48 h of fracture. The overall time to surgery can be decreased significantly resulting in improved outcomes for patients and decreased costs to patients and health systems.

22.2.2 Establishing Goals of Care Prior to Operating

It is extremely important to understand the patient's overall goals of care while completing the workup and optimizing a fragility fracture patient for surgery. Different approaches to patient management may be indicated depending on the patient's goals of care, level of pre-fracture independence, and level of pain. All of these factors should be considered carefully. As one study with 357 participants from senior centers and assisted living facilities illustrated, only 11% of participants ranked "Staying Alive" as their highest priority when compared with "Independence," "Pain Relief," and "Symptom Relief" [18].

Additionally, before surgery it is important to understand whether the patient's goals of care include specific orders such as Do Not Resuscitate and Do Not Intubate. Communication with the geriatrician, hospitalist, or primary care provider who is involved with the patient's care team can help develop an understanding of the goals of care for each patient.

22.2.3 Weight-Bearing on Postoperative Day 1

With the prevailing goal of allowing the patient to bear weight immediately after hip fracture surgery, careful selection of the most appropriate surgical procedure is of utmost importance. The geriatric population may struggle with limited weight bearing and mobility restrictions for multiple reasons including underlying dementia, postoperative delirium, pre-existing functional limitations, and overall frailty [8]. Therefore, choosing a procedure that allows a patient "weight-bearing as tolerated" status on the repaired limb is optimal and associated with better mobilization and recovery over time [19]. Immobility after surgery can be detrimental and can result in irreversible muscle loss in the geriatric population [14].

To achieve the goal of "weight-bearing as tolerated" status immediately after surgical repair, clear communication must exist between the orthopedic surgeon performing the procedure, the geriatrician or hospitalist co-manager, therapists, and the nursing staff caring for the patient. Restoring early mobility represents a key principle in orthogeriatric management allowing the patient to regain pre-injury function and decrease morbidity [20].

Even in non-hip fragility fractures, function and mobility remain a major goal in management. For example, in some cases such as proximal humerus fractures where patients are wheelchair dependent, operating in a timely manner and choosing a surgical technique that allows patients to weight-bear on the repaired limb is vitally important to minimize post-surgical complications and regain pre-injury functional status.

22.3 A System Perspective

Three common models of care in fragility fracture inpatient management are Traditional Care, a Consultant Team under Orthopaedic Leadership, and Comanaged Care [21]. Each system of care presents different challenges in meeting the goals of care for a fragility fracture, namely getting a patient to surgery within 24–48 h of their fracture, weight-bearing as tolerated status on postoperative day 1, decreasing functional loss, and decreasing length hospital stay. Improvements to the systems of care for fragility fractures can produce better outcomes for patients [12]. This section will detail each of these common models and will highlight the advantages and disadvantages of each.

22.3.1 Traditional Care Model

The traditional model of care in fracture management begins in the emergency department. Overcrowding of the emergency department is commonplace. Evidence suggests that over 90% of emergency departments experience overcrowding several times per week, resulting in long wait times and full beds [22]. Fragility fracture patients in the emergency department usually present as an obvious diagnosis, but often are triaged into the less acute areas of the emergency department due to underreported pain, higher acuity cases, and overcrowding [8]. Patients sustaining ground level falls with trauma activation in the emergency department regularly undergo a full-body CT once determined to have stable vital signs.

During the admission process of a fragility fracture patient, there may be disagreement about who should ultimately admit the patient, the medical team, or the surgical team. Such "turf wars" delay the patient's admission and time to surgery and cause discord between two teams that need to have a strong interdisciplinary relationship to efficiently and effectively manage fragility fractures. In the most traditional models of care, a fragility fracture patient would be admitted under the care of the orthopedic surgeon and assessed for surgery. Further medical evaluation would be provided by the hospitalist or required medical subspecialist in a consultative manner under the direction of the orthopedic surgeon.

Medical physicians may feel uncomfortable with the process of optimizing a patient for early surgery, especially if this is not a common type of assessment for the consultant. Often, this care model results in excessive consultations and unnecessary testing, resulting in delayed surgery for fragility fracture patients [23]. Once the patient has been optimized by the surgical and medical teams, the anesthesia team will complete their assessment. Limited preoperative testing and consultation may make the anesthesiologist uncomfortable with proceeding to surgery, resulting in further delays or cancellations. These asynchronous and siloed evaluations waste valuable time. Simple protocols for fragility fracture management and better communication between the medical, surgical, and anesthesia teams can help reduce these delays.

Once the patient undergoes surgery, the orthopedic surgeon remains in charge of postoperative management, and in traditional models this portion of management usually takes place in the orthopedic ward. As previously discussed, one of the goals of fragility fracture management is to get the patient to "weight bearing as tolerated" status within 24 h of operating. However, other comorbidities may restrict the patient's weight-bearing ability and can contribute to the development of pressure ulcers. In other models of care, interdisciplinary leadership may identify and address these comorbidities more accurately and decrease the risk of consequential complications.

Newer care models represent successive improvements to the Traditional Model of fragility fracture care [24]. The variations that have been described and examined appear as early as 1988 in the literature, and have continued to evolve progressively toward more team-based care over the last three decades [21, 25]. While these developed slowly with only small changes made to the models over time, this chapter will focus on two of the more widely used and studied approaches.

22.3.2 Consultant Team Under the Leadership of Orthopedics

The addition of consultants to the care team of fragility fracture patients was one of the earlier changes made to the Traditional Model of Care. In this updated model, a team of medical consultants from a variety of subspecialties provides recommendations for particular components of the patient's care while still under the direction of an orthopedic surgeon [26]. The orthopedic surgeon still assumes the decision-making responsibility of patient care from hospital admission, through peri- and postoperative care, and coordinates the patients discharge. The medical specialists discuss individual cases with the orthopedic team and provide valuable input for the orthopedic surgeon's decision-making, but this model again relies heavily on a single physician as the leader of the care team (in this case the orthopedist) [21].

This consultant model provides inconsistent benefits. In detailing the published results of this model of fragility fracture care, Giusti et al. have highlighted the differences in benefit based on timing of consultation [21]. If the consultation occurred postoperatively, no significant differences were reported between the traditional model of care and the consultant model [25, 26]. However, when the consultant team became involved preoperatively with daily visits, there was a slight decrease in hospital length of stay when compared with the Traditional Model of fragility fracture care [27, 28].

It is important to realize that the benefits seen here are likely from the involvement of multiple disciplines, albeit in a limited approach. Ultimately, while there are slight benefits to this "consultant" model of care, successive more progressive models have provided greater benefits both in the short and long term and for the patient and system at large [29]. These more complex models of care seek to build on this teamwork and apply it under different leadership strategies, namely a shared leadership between an orthopedic surgeon and a geriatrician [12].

22.3.3 Comanaged Care: Assuming Co-Leadership in Fragility Fracture Management

The comanaged care model in the inpatient management of fragility fractures is a truly interdisciplinary approach that involves complex and advanced teamwork. It evolved from many iterations of approaches that stemmed from the Traditional Model of management and continued to involve multiple specialties as consultants in patient management [21, 25]. In the comanaged care model, leadership of the patient's care team is shared equally between an orthopedic surgeon and a geriatrician (or generalist/hospitalist who specializes in the care of elderly patients). This shared leadership presents several challenges in patient care and demands that those individuals involved in this approach communicate effectively with one another.

Equally shared patient care responsibility between the orthopedist and geriatrician remains the most important guiding principle of the comanaged care model for fragility fracture management [29]. Simply put, both specialties share responsibility for seeing the patient, writing their own orders for the patient, and communicating with each other regarding management. Because the orthopedic surgeon and geriatrician are working in cooperation, but both fully responsible for their own orders, this results in a more efficient and less error prone system of patient management [12, 29].

When a patient with a fragility fracture is admitted under the comanaged care model, the orthopedic surgeon and geriatrician will have consistent communication regarding the subsequent steps in patient care, namely in optimizing a patient for surgery and making a surgical determination. Because the two specialties work together in a collaborative setting, there should be no delays in admission (or turf wars") while trying to determine which service will admit as primary team [29].

The comanaged care model of the inpatient management of fragility fractures is described as patient-centered, protocol-driven, standardized care [29]. The comanaged model uses standard orders and procedures at each step of patient management, while still recognizing the importance of a patient-centered approach. In other words, each patient will follow the same pathway and steps throughout their admission, but changes are made based on their individual needs. The preoperative stage of the comanaged care model also involves a "comprehensive geriatric consultation" [29, 30]. This comprehensive consultation will be discussed in detail in the Sect. 22.6 later in this chapter.

The benefits in outcomes of fragility fractures under the comanaged care model have been extensively reported. Friedman et al. followed 193 patients with femoral fractures through a comanaged care model at the University of Rochester comparing outcomes to 121 patients treated without a comanaged care model at a local hospital, one which shares some faculty and staff with the University of Rochester [12]. Although the patients admitted to the comanaged care system were significantly older and had more comorbidities, the comanaged model was still associated with greater benefits [12]. The mean length of time from admission to surgery decreased from 37 h (standard deviation = 64 h) in the local hospital to 24 h (SD = 17 h) in the comanaged care model at the University of Rochester ($p = 0.02$) [12] (see Table 22.1). Additionally, the mean length of hospital stay decreased from 8.3 days (SD = 6.3) at the local hospital to 4.6 days (SD = 3.3) under comanaged care ($p < 0.001$) [12]. Decreasing time to surgery, as previously discussed, is associated with numerous benefits to the patient and the system in the management of fragility fractures, and decreasing the hospital length of stay provides cost-saving advantages for the comanaged care model over previous systems [13–16]. Additional studies have also shown that the comanaged care model decreases major medical complications, decreases length of stay, decreases in hospital mortality, and has favorable survival curves in comparison to the consultant and traditional models [31–33].

Table 22.1 shows the outcomes (length of stay and time to surgery) of a comanaged care program compared to a local hospital using usual care (non-comanaged care).

Given the successes of the comanaged model for fragility fractures, both orthopedists and geriatricians should commit to implementation in the United States and abroad. This model can be implemented in most hospitals in the United States with the commitment of a small group of orthopedic surgeons and geriatricians who demonstrate a willingness to communicate and work together toward a common goal [21].

Table 22.1 Comparison of a Comanaged Care Program with usual care in Rochester, NY

	Comanaged care model at University of Rochester	Local hospital without comanaged care	*p* value
Mean time from admission to surgery	24 h (SD = 64)	37 h (SD = 17)	0.02
Mean length of hospital stay	4.6 days (SD = 3.3)	8.3 days (SD = 6.3)	<0.001

22.4 Interdisciplinary Management: The Importance of Teamwork

The aging population has been met with a call for increased geriatric education at both the medical school and graduate levels. There is evidence to suggest that most medical schools have responded to the call by developing dedicated geriatric initiatives during training. Unfortunately, studies suggest that exposure between geriatric faculty and learners remains low with as little as 7.8% of geriatricians on faculty at medical schools participating in those educational initiatives [34, 35]. As mentioned earlier, many disciplines beyond the geriatrician are needed to effectively manage an orthogeriatric patient including primary care physicians, emergency physicians, hospitalists, generalists, internal medicine subspecialists, and surgeons. With limited medical education in geriatrics, many inexperienced physicians may be unfamiliar or uncomfortable with their role in the management of elderly patients.

In hopes of curbing the expected rise in the number of fragility fractures as the population ages, orthopedic surgeons and geriatricians will need to assume leadership positions not only in the management of this population, but also in the education of those who will be part of the care team [1]. The fragility fracture management principles should not only be taught at the medical school level but also be reinforced at the GME level.

When managing patients with fragility fractures, each member of the team must share the same goals. Establishing protocols and holding brief interdisciplinary meetings with leaders from other specialties to refine those protocols is an imperative first step that should be taken toward optimizing inpatient management. For example, the importance of operating within 24–48 hours of fracture, as well as allowing a fragility fracture patient to "weight-bear as tolerated" immediately after surgery should be understood and accepted across disciplines and specialties. Additionally, allowing leaders of other disciplines to ask questions and express concerns about their specialty's role in this process is an important step that should take place here to facilitate buy-in to the system moving forward. It is advised to have the involvement of a geriatrician in these interdisciplinary meetings, offering expertise on the inpatient management of elderly patients. As described in the comanaged care model, there are significant benefits to a co-led team by an orthopedic surgeon and geriatrician in the management of fragility fractures [29]. Having input from geriatricians in early meetings to establish protocol will facilitate further interdisciplinary relationships and ensure that the needs of elderly patients are being met. To achieve the goal of early surgery for patients with fragility fractures, early admission to the hospital and avoidance of unnecessary testing are essential preoperative steps. The uncertainty that may exist around necessary vs. unnecessary preoperative testing for optimization for surgery may also be alleviated by involving a geriatrician in these early meetings.

22.5 Fragility Fractures: Emergency Department to Hospital Admission

Working with physicians in the emergency department to establish protocols and meet the goals of fragility fracture management is essential to avoid undergoing an extended workup that can significantly delay the time to surgery. Implementing a system that uses standardized orders and calls for minimal testing is often counterintuitive to the usual training in this setting. This process requires dedication, communication, and patience from the leadership of orthopedic surgery, geriatrics, and the emergency department team.

When a fragility fracture patient presents to the emergency department, emergency medical physicians first identify the fracture based on presentation. A clear description of the injury event should be taken to identify the case as a fragility fracture, often occurring from a ground-level fall. It is important to note that a fragility fracture from a ground-level fall does not warrant the same protocols as a fully traumatized patient, such as a patient with fractures due to a motor vehicle accident or a fall from significant height. If the patient is deemed stable by the emergency medicine physician, a standardized order set should be activated, allowing the patient to be admitted under the co-leadership of the orthopedic surgeon and the geriatrician [29].

A clear and accurate history is also essential once the fracture has been identified as a fragility fracture. Clear communication and transfer of records if available when the patient presents in the emergency department is paramount. Many geriatric patients that have sustained a fragility fracture are transferred to the hospital from nursing homes or assisted living facilities; records from these facilities should arrive with the patient but occasionally are not sent [36, 37]. Records are helpful in ascertaining the patient's pre-injury functional status, determining any history of cognitive issues which may increase the risk of delirium, and providing an accurate medication list to reconcile. Having accurate records can guide decision making throughout the patient's hospital stay and help determine goals, especially trying to regain pre-injury functional status and independence.

Beyond having records that outline the patient's co-morbidities, pre-hospital functional and cognitive status, having a complete record of the patient's medication list is imperative. During the comprehensive geriatric assessment on admission, the medication list is reconciled and reviewed as medications can contribute to falls, fractures, and the unintended and unwanted sequela of the inpatient admission such as delirium. An effective geriatric assessment has been shown to decrease delirium by over one-third [29, 38].

Common pitfalls befalling timely admission to orthopedic surgery and geriatrics include unnecessary testing in the emergency department and "turf wars" in models that do not have defined co-leadership in the management of fragility fractures. Overuse of imaging is a common example of unnecessary testing in fragility fractures of the hip. A plain X-ray of the hip is most often sufficient in making a surgical determination for these patients and should be taken instead of a CT scan if the patient is deemed to be stable and is suspected to have a fragility fracture of the hip [8].

As stated, under a comanaged care model of fragility fracture management, the patient would be admitted to a team led by an orthopedic surgeon and a geriatrician to meet the goal of operating within 24–48 h after a fragility fracture [29]. Given the defined co-leadership and cooperation between the surgeon and geriatrician in the comanaged care model, no one specialty needs to rationalize, explain, or authorize, to which service the patient will ultimately be admitted. However, in systems other than comanaged care, these types of disagreements occur routinely.

22.6 Efficiency and Safety in the Preoperative Assessment

Once admitted, safe and efficient optimization of the fragility fracture patient for surgery should take place. Within the comanaged care model, the orthopedic surgeon and geriatrician may submit their own orders during this time to reduce iatrogenic errors; however, a standardized order set is used to reduce unnecessary tests and wasted time in the optimization of the patient [29, 30]. These standardized order sets avoid medications that cause delirium, while providing a guide for medical management using generic medications to reduce cost [29]. It is important to note that the comanaged care model is "patient-centered," meaning at any point during this workup, the protocols can be adjusted to meet the individual needs of the patient.

Anesthesia management will be detailed in a later section, but it is important to note that early communication with the anesthesia team during the preoperative period can help reduce delays before surgery after a patient is optimized [8].

The "comprehensive geriatric assessment" is an integral step in the comanaged care of fragility fractures [30]. During this encounter, the geriatrician will see the patient and provide a comprehensive assessment including reconciliation of medications. Given the prevalence of polypharmacy, increasing rates of adverse drug events, including drug–drug interactions medications may be held prior to surgery or stopped completely [39, 40]. Additionally, the geriatrician working with the patient may add medications at this visit that will help optimize the patient or manage pain appropriately without inducing delirium.

During this same encounter, the geriatrician will perform a mental status exam, functional status exam, and determine goals of care with the patient [29]. Ideally the mental status exam will identify patients with underlying cognitive impairment with or without superimposed delirium. Hip fracture patients commonly develop delirium, with a prevalence estimated at up to 61% [41]. As mentioned, identifying medications that could contribute to the development of delirium is imperative. Because pre-injury functional status is a predictor of patient outcomes, determining the patient's pre-hospital functional status is a necessary part of the geriatric assessment. Evidence suggests that patients with low functional status may be 1.7 times more likely to die after hip fracture [42]. The patient's pre-injury functional status will also help inform the surgeon when selecting a surgical technique or implant to best regain function [29, 43]. The geriatrician will also determine if the patient has specific goals of care such as Do Not Resuscitate and Do Not Intubate. Patient's goals vary; as a leader in orthogeriatric management, understanding a patient's expectations and respecting their goals is vitally important to providing compassionate care to patients with fragility fracture [18]. It is essential that the care team does not lose focus of this tenant while optimizing a fracture program.

Reviewing additional tests should be the responsibility of both the orthopedic surgeon and the geriatrician in the comanaged care model. This requires constant communication so that each physician is aware of the tests the other orders and the reasoning behind them [21]. Commonly the tests ordered during the workup of these fractures include a Basic Metabolic Panel, Complete Blood Count (CBC), Prothrombin Time (PT), Partial Thromboplastin Time (PTT), and Hematocrit (Hct) [8]. It is important to limit the number of tests ordered to decrease time to surgery, but these standard tests should be ordered for every patient and need to be included in the standard order sets in the comanaged care model.

The patient should be screened for anemia with a CBC. The anemia may be corrected before surgery if the hemoglobin is below 10 g, and the patient is at risk for excessive blood loss during the surgical repair. Should the patient present with a hemoglobin below 10 g, the co-led care team should consider a transfusion to minimize blood loss [8]. Significant electrolyte abnormalities should be corrected before surgery. Geriatric patients often present with dehydration after laying on the ground for extended time after a fall and should be adequately hydrated. In fact, evidence suggests that greater than one-third of older patients presenting to the hospital with medical emergencies suffer from hyperosmolar dehydration [44].

The prothrombin time (INR) and partial thromboplastin time should also be measured in the preoperative assessment to evaluate for coagulopathies and determine the risk of excessive blood loss during operation. Many geriatric patients take medication such as warfarin for anti-coagulation, and thus the INR is often elevated. The goal in preoperative management is to lower the INR to below 1.5. However, this goal is not without controversy; variation has been shown in the management of semi-urgent hip fracture patients on warfarin with INR higher than 1.5 [45, 46]. Usually though, early reversal of anticoagulation is feasible and will allow for earlier surgery and the observed benefits of operation within 24–48 h [17, 47]. Oral vitamin K should be used to lower the INR preoperatively, and fresh frozen plasma may be infused perioperatively during the operation to further reduce blood loss in patients with elevated INR.

A urinalysis should be performed if the patient displays any symptoms of infection. Having a urinary tract infection has been shown to increase the relative risk of a superficial wound infection for patients undergoing orthopedic surgery by a 2:1 ratio [48]. Even patients with asymptomatic urinary tract colonization have been shown to have higher rates of superficial wound infection in orthopedic surgery [48].

If indicated based on presentation, the geriatrician managing the patient may order an electrocardiogram to review for abnormalities or changes from previous tracings to rule out a myocardial infarction. However, extensive cardiovascular testing that does not provide immediate benefit to the patient or increase safety in the surgical procedure should be avoided otherwise, as it can delay time to surgery [8]. If the geriatrician does not feel that an electrocardiogram is essential for care during the preoperative stage, it is not necessary [30]. Additionally, patients with high cardiovascular risk factors already on beta-blockers will likely continue that class of medication during the perioperative period to help mitigate adverse cardiovascular events [49, 50].

Under the comanaged care model, very few consultations other than the comprehensive geriatric assessment take place for most patients. Once the patient has been evaluated, they are categorized into "low, medium, high, and very high" risk groups [29]. As soon as the patient is considered optimized for surgery by the geriatrician and the orthopedic surgeon under the comanaged care model, surgery should be scheduled. If the patient is at very high risk for surgery and the case is complicated, the surgery should be completed when a full support team is present. Patients should also be started on antibiotic treatment within 1 h of incision, and stopped <24 h after the surgical procedure is completed to decrease the risk of wound infection [8].

22.7 Anesthesia Management for Fragility Fractures

The anesthesia team should be informed of the patient's case early in management and notified of scheduling of surgery as soon as it takes place. Communication between the anesthesia team and the leadership of each case will help eliminate delays and cancellations. In complex cases, early involvement allows for the anesthesiologist to express concerns and work with the patient's leadership team to promptly address them preoperatively. Additionally, the anesthesia team should be informed of the results of the comprehensive geriatric assessment to address any issues well before the operation takes place. This model requires strong interdisciplinary relationships which can be formed through early involvement in cases, clear communication, and respect. Departmental leadership in all disciplines involved can help facilitate these relationships both through organized meetings and personal mentorship and counseling.

There is some debate on the optimal anesthesia technique for the management of fragility fractures. Many decisions on anesthesia management will vary depending on the type of fracture the patient presents with, as well as the recommendations of the geriatrician and the anesthesiologist involved. However, there is evidence that regional anesthesia be associated with decreased complications and even decreased mortality rates for some fragility fractures. In a study of New York state hospitals following patients with hip fractures performed by Neuman et al., regional anesthesia was found to have a 29% decreased adjusted odds of mortality over general anesthesia, and a 24% decreased adjusted odds of inpatient pulmonary complications [51]. It should be noted that these benefits significantly varied with the type of fracture, with intertrochanteric fractures displaying the above significant differences but femoral neck fractures not showing similar associations with mortality or inpatient pulmonary complications. In other potential benefits, regional anesthesia has also been shown to decrease delirium, and thus a neuraxial blockade should be used when possible for patients at increased risk [52]. Again, fragility fracture management should be patient-centered, and therefore adjustments can be made to standardized protocols to fit the needs of each patient depending on comorbidities or differing goals of care.

For more detailed information on anesthesia, see "Functional Recovery After Hip Fracture" (Chap. 37). For more information on delirium, see "Functional Recovery After Hip Fracture" (Chap. 37).

22.8 Guiding Principles in Choosing a Surgical Technique

The vast majority of fragility fractures will require surgical intervention. Infrequently, however, a patient will present with a non-displaced fragility fracture that can be managed nonoperatively. When possible, these fractures should be managed without surgery if the patient is expected to regain pre-injury functional status. Again, the patient's goals of care and functional status should be ascertained prior to this determination.

Returning to pre-fracture level of function through early intervention and immediate weight bearing as tolerated remains the primary goal in the surgical intervention of fragility fractures, especially fragility fractures of the hip. A surgical technique should be chosen that allows for weight-bearing as tolerated on the joint [53]. Fully defining this goal for each patient requires a full understanding of the patient's functional status before the fracture, and again highlights the importance of the comprehensive geriatric assessment, including a functional status assessment.

If the fracture is stable and non-displaced, often this can be treated with fixation. However, this is joint, fracture, and patient specific; comorbidities and goals should be weighed during surgical determination. Fixation is also more often used in younger patients, or patients with high pre-injury function. For fractures that are irreparable or with a high likelihood of failure in fixation, arthroplasty may be indicated. The choice of surgical technique should also be guided by the skill of the surgeon, meaning that orthopedic surgeons who are more familiar with joint replacements may be more likely to perform that procedure, and surgeons who are less familiar with total joint replacement may opt for hemiarthroplasty [8].

Ultimately, "weight-bearing as tolerated" status within 1 day of surgery and maintaining functional status remain guiding principles when choosing a surgical technique in a fragility fracture patient. Once the fracture has been repaired and confirmatory imaging has been completed, geriatric patients should be allowed to bear weight immediately to aid in recovery [19]. Many elderly patients may use assistive devices such as canes, walkers, and wheelchairs to help maintain functional independence. Therefore, including fractures of the humerus and wrist in this discussion is necessary as the ability to bear weight postoperatively on the repaired upper limb will impact early mobilization in these patients.

Specifics of surgical techniques are largely outside the scope of this chapter; for more information please see "Functional Recovery After Hip Fracture" (Chap. 37).

22.9 Effective Postoperative Management

Within a comanaged care fracture program, the leading orthopedic surgeon and geriatrician provide the standardized order sets specific to the institution [12]. These standard order sets are established to decrease the incidence of delirium in the postoperative period and should not include "deliriogenic" medications. The standardized order sets should also address bone health as GLFs or low energy hip fractures indicate osteoporosis. As a first step a Vit D level should be checked [8]. Antibiotics initiated perioperatively should be stopped within 24 h after the procedure [8]. Postoperatively each physician continues to write their own orders and communicate frequently with the other physician to decrease iatrogenic errors [12]. Beyond physician orders, standardized nursing care plans should be used, and both the orthopedic surgeon and the geriatrician continue to assume a shared responsibility for the patient's care.

Immediately after surgery, the patient should start bearing weight on the limb as tolerated. Often it is not possible for elderly patients to limit their weight-bearing status, and early mobilization is essential to regain pre-injury functional status [29]. Mobilization is not only necessary for functional outcomes, but to help mitigate delirium as well. For each day a patient does not ambulate after a hip fracture, they have an increased risk of developing postoperative delirium [54]. Each member of the postoperative care team including nursing, therapies, care partners, and providers must understand this crucial component to recovery and work together to mobilize patients.

Other prevention strategies to decrease the risk of postoperative delirium include family or friends at bedside [40] and removal of all restraints and tethers as soon as possible, including catheters, nasal cannula, and IVs. Patients should be allowed and encouraged to wear their glasses and hearing-aids during their entire hospital stay, as this has also been shown to decrease the risk of delirium [38, 55]. The patient should also undergo a daily evaluation by the geriatrician to identify whether they are at increased risk of delirium or exhibiting signs of delirium. Medications with an increased risk for causing delirium should be avoided during this period as well. For more on avoiding delirium in the management of fragility fractures, please see "Functional Recovery After Hip Fracture" (Chap. 37).

It can be difficult to accurately quantify a fragility fracture patient's pain postoperatively. Elderly patients have been shown to have a higher pain threshold and have a tendency to not accurately report their pain [56, 57]. While there is some conflicting evidence regarding pain management in elderly patients, especially those with fragility fractures of the hip, a few guiding principles do exist. Low doses of opioids as needed may be used in conjunction with consistent acetaminophen as an effective strategy with minimal side effects. The side effects of non-steroidal anti-inflammatory medications (NSAIDs) are well documented and can include acute kidney injury, gastrointestinal bleeding, and the development of delirium [58]. However, there is also evidence that NSAIDs reduce the opioid dose needed to control pain and opioid side-effects, and therefore may be considered in selected patients [59]. All deliriogenic medications should be avoided in managing pain and postoperative symptoms. Certain muscle relaxants and neuropathic pain agents may be contraindicated, and the Beers Criteria should be reviewed to help determine the appropriate medications [60].

Patients undergoing surgical treatment of fragility fractures should be treated with anticoagulants postoperatively to avoid complications such as deep venous thrombosis, stroke, or pulmonary embolism. Rapid anticoagulative agents such as unfractionated heparin and low molecular weight heparins can be considered. Complications associated with heparin include bleeding from the incision site, risk of heparin-induced thrombocytopenia (HIT), and risk of heparin-induced thrombocytopenia with thrombosis (HITT). Therefore, patients who receive unfractionated heparin should be monitored closely. Low molecular weight heparins are a good alternative to unfractionated heparin as they have a lower risk of HIT and do not require the same intensity in monitoring. However, low molecular weight heparins are often expensive and are injected subcutaneously, which can be cumbersome [8]. Fondaparinux is another expensive anticoagulant that primarily inhibits factor Xa in the coagulation cascade. Despite the expense, fondaparinux is an effective medication for thromboembolic prophylaxis and therefore should be considered in patients undergoing surgical management of fragility fractures.

Warfarin is an inexpensive medication that can be used as thromboprophylaxis in patients undergoing surgery for a fragility fracture. As an oral medication, this is an easily administered anticoagulant, but also presents a risk for bleeding and warfarin-induced skin necrosis. Patients taking warfarin should be closely monitored by following the INR to assess the risk of bleeding and other complications. Additionally, warfarin takes 72–96 h to reach a peak plasma level, which is significantly longer than unfractionated heparin and the low molecular weight heparins [61]. This time frame is not ideal for patients undergoing a surgery for fragility fracture. Newer anticoagulative agents such as coagulation factor Xa inhibitors are also commonly used in as thromboprophylaxis in the postoperative period. These medications include apixaban and rivaroxaban and have proven effective at minimizing postoperative complications such as deep vein thrombosis and pulmonary embolism [62]. The benefits, costs, and side effects of each medication should be discussed between the fragility fracture co-leadership team to reach a consensus for thromboprophylaxis.

In fragility fracture patients, pressure sores are a painful and detrimental consequence and can lead to infection and subsequent complications. As discussed, patients undergoing fragility fracture management should be weight-bearing within 24 h of operation. This should help effectively minimize the development of pressure sores after operation, but additional measures should also be taken. Frequent repositioning postoperatively, pressure-reducing mattresses, and avoidance of compression clothing are important ways that the care team should avoid pressure sore development in fragility fracture patients. There is also evidence that the risk of pressure sore development may also be decreased by nutritional supplements and moisturizing sacral skin [63]. Delirium has also been associated with the development of pressure sores [64]. Therefore, minimizing medications that may cause delirium and adhering to protocols discussed earlier (no restraints to the bed, etc.) are additional methods of reducing the incidence of pressure sores.

Management of the patient's osteoporosis and prevention of a secondary fragility fracture are discussed in a later section. However, it should be noted here that it is the role of both the orthopedic surgeon and the geriatrician as a team to counsel the patient regarding bone health and the need for follow up. Fragility fractures are the result of suboptimal bone health, and therefore patients are at risk for sustaining another fragility fracture. The postoperative period is a time when physicians involved in inpatient management have an opportunity to intervene in this cycle.

The vast majority of fragility fracture patients will continue rehabilitation at a Skilled Nursing Facility following discharge [12, 30]. In the comanaged model, the patient (and SNF staff) should be given standard instructions and their final medication list. The orthopedic surgeon and geriatrician should have both reviewed this list, discontinuing potentially harmful medications or medications that may have had drug–drug interactions due to "polypharmacy" [29, 40]. The orthopedic surgeon should follow-up with the patient regarding their bone health and their rehabilitation; after a successful discharge from the skilled nursing facility patients usually return to their previous primary care home and do not require formal follow up with the geriatrician [29].

22.10 Secondary Prevention of Fragility Fractures: The Role of a Fragility Fracture Care Team

Sustaining a fragility fracture of any kind is a major risk factor for the development of another fragility fracture. A patient's risk of sustaining a major osteoporotic fracture increases 2.7-fold in the first year after sustaining a first major osteoporotic fracture, with the risk declining over time [65]. Immediate and long-term interventions are essential to help decrease the risk of a secondary fracture due to poor bone health. Studies suggest that many patients with these fractures are not being effectively evaluated and treated for osteoporosis [66, 67]. Within the comanaged model of a fragility fracture, there are steps that the care team can take to decrease the patient's risk of sustaining a second fragility fracture and ensure the patient understands the importance of following up on their bone health.

While the specifics of secondary prevention of fragility fractures are largely outlined in the Chaps. 36 and 37, the role that orthopedic surgeons and geriatricians should take in prevention will be outlined here. This is an opportunity for those managing the fragility fracture to have an impact other than direct treatment. Although the patient should be started on vitamin D therapy during inpatient management as a first step for the treatment of osteoporosis, stressing to the patient that they should closely monitor their bone health with their primary care physician is an important step in management and can be undertaken by either the orthopedic surgeon or the geriatrician leading the patient's care team [29].

22.11 Leadership in Implementing a Fragility Fracture Program

The co-managed care model has been studied and proven to be an effective model given due to the extensive benefits shown in patient outcome and cost-reduction [12, 29, 30, 68]. However, based on local practice patterns and established relationships, these leadership tenants may be used to optimize other systems of management already in place.

22.11.1 Individual Counseling

The new fragility fracture protocol may represent a drastic change to the way the institution manages these cases and may be very different than how physicians involved in the new program were initially trained in the management of these patients. Orthopedic and geriatric leadership need to be aware that such a change may be very difficult for some physicians if they feel previous handling of these fractures provided better care. In these situations, one-on-one counseling can make a major difference for physicians. These are not meant to be meetings where physicians feel forced into a new protocol that they are uncomfortable with. Rather, they should be an open dialogue between the leadership of the specialty involved and the individual physician. The goal is to understand why an individual may feel strongly about how they have previously handled these fractures and address differences. These counseling sessions build rapport between people involved in these fragility fracture programs and will help facilitate communication and respect between all involved.

22.11.2 Patience

Sweeping changes to conventional hospital protocol take significant time to solidify and produce results, even when they are within one department. Given the degree of interdisciplinary dependence and teamwork involved in implementing an effective fragility fracture protocol, this process may take longer than expected for each specialty to consistently make the necessary changes. Having an awareness of this opposition to change and setting smaller achievable goals should help the adoption and acceptance of the comanaged fragility fracture program over time.

Working toward manageable goals is an effective way to ensure that everyone is participating in the program. For example, ensuring that 90% of fragility fracture patients will have a comprehensive geriatric consult within 6 h of admission would be a good starting point to ensure geriatricians are fully involved in the fragility fracture program. Early notification of the anesthesiology team within 6 h of fragility fracture patient's hospital admission with the goal to decrease delays and cancellations due to uncertainty in the anesthesia decision-making will help garner support from the anesthesia team.

Regardless of how the short-term goals are set, the overall objective remains the same in orthogeriatric inpatient comanagement: implement a patient-centered, protocol-driven, standardized care program for fragility fractures. Operating this system with compassion and adjusting for the patient's functional status and overall goals allow for the optimal care of a wide variety of patients with fragility fractures.

References

1. Cooper C, Campion G, Melton LJ 3rd. Hip fractures in the elderly: a world-wide projection. Osteoporos Int. 1992;2:285–9.
2. Haentjens P, Magaziner J, Colon-Emeric CS, et al. Meta-analysis: excess mortality after hip fracture among older women and men. Ann Intern Med. 2010;152:380–90.
3. Schemitsch EH, Sprague S, Heetveld MJ, et al. Loss of independence after operative management of femoral neck fractures. J Orthop Trauma. 2019;33:292–300.
4. Tang VL, Sudore R, Cenzer IS, et al. Rates of recovery to pre-fracture function in older persons with hip fracture: an observational study. J Gen Intern Med. 2017;32:153–8.
5. Youm T, Koval KJ, Zuckerman JD. The economic impact of geriatric hip fractures. Am J Orthop. 1999;28:423–8.
6. Friedman SM, Mendelson DA. Epidemiology of fragility fractures. Clin Geriatr Med. 2014;30:175–81.
7. Wallman K. Older Americans—key indicators of well-being. In: Federal Interagency Forum on Aging Related Statistics; 2016.
8. Mears SC, Kates SL. A guide to improving the care of patients with fragility fractures, edition 2. Geriatr Orthop Surg Rehabil. 2015;6:58–120.
9. Johnell O, Kanis JA. An estimate of the worldwide prevalence and disability associated with osteoporotic fractures. Osteoporos Int. 2006;17:1726–33.
10. Melton LJ 3rd, Chrischilles EA, Cooper C, et al. Perspective. How many women have osteoporosis? J Bone Miner Res. 1992;7:1005–10.
11. Kling JM, Clarke BL, Sandhu NP. Osteoporosis prevention, screening, and treatment: a review. J Womens Health (Larchmt). 2014;23:563–72.
12. Friedman SM, Mendelson DA, Bingham KW, et al. Impact of a comanaged Geriatric Fracture Center on short-term hip fracture outcomes. Arch Intern Med. 2009;169:1712–7.
13. Al-Ani AN, Samuelsson B, Tidermark J, et al. Early operation on patients with a hip fracture improved the ability to return to independent living. A prospective study of 850 patients. J Bone Joint Surg Am. 2008;90:1436–42.
14. Orosz GM, Magaziner J, Hannan EL, et al. Association of timing of surgery for hip fracture and patient outcomes. JAMA. 2004;291:1738–43.
15. Pioli G, Frondini C, Lauretani F, et al. Time to surgery and rehabilitation resources affect outcomes in orthogeriatric units. Arch Gerontol Geriatr. 2012;55:316–22.
16. Simunovic N, Devereaux PJ, Sprague S, et al. Effect of early surgery after hip fracture on mortality and complications: systematic review and meta-analysis. CMAJ. 2010;182:1609–16.
17. Moja L, Piatti A, Pecoraro V, et al. Timing matters in hip fracture surgery: patients operated within 48 hours have better outcomes. A meta-analysis and meta-regression of over 190,000 patients. PLoS One. 2012;7:e46175.
18. Fried TR, Tinetti ME, Iannone L, et al. Health outcome prioritization as a tool for decision making among older persons with multiple chronic conditions. Arch Intern Med. 2011;171:1854–6.
19. Hoffmann RH, Np. Femur:proximal. In: Ruedi TP, Murphy WM, editors. AO principles of fracture management. New York: Thieme; 2000. p. 441–54.
20. Siu AL, Penrod JD, Boockvar KS, et al. Early ambulation after hip fracture: effects on function and mortality. Arch Intern Med. 2006;166:766–71.
21. Giusti A, Barone A, Razzano M, et al. Optimal setting and care organization in the management of older adults with hip fracture. Eur J Phys Rehabil Med. 2011;47:281–96.
22. Derlet R, Richards J, Kravitz R. Frequent overcrowding in U.S. emergency departments. Acad Emerg Med. 2001;8:151–5.
23. Katz RI, Cimino L, Vitkun SA. Preoperative medical consultations: impact on perioperative management and surgical outcome. Can J Anaesth. 2005;52:697–702.
24. Pioli G, Giusti A, Barone A. Orthogeriatric care for the elderly with hip fractures: where are we? Aging Clin Exp Res. 2008;20:113–22.
25. Gilchrist WJ, Newman RJ, Hamblen DL, et al. Prospective randomised study of an orthopaedic geriatric inpatient service. BMJ. 1988;297:1116–8.
26. Naglie G, Tansey C, Kirkland JL, et al. Interdisciplinary inpatient care for elderly people with hip fracture: a randomized controlled trial. CMAJ. 2002;167:25–32.
27. Khasraghi FA, Christmas C, Lee EJ, et al. Effectiveness of a multidisciplinary team approach to hip fracture management. J Surg Orthop Adv. 2005;14:27–31.
28. Swanson CE, Day GA, Yelland CE, et al. The management of elderly patients with femoral fractures. A randomised controlled trial of early intervention versus standard care. Med J Aust. 1998;169:515–8.
29. Kates SL, Mendelson DA, Friedman SM. Co-managed care for fragility hip fractures (Rochester model). Osteoporos Int. 2010;21:S621–5.
30. Friedman SM, Mendelson DA, Kates SL, et al. Geriatric co-management of proximal femur fractures: total quality management and protocol-driven care result in better outcomes for a frail patient population. J Am Geriatr Soc. 2008;56:1349–56.
31. Barone A, Giusti A, Pizzonia M, et al. A comprehensive geriatric intervention reduces short- and long-term mortality in older people with hip fracture. J Am Geriatr Soc. 2006;54:711–2.
32. Gonzalez-Montalvo JI, Alarcon T, Mauleon JL, et al. The orthogeriatric unit for acute patients: a new model of care that improves efficiency in the management of patients with hip fracture. Hip Int. 2010;20:229–35.
33. Vidan M, Serra JA, Moreno C, et al. Efficacy of a comprehensive geriatric intervention in older patients hospitalized for hip fracture: a randomized, controlled trial. J Am Geriatr Soc. 2005;53:1476–82.

34. Eleazer GP, Doshi R, Wieland D, et al. Geriatric content in medical school curricula: results of a national survey. J Am Geriatr Soc. 2005;53:136–40.
35. Warshaw GA, Bragg EJ, Shaull RW, et al. Academic geriatric programs in US allopathic and osteopathic medical schools. JAMA. 2002;288:2313–9.
36. Jones JS, Dwyer PR, White LJ, et al. Patient transfer from nursing home to emergency department: outcomes and policy implications. Acad Emerg Med. 1997;4:908–15.
37. Sweitzer BJ. Preoperative screening, evaluation, and optimization of the patient's medical status before outpatient surgery. Curr Opin Anaesthesiol. 2008;21:711–8.
38. Marcantonio ER, Flacker JM, Wright RJ, et al. Reducing delirium after hip fracture: a randomized trial. J Am Geriatr Soc. 2001;49:516–22.
39. Baranzini F, Diurni M, Ceccon F, et al. Fall-related injuries in a nursing home setting: is polypharmacy a risk factor? BMC Health Serv Res. 2009;9:228.
40. Jyrkka J, Enlund H, Korhonen MJ, et al. Polypharmacy status as an indicator of mortality in an elderly population. Drugs Aging. 2009;26:1039–48.
41. Inouye SK, Westendorp RG, Saczynski JS. Delirium in elderly people. Lancet. 2014;383:911–22.
42. Berry SD, Samelson EJ, Bordes M, et al. Survival of aged nursing home residents with hip fracture. J Gerontol A Biol Sci Med Sci. 2009;64:771–7.
43. Robinson TN, Eiseman B, Wallace JI, et al. Redefining geriatric preoperative assessment using frailty, disability and co-morbidity. Ann Surg. 2009;250:449–55.
44. El-Sharkawy AM, Watson P, Neal KR, et al. Hydration and outcome in older patients admitted to hospital (The HOOP prospective cohort study). Age Ageing. 2015;44:943–7.
45. Ashouri F, Al-Jundi W, Patel A, et al. Management of warfarin anticoagulation in patients with fractured neck of femur. ISRN Hematol. 2011;2011:294,628.
46. Cohn MR, Levack AE, Trivedi NN, et al. The hip fracture patient on warfarin: evaluating blood loss and time to surgery. J Orthop Trauma. 2017;31:407–13.
47. Gleason LJ, Mendelson DA, Kates SL, et al. Anticoagulation management in individuals with hip fracture. J Am Geriatr Soc. 2014;62:159–64.
48. Ollivere BJ, Ellahee N, Logan K, et al. Asymptomatic urinary tract colonisation predisposes to superficial wound infection in elective orthopaedic surgery. Int Orthop. 2009;33:847–50.
49. Van Klei WA, Bryson GL, Yang H, et al. Effect of beta-blocker prescription on the incidence of postoperative myocardial infarction after hip and knee arthroplasty. Anesthesiology. 2009;111:717–24.
50. Wallace AW, Au S, Cason BA. Association of the pattern of use of perioperative beta-blockade and postoperative mortality. Anesthesiology. 2010;113:794–805.
51. Neuman MD, Silber JH, Elkassabany NM, et al. Comparative effectiveness of regional versus general anesthesia for hip fracture surgery in adults. Anesthesiology. 2012;117:72–92.
52. Sieber FE, Zakriya KJ, Gottschalk A, et al. Sedation depth during spinal anesthesia and the development of postoperative delirium in elderly patients undergoing hip fracture repair. Mayo Clin Proc. 2010;85:18–26.
53. Koval KJ, Sala DA, Kummer FJ, et al. Postoperative weight-bearing after a fracture of the femoral neck or an intertrochanteric fracture. J Bone Joint Surg Am. 1998;80:352–6.
54. Kamel HK, Iqbal MA, Mogallapu R, et al. Time to ambulation after hip fracture surgery: relation to hospitalization outcomes. J Gerontol A Biol Sci Med Sci. 2003;58:1042–5.
55. Inouye SK. Delirium after hip fracture: to be or not to be? J Am Geriatr Soc. 2001;49:678–9.
56. Chai E, Horton JR. Managing pain in the elderly population: pearls and pitfalls. Curr Pain Headache Rep. 2010;14:409–17.
57. Gibson SJ, Helme RD. Age-related differences in pain perception and report. Clin Geriatr Med. 2001;17:433–56, v–vi.
58. Wongrakpanich S, Wongrakpanich A, Melhado K, et al. A comprehensive review of non-steroidal anti-inflammatory drug use in the elderly. Aging Dis. 2018;9:143–50.
59. Marret E, Kurdi O, Zufferey P, et al. Effects of nonsteroidal antiinflammatory drugs on patient-controlled analgesia morphine side effects: meta-analysis of randomized controlled trials. Anesthesiology. 2005;102:1249–60.
60. By the American Geriatrics Society Beers Criteria Update Expert P. American Geriatrics Society 2019 updated AGS beers criteria(R) for potentially inappropriate medication use in older adults. J Am Geriatr Soc. 2019;67:674–94.
61. Ansell J. Warfarin versus new agents: interpreting the data. Hematology Am Soc Hematol Educ Program. 2010;2010:221–8.
62. Fisher WD, Eriksson BI, Bauer KA, et al. Rivaroxaban for thromboprophylaxis after orthopaedic surgery: pooled analysis of two studies. Thromb Haemost. 2007;97:931–7.
63. Reddy M, Gill SS, Rochon PA. Preventing pressure ulcers: a systematic review. JAMA. 2006;296:974–84.
64. Remaley DT, Jaeblon T. Pressure ulcers in orthopaedics. J Am Acad Orthop Surg. 2010;18:568–75.
65. Johansson H, Siggeirsdottir K, Harvey NC, et al. Imminent risk of fracture after fracture. Osteoporos Int. 2017;28:775–80.
66. Ekman EF. The role of the orthopaedic surgeon in minimizing mortality and morbidity associated with fragility fractures. J Am Acad Orthop Surg. 2010;18:278–85.
67. Hooven F, Gehlbach SH, Pekow P, et al. Follow-up treatment for osteoporosis after fracture. Osteoporos Int. 2005;16:296–301.
68. Kates SL, Mendelson DA, Friedman SM. The value of an organized fracture program for the elderly: early results. J Orthop Trauma. 2011;25:233–7.

Comanagement Admission and Timing of Surgery

23

Valentin Neuhaus and Carina Pothmann

23.1 Introduction

The main goal in geriatric trauma is to achieve positive outcomes for patients. Typical outcome measures in geriatric trauma are mortality, postoperative delirium, or patients returning home. Many factors influence these outcomes. Lisa Lezzoni, a Harvard Medical School professor, wrote the book "Risk Adjustment for Measuring Health Care Outcomes" [1]. She presented the formula in which "outcome equals patient factors plus effectiveness of care plus random events." Comanagement admission and the timing of surgery affect and interact with all factors and have a paramount influence on outcomes, particularly mortality. An increasing number of studies on the geriatric and surgical comanagement of elderly trauma patients have been published, showing a positive synergistic effect. Most studies on the timing of surgery were performed in patients with hip fractures. Early hip surgery was associated with lower mortality and morbidity, especially fewer pressure ulcers, cases of urinary tract infection, and cases of pneumonia [2, 3]. Consequently, many national and international guidelines recommend early surgery in patients with hip fractures for better outcomes. However, there are some controversies [4, 5]. Some studies have also shown a favorable outcome with delayed surgery in distinct patient groups. Hence, more factors must be included in such disclosures. Analogous to Lisa Lezzoni's formula, we propose the formula in which "timing depends on patient factors, medical care, and random events":

- Patient-Related Factors
  - Sustained injuries, life- or limb-threatening, multiple or isolated
  - Comorbidities that can or cannot be improved
  - Current medication
  - Patient's will
- Medical Care
  - Surgeons, including those who have completed training
  - Hospital (e.g., operating room availability)
  - Need for special implants/prosthesis/material
- Random Events

V. Neuhaus (✉) · C. Pothmann
Department of Trauma Surgery, University Hospital of Zurich, Zurich, Switzerland
e-mail: valentin.neuhaus@usz.ch; carina.pothmann@usz.ch

H.-C. Pape et al. (eds.), *Senior Trauma Patients*, https://doi.org/10.1007/978-3-030-91483-7_23

23.2 Patient-related Factors

23.2.1 Injuries

23.2.1.1 Life- or Limb-Threatening Injuries

Life-threatening and potentially life-threatening injuries must be addressed immediately. We are hunting for airway obstruction, tension pneumothorax, open pneumothorax, massive hemothorax, flail chest, and hemodynamic instability due to hemorrhage [6]. Usually, a heart rate >100 per minute and a systolic blood pressure <90 mmHg are the cut-offs for defining hemodynamic instability. These values are probably not ideal in geriatric trauma patients due to some effects of aging on physiologic and pathophysiologic responses. Some studies suggest using a higher systolic blood pressure of 110 mmHg as a threshold [7]. After life-saving procedures are performed, open fractures, compartment syndrome, and injuries with compromised arterial supply, or *limb-threatening* injuries, must be treated. The timing of the treatment of life- and limb-threatening injuries is not under debate. They must be treated as soon as they are diagnosed.

23.2.1.2 Multiple or Isolated Injuries

Multiple injuries often warrant a damage control procedure in unstable or extremis patients. Several factors are used to distinguish stable, unstable, or extremis patients [8–11]. The presence of shock, coagulopathy, hypothermia, and distinct chest, abdominal, or pelvic injuries are the main parameters. Age is not a specific risk factor for classification as unstable or in extremis. Current research is ongoing about this topic. One question is how well elderly patients endure the second hit and, consequently, if this hit must be further minimized in elderly patients. Because of missing evidence, the sequencing of treatment and fracture care remains the same as in younger individuals.

Fractures in the lower extremity cause pain and immobility. It seems obvious that early surgery will allow earlier mobilization and, as a consequence, fewer complications. The association between timing of surgery and outcome is best studied in hip fractures, since fractures of the hip are very common. Many national guidelines recommend early surgery within 24 or 48 h. Lewis and Waddell performed an intensive literature review and concluded that the goal is to achieve painless mobilization with a low rate of morbidity and mortality [4]. While the goal is obvious, it is less clear which outcome parameters are the best measures. Looking at the most often used outcome parameters (mortality, pressure ulcers, urinary tract infection, and pneumonia), they concluded that a healthy elderly patient with a hip fracture should be operated on as soon as possible. They also concluded that in the case of significant reversible comorbidities, it seems advisable to improve the patients' health status for one or two days and consequently perform the operation in a healthier individual. One-year mortality is 20% in hip fracture patients [12]; however, mortality can be decreased by improving comorbidity in these patients [13]. Typical examples are patients with decompensated heart failure or with coronary heart disease, which must be treated with a stent or a coronary artery bypass first. In brief, healthy patients must be treated in a timely manner, and a nonmedical delay must be avoided. If a comorbidity represents a significant risk factor for mortality or morbidity and can be improved, then a delay of one or two days is acceptable to treat this disease. Prophylactic decubitus measures must be started simultaneously. Especially in these patients with a medical delay, the comanagement among geriatric specialists, internal specialists, and trauma surgeons is of exceptional importance [14, 15]. A comprehensive and multidisciplinary approach is indicated in these patients, along with standardized operating procedures. Early evaluation and assessment in the emergency department, medical comanagement if necessary, and surgery as soon as possible to keep door-to-knife time as short as possible must be the goal. All these actions improve mortality, shorten the length of stay, and lower the postoperative complication rates.

Fragility fractures of the pelvis or the spine are often treated nonoperatively, depending on the type of fracture [16, 17]. After failed nonoperative treatment, mostly because patients cannot be mobilized due to pain, a surgical approach is offered. The duration of nonoperative treatment is disputable; some surgeons offer surgery within days [18], while other surgeons wait more than one to two weeks [19] to proceed with surgery. Spinal injuries have a higher impact on negative outcomes [20] and should be performed earlier.

The timing of surgery in fractures of the upper extremity usually does not represent a major issue or a risk factor for mortality and morbidity. Similar to cases of fractures in the lower extremity, we tend to operate as soon as the patient is fit for the operation. An earlier operation, especially at the proximal humerus, can be associated with better outcomes and fewer complications, and patients can be mobilized and discharged earlier [21, 22].

23.2.2 Comorbidities

Polymorbidity is a normal part of the aging process [23, 24] and geriatric trauma care. It can even be the reason for falls. Cardiovascular assessment in the emergency department is essential to rule out low blood pressure or arrhythmia as the cause of the fall. Nevertheless, polymorbidity causes an immense delay and the need for specialist involvement [25]. We are facing an increasing number of patients with a disease causing falls; the disease needs to be treated immediately, either operatively or nonoperatively. Typical examples are acute stroke or myocardial infarction. The medical consequences are often the use of anti-aggregative medication with a higher risk for perioperative complications. Another problem is a patient having a disease (e.g., decompensated heart failure), which has an important effect on outcomes and can be improved with simple maneuvers. All these interventions cause a delay in the treatment of injuries; however, geriatric comanagement helps to improve the current patient's health status and consequently lowers mortality and morbidity [26]. Standardized protocols with clear pre- and postoperative diagnostic and treatment algorithms and the involvement of specialists, if needed, can improve the outcomes of geriatric trauma patients [27]. The prioritization is a multidisciplinary decision involving the trauma surgeon, intensivists, and diverse specialists in geriatrics, cardiology, neurology, and other disciplines.

23.2.3 Current Medication

Polypharmacy is common and causes many dangerous problems [28, 29]. The cessation of acetylsalicylic acid (aspirin) and other medications is very common to lower the risk of operation. However, the cessation of certain medications can cause the recurrence of certain diseases or symptoms. Currently, there is quite a high discordance between daily practice and some guideline recommendations [30]. We tend to continue aspirin, especially in patients with stents.

New oral anticoagulants (NOACs), as an alternative to vitamin K antagonists, are emerging into the market. Typical agents are rivaroxaban and apixaban. They are very potent, convenient, and sometimes safer; however, they are not ideal in patients needing surgery [31]. Many national guidelines recommend ceasing NOACs for at least 24 h before invasive or surgical procedures without bridging during cessation. NOACs should be stopped for at least 48 h in cases of high-risk procedures (e.g., brain, spinal cord). As an alternative, the assessment of their blood level can be helpful in distinct situations.

23.3 Medical Care

23.3.1 Surgeons

Orthogeriatric trauma care is becoming increasingly specialized. The bone quality and the aim of the operation (full weight-bearing as soon as possible) warrant special considerations and techniques. A "one-shot surgery" is the main goal. There are many courses and meetings only about orthogeriatric trauma care, which help surgeons become familiar with these issues.

In parallel, politicians are regulating the health care sector. These regulations (e.g., being allowed to perform or being prohibited from performing distinct procedures) can result in a certain nonmedical delay in early treatment.

23.3.2 Hospital

Delays in treating patients with hip fractures are quite common. In many hospitals, orthogeriatric trauma care is performed during the nights or weekends. Fracture care has a lower priority. Accordingly, the outcomes can be negative. The organization of an emergency theatre in the case of limited operating room capacity to get the patients into the OR as quickly as possible could improve the outcomes [32]. The goal must be early surgery. Another issue is that most of the nonmedical delays are due to hospital factors [33], which could be improved by organizational actions.

As a further step, the presence of an orthogeriatric service, characterized by a collaboration between trauma surgeons and geriatric specialists focusing on the early and professional assessment and treatment of elderly trauma patients, improves the mortality and morbidity of these patients [34]. Such services usually also prioritize elderly patients before younger and healthier patients.

23.3.3 Need for Special Implants/ Prosthesis

As patients grow older, we also see older prostheses and implant models, which can cause further problems. The local availability of many different implants and prostheses is no longer possible—there is the pressure of high costs, and the outsourcing of materials is common.

References

1. Iezzoni LI. Risk adjustment for measuring health care outcomes. 3rd ed. Chicago, IL: Health Administration Press; 2003. p. 508.
2. Klestil T, Roder C, Stotter C, et al. Impact of timing of surgery in elderly hip fracture patients: a systematic review and meta-analysis. Sci Rep. 2018;8(1):13933.
3. Klestil T, Roder C, Stotter C, et al. Immediate versus delayed surgery for hip fractures in the elderly patients: a protocol for a systematic review and meta-analysis. Syst Rev. 2017;6(1):164.
4. Lewis PM, Waddell JP. When is the ideal time to operate on a patient with a fracture of the hip?: a review of the available literature. Bone Joint J. 2016;98-B(12):1573–81.
5. Hagino T, Ochiai S, Senga S, et al. Efficacy of early surgery and causes of surgical delay in patients with hip fracture. J Orthop. 2015;12(3):142–6.
6. Galvagno SM Jr, Nahmias JT, Young DA. Advanced trauma life support((R)) update 2019: management and applications for adults and special populations. Anesthesiol Clin. 2019;37(1):13–32.
7. Eastridge BJ, Salinas J, McManus JG, et al. Hypotension begins at 110 mm Hg: redefining "hypotension" with data. J Trauma. 2007;63(2):291–7. discussion 297-299
8. Pape HC, Giannoudis P, Krettek C. The timing of fracture treatment in polytrauma patients: relevance of damage control orthopedic surgery. Am J Surg. 2002;183(6):622–9.
9. Pape HC, Giannoudis PV, Krettek C, et al. Timing of fixation of major fractures in blunt polytrauma: role of conventional indicators in clinical decision making. J Orthop Trauma. 2005;19(8):551–62.
10. Pape HC, Halvachizadeh S, Leenen L, et al. Timing of major fracture care in polytrauma patients – an update on principles, parameters and strategies for 2020. Injury. 2019;50(10):1656–70.
11. Pape HC, Tornetta P 3rd, Tarkin I, et al. Timing of fracture fixation in multitrauma patients: the role of early total care and damage control surgery. J Am Acad Orthop Surg. 2009;17(9):541–9.
12. Leibson CL, Tosteson AN, Gabriel SE, et al. Mortality, disability, and nursing home use for persons with and without hip fracture: a population-based study. J Am Geriatr Soc. 2002;50(10):1644–50.
13. Elkbuli A, Eily A, Polcz V, et al. Isolated hip fracture in the elderly and time to surgery: is there an outcome difference? Trauma Surg Acute Care Open. 2018;3(1):e000212.
14. Friedman SM, Mendelson DA, Kates SL, et al. Geriatric co-management of proximal femur fractures: total quality management and protocol-driven care result in better outcomes for a frail patient population. J Am Geriatr Soc. 2008;56(7):1349–56.
15. Middleton M. Orthogeriatrics and hip fracture care in the UK: factors driving change to more integrated models of care. Geriatrics (Basel). 2018;3(3)
16. Krappinger D, Kammerlander C, Hak DJ, et al. Low-energy osteoporotic pelvic fractures. Arch Orthop Trauma Surg. 2010;130(9):1167–75.
17. Rommens PM, Arand C, Hofmann A, et al. When and how to operate fragility fractures of the pelvis? Indian J Orthop. 2019;53(1):128–37.
18. Rommens PM, Ossendorf C, Pairon P, et al. Clinical pathways for fragility fractures of the pelvic ring: personal experience and review of the literature. J Orthop Sci. 2015;20(1):1–11.

19. Tosounidis G, Wirbel R, Culemann U, et al. Misinterpretation of anterior pelvic ring fractures in the elderly. Unfallchirurg. 2006;109(8):678–80.
20. Liem IS, Kammerlander C, Raas C, et al. Is there a difference in timing and cause of death after fractures in the elderly? Clin Orthop Relat Res. 2013;471(9):2846–51.
21. Abdelhady AM. Timing of shoulder arthroplasty in comminuted proximal humerus fracture, how much does it matter? Eur J Orthop Surg Traumatol. 2013;23(5):515–9.
22. Siebenburger G, Van Delden D, Helfen T, et al. Timing of surgery for open reduction and internal fixation of displaced proximal humeral fractures. Injury. 2015;46(Suppl 4):S58–62.
23. Faner R, Cruz T, Lopez-Giraldo A, et al. Network medicine, multimorbidity and the lung in the elderly. Eur Respir J. 2014;44(3):775–88.
24. Foreman KJ, Marquez N, Dolgert A, et al. Forecasting life expectancy, years of life lost, and all-cause and cause-specific mortality for 250 causes of death: reference and alternative scenarios for 2016-40 for 195 countries and territories. Lancet. 2018;392(10159):2052–90.
25. Wei J, Zeng L, Li S, et al. Relationship between comorbidities and treatment decision-making in elderly hip fracture patients. Aging Clin Exp Res. 2019;31(12):1735–41.
26. Swart E, Kates S, McGee S, et al. The case for comanagement and care pathways for osteoporotic patients with a hip fracture. J Bone Joint Surg Am. 2018;100(15):1343–50.
27. Grigoryan KV, Javedan H, Rudolph JL. Orthogeriatric care models and outcomes in hip fracture patients: a systematic review and meta-analysis. J Orthop Trauma. 2014;28(3):e49–55.
28. Carroll C, Hassanin A. Polypharmacy in the elderly-when good drugs lead to bad outcomes: a teachable moment. JAMA Intern Med. 2017;177(6):871.
29. Gleich J, Pfeufer D, Zeckey C, et al. Orthogeriatric treatment reduces potential inappropriate medication in older trauma patients: a retrospective, dual-center study comparing conventional trauma care and co-managed treatment. Eur J Med Res. 2019;24(1):4.
30. Plumer L, Seiffert M, Punke MA, et al. Aspirin before elective surgery-stop or continue? Dtsch Arztebl Int. 2017;114(27-28):473–80.
31. Yeh CH, Hogg K, Weitz JI. Overview of the new oral anticoagulants: opportunities and challenges. Arterioscler Thromb Vasc Biol. 2015;35(5):1056–65.
32. Bhattacharyya T, Vrahas MS, Morrison SM, et al. The value of the dedicated orthopaedic trauma operating room. J Trauma. 2006;60(6):1336–40. discussion 1340-1331
33. Cha YH, Ha YC, Yoo JI, et al. Effect of causes of surgical delay on early and late mortality in patients with proximal hip fracture. Arch Orthop Trauma Surg. 2017;137(5):625–30.
34. Stenqvist C, Madsen CM, Riis T, et al. Orthogeriatric service reduces mortality in patients with hip fracture. Geriatr Orthop Surg Rehabil. 2016;7(2):67–73.

24 Diagnostic Procedures: Coagulation

Jan-Dirk Studt, Alexander Kaserer, and Donat R. Spahn

Oral anticoagulants (OAC) are prescribed to a significant proportion of the population. The main indications are the therapy and secondary prophylaxis of venous thromboembolism, the prevention of stroke and systemic embolism in non-valvular atrial fibrillation, and thromboprophylaxis after hip and knee replacement. These entities affect predominantly older patients in whom comorbidities with an impact on OAC excretion and bleeding risk occur more frequently. Substances used for oral anticoagulation are vitamin K antagonists (VKA) such as phenprocoumon, acenocoumarol, or warfarin and the newer direct oral anticoagulants (DOAC). Available DOAC include the thrombin (factor IIa) antagonist dabigatran etexilate, and the factor Xa antagonists rivaroxaban, apixaban, and edoxaban. Betrixaban is another factor Xa antagonist with a longer half-life which is currently not available in Europe (Table 24.1).

In trauma patients, a significant residual OAC effect promotes hemorrhage, delays surgery, and may trigger the administration of an antidote. Trauma patients are often unable to indicate whether they are taking an OAC. Also, the type of OAC often remains unknown as well as the indication for anticoagulant treatment or the time of its last ingestion. In addition, potentially interacting co-medication is frequent. Fast and reliable determination of an OAC's plasma level is therefore essential for the clinical management of these patients, and is recommended by the latest European Trauma Treatment Guidelines [1]. Accordingly, we give an overview on how OAC affect routine coagulation assays, and which assays are useful for discriminating between the different substances and for monitoring their plasma level.

24.1 Oral Anticoagulants and Routine Assays of Coagulation

Whether routine assays of coagulation (prothrombin time [PT/Quick test] and international normalized ratio [INR], activated partial thromboplastin time [aPTT], thrombin time, and fibrinogen according to *Clauss* as a thrombin time-derived test) are affected by an OAC and to what extent depends on several factors. The most important of these are:

- The OAC's mechanism of action and target: decreased synthesis of vitamin K-dependent coagulation factors, thrombin inhibition, or factor Xa inhibition.
- The OAC's dosage and pharmacokinetics, and the interval between its last ingestion and

J.-D. Studt (✉)
Division of Medical Oncology and Hematology, University of Zürich and University Hospital Zürich, Zürich, Switzerland
e-mail: jan-dirk.studt@usz.ch

A. Kaserer · D. R. Spahn
Institute of Anesthesiology, University of Zürich and University Hospital Zürich, Zürich, Switzerland

H.-C. Pape et al. (eds.), *Senior Trauma Patients*, https://doi.org/10.1007/978-3-030-91483-7_24

Table 24.1 Characteristics and monitoring of direct oral anticoagulants (DOAC). If assays with DOAC-specific calibration (preferred) are not available, routine assays serve for detecting a clinically relevant residual plasma concentration (exclusion)

Substance	Dabigatran	Rivaroxaban	Apixaban	Edoxaban
Trade name	Pradaxa®	Xarelto®	Eliquis®	Lixiana®
Target	Factor IIa (thrombin)	Factor Xa	Factor Xa	Factor Xa
T_{max} (h)	0.5–2	2–4	3–4	1–2
$T_{1/2}$ (h)	12–14	5–9 (young) 11–13 (elderly)	12	10–14
Preferred assay for monitoring	Calibrated anti-IIa	Calibrated anti-Xa	Calibrated anti-Xa	Calibrated anti-Xa
Assay for exclusion	Thrombin time	Anti-Xa (heparin)	Anti-Xa (heparin)	Anti-Xa (heparin)

Table 24.2 Discrimination between oral anticoagulants using three routine coagulation assays

	PT/INR	Thrombin time	Anti-Xa assay
VKA	⬆	0	0
Dabigatran	Variable	⬆	0
Factor Xa antagonists	Variable	0	⬆

PT/INR prothrombin time/international normalized ratio, *VKA* vitamin K antagonists, ⬆ strong effect, *0* no effect

blood sampling all affecting plasma concentration.

- The assay's or reagent's sensitivity to the respective OAC.

VKA affect primarily PT/Quick test and INR, which serve for their monitoring. VKA have no effect on thrombin time and fibrinogen *(Clauss)*.

In contrast, the thrombin antagonist dabigatran significantly prolongs the thrombin time. Fibrinogen (*Clauss*) which is determined by a thrombin time-derived test may be underestimated in the presence of a high dabigatran plasma concentration. PT/INR is prolonged to a lesser extent, and for some reagents only in the presence of a high dabigatran plasma concentration.

Factor Xa antagonists (rivaroxaban, apixaban, edoxaban) may affect PT/INR but have no effect on thrombin time or fibrinogen (*Clauss*). They are the only class of OAC with an impact on anti-Xa activity assays.

Because of such differences among the OAC, their fast and reliable discrimination in the emergency setting is achieved by combining three routine assays of coagulation: PT/INR, thrombin time, and anti-Xa assay (Table 24.2).

The higher the dose and the plasma concentration of an anticoagulant, the more pronounced is its effect on coagulation assays. Equally important is the OAC's pharmacokinetics and the interval between its ingestion and the blood sampling.

- VKA have a long half-life (e.g., phenprocoumon approximately 160 h) so that their effect on coagulation assays will not change significantly during a day.
- In contrast, DOAC reach peak plasma level with a maximal impact on coagulation assays approximately 1–4 h after ingestion (dabigatran 0.5–2 h, rivaroxaban 2–4 h, apixaban 3–4 h, and edoxaban 1–2 h). Trough levels with no or only minor impact on coagulation assays are observed after 12–24 h.

24.2 Assays for DOAC

Different assays and types of reagents show a different sensitivity for DOAC [2]. Therefore, PT/INR within the normal range do not exclude a clinically significant residual DOAC plasma concentration. For a precise quantitation of their plasma concentration, assays calibrated for the respective DOAC are used [3, 4].

- Thrombin time-derived assays calibrated for dabigatran for the quantitation of the thrombin (FIIa)-antagonist dabigatran ("anti-factor IIa activity assay"). If not available, a thrombin time that is not prolonged serves for excluding a clinically significant dabigatran plasma concentration.
- Anti-FXa activity assays calibrated for rivaroxaban, apixaban, or edoxaban for the quantitation of the respective DOAC's plasma concentration. If DOAC-calibrated assays are not available, a universal anti-FXa activity assay calibrated for low molecular weight-heparin (LMWH) serves for excluding a clinically significant plasma concentration. Due to its correlation with DOAC-specific assays, it allows a quantitative estimation, in addition.

It is important to remember that anti-factor IIa and anti-factor Xa assays are affected not only by DOAC but also by coadministration of unfractionated or LMWH. Unless an assay contains a heparin-neutralizing agent (such as the Biophen DiXaI assay [Hyphen Biomed, Neuville-sur-Oise, France]) it is not possible to discriminate the respective contributions of DOAC and coadministered heparin.

Anesthesiological guidelines provide recommendations on standard preoperative intervals after the last ingestion of DOAC. However, the perioperative bleeding risk associated with DOAC has not been systematically investigated and at present, different recommendations on preoperative cut-off concentrations are proposed. The Swiss Society of Anaesthesiology and Resuscitation Guidelines recommend a residual rivaroxaban plasma level of <50 ng/ml for elective surgery as it was shown that this concentration does not exacerbate ongoing hemorrhage. The International Society on Thrombosis and Haemostasis and the French Working Group on Perioperative Haemostasis recommend a DOAC plasma concentration of <30 ng/ml for surgery with a high bleeding risk.

Factors should be considered that can result in a higher-than-expected residual DOAC plasma level. We retrospectively investigated 518 measurements in 368 patients and identified amiodarone co-medication and impaired renal function with a glomerular filtration rate of <60 ml/min as such factors. In these patients, preoperative determination of DOAC plasma level would be advisable even when routine preoperative intervals are observed [5].

References

1. Spahn DR, Bouillon B, Cerny V, Duranteau J, Filipescu D, Hunt BJ, Komadina R, Maegele M, Nardi G, Riddez L, Samama CM, Vincent JL, Rossaint R. The European guideline on management of major bleeding and coagulopathy following trauma. Fifth edition. Crit Care. 2019;23:98.
2. Samama MM, Martinoli JL, LeFlem L, Guinet C, Plu-Bureau G, Depasse F, Perzborn E. Assessment of laboratory assays to measure rivaroxaban-an oral, direct factor Xa inhibitor. Thomb Haemost. 2010;3:815–25.
3. Baglin T, Hillarp A, Tripodi A, Elalamy I, Buller H, Ageno W. Measuring oral direct inhibitors of thrombin and factor Xa: a recommendation from the Subcommittee on Control of Anticoagulation of the Scientific and Standardization Committee of the International Society on Thrombosis and Haemostasis. J Thromb Haemost. 2013;11:756–60.
4. Kitchen S, Gray E, Mackie I, Baglin T, Makris M. Measurement of non-Coumarin anticoagulants and their effects on tests of haemostasis: guidance from the British Committee for Standards in Haematology. Br J Haematol. 2014;166:830–41.
5. Kaserer A, Schedler A, Jetter A, Seifert B, Spahn DR, Stein P, Studt JD. Risk factors for higher-than-expected residual rivaroxaban plasma concentrations in real-life patients. Thromb Haemost. 2018;118:808–17.

Prevention and Management of Infections in Elderly

25

F. Ziegenhain, G. N. Jukema, and H. Sax

25.1 Background

25.1.1 Infectious Complications

Infectious complications in trauma patients are one of the major adverse events in trauma patients and affect the primary outcome [2, 3]. They lead to a significant increase in length of stay and costs as well as morbidity and mortality [4, 5]. The four most important healthcare-associated infections (HAI) are pneumonia, catheter-associated urinary tract infection (CAUTI), central line-associated bloodstream infections (CLABSI), and surgical site infections (SSI). They all have in common, that, in theory, most of them would be preventable [6–8]. A reduction of these infections thanks to the implementation of preventive measures could be obtained over the last few years, yet there is still considerable room for improvement [9]. Over the last 15 years, it has become increasingly clear that insights from implementation science [10], social sciences, and human factors engineering [11, 12] are needed to achieve safer hospitals, including the eradication of the preventable proportion of HAI. The World Health Organization (WHO) is producing ample guidance and tools in this approach [13]

The definition of the four most common HAIs according to the latest version of the European Centers for Disease Prevention and Control are listed in Table 25.1 [14]

25.1.2 Hospital-Acquired Pneumonia

Hospital-acquired pneumonia (HAP) is subdivided in two groups, ventilator-associated pneumonia (VAP) and non-ventilator-associated hospital-acquired pneumonia (nvHAP) [15]. Pneumonia is one of the most common HAI in general [16]. Many of the elderly patients are especially vulnerable for these HAP due to pre-existing conditions like dysphagia, dementia, and neurological conditions [17, 18].

25.1.3 Catheter-Associated Urinary Tract Infections

Between 75% and 80% of urinary tract infections that occur in hospitals are associated with the use of indwelling catheters [19, 20]. If the patient develops an urosepsis, mortality rates are as high as 20–40% [21, 22]. Approximately a quarter of all patients are catheterized during their hospital

F. Ziegenhain (✉) · G. N. Jukema
Department of Trauma, University Hospital Zurich, Zurich, Switzerland
e-mail: franziska.ziegenhain@usz.ch; gerroltnico.jukema@usz.ch

H. Sax
Department of Infectious Diseases and Hospital Epidemiology, University Hospital Zurich, Zurich, Switzerland
e-mail: hugo.sax@mac.com

H.-C. Pape et al. (eds.), *Senior Trauma Patients*, https://doi.org/10.1007/978-3-030-91483-7_25

Table 25.1 Definition of the four most common healthcare-associated infections

Hospital-acquired pneumonia	Two or more serial chest X-rays or CT-scans with a suggestive image of pneumonia for patients with underlying cardiac or pulmonary disease(in patients without underlying cardiac or pulmonary disease one definitive chest X-ray or CT-scan is sufficient), and at least one of the following: • fever >38°C with no other cause; • leukopenia (<4000 WBC/mm³) or leucocytosis (≥12,000 WBC/mm³);and at least one of the following(or at least two if clinical pneumonia only = PN 4 and PN 5): • New onset of purulent sputum, or change in character of sputum (colour, odour, quantity, consistency); • cough or dyspnoea or tachypnoea; • Suggestive auscultation (rales or bronchial breath sounds), rhonchi, wheezing; • Worsening gas exchange (e.g. O_2 desaturation or increased oxygen requirements or increased ventilation demand); and according to the used diagnostic method: (a) bacteriologic diagnostic test performed by: • Positive quantitative culture from minimally contaminated LRT (lower respiratory tract) specimen (PN 1):-broncho-alveolar lavage (BAL) with a threshold of >104 CFU²/ml or ≥5% of BAL obtained cells contain intracellular bacteria on direct microscopic exam (classified on the diagnostic category BAL);-protected brush (PB Wimberley) with a threshold of >103 CFU/ml;-distal protected aspirate (DPA) with a threshold of >103 CFU/ml. • Positive quantitative culture from possibly contaminated LRT specimen (PN 2):-quantitative culture of LRT specimen (e.g. endotracheal aspirate) with a threshold of 106 CFU/mlb) Alternative microbiology methods (PN 3): • Positive blood culture not related to another source of infection; • Positive growth in culture of pleural fluid; • pleural or pulmonary abscess with positive needle aspiration; • Histologic pulmonary exam shows evidence of pneumonia; • Positive exams for pneumonia with virus or particular germs (Legionella, Aspergillus, mycobacteria, mycoplasma, Pneumocystis carinii):-positive detection of viral antigen or antibody from respiratory secretions (e.g. EIA, FAMA, shell vial assay, PCR);-positive direct exam or positive culture from bronchial secretions or tissue; -seroconversion (e.g. influenza viruses, Legionella,Chlamydia);-detection of antigens in urine (Legionella). (c) Others: • Positive sputum culture or non-quantitative LRT specimen culture (PN 4); • No positive microbiology (PN 5).
Catheter-associated urinary tract infection	UTI-A: Microbiologically confirmed symptomatic UTI • Patient has at least one of the following signs of symptoms with no other recognized cause: Fever (>38°C), urgency, frequency, dysuria, or suprapubic tenderness and • patient has a positive urine culture, that is, ≥105 microorganisms per ml of urine with no more than two species of microorganisms. UTI-B: Not microbiologically confirmed symptomatic UTI • Patient has at least two of the following with no other recognized cause: Fever (> 38°C), urgency, frequency, dysuria, or suprapubic tenderness, and • At least one of the following: Positive dipstick for leukocyte esterase and/or nitrate;-pyuria urine specimen with ≥10 WBC/ml or ≥3 WBC/high-power field of unspun urine;-organisms seen on gram stain of unspun urine;-at least two urine cultures with repeated isolation of the same uropathogen (gram-negative bacteria or *S. saprophyticus*) with ≥102 colonies/ml urine in non-voided specimens;-≤105 colonies/ml of a single uropathogen (gram-negative bacteria or *S. saprophyticus*) in a patient being treated with effective antimicrobial agent for a urinary infection;-physician diagnosis of a urinary tract infection;-physician institutes appropriate therapy for a urinary infection. UTI-C: Asymptomatic bacteriuria: • Patient has no fever (>38°C), urgency, frequency, dysuria, or suprapubic tenderness and either of the following criteria: • Patient has had an indwelling urinary catheter within seven days before urine is cultured, and • Patient has a urine culture, that is, ≥ 10e5 microorganisms per ml of urine with no more than two species of microorganisms; • Patient has not had an indwelling urinary catheter within seven days before the first positive culture; and • Patient has had at least two positive urine cultures ≥ 105 microorganisms per mm3 of urine with repeated isolation of the same microorganism and no more than two species of microorganisms. * Note: Bloodstream infections secondary to asymptomatic bacteriuria are reported as BSI with source (origin) S-UTI

Central line-associated bloodstream infection	• One positive blood culture for a recognized pathogen or • Patient has at least one of the following signs or symptoms: Fever (> 38°C), chills, or hypotension and • Two positive blood cultures for a common skin contaminant (from two separate blood samples, usually within 48 hours).Skin contaminants = coagulase-negative staphylococci, Micrococcus sp., Propionibacterium acnes, Bacillus sp., Corynebacterium sp. Note: This definition corresponds to the former HELICS BSI-A definition; BSI-B (single blood culture for skin contaminants in patients with central vascular catheter and adapted treatment) was deleted following recommendations at an ECDC expert meeting in January 2009 and subsequent confirmation at the annual meeting. Sources of bloodstream infection: • Catheter-related: The same microorganism was cultured from the catheter or symptoms improve within 48hours after removal of the catheter (C-PVC: Peripheral catheter, C-CVC: Central vascular catheter). Important: Report C-CVC or C-PVC BSI as CRI3-CVC or CRI3-PVC respectively if microbiologically confirmed; see CRI3 definition. • Secondary to another infection: The same microorganism was isolated from another infection site, or strong clinical evidence exists that bloodstream infection was secondary to another infection site, invasive diagnostic procedure or foreign body:-pulmonary (S-PUL);-urinary tract infection (S-UTI);-digestive tract infection (S-DIG);-surgical site infection (S-SSI);-skin and soft tissue (S-SST);-other (S-OTH). • Unknown origin (UO): None of the above, bloodstream infection of unknown origin (verified during survey and no source found) • Unknown (UNK): No information available about the source of the bloodstream infection or information missing note: Primary bloodstream infections include catheter-related BSI and BSI of unknown origin. CRI3-CVC: Microbiologically confirmed CVC-related bloodstream infection • BSI occurring 48hours before or after catheter removal (if any) and • Positive culture with the same microorganism of either:-quantitative CVC culture ≥103CFU/ml or semi-quantitative CVC culture >15 CFU;-quantitative blood culture ratio CVC blood sample/peripheral blood sample > 5 [3];-differential delay of positivity of blood cultures [4]: CVC blood sample culture positive two hours or more before peripheral blood culture (blood samples drawn at the same time);-positive culture with the same microorganism from pus from insertion site.
Surgical site infection	Superficial incisional (SSI-S) infection occurs within 30 days after the operation and infection involves only skin and subcutaneous tissue of the incision and at least one of the following: • Purulent drainage with or without laboratory confirmation, from the superficial incision. • Organisms isolated from an aseptically obtained culture of fluid or tissue from the superficial incision. • At least one of the following signs or symptoms of infection: pain or tenderness, localized swelling, redness, or heat, and superficial incision is deliberately opened by surgeon, unless incision is culture-negative. • Diagnosis of superficial incisional SSI made by a surgeon or attending physician. Deep incisional (SSI-D)infection occurs within 30 days after the operation if no implant is left in place, or within 90 days if implant is in place and the infection appears to be related to the operation and infection involves deep soft tissue (e.g. fascia, muscle) of the incision and at least one of the following: • Purulent drainage from the deep incision but not from the organ/space component of the surgical site. • A deep incision spontaneously dehisces or is deliberately opened by a surgeon when the patient has at least one of the following signs or symptoms: Fever (> 38 °C), localized pain or tenderness, unless incision is culture-negative. • An abscess or other evidence of infection involving the deep incision is found on direct examination, during reoperation, or by histopathologic or radiologic examination. • Diagnosis of deep incisional SSI made by a surgeon or attending physician. Organ/space (SSI-O)infection occurs within 30 days after the operation if no implant is left in place, or within 90 days if implant is in place and the infection appears to be related to the operation and infection involves any part of the anatomy (e.g. organs and spaces) other than the incision which was opened or manipulated during an operation, and at least one of the following: • Purulent drainage from a drain that is placed through a stab wound into the organ/space; • Organisms isolated from an aseptically obtained culture of fluid or tissue in the organ/space; • An abscess or other evidence of infection involving the organ/space that is found on direct examination, during reoperation, or by histopathologic or radiologic examination; • Diagnosis of organ/space SSI made by a surgeon or attending physician.

The reproduced definitions are according to the European Centers for Disease Prevention and Control (ECDC) [14]

Table 25.2 Preventive measures against non-ventilator-associated hospital-acquired pneumonia

Basic steps	Oral hygiene Eating and drinking in upright position Assessment and treatment for dysphagia
Physiotherapy	Respiratory therapy Early mobilization
Medication	Avoid Sedativa Re-evaluation of PPI and antiacids

stay with even a higher proportion among the elderly [23, 24]. Prevention of CAUTI is crucial to improve the outcome in trauma patients. Taking steps to educate the medical staff and implementing basic measurements can significantly reduce the number of urinary tract infections [20].

25.1.4 Central Line-Associated Bloodstream Infections (CLABSI)

The use of a central venous catheter is often inevitable in patients after severe trauma. However, they entail the risk of serious infectious complications. Risk of infection increases with every day the central line stays in place. CLABSI are associated with higher mortality and prolonged hospital stay [25–27].

25.1.5 Surgical Side Infections

SSI is defined as an infection that occurs after a surgical intervention and is located at the surgical site [28]. They can be further divided into superficial and deep wound or organ space infections. The criteria of diagnosis include local signs of infection, purulent secretion from the wound, positive cultures from the wound, spontaneous or surgical wound reopening [29]. Cases with implanted foreign material tend to be more difficult to treat, as a biofilm forms on the implants with reduced antibiotic penetration [1]. In traumatology, implant-associated surgical site infects still pose one of the most difficult problems to solve. Especially when the implanted material cannot be removed, controlling the infection often confronts the medical team with serious challenges [30]. In that particular situation a new challenging treatment modality, so-called 'negative pressure wound therapy with instillation technique' can be helpful to treat infection to retain implants. This treatment is highly effective if applied within 90 days after implant of (metal) hardware [31, 32].

25.1.6 Comorbidities

Elderly patients often have more comorbidities then their younger counterparts [33]. These pre-existing conditions make them more vulnerable for infections. Especially frail patients are at risk for developing complications and therefor adverse outcomes [34–36]. Medical staff dealing with elderly trauma patients need to assess that risk and emphasize it.

25.2 Prevention

25.2.1 Hand Hygiene

Hand hygiene is the most effective way in preventing the spread of virulent or multi-resistant pathogens [37, 38]. An internationally established ruleset exists in the 'My five moments for hand hygiene' for hand hygiene indications [39]. Yet, the use of this simple preventive measure by healthcare providers is still substandard [40]. This topic should be especially emphasized as this basic measurement can significantly reduce the incidence of all nosocomial infections [1, 6, 37, 38, 41]. The WHO has issued guidance and tools for the successful implementation of hand hygiene rules on the institutional and national level [42] based on 'five avenues of action': (1) system change, i.e. an adequate infrastructure with the availability of alcohol-based handrub at the bedside; (2) monitoring of hand hygiene performance and feedback to those concerned; (3) education and training of all healthcare providers; (4) visual reminders at the workplace; and, (5) institutional patient safety culture and leadership [43].

25.2.2 Pneumonia

For prevention of pneumonia several interventions have proven effective [15, 44–46]. The most effective measures for nvHAP are listed in Table 25.2 below. The prevention of VAP follows the well-established principles. Especially the assessment and treatment of dysphagia, oral hygiene, and early mobilization should be emphasized in older patients.

25.2.3 Catheter-Associated Urinary Tract Infections

The use of indwelling urinary catheters is one of the most important risk factors for developing a urinary tract infection. Elderly patients are more likely to be catheterized during their hospital stay [23]. The risk of infections increases with every day the catheter stays in place [24]. Therefore, indwelling catheters should only be used for defined indications and removed as soon as they are not indicated anymore. These include surgical procedures of long durations, acute bladder retention, immobilization (e.g. in patients with unstable spine injuries), critically ill patients who need an exact monitoring of urinary output, and decubital ulcera in incontinent patients and palliative care [19]. In incontinent patients, other options like urinary condoms in men and diapers should be the first choice. Strategies for the successful implementation of preventive measures have been established, including daily reminders to re-evaluate the indication for catheterization, attributing the responsibility for removal to nursing staff, standardization and training of staff on the aseptic catheterization [47]. If an infection is suspected, the system whole system should be changed under antibiotic treatment since biofilm is likely to form that jeopardizes treatment success [1, 48].

25.2.4 Central Line-Associated Bloodstream Infections

Similar to CAUTI, the risk of CLABSI increases with every day the catheter stays in place [27]. Therefore, the same preventive strategies apply, including aseptic handling of insertion site and hubs, aseptic insertion using maximal barrier precautions. Additionally, the femoral insertion site should be avoided, and chlorhexidine-patches applied at the insertion site [26] The handling of the system must be exclusively done by trained medical staff. The insertion side should be checked regularly for signs of infection (swelling, pain, purulent secretion). If there is any suspicion of infection, the catheter should be removed and the tip sent in for microbiological testing [25, 26]. Blood cultures taken simultaneously through the central line and from a peripheral vein allow for the assessment of the differential time-to-positivity to distinguish a line infection from another reason for the bloodstream infection.

25.3 Treatment of Healthcare-Associated Infections

Antibiotics should be administered when a HAI is clearly suspected on the basis of a thorough clinical and laboratory evaluation. The primary choice should be active against the range of expected bacteria compatible with the clinical suspicion(s). Adequate microbiologic sampling should always be done prior to the first dose of antibiotics. As soon as the results of the sampling are available, antibiotics should be targeted to match the identified compartment, bacteria and antibiotic resistance profile. Pre-existing conditions should be considered before administering antibiotics, especially chronic renal insufficiency, liver diseases, and allergies to establish the right choice and dose of the anti-infective therapy. Especially in elderly patients with polypharmacy, drug interactions have to be considered.

For SSI, the common rule is that the best therapy in most of the cases is a primary surgical approach. In infected wounds, a thorough debridement should be performed [30]. In addition to surgical therapy, negative pressure wound therapy has been proven highly effective to limit the number of surgical procedures needed to treat infection and to reduce the risk for later recurrences [49]. Whenever possible, foreign material should be removed. In traumatology, this is often not possible. In these cases, an interdisciplinary approach should be pursued to ensure the best possible outcome for the patient.

25.4 Summary

Even today, HAI are still being responsible for unnecessary morbidity, mortality, costs, and prolonged duration of hospital stay. Especially the vulnerable population of elderly patients is at increased risk for enduring these adverse outcomes. When initializing treatment, pre-existing conditions such as kidney and renal diseases should be considered. Sampling should always be done prior to administering antibiotics. As a large proportion of these infections are avoidable, healthcare providers should especially emphasize on the prevention of these adverse events. Evidence-based preventive measures have been well established and should be implemented using best practice from implementation science.

References

1. Schreiber PW, Sax H, Wolfensberger A, Clack L, Kuster SP. The preventable proportion of healthcare-associated infections 2005–2016: systematic review and meta-analysis. Infect Control Hosp Epidemiol. 2018;39(11):1277–95.
2. Cole E, Davenport R, Willett K, Brohi K. The burden of infection in severely injured trauma patients and the relationship with admission shock severity. J Trauma Acute Care Surg. 2014;76(3):730–5.
3. Lazarus HM, Fox J, Burke JP, Lloyd JF, Snow GL, Mehta RR. Trauma patient hospital-associated infections: risks and outcomes. J Trauma Acute Care Surg [Internet]. 2005;59(1) Verfügbar unter: https://journals.lww.com/jtrauma/Fulltext/2005/07000/Trauma_Patient_Hospital_Associated_Infections_.31.aspx
4. Salmanov A, Litus V, Vdovychenko S, Litus O, Davtian L, Ubogov S. Healthcare-associated infections in intensive care units. Wiad Lek. 2019;72(5 cz 2):963–9.
5. Glance LG, Stone PW, Mukamel DB, Dick AW. Increases in mortality, length of stay, and cost associated with hospital-acquired infections in trauma patients. Arch Surg. 2011;146(7):794–801.
6. van der Kooi T, Sax H, Pittet D, van Dissel J, van Benthem B, Walder B. Prevention of hospital infections by intervention and training (PROHIBIT): results of a pan-European cluster-randomized multicentre study to reduce central venous catheter-related bloodstream infections. Intensive Care Med [Internet]. 2018;44(1):48–60Verfügbar unter:. https://doi.org/10.1007/s00134-017-5007-6.
7. NCDC 2030. NCD countdown 2030: worldwide trends in non-communicable disease mortality and progress towards sustainable development goal target 3.4. Lancet (London, England) [Internet]. 2018;392(10152):1072–88. Verfügbar unter: https://www.ncbi.nlm.nih.gov/pubmed/30264707
8. Zarb P, Coignard B, Griskeviciene J, Muller A, Vankerckhoven V, Weist K. The european Centre for disease prevention and control (ECDC) pilot point prevalence survey of healthcare-associated infections and antimicrobial use. Bd. 17. Eur Secur. 2012:1–16.
9. Centers for Disease Control and Prevention. 2018 National and State Healthcare-Associated Infections Progress Report. 2019;(CDC):1–13.
10. Gilmartin HM, Hessels AJ. Dissemination and implementation science for infection prevention: a primer. Am J Infect Control [Internet]. 2019;47(6):688–92. Verfügbar unter: http://www.sciencedirect.com/science/article/pii/S0196655319300641
11. Pennathur PR, Herwaldt LA. Role of human factors engineering in infection prevention: gaps and opportunities. Curr Treat Options Infect Dis. 2017;9(2):230–49.
12. Drews FA, Visnovsky LC, Mayer J. Human factors engineering contributions to infection prevention and control. Hum Factors. 2019;61(5):693–701.
13. Core Components for IPC. Implementations tools and resources. https://www.who.int/infection-prevention/tools/cor.
14. ECDC. Point prevalence survey of healthcare-associated infections and antimicrobial use in European acute care hospitals 2011–2012. 2013
15. Mitchell BG, Russo PL, Cheng AC, Stewardson AJ, Rosebrock H, Curtis SJ. Strategies to reduce non-ventilator-associated hospital-acquired pneumonia: a systematic review. Infect Dis Heal [Internet]. 2019;24(4):229–39Verfügbar unter:. https://doi.org/10.1016/j.idh.2019.06.002.
16. Magill SS, Edwards JR, Bamberg W, Beldavs ZG, Dumyati G, Kainer MA. Multistate point-prevalence survey of health care–associated infections for the emerging infections program healthcare-associated infections and antimicrobial use prevalence survey team * Centers for Disease Control and Prevention St Paul (RL). Connect Dep Public Heal Oakl JN Decatur SMR [Internet]. 2014;370(13):1198–208. Verfügbar unter: https://www.ncbi.nlm.nih.gov/pmc/articles/PMC4648343/pdf/nihms736784.pdf
17. Sue EE. Dysphagia and aspiration pneumonia in older adults. J Am Acad Nurse Pract. 2010;22(1):17–22.
18. Janssens JP, Krause KH. Pneumonia in the very old. Lancet Infect Dis. 2004;4(2):112–24.

19. Carolyn V, Gould, Umscheid CA, Agarwal RK, Kuntz G, Pegues DA, M and the HICPAC. Guideline for prevention of catheter-associated urinary tract infections 2009. Cent Dis Control Prev [Internet]. 2009;(2009):1–61. Verfügbar unter: https://www.cdc.gov/infectioncontrol/pdf/guidelines/cauti-guidelines-H.pdf%0Ahttps://www.cdc.gov/infectioncontrol/guidelines/cauti/
20. Elkbuli A, Miller A, Boneva D, Puyana S, Bernal E, Hai S. Targeting catheter-associated urinary tract infections in a trauma population: a 5-S bundle preventive approach. J Trauma Nurs|JTN [Internet]. 2018;25(6) Verfügbar unter: https://journals.lww.com/journaloftraumanursing/Fulltext/2018/11000/Targeting_Catheter_Associated_Urinary_Tract.9.aspx
21. Wagenlehner FM, Lichtenstern C, Rolfes C, Mayer K, Uhle F, Weidner W. Diagnosis and management for urosepsis. Int J Urol. 2013;20(10):963–70.
22. Dreger NM, Degener S, Ahmad-Nejad P, Wöbker G, Roth S. Urosepsis - Ursache, diagnose und therapie. Dtsch Arztebl Int. 2015;112(49):837–47.
23. Hazelett SE, Tsai M, Gareri M, Allen K. The association between indwelling urinary catheter use in the elderly and urinary tract infection in acute care. BMC Geriatr. 2006;6:1–7.
24. Letica-Kriegel AS, Salmasian H, Vawdrey DK, Youngerman BE, Green RA, Furuya EY. Identifying the risk factors for catheter-associated urinary tract infections: a large cross-sectional study of six hospitals. BMJ Open. 2019;9(2):1–7.
25. Ziegler MJ, Pellegrini DC, Safdar N. Attributable mortality of central line associated bloodstream infection: systematic review and meta-analysis. Infection. 2014;43(1):29–36.
26. Marschall J, Mermel LA, Fakih M, Hadaway L, Kallen A, O'Grady NP. Strategies to prevent central line–associated bloodstream infections in acute care hospitals: 2014 update. Infect Control Hosp Epidemiol. 2014;35(7):753–71.
27. Teeple E, Collins J, Shrestha S, Dennerlein J, et al. Prevention of central line-associated bloodstream infections. Physiol Behav. 2018;176(1):139–48.
28. Centers for Disease Control and Prevention. Healthcare associated infections [Internet]. Verfügbar unter: https://www.cdc.gov/hai/ssi/ssi.html
29. Horan TC, Gaynes RP, Martone WJ, Jarvis WR, Emori TG. CDC definitions of nosocomial surgical site infections, 1992: a modification of CDC definitions of surgical wound infections. Infect Control Hosp Epidemiol [Internet]. 1992;13(10):606–8. Verfügbar unter: https://www.cambridge.org/core/article/cdc-definitions-of-nosocomial-surgical-site-infections-1992-a-modification-of-cdc-definitions-of-surgical-wound-infections/C14E2711020EE8FBADAEB574DFEB0E1C
30. Ochsner PE, Borens O, Bodler P-M, Broger I, Eich G, Hefti F. Infektionen des Bewegungsapparates: Grundlagen, Prophylaxe, Diagnostik und Therapie. Eigenverlag swiss orthopaedcs; 2015.
31. Timmers MS, Graafland N, Bernards AT, Nelissen RGHH, Van Dissel JT, Jukema GN. Negative pressure wound treatment with polyvinyl alcohol foam and polyhexanide antiseptic solution instillation in posttraumatic osteomyelitis. Wound Repair Regen. 2009;17(2):278–86.
32. Lehner B, Fleischmann W, Becker R, Jukema GN. First experiences with negative pressure wound therapy and instillation in the treatment of infected orthopaedic implants: a clinical observational study. Int Orthop. 2011;35(9):1415–20.
33. Calcagno C, Lobatto ME, Robson PM, Millon A. Ageing and the epidemiology of multimorbidity Miguel. Eur Respir J. 2016;28(10):1304–14.
34. Chen C-L, Chen C-M, Wang C-Y, Ko P-W, Chen C-H, Hsieh C-P. Frailty is associated with an increased risk of major adverse outcomes in elderly patients following surgical treatment of hip fracture. Sci Rep [Internet]. 2019;9(1):19135. Verfügbar unter: https://www.ncbi.nlm.nih.gov/pubmed/31836751
35. Brooks SE. Evidence – based C are of geriatric trauma patients. 2017;97:1157–1174.
36. Clegg A, Young J, Iliffe S, Rikkert MO, Rockwood K. Frailty in elderly people. Lancet. 2013;381(9868):752–62.
37. Boyce J, Chartier Y, Chraiti M, Cookson B, Damani N, Dharan S. WHO guidelines on hand hygiene in health care. Geneva World Heal Organ. 2009;
38. Allegranzi B, Pittet D. Role of hand hygiene in healthcare-associated infection prevention. J Hosp Infect [Internet]. 2009;73(4):305–15. Verfügbar unter: https://doi.org/10.1016/j.jhin.2009.04.019
39. Sax H, Allegranzi B, Uçkay I, Larson E, Boyce J, Pittet D. "My five moments for hand hygiene": a user-centred design approach to understand, train, monitor and report hand hygiene. J Hosp Infect. 2007;67(1):9–21.
40. Pittet D, Boyce JM. Hand hygiene and patient care: pursuing the Semmelweis legacy. Lancet Infect Dis [Internet]. 2001;1(April):9–20. Verfügbar unter: https://doi.org/10.1016/S1473-3099(09)70295-6
41. Hansen S, Schwab F, Gastmeier P, Pittet D, Zingg W, Sax H. Provision and consumption of alcohol-based hand rubs in European hospitals. Clin Microbiol Infect. 2015;21(12):1047–51.
42. WHO. WHO guidelines on hand hygiene in health care first global patient safety challenge clean care is safer care. 2009;30(1):270. Verfügbar unter: http://whqlibdoc.who.int/publications/2009/9789241597906_eng.pdf
43. WHO. WHO clean care is safer care [Internet]. Verfügbar unter: https://www.who.int/gpsc/5may/tools/en/
44. Woodhead M, Blasi F, Ewig S, Garau J, Huchon G, Ieven M. Guidelines for the management of adult lower respiratory tract infections - Full version. Clin Microbiol Infect [Internet]. 2011;17:E1–59. Verfügbar unter: https://doi.org/10.1111/j.1469-0691.2011.03672.x

45. Komission für Krankenhaushygiene und Infektionsprävention am Robert Koch-Insitut. Prävention der nosokomialen Pneumonie. Intensivmed und Notfallmedizin. 2000;37(7):653–61.
46. Torres A, Niederman MS, Chastre J, Ewig S, Fernandez-Vandellos P, Hanberger H. International ERS/ESICM/ESCMID/ALAT guidelines for the management of hospital-acquired pneumonia and ventilator-associated pneumonia. Eur Respir J [Internet]. 2017;50(3). Verfügbar unter: https://doi.org/10.1183/13993003.00582-2017
47. Lo E, Nicolle LE, Coffin SE, Gould C, Maragakis LL, Meddings J. Strategies to prevent catheter-associated urinary tract infections in acute care hospitals: 2014 update. Infect Control Hosp Epidemiol [Internet]. 2014;35(5):464–79. Verfügbar unter: https://www.cambridge.org/core/product/identifier/S0899823X00191664/type/journal_article
48. Infektionsprä- K. Prävention und Kontrolle Katheter-assoziierter Harnwegsinfektionen: Empfehlung der Kommission für Krankenhaushygiene und Infektionsprävention (KRINKO) beim Robert Koch-Institut. Bundesgesundheitsblatt – Gesundheitsforsch – Gesundheitsschutz. 2015;58(6):641–50.
49. Osterhoff G, Zwolak P, Krüger C, Wilzeck V, Simmen HP, Jukema GN. Risk factors for prolonged treatment and hospital readmission in 280 cases of negative-pressure wound therapy. J Plast Reconstr Aesthetic Surg. 2014;67(5):629–33.

Part VI

Surgical Management of Major Fractures

Preparation for Surgery: What to Consider

26

Markus Gosch

Fragility fracture patients are at high risk of surgical procedures and anesthesia. However, most of them will benefit from early surgery. The goal is to reduce mortality as well as pre-, peri-, and postoperative complications and maintain quality of life and independency. The first step is to consider whether it is an urgent indication, probably life-threatening trauma, like a hip fracture, or an elective indication (e.g., like the most proximal humerus fractures or wrist fractures). If we have to deal with an urgent indication, the focus should be on a smart preoperative process to avoid an unnecessary delay of surgery. In this case, the benefit of early surgery exceeds the benefits of a comprehensive preoperative evaluation of older patients. There are only very few cases, where a preoperative optimization is indicated. If we go for preoperative optimization, we need to fix a clear goal and start a coordinated interdisciplinary process including regular check-ups. In contrast, in elective surgery, we have to weigh all risks and benefits. Therefore, it could be necessary to go for a more comprehensive evaluation of the patients and their comorbidities.

26.1 Anamnesis

Each assessment of an older patient has to start with a short face-to-face interview. It is very helpful to get detailed information about the trauma occurrence and the medical history of the patient. In case of an impaired communication due to a reduced consciousness or a cognitive decline, family members or other related persons, like nursing staff, should be contacted as soon as possible. Both aspects are useful to estimate very early in the process the risk of your older patient.

Regarding the trauma itself, we must have a closer look at the event of the accident. On one hand, we have to search for underlying diseases (e.g., severe aortic stenosis, acute myocardial infarction, acute heart failure decompensation, intercerebral bleeding or ischemia, and sepsis). Relevant findings could lead to an indication for a delay of surgery or even to a contraindication, particularly in elective cases. Acute heart failure decompensation would induce an indication for a preoperative optimization, whereas an intracerebral bleeding is a contraindication for surgery. Severe aortic stenosis is relevant to know and has an impact on the choice of anesthesia and treatment. However, it is not a contraindication or a reason to postpone surgery. On the other hand, place and circumstances of the trauma help us to evaluate patient's risk. Among older adults, up to 90% of all falls occur at home or in institutions, like nursing homes. Predominantly affected are older adults with

M. Gosch (✉)
Department for Geriatric Medicine, Paracelsus Private Medical University, General Hospital Nuremberg, Nuremberg, Germany
e-mail: markus.gosch@pmu.ac.at

H.-C. Pape et al. (eds.), *Senior Trauma Patients*, https://doi.org/10.1007/978-3-030-91483-7_26

already existing functional impairments. The reduced mobility hinders these people to walk outside or go shopping, as a consequence they spend most of their time at home or in their institution. In contrast, we have a small proportion of older and very old people who are still mobile, able to go out for shopping or visit a restaurant. They are less affected by their morbidities, except osteoporosis and functionality. Thus, this group of patients has a reduced perioperative risk compared to the others. This fact is also reflected in the literature and results in higher mortality after sustaining a fracture at home compared to a car accident [1]. Concordant to that, the place of living is a strong predictor for poor outcomes. Nursing home residents have a significant higher short- and long-term mortality and a higher risk for complications [2, 3]. Comorbidities and polypharmacy are other risk factors which can be easily recognized by enquiring patient's history. A preexisting dementia or a prior delirium are very strong risk factors for further delirium [4]. Besides cognition, other functional impairments like impaired mobility have also a negative impact on the outcome of older fragility fracture patients [2, 5].

Multimorbidity is very frequent in older adults. Thirty-five percent of all hip fracture patients have at least one comorbidity, 17% two, and 7% three or more [6]. Especially, the last group has the highest in-hospital mortality and the highest risk of complications [6]. The most frequent comorbidities are cardiovascular diseases (24%), pulmonary diseases (14%), stroke (13%), diabetes (9%), cancer (8%), and renal failure [6]. In clinical practice, scores may help to assess the comorbidities and to estimate the risk of the patient. Frequently used is the Charlson Comorbidity Index (CCI) [7]. It's a simple score based on 17 items. An assessment of the severity of a single disease is missing. However, the sum shows a strong correlation with short- and long-term mortality [2]. The advantage of the CCI is the simple use and also the possibility of retrospective application. More complex is the Modified Cumulative Illness Rating Scale (CIRS) [8]. Comparable to the CCI the CIRS is designed to meet the need for a brief, comprehensive and reliable instrument for assessing multimorbidity. The scale format provides for 13 relatively independent areas grouped under body systems. Ratings are made on a 5-point "degree of severity" scale.

A coordinated assessment of multimorbidity should be done regularly in all older trauma patients, regardless of the pressure of surgery. The assessment is one of the basic information for further treatment goals and plans.

Comorbidities and their impact on outcome [9]:

- Heart failure → 63% increased risk of mortality and readmission
- Myocardial infarction → 70% increased risk of myocardial infarction
- Atrial fibrillation → 200% increased risk of mortality
- Stroke → absolute risk 1% peri-operatively
- COPD → higher risk of readmission rate and pneumonia, length of stay
- Thromboembolism → risk of pulmonary embolism 10–14%, for deep venous thrombosis 19–91%
- Chronic renal failure → no data available
- Anemia → hemoglobin < 8 g/dl increases postoperative mortality, <10 g/dl increased risk of myocardial infarction
- Dementia/Delirium → increases mortality and risk for long-term care
- Polypharmacy → increases mortality and morbidity

Polypharmacy is often a result of an existing multimorbidity. Adverse drug reactions are a common phenomenon in older adults. The incidence of adverse drug reactions is up to 5% among in-hospital patients and increases up to 30% in older emergency patients [10, 11]. The most important risk factor of adverse drug reactions is the absolute number of prescriptions [12]. Accurate and comprehensive documentation of the medication is essential to minimize the risk. Medication should be checked for potential inappropriate medication (PIM) for older adults. Different tools are available, like the Beer's list or STOPP and START criteria, and may help to improve the quality of medication as well as the outcome of older fragility fracture patients [13–15].

Impaired activities of daily living and mobility are very common in older fragility fracture patients and they have a significant impact on the outcome. A high level of dependency preoperatively is the strongest predictor for six-month mortality [16]. Furthermore, reduced mobility is associated with the risk of postoperative delirium, institutionalization, and nosocomial infections, like MRSA [17–20]. The preoperative assessment of the functional status and mobility is an essential part of the preoperative evaluation in older adults. Assessment instruments have to be chosen consistent with the clinical situation and the special setting. In contrast to elective surgery, in an emergency case, we can predominantly use only anamnestic data. According to the guidelines of the American Geriatric Society (AGS) all older patients should be screened for functional and mobility impairments [21]. AGS recommends four questions as a short simple screening test for functional assessment:

- Can you get out of bed or chair yourself?
- Can you dress and bath yourself?
- Can you make your own meals?
- Can you do your own shopping?

If the patient's answer is NO to any of these questions, a more in-depth evaluation should be performed.

All patients should be assessed for their ability to perform daily activities. Usually we use the Barthel-Index [22], including the following items: urinary and fecal incontinence, grooming, toilet use, feeding, transfers, walking, dressing, climbing stairs, and bathing. In this special setting, daily activities are assessed by a short interview of the patient. In case of a relevant cognitive impairment, relatives or staff members of the nursing home should be involved.

Even, the Timed Up&Go is a simple to perform and validated tool. It is not appropriate for emergency patients [23]. This mobility test can be performed preoperatively in elective surgery. A pathological result is a strong predictor for postoperative mortality and institutionalization [16]. For acute settings, Parker Mobility Score (PMS) is recommended [24]. Again, this test is based on the patient's statements. However, the score is quite simple, can be done by everyone. A low PMS has a strong correlation with postoperative mortality and morbidity [5]

Parker Mobility Score (PMS):

Mobility	No difficulty	With an aid	With help from another person	Not at all
Able to get about the house	3	2	1	0
Able to get out of the house	3	2	1	0
Able to go shopping	3	2	1	0

Older fragility fracture patients are characterized by a high complexity. This leads to the fact, that the interdisciplinary team is focused on many different medical problems and we have to be aware not to neglect the patient's will. Not only for ethical aspects, but also for adherence, the patient's will has to be integrated in the treatment process.

26.2 Physical Assessment

The basic assessment includes a check of vital parameters (blood pressure, heart rate, oxygen saturation) and a global clinical impression. From the geriatric point of view, frailty and sarcopenia are of special interest. However, in case of emergency patients, a clear diagnostic process according to current literature for both syndromes is not really realizable. It remains the only expertise of geriatrician to diagnose them [25].

Besides injuries, physical assessment of older trauma patient covers cardiopulmonary assessment, evaluation of hydration (edema or signs of dehydration), assessment of skin (vulnerability, hematoma), and cognition.

An auscultation is quickly available and quite simple. It may help to detect a heart murmur or an edema of the lung. Aortic stenosis is frequent in older adults. It could be a reason for a syncope and may have an impact on the kind of anesthesia. Hydration is recommended in all patients, except when there are signs of heart failure decompensation, like breathlessness or edema.

Delirium is very frequent among older adults undergoing surgery. Some of the patients have already delirium at admission, but most of them are developing a delirium during their hospital stay. Acute onset is probably the most important diagnostic aspect. Therefore, cognition ad admission is essential to detect delirium. A comprehensive cognitive assessment is not appropriate for emergency patients, but still a short screening is recommended. One option is the Mini-Cog [26]. It takes only a few minutes and is able to detect an existing cognitive impairment. Another option is the Confusion Assessment Method (CAM) Score [27]. A pharmacological prevention, even for high-risk patients, is not recommended, but all older patients should receive non-pharmacological measures to prevent or reduce the risk of delirium.

26.3 Medical Examinations

An electrocardiogram (ECG) is no longer recommended routinely for preoperative screening, particularly in patients with a low risk [28]. It is still recommended for operation with an intermediate risk and vascular surgery, and for all patients with cardiovascular diseases, diabetes, renal failure, and pulmonary diseases [28]. Regarding the high prevalence of these diseases among old and very old patients, it is reasonable to keep a preoperative ECG as a standard procedure.

Similar are the recommendations regarding a preoperative chest X-ray. A benefit of a routine preoperative application of chest X-ray is not proven, but it is recommended for patients with a suspected lung disease, smoking, asthma, COPD, age older than 70 years, chronical cardiopulmonary disease, major surgery, and higher risk for postoperative ICU stay [28]. For older fragility patients, the chest X-ray should be part of the preoperative assessment.

The role of preoperative echocardiography is still discussed controversially. In most departments, the need for a transthoracic echocardiography leads to a significant delay of surgery [29, 30]. Furthermore, the impact of a preoperative echocardiography on the outcome and on the further management of patients seems to be very weak, including patients with a significant heart murmur [30, 31]. Even hip fracture patients with severe aortic stenosis did not have an increased perioperative mortality or morbidity risk [32]. Another retrospective trial from Australia showed a positive impact of preoperative echocardiography on the outcome and no delay of surgery [33]. In conclusion, transthoracic echocardiography might be useful in older fragility fracture patients with known or suspected heart disease. But it's not worth accepting a delay of surgery for more than 24–48 h. If preoperative echocardiography is required, it should be available immediately.

26.4 Lab Tests

Each older fragility fracture patient should receive a blood draw. In emergency cases, blood count, creatinine, electrolytes, and coagulations tests are routinely recommended [28]. More blood tests are related to anamnesis and comorbidities. Urine testing is recommended only if there are signs of a clinically relevant urinary tract infection.

26.5 Preoperative Medical Care

There are only very few fragility fracture patients without pain at admission. Therefore, pain management is an essential part of preoperative care. Insufficient pain control has negative effects on physiology and clinical outcomes. Poor pain control in older hip fracture patients leads to an increased rate of postoperative delirium, length of stay, and poor participation in therapy [34]. In the preoperative phase, low to modest doses of intravenous opioids are typically necessary to achieve rapid and sufficient pain control. Additional nerve blocks are appropriate, especially in the preoperative setting. Nerve blocks are able to reduce opioid dose and risk of delirium [35].

Another important part is hydration. Older fragility fracture patients are often dehydrated or are getting dehydrated by waiting for surgery. In a recent study, a total of 21.8% of older patients undergoing orthopedic surgery are dehydrated and 35.2% are defined as at risk of dehydration [36]. There were significantly more patients in the dehydrated group were female, having diuretic medication, swallowing difficulty, edema, tube feeding, diaper or urinary catheter use, with postoperative complications in respiratory, gastrointestinal, and hematological systems, and died within 30 days than those in the euhydrated group [36].

Besides an early diagnosis of delirium, it is important to maximize non-pharmacological attempts to prevent or minimize delirium by all healthcare providers. Early surgery and proactive management are crucial.

Preparation for surgery:
– Basic measures of preoperative preparation
– Analgesia
– Hydration
– Stabilization of vital signs
– Non-pharmacological delirium prevention
Preoperative assessment:
– What happened?—comprehensive anamnesis
– Assess cognition and patient's will
– Assess functional status and pre-fracture mobility
– Identify geriatric syndromes, like frailty, sarcopenia, malnutrition
– Assess comorbidities and polypharmacy
– Identify risk factors for delirium
– Do a physical examination
– Go for an ECG and chest X-ray
– Do lab test as recommended
– Set a treatment goal
In case of optimization
– Set a clear goal
– Find an interdisciplinary consent on required tests
– Set a timeframe
– Organize a regularly check-up

References

1. Sampalis JS, Nathanson R, Vaillancourt J, Nikolis A, Liberman M, Angelopoulos J, et al. Assessment of mortality in older trauma patients sustaining injuries from falls or motor vehicle collisions treated in regional level I trauma centers. Ann Surg. 2009;249(3):488–95.
2. Kammerlander C, Gosch M, Kammerlander-Knauer U, Luger TJ, Blauth M, Roth T. Long-term functional outcome in geriatric hip fracture patients. Arch Orthop Trauma Surg. 2011;131(10):1435–44.
3. Fleischman RJ, Adams AL, Hedges JR, Ma OJ, Mullins RJ, Newgard CD. The optimum follow-up period for assessing mortality outcomes in injured older adults. J Am Geriatr Soc. 2010;58(10):1843–9.
4. Raats JW, van Eijsden WA, Crolla RM, Steyerberg EW, van der Laan L. Risk factors and outcomes for postoperative delirium after major surgery in elderly patients. PLoS One. 2015;10(8):e0136071.
5. Gosch M, Druml T, Nicholas JA, Hoffmann-Weltin Y, Roth T, Zegg M, et al. Fragility non-hip fracture patients are at risk. Arch Orthop Trauma Surg. 2015;135(1):69–77.
6. Roche JJ, Wenn RT, Sahota O, Moran CG. Effect of comorbidities and postoperative complications on mortality after hip fracture in elderly people: prospective observational cohort study. BMJ. 2005;331(7529):1374.
7. Charlson ME, Pompei P, Ales KL, MacKenzie CR. A new method of classifying prognostic comorbidity in longitudinal studies: development and validation. J Chronic Dis. 1987;40(5):373–83.
8. Salvi F, Miller MD, Grilli A, Giorgi R, Towers AL, Morichi V, et al. A manual of guidelines to score the modified cumulative illness rating scale and its validation in acute hospitalized elderly patients. J Am Geriatr Soc. 2008;56(10):1926–31.
9. Gosch M. Multimorbidität. In: Gosch S, Böcker K, editors. Alterstraumatologie. Stuttgart – New York: Georg Thieme Verlag; 2019. p. 18–26.
10. Lazarou J, Pomeranz BH, Corey PN. Incidence of adverse drug reactions in hospitalized patients: a meta-analysis of prospective studies. JAMA. 1998;279(15):1200–5.
11. Leendertse AJ, Egberts AC, Stoker LJ, van den Bemt PM, Group HS. Frequency of and risk factors for preventable medication-related hospital admissions in the Netherlands. Arch Intern Med. 2008;168(17):1890–6.
12. Laroche ML, Charmes JP, Nouaille Y, Picard N, Merle L. Is inappropriate medication use a major cause of adverse drug reactions in the elderly? Br J Clin Pharmacol. 2007;63(2):177–86.
13. Beers MH, Ouslander JG, Rollingher I, Reuben DB, Brooks J, Beck JC. Explicit criteria for determining inappropriate medication use in nursing home residents. UCLA division of geriatric medicine. Arch Intern Med. 1991;151(9):1825–32.

14. O'Mahony D, O'Sullivan D, Byrne S, O'Connor MN, Ryan C, Gallagher P. STOPP/START criteria for potentially inappropriate prescribing in older people: version 2. Age Ageing. 2015;44(2):213–8.
15. Gosch M, Wortz M, Nicholas JA, Doshi HK, Kammerlander C, Lechleitner M. Inappropriate prescribing as a predictor for long-term mortality after hip fracture. Gerontology. 2014;60(2):114–22.
16. Robinson TN, Eiseman B, Wallace JI, Church SD, McFann KK, Pfister SM, et al. Redefining geriatric preoperative assessment using frailty, disability and co-morbidity. Ann Surg. 2009;250(3):449–55.
17. Dasgupta M, Dumbrell AC. Preoperative risk assessment for delirium after noncardiac surgery: a systematic review. J Am Geriatr Soc. 2006;54(10):1578–89.
18. Brouquet A, Cudennec T, Benoist S, Moulias S, Beauchet A, Penna C, et al. Impaired mobility, ASA status and administration of tramadol are risk factors for postoperative delirium in patients aged 75 years or more after major abdominal surgery. Ann Surg. 2010;251(4):759–65.
19. Chen TY, Anderson DJ, Chopra T, Choi Y, Schmader KE, Kaye KS. Poor functional status is an independent predictor of surgical site infections due to methicillin-resistant *Staphylococcus aureus* in older adults. J Am Geriatr Soc. 2010;58(3):527–32.
20. Anderson DJ, Chen LF, Schmader KE, Sexton DJ, Choi Y, Link K, et al. Poor functional status as a risk factor for surgical site infection due to methicillin-resistant *Staphylococcus aureus*. Infect Control Hosp Epidemiol. 2008;29(9):832–9.
21. Chow WB, Rosenthal RA, Merkow RP, Ko CY, Esnaola NF, American College of Surgeons National Surgical Quality Improvement P, et al. Optimal preoperative assessment of the geriatric surgical patient: a best practices guideline from the American College of Surgeons National Surgical Quality Improvement Program and the American Geriatrics Society. J Am Coll Surg. 2012;215(4):453–66.
22. Lawton MP, Brody EM. Assessment of older people: self-maintaining and instrumental activities of daily living. Gerontologist. 1969;9(3):179–86.
23. Podsiadlo D, Richardson S. The timed "Up & Go": a test of basic functional mobility for frail elderly persons. J Am Geriatr Soc. 1991;39(2):142–8.
24. Parker MJ, Palmer CR. A new mobility score for predicting mortality after hip fracture. J Bone Joint Surg Br. 1993;75(5):797–8.
25. Liem IS, Kammerlander C, Suhm N, Blauth M, Roth T, Gosch M, et al. Identifying a standard set of outcome parameters for the evaluation of orthogeriatric co-management for hip fractures. Injury. 2013;44(11):1403–12.
26. Borson S, Scanlan J, Brush M, Vitaliano P, Dokmak A. The mini-cog: a cognitive 'vital signs' measure for dementia screening in multi-lingual elderly. Int J Geriatr Psychiatry. 2000;15(11):1021–7.
27. Inouye SK, Kosar CM, Tommet D, Schmitt EM, Puelle MR, Saczynski JS, et al. The CAM-S: development and validation of a new scoring system for delirium severity in 2 cohorts. Ann Intern Med. 2014;160(8):526–33.
28. Guidelines ANA. Optimal preoperative assessment of the geriatric surgical patients 2016. Available from: https://www.facs.org/-/media/files/quality-programs/geriatric/acs-nsqip-geriatric-2016-guidelines.ashx?la=en.
29. O'Heireamhoin S, Beyer T, Ahmed M, Mulhall KJ. The role of preoperative cardiac investigation in emergency hip surgery. J Trauma. 2011;71(5):1345–7.
30. Ricci WM, Della Rocca GJ, Combs C, Borrelli J. The medical and economic impact of preoperative cardiac testing in elderly patients with hip fractures. Injury. 2007;38(Suppl 3):S49–52.
31. Jettoo P, Kakwani R, Junejo S, Talkhani I, Dixon P. Pre-operative echocardiogram in hip fracture patients with cardiac murmur--an audit. J Orthop Surg Res. 2011;6:49.
32. Leibowitz D, Rivkin G, Schiffman J, Rott D, Weiss AT, Mattan Y, et al. Effect of severe aortic stenosis on the outcome in elderly patients undergoing repair of hip fracture. Gerontology. 2009;55(3):303–6.
33. Canty DJ, Royse CF, Kilpatrick D, Bowyer A, Royse AG. The impact on cardiac diagnosis and mortality of focused transthoracic echocardiography in hip fracture surgery patients with increased risk of cardiac disease: a retrospective cohort study. Anaesthesia. 2012;67(11):1202–9.
34. Morrison RS, Magaziner J, McLaughlin MA, Orosz G, Silberzweig SB, Koval KJ, et al. The impact of post-operative pain on outcomes following hip fracture. Pain. 2003;103(3):303–11.
35. Abou-Setta AM, Beaupre LA, Rashiq S, Dryden DM, Hamm MP, Sadowski CA, et al. Comparative effectiveness of pain management interventions for hip fracture: a systematic review. Ann Intern Med. 2011;155(4):234–45.
36. Chan HYL, Cheng A, Cheung SSS, Pang WW, Ma WY, Mok LC, et al. Association between dehydration on admission and postoperative complications in older persons undergoing orthopaedic surgery. J Clin Nurs. 2018;27(19–20):3679–86.

Management of Anemia

27

Julian Rössler, Jan Breckwoldt, and Donat R. Spahn

Exsanguination is one of the leading causes of death in trauma patients [1]. In a geriatric patient, physiological reserves decline and comorbidities become more frequent. For example, in addition to traumatic blood loss, in more than a third of all elderly patients, anemia is already prevalent before the injury. Other comorbidities, like cardiovascular disease, put crucial tissues at greater risk of hypoxia. This renders the management of posttraumatic anemia within the elderly population a challenging topic [2].

27.1 Allogenic Blood Transfusions

While the risk of death increases with the severity of anemia, a liberal treatment with allogenic red blood cell (RBC) transfusions, does more harm than good [3]. Still, RBC transfusions remain one of the most common medical interventions. However, their use is steadily declining with growing evidence regarding adverse events of transfusions and the advantages of restrictive transfusion thresholds. RCBs, like all biological blood components, are living human tissues, making every transfusion a liquid organ transplantation. Thus, they are associated with a number of short- and long-term immunomodulatory adverse events, as well as a variety of serious non-immunological complications. Protecting patients from these risks requires the prevention of inappropriate transfusions [4].

An RBC transfusion is appropriate when oxygen demand exceeds supply in a way that can only be adequately restored by the immediate administration of oxygen carriers. While this is basically a pathophysiologic condition, the threshold for an RBC transfusion is usually defined by a hemoglobin level, also called a transfusion trigger. Based on basic physiological models, these thresholds (triggers) used to be rather liberal and encouraged premature intervention. In the last two decades, however, supported by substantial scientific evidence, transfusion triggers became more restrictive. Most commonly, the restrictive transfusion threshold now is set at a hemoglobin level of 7 g/dL or 8 g/dL to trigger transfusion, while the liberal transfusion threshold implies a higher hemoglobin level of 9–10 g/dL.

In the general surgical population, definitive evidence has been provided that a restrictive approach to RBC transfusion not only reduces blood use but also does not cause harm. With mounting evidence, in 2016, a large meta-analysis by the Cochrane Collaboration analyzed more than 12,000 patients from 31 trials investigating liberal vs. restrictive transfusion triggers [5]. Of these trials, six were conducted in orthopedic surgery. Primarily, the restrictive transfusion strategy more than halved the risk of

J. Rössler · J. Breckwoldt · D. R. Spahn (✉)
Institute of Anesthesiology, University of Zurich and University Hospital Zurich, Zurich, Switzerland
e-mail: donat.spahn@usz.ch

H.-C. Pape et al. (eds.), *Senior Trauma Patients*, https://doi.org/10.1007/978-3-030-91483-7_27

receiving an RBC transfusion. Further, overall as well as in the orthopedic surgery subgroup, there was no significant difference between the two triggers regarding clinical outcomes. Most importantly, 30-day mortality did not differ between the two approaches. Additionally, restrictive transfusion thresholds did not affect any of the other assessed outcomes including myocardial infarction or other cardiac events, stroke, thromboembolism, or infection. If these patients do not benefit clinically from a liberal transfusion threshold, there is no indication for transfusion above a hemoglobin concentration of 7–8 g/dL. Thus, applying restrictive triggers does not mean withholding treatment, but reasonably avoiding an unnecessary intervention with many adverse events.

Moreover, restrictive transfusion triggers may even be beneficial in certain situations or populations. In the meta-analysis, three studies cumulating more than 1500 patients suffering acute blood loss, were analyzed as a separate group. Here, a restrictive approach to transfusion triggers reduced 30-day mortality with a risk ratio of 0.65 (95% confidence interval (CI) 0.43–0.97). Importantly, in the largest trial from this subgroup the mean patient age was 65 years, which is a frequent cut-off value for geriatric research. This study in itself also favored a restrictive approach [6].

It has been argued—but wrongfully so—that due to limited physiological reserves, an elderly patient may require a liberal transfusion threshold. In a large prospective trial, over 2000 geriatric patients at high cardiovascular risk after hip replacement surgery were randomly assigned to either a restrictive (8 g/dL) or a liberal (10 g/dL) transfusion regimen. The mean patient age was an astonishing 82 years and all patients had either clinical evidence of or risk factors for cardiovascular disease. The first results were reported after a 60-day follow-up, where the liberal transfusion strategy, as compared with a restrictive strategy, did not reduce rates of death or inability to walk independently on 60-day follow-up [7]. Later, after a long-term follow-up of 3 years, no difference in mortality or cause of death was found [8]. This may be because the original idea that reduced physiological reserves would compromise the ability to tolerate acute anemia was incorrect. In fact, an increase in cardiac output due to anemia does not decrease with increasing age and consequently, neither does the ability to deliver oxygen [9]. While the present evidence already clearly favors a restrictive approach, in order to dispel last doubts, the Liberal trial (clinicalTrials.gov identifier: NCT03369210) is currently recruiting patients over 70, assigning them to either a 9 g/dL or 7.5 g/dL transfusion threshold, and evaluating mortality as well as anemia associated ischemic events (e.g., acute myocardial infarction or acute ischemic stroke) in a 90-day follow-up.

A transfusion threshold of 7–8 g/dL has become the standard of care in a geriatric patient. Allogenic RBC transfusions are of no benefit in hemodynamically stable patients with a hemoglobin concentration above 7 g/dL and should be avoided to minimize adverse events. If a normovolemic patient is hemodynamically unstable or shows signs of inadequate oxygenation despite exhausted respiratory and circulatory support, a new transfusion trigger may be set at 8 g/dL. Importantly, a low hemoglobin value on itself does not require a transfusion. The patient's clinical state and individual needs should always be considered in the decision.

27.2 Alternative Treatments

Allogenic transfusions should be applied very restrictively. However, because of the risks associated with anemia, physicians should be familiar with alternative treatments. For this reason, the U.S. Food and Drug Administration container label extension for RBC units states the following contraindication: "Red-cell-containing components should not be used to treat anemias that can be corrected with specific hematinic medications such as iron, vitamin B12, folic acid, or erythropoietin" [10]. In the geriatric population, two scenarios must be considered.

First, next to traumatic blood loss, other etiologies of anemia may have already been prevalent before the injury. Often, laboratory investigation

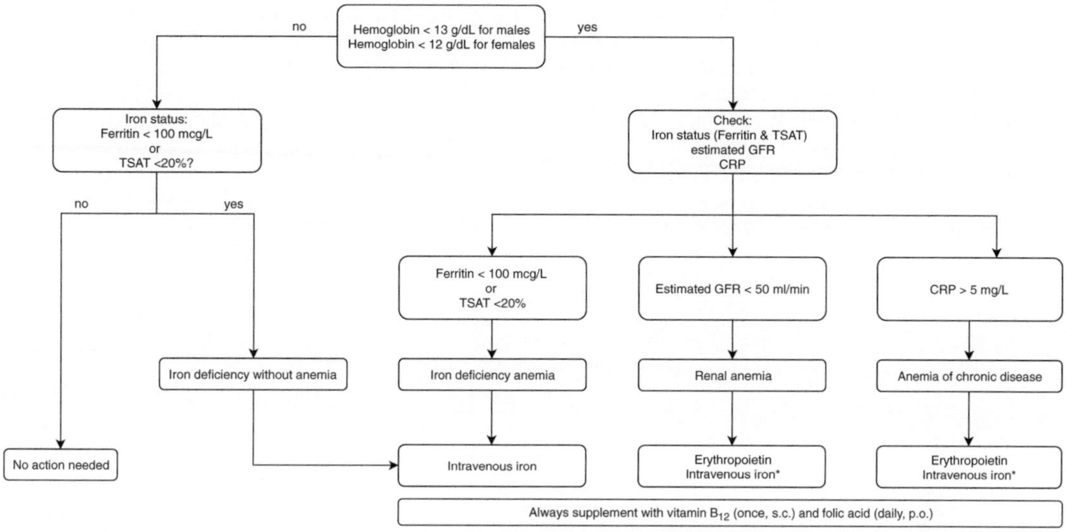

Fig. 27.1 Goal-directed algorithm for the detection, assessment, and management of posttraumatic anemia. *Asterisk* only if Ferritin <1000 mcg/L

can lead to the correct diagnosis, making management largely dependent on the underlying etiology. In these cases, anemia can be corrected by a goal-directed treatment with, for example, parenteral iron substitution in case of iron deficiency or vitamin B12 and folate. An erythropoietin deficiency with or without exocrine kidney insufficiency, or chronic inflammation, is also quite prevalent in older persons and may be treated with erythropoiesis-stimulating agents, depending on local regulations (Fig. 27.1).

Secondly, in the case of acute traumatic blood loss, a fast combination treatment may be the key—regardless of underlying conditions. A landmark study in cardiac surgery patients with preoperative anemia or iron deficiency was able to show that combination treatment with intravenous iron, subcutaneous erythropoietin alpha, vitamin B12, and oral folic acid only on the day before surgery, reduced allogeneic blood product transfusions without significant side effects [11]. If this ultra-short-term treatment succeeds in such a high-risk group of patients, it may very well also improve transfusion regimens for geriatric trauma patients.

References

1. Spahn DR, Bouillon B, Cerny V, Duranteau J, Filipescu D, Hunt BJ, et al. The European guideline on management of major bleeding and coagulopathy following trauma: fifth edition. Crit Care. 2019 Mar 27;23(1):98.
2. Stauder R, Valent P, Theurl I. Anemia at older age: etiologies, clinical implications, and management. Blood. 2018;131(5):505–14.
3. LaPar DJ, Hawkins RB, McMurry TL, Isbell JM, Rich JB, Speir AM, et al. Preoperative anemia versus blood transfusion: which is the culprit for worse outcomes in cardiac surgery? J Thorac Cardiovasc Surg. 2018 Jul;156(1):66–74.e2.
4. Carson JL, Triulzi DJ, Ness PM. Indications for and adverse effects of red-cell transfusion. N Engl J Med. 2017;377(13):1261–72.
5. Carson JL, Stanworth SJ, Roubinian N, Fergusson DA, Triulzi D, Doree C, et al. Transfusion thresholds and other strategies for guiding allogeneic red blood cell transfusion. Cochrane Database Syst Rev 2016;10:CD002042.
6. Villanueva C, Colomo A, Bosch A, Concepción M, Hernandez-Gea V, Aracil C, et al. Transfusion strategies for acute upper gastrointestinal bleeding. N Engl J Med. 2013;368(1):11–21.
7. Carson JL, Terrin ML, Noveck H, Sanders DW, Chaitman BR, Rhoads GG, et al. Liberal or restrictive transfusion in high-risk patients after hip surgery. N Engl J Med. 2011;365(26):2453–62.

8. Carson JL, Sieber F, Cook DR, Hoover DR, Noveck H, Chaitman BR, et al. Liberal versus restrictive blood transfusion strategy: 3-year survival and cause of death results from the FOCUS randomised controlled trial. Lancet. 2015;385(9974):1183–9.
9. Casutt M, Seifert B, Pasch T, Schmid ER, Turina MI, Spahn DR. Factors influencing the individual effects of blood transfusions on oxygen delivery and oxygen consumption. Crit Care Med. 1999;27(10):2194–200.
10. AABB. Circular of Information for the Use of Human Blood and Blood Components [Internet]. 2017 [cited 2019 Jul 31]. Available from: http://www.aabb.org/tm/coi/Documents/coi1017.pdf
11. Spahn DR, Schoenrath F, Spahn GH, Seifert B, Stein P, Theusinger OM, et al. Effect of ultra-short-term treatment of patients with iron deficiency or anaemia undergoing cardiac surgery: a prospective randomised trial. Lancet. 2019;393(10187):2201–12.

Specifics of Surgical Management: Proximal Femur Fractures

28

Abhishek Ganta and Kenneth A. Egol

28.1 Introduction to Geriatric Proximal Femur Fractures

Proximal femur fractures are significant injuries that affect the geriatric population from a medical and a financial standpoint. They remain one of the most common injuries in this age group and are expected to rise in frequency over the next few decades [1]. By 2025, the number of hip fractures worldwide is to rise to 2.6 million and 6.25 million by 2050 [2, 3]. Along with an increase in the number of these fractures, they represent a large financial burden in the USA with annual treatment costs at approximately $6 billion USD [4].

Proximal femur fractures can be classified as either intracapsular such as femoral neck fractures or extracapsular such as pertrochanteric or subtrochanteric femur fractures. Treatment of these injuries in this patient population is challenging due to poor bone quality, medical comorbidities, and patient frailty. The overall goal for any orthopedic intervention is to return patients to their pre-injury level of function; however, this may be impacted by the patient's reliance on assistive devices, chronic systemic diseases, perioperative cognitive disorders, and the development of any postoperative complications. The hospital mortality rate is around 15% with 1-year mortality rate at around 30% [5]. This risk is increased with dependency, loss of walking capacity, preexisting cognitive decline, increased ASA classification, and severity of medical comorbidities [6]. Patients with higher ISS scores were noted to have higher mortality rates than previously quoted, and these rates increase with patient age [7, 8]. Risk stratified scores have now been developed in geriatric trauma patients to identify patients with higher mortality rates [9, 10].

Ultimately, patients fall into one of three categories: those who are independent ambulators without significant medical comorbidities, frail patients with multiple medical comorbidities who can perform activities of daily living but demonstrate difficulty with instrumental activities of daily living, and lastly dependent patients that require daily assistance and live in an institution [11]. Understanding and identifying patients' pre-injury level of function and comorbid status can lead to improved perioperative management and decrease the risk of postoperative complications. While the ultimate goal following operative management of these injuries is to restore pre-injury level of function, the elderly patient's ability to cope with the metabolic and physio-

A. Ganta (✉)
Division of Orthopedic Trauma Surgery, Department of Orthopedic Surgery, NYU Langone Health, NYU Langone Orthopedic Hospital, New York, NY, USA
e-mail: abhishek.ganta@nyulangone.org

K. A. Egol
Department of Orthopedic Surgery, NYU School of Medicine, NYU Langone Health, NYU Langone Orthopedic Hospital, New York, NY, USA
e-mail: Kenneth.egol@nyulangone.org

H.-C. Pape et al. (eds.), *Senior Trauma Patients*, https://doi.org/10.1007/978-3-030-91483-7_28

logic demands from these injuries may reduce their level of function and independence [12].

28.2 Radiographic Workup

In order to fully evaluate the fracture characteristic, the authors recommend an AP pelvis radiograph with dedicated AP and lateral views of the affected hip and femur. A traction internal rotation view of the ipsilateral hip can assist with defining fracture pattern further [13]. The view is obtained by shooting an AP hip radiograph as the physician pulls traction at the ankle and internally rotates the hip 15 degrees (based on the average amount of anteversion seen in the adult femoral neck). Care should be taken to avoid shearing of the skin in the lower extremity while performing this maneuver.

It is important to assess the patient's native femoral neck coronal alignment and as well as the presence of any excessive femoral bow on either view [14]. A cross-table lateral view of the injured hip is recommended over a frog lateral as this may not only mitigates discomfort but also prevents a non-displaced fracture from displacing.

In the setting of hip pain and difficulty/ inability to ambulate, patients may have sustained an occult femoral neck or intertrochanteric fracture. Patients may complain of pain slight pain in the groin, thigh or referred pain along the medial side of the knee. These fractures may not be recognized on initial radiographs and failure to diagnose them may lead to displacement following weight-bearing. Advanced imaging such as bone scans, CT, or MRI may be required for diagnosis. MRI has the highest accuracy, is simple to perform, and can diagnose injuries more acutely [15, 16]. Having adequate and appropriate radiographic information will allow the treating surgeon to not only fully understand the fracture pattern, but also choose the appropriate surgical technique for treatment.

28.3 Intracapsular Fractures (Femoral Neck Fractures)

Femoral neck fractures are uncommon in young patients and are usually the result of high-energy trauma. It is generally considered that femoral neck fractures in the geriatric population are "pathologic" secondary to osteoporosis/osteomalacia. Osteoporosis/osteomalacia in this region causes bone to lose its normal trabecular architecture [17]. As a consequence, there can be an increased amount of posterior comminution associated with fractures and this has been postulated to increase rates of failure of internal fixation [18]. Swinontkowski noted that the critical element in the stability of fixation of displaced femoral neck fractures is the quality of the bone [19].

The Garden classification is commonly used to describe femoral neck fractures based on the displacement of the fracture fragments. Garden 1 corresponds with a valgus impacted fracture, Garden 2 corresponds with a non-displaced fracture, Garden 3 and 4 corresponds to complete fractures with the Garden 4 having 100% displacement. Other descriptive methods include the direction of the fracture angle as well as the anatomic location of the fracture. While the Garden classification has poor interobserver reliability, it can be used to communicate whether or not the fractures are valgus impacted/ minimally displaced or completely displaced [20]. Most have gone to using displaced and non-displaced as terminology. Despite this, Garden's original classification continues to be utilized to guide treatment.

Fixation options range from parallel cannulated screws (2, 3, or 4), sliding hip screw (SHS) construct, hemiarthroplasty, and total hip arthroplasty (THA) depending upon the degree of fracture displacement. Arthroplasty options may be either cemented or press-fit depending on surgeon preference. Ultimately the treatment question becomes whether to fix the femoral neck fracture or perform an arthroplasty procedure [21]. Garden I and II Fractures (non-displaced) are typically treated with fixation in situ with cannulated screws (Fig. 28.1a–d). The inverted triangle position is the most common configuration; however, is conflicting evidence about number of pins and also the configuration of pin [22].

28.4 Internal Fixation of Femoral Neck Fractures

Placement of cannulated screws can be performed on either a radiolucent flat top table or a fracture (traction) table; the authors prefer to use

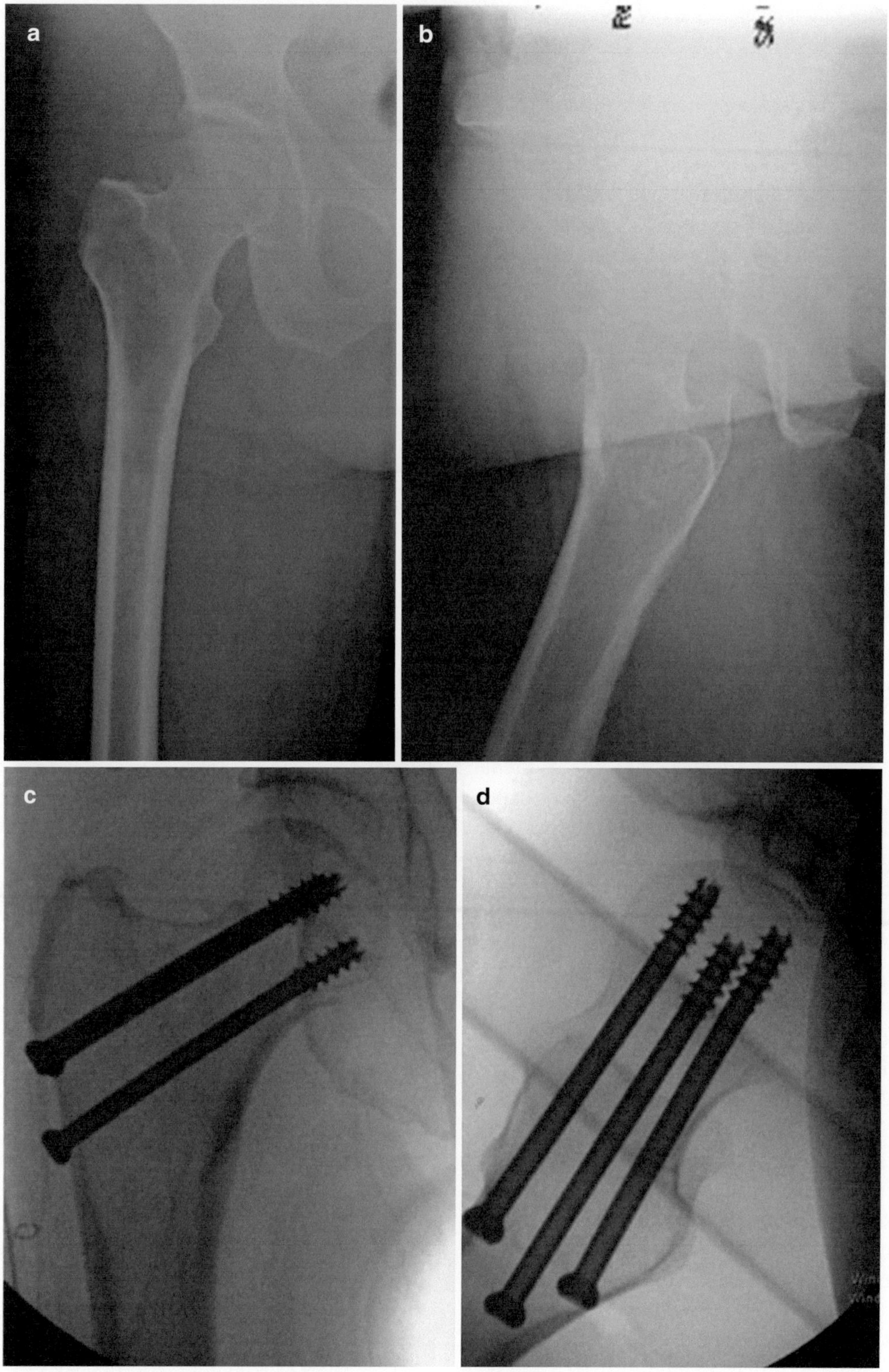

Fig. 28.1 (**a**) AP radiograph demonstrates a valgus impacted fracture of the femoral neck (Sacks). (**b**) Lateral radiograph demonstrates a valgus impacted fracture of the femoral neck, note the lack of posterior comminution. (**c**) Postoperative AP radiograph of an inverted triangle cannulated screw configuration. (**d**) Postoperative Lateral radiograph of an inverted triangle cannulated screw configuration

a fracture table as it can apply traction if needed and also holds the leg in a constant position negating the use of an assistant and allows for changes in fluoroscopy position without rotation of the affected leg (Fig. 28.2). It is important to screen the fluoroscopy after positioning to confirm that the fracture has not displaced in the interim. A small open incision is made laterally and the IT band is incised inferior to the vastus ridge for all wires or a percutaneous nick can be made for each wire separately. Guidewires are then introduced into the femoral neck using fluoroscopy. For the inverted triangle configuration, one guidewire is placed central and inferior along the calcar. The remaining two are then placed in a posterior superior and anterior superior position. The goal is to obtain spread; however, caution must be taken to ensure that the posterior superior screw which may look intraosseous on fluoroscopy could potentially be "in out in". While the clinical implication of this is unknown, this screw is in close proximity to the vascular supply to the femoral head [23]. If a fourth screw is to be added, it should be placed posteriorly to support posterior comminution; typically, this is done for displaced fractures that require a reduction [24]. The most inferior screw should not be placed distal to the level of the lesser trochanter as this may create a stress riser in the subtrochanteric region [25].

If two cannulated screws are to be used, one screw should be placed in the inferior/central along the calcar and the second screw placed more proximal in the femoral neck and in the central or posterior segment on the lateral position [26].

While used more often in younger patients, a SHS construct can be used for femoral neck fractures in the elderly. This implant is more than often used for basicervical fracture patterns. A de-rotational screw placed superior and parallel to the lag screw could be used to prevent rotation of the [27] neck during insertion of the large central lag screw [28] (Fig. 28.3a–c). The FAITH trial randomized large cohorts of patients to SHS or cannulated screws in both displaced and non-displaced femoral neck fractures [27]. Patients were included only if the surgeon felt that fixation was a better option than replacement. Overall, there was no significant difference in nonunion, implant failures, and infection. The reoperation rate was noted to be 14% for all causes in this large multinational observational study [27].

28.5 Hemiarthroplasty and Total Hip Arthroplasty for Displaced Femoral Neck Fractures

There is a defined rate of revision surgery that occurs following internal fixation of femoral neck fractures even if non-displaced. Hemiarthroplasty, while associated with greater intraoperative time, higher blood loss, and greater complication rate, has a significantly lower rate of revision surgery after internal fixation of displaced femoral neck fractures in the elderly [29].

The higher the amount of displacement, the higher the likely hood of nonunion and fixation failure in the elderly population [30, 31]. Arthroplasty options include unipolar or bipolar hemiarthroplasty or THA. Each of these stems may be cemented or press fit. The surgical approach for an arthroplasty procedure can be either an anterior approach, anterolateral, or posterolateral (Table 28.1). The choice of approach is ultimately based on surgeon comfort, with the anterior-based approaches having a lower dislocation rate due to preservation of the posterior capsular structures [32].

Hemiarthroplasty may be performed with either a bipolar or unipolar implant. A bipolar hemiarthroplasty has a dual articulation between the inner head and shell and the shell and the acetabulum. In comparison, a unipolar hemiarthroplasty has a single articulation between the shell and the acetabulum (Fig. 28.4). The theoretical advantage of this dual articulation is to reduce wear and decrease acetabular protrusion; however, studies have demonstrated that this dual articulation ceases to function over time and the stem behaves as a unipolar arthroplasty [33–36]. Due to this, the bipolar hemiarthroplasty may not be as cost-effective as a unipolar arthroplasty.

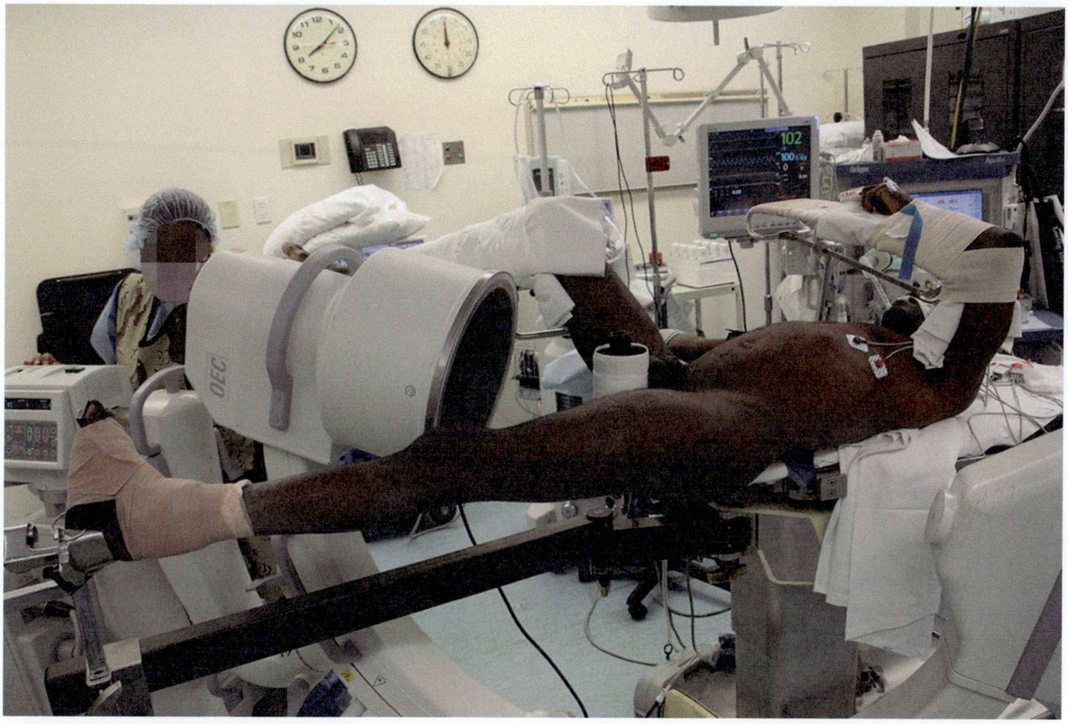

Fig. 28.2 Fracture table set up

While these implants are available in cemented and non-cemented designs, controversy regarding fixation strategy remains. In a large metanalysis by Parker et al., cemented prostheses were associated with less pain and improved mobility at 1 year [37]. Furthermore, other studies have demonstrated a lower risk of peri-prosthetic fracture with the use of a cemented implant [38]. Ultimately, if the patient has thick femoral cortices a press fit stem may be used; however, in the setting of most of these fractures, the patulous bone often suggests the use of a cemented stem [39]. The ultimate goal is to restore femoral neck offset, leg length, and adequately tension the hip abductors. Achieving these goals ensures a low rate of dislocation and restores hip mechanics [40]. Unlike, elective hip arthroplasty, restoration of leg lengths may be difficult because the neck cut is dictated by the fracture (Fig. 28.5a, b).

While hemiarthroplasty performs well in the postoperative period; THA has been noted to have improved functional outcomes that surpass hemiarthroplasty [41] (Fig. 28.6a). THA is associated with increased cost, a greater magnitude of surgery, increased blood loss, and also an increased dislocation rate in patients with a femoral neck fracture [42]. It does play a definitive role in patients who have eroded through the acetabulum with a hemiarthroplasty prosthesis, patients with antecedent symptomatic hip arthritis, and salvage after nonunion or AVN of the femoral head after internal fixation [43, 44]. It is now recommended to be used in patients who are highly active and would potentially survive greater than 10 years.

Internal fixation should be used with caution in treating displaced fractures in this cohort of patients as there is a significant rate of requiring revision surgery, up to 30–40%. This procedure should be reserved for the Garden 1 and 2 fractures in this patient population. Specific age cutoffs to define the elderly do not exist and decisions should be made on a case-by-case basis. Hemiarthroplasty is a reliable and predicable procedure in the treatment of displaced femoral neck fractures; however, in patients with preexisting arthritis and highly active patients, a THA can be a cost-effective treatment with improved long-term outcomes [45, 46].

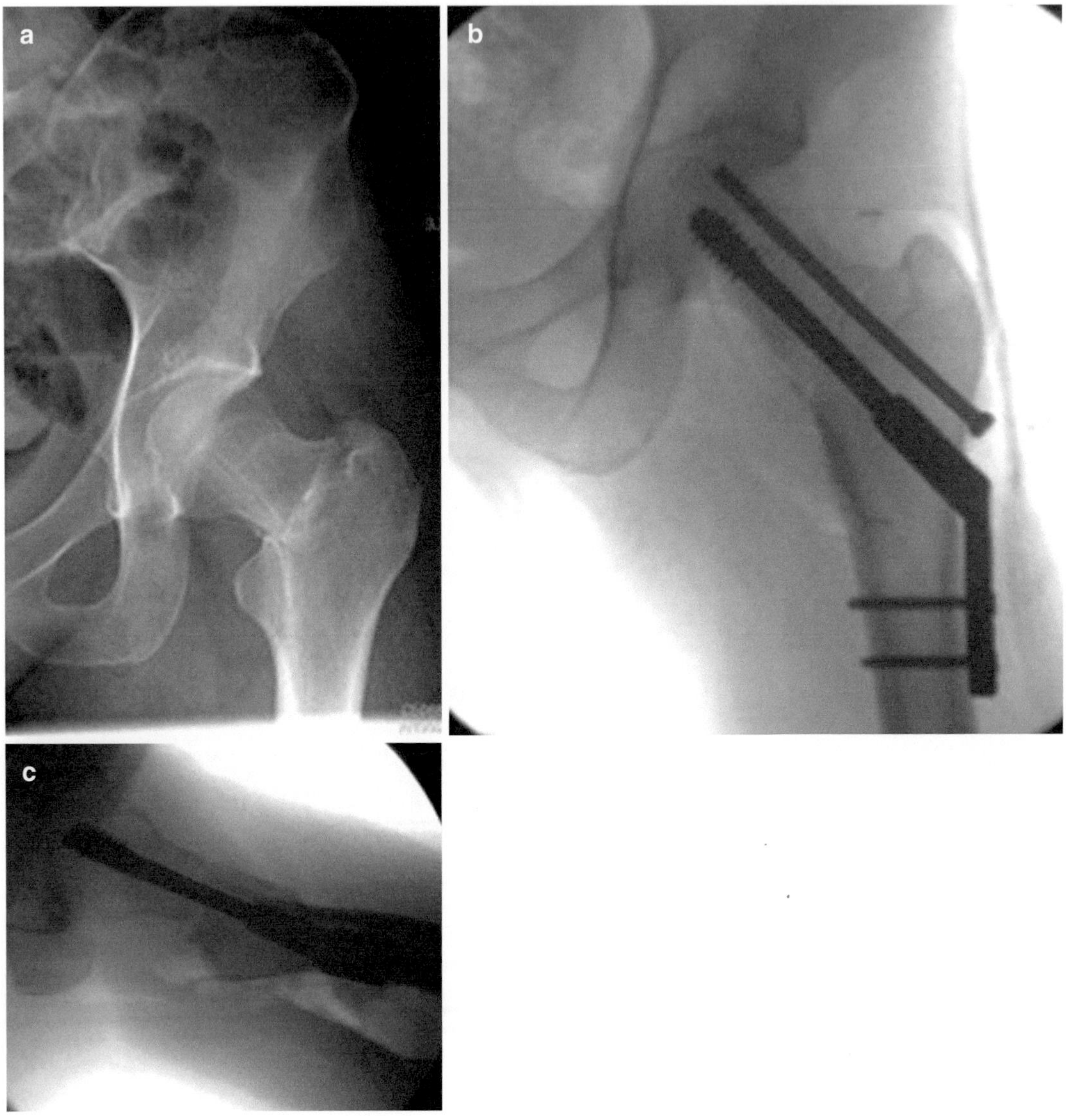

Fig. 28.3 (**a**) AP Pelvis radiograph of a basicervical fracture pattern. (**b**) AP radiograph of a SHS with de-rotational screw. (**c**) Lateral radiograph of a SHS with de-rotational screw

28.6 Pertrochanteric Femur Fracture

Pertrochanteric hip fractures are extracapsular and are located distal to the femoral neck between the greater and lesser trochanters. Patients with these injuries tend to be older and more frail than those with intracapsular hip fractures with mortality rates similar or slightly lower than femoral neck fractures [47, 48]. Due to their anatomical location, these fractures have an abundant vascular supply leading to fewer healing complications relative to intracapsular femoral neck fractures.

28.7 Determining Stability

While there are a number of classification systems used to describe these fractures, the AO/OTA classification has an acceptable method of both intra- and interobserver reliability [49].

Table 28.1 Surgical approaches for femoral neck fractures

Approach	Interval
Anterior (Hueter)	Superficial: TFL/Sartorious Deep: Recuts/gluteus Medius
Anterolateral (Hardinge)	TFL/gluteus Medius/Minimus
Direct lateral (Watson Jones)	Superficial: TFL Split Deep: Gluteus medius split
Posterolateral	Superficial: Gluteus Maximus Split Deep: Division of the short external rotators

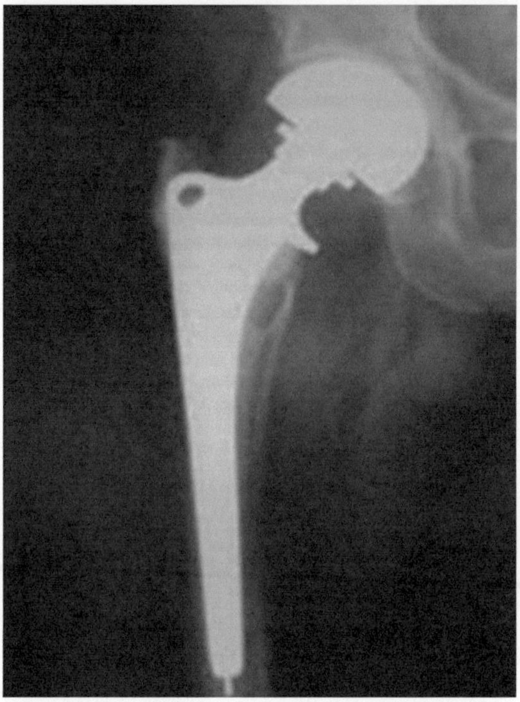

Fig. 28.4 AP Radiograph of a bipolar hemiarthroplasty

Intertrochanteric fractures are all described as 31 due to anatomical location. They are further subdivided by A1, A2, and A3. A1 fractures are two-part fractures and are considered stable. A2 fractures are comminuted and unstable and A3 fractures include subtrochanteric extension as well as reverse obliquity patterns.

Determining stability is dependent on multiple variables. A1 fractures are considered stable as they can have interdigitation of the fracture site following fixation. A2 fractures are considered unstable as they are multi-fragmentary and have compromised the medial buttress (Fig. 28.7a–e). A3 fractures have subtrochanteric extension or reverse obliquity fracture patterns. Ultimately, since both posteromedial and lateral buttresses are lacking, they may behave like subtrochanteric fractures.

An A2 subtype exists where the lateral cortex is incompetent and should be recognized. An intact lateral wall acts as a buttress to prevent excessive medialization and subsequent failure. Thickness of the lateral wall, measured 3 cm distal to the vastus ridge, should be greater than 20.5 mm if the surgeon plans on using a SHS device [50]. Lateral cortices thinner than this are prone to intraoperative fracture when reaming for the insertion of the lag screw in a SHS [51–53]. In summary, unstable fractures radiographically contain increasing number of parts, a reverse obliquity orientation, increasing degree of posterior medial comminution, and decreased thickness of the lateral cortical buttress under the vastus ridge.

This classification is not only useful for describing the injury but can also guide implant decision. These injuries are treated with either intramedullary fixation with a cephalomedullary implant (CMN) or extramedullary fixation with a SHS (Fig. 28.8a–d).

28.8 Surgical Management

The authors prefer to use a fracture (traction) table for the treatment of these injuries. The fracture table will provide sustained traction without the use of an assistant. Positioning on the fracture table is of utmost importance as improper positioning can hinder obtaining an adequate reduction. The perineal post can act as a lever pushing the fracture into varus. The operative site should be shifted away from the post with the buttock hanging off the side of the table. The good leg should be in a heel-to-toe position to prevent the ipsilateral hemipelvis from rotating toward the post while traction is being pulled. Attention to detail in during this process will mitigate positioning-related malreductions.

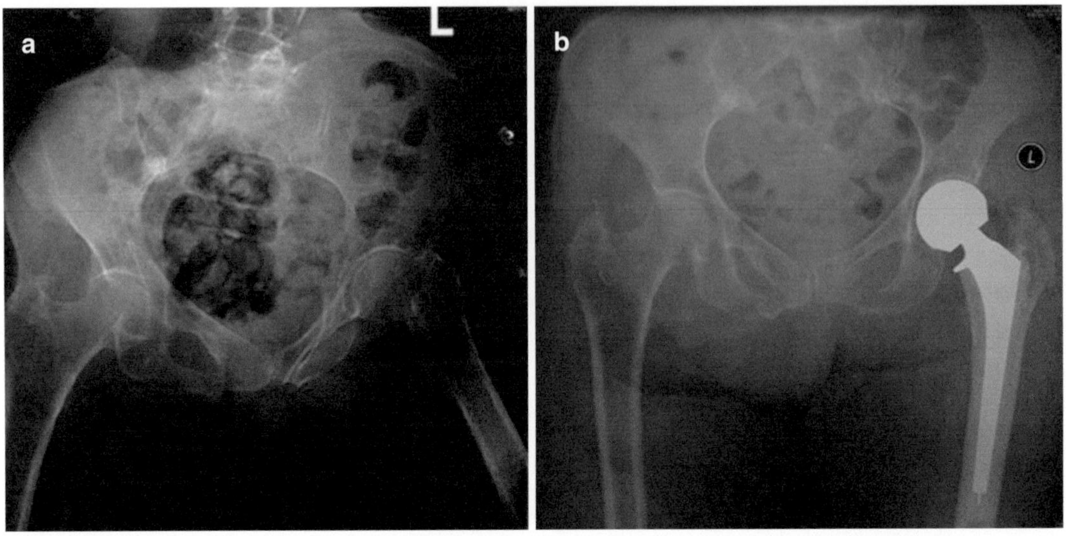

Fig. 28.5 (**a**) AP pelvis of displaced femoral neck fracture. (**b**) AP pelvis of unipolar hemiarthroplasty

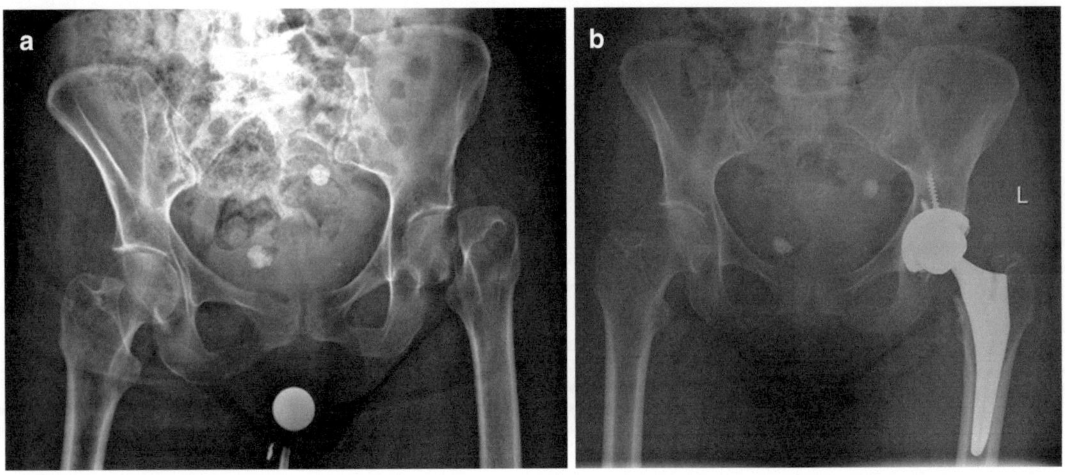

Fig. 28.6 (**a**) AP pelvis of displaced femoral neck fracture. (**b**) AP pelvis of THA after a femoral neck fracture

28.9 CMN Versus Sliding Hip Screw

There has been an increasing trend in the use of intramedullary nailing devices (Fig. 28.9a, b) in the preference to SHSs for the treatment of intertrochanteric hip fracture, despite robust quality evidence to support their use [54]. Fracture stability has been used as a surrogate to guide implant choice [55]. As discussed in the prior section, a stable fracture is mainly comprised of two parts that once reduced can compress against one another and is able to withstand the forces of a single leg stance after fixation [56].

With the more unstable fracture patterns, the implant must bear more load to avoid loss of reduction through collapse. Implant options for fixation of intertrochanteric fractures include SHS with or without a trochanteric stabilization plate, short intramedullary nails, and long intramedullary nails. Intramedullary nails offer the advantage of less soft tissue disruption at the fracture site, potentially less operative time, and increased biomechanical superiority, most notably in unstable fracture patterns [57–59]. However, despite this, a large number of randomized controlled trials have failed to demonstrate any differences in outcomes between SHSs and intramedullary devices [60, 61].

Caution should be taken in A2 fractures with a thin lateral wall with the use of a SHS construct. In a retrospective series of 214 patients, there was a significantly higher rate of reoperation (22%) with postoperative findings of a fractured lateral wall. Furthermore, lateral wall incompetency was radiographically identified in more unstable fracture patterns per the AO/OTA classification (palm JBJS 2007). Even with an adequate TAD and reduction, lateral wall incompetence could potentially lead to catastrophic failure with incor-

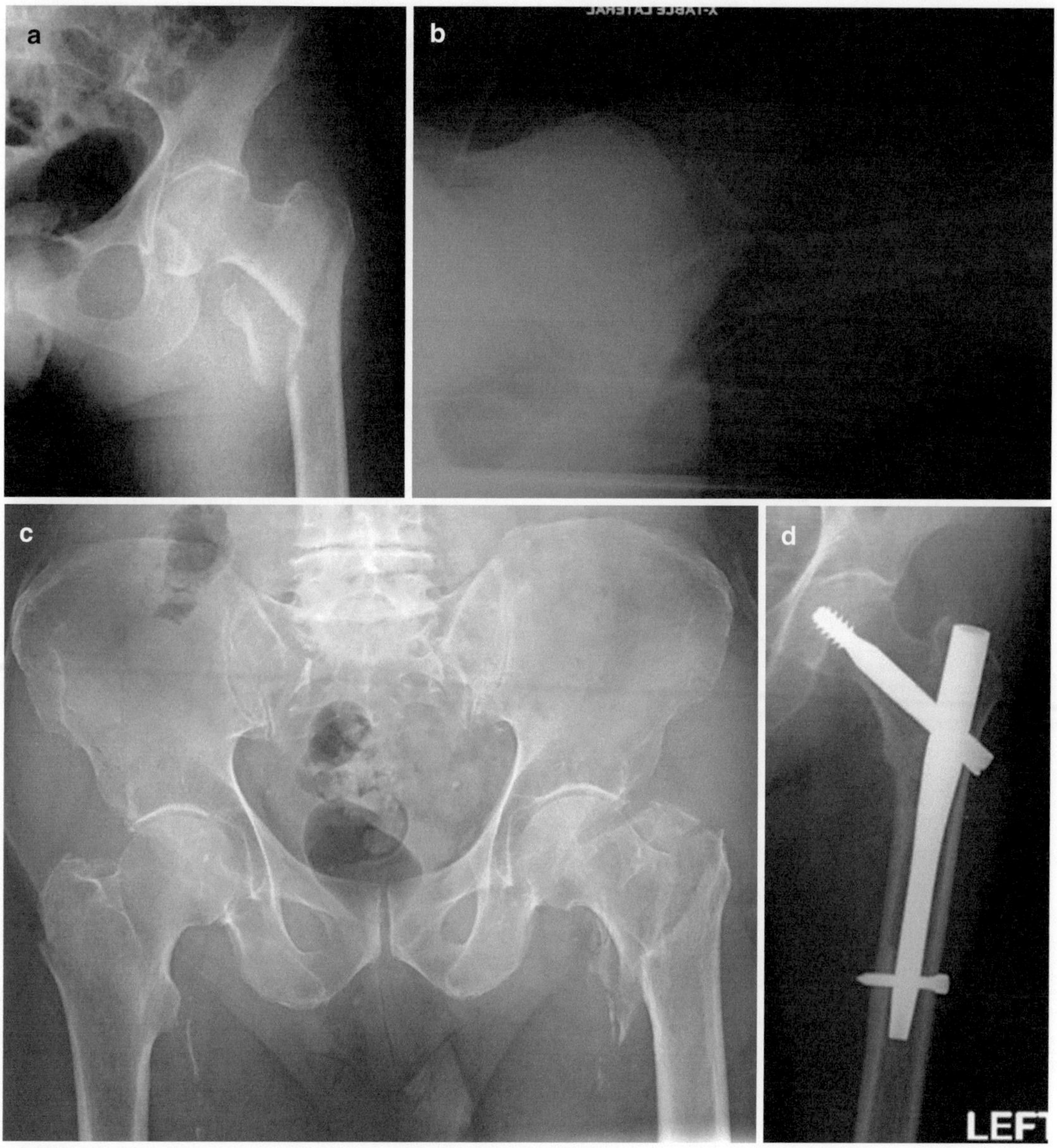

Fig. 28.7 (**a**) AP hip radiograph of an unstable intertrochanteric femur fracture. (**b**) Lateral hip radiograph of an unstable intertrochanteric femur fracture. (**c**) AP radiograph of an intertrochanteric femur fracture with an incompetent lateral wall. (**d**) AP hip radiograph of an unstable intertrochanteric femur fracture treated with an IMN. (**e**). Lateral hip radiograph of an unstable intertrochanteric femur fracture treated with an IMN

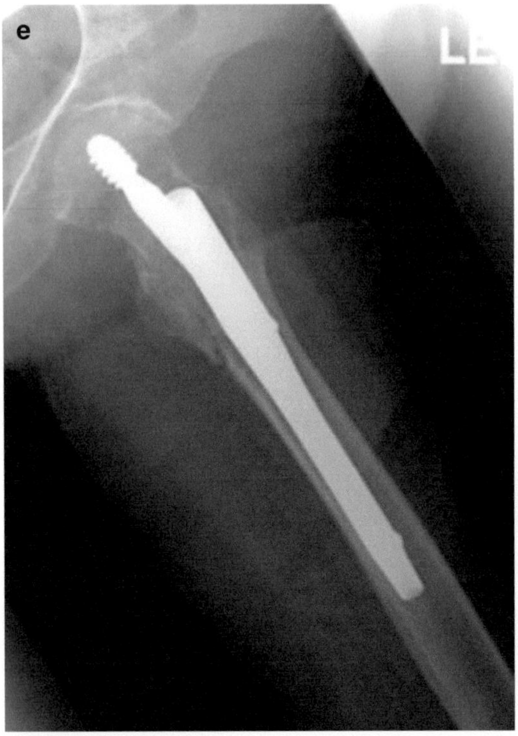

Fig. 28.7 (continued)

rect implant choice. If a SHS is to be used, studies have shown decreased failure rates with the addition of a trochanteric stabilization plate which can act as a lateral buttress [62].

Intramedullary fixation of these fractures does prevent excessive collapse as the nail acts as a lateral buttress and by doing so, has less femoral neck shortening, shorter leg length discrepancy, and medialization of the shaft [63, 64]. Femoral medialization and excessive collapse have been demonstrated to alter hip biomechanics which can theoretically impair mobility; however, the results from clinical studies regarding this are conflicting [65, 66]. Regardless of implant choice, it is imperative to have an exacting reduction and mitigate technical errors in implant technique.

28.10 Cephalomedullary Fixation

Both intramedullary and extramedullary implants have cephalomedullary fixation with either a helical blade, a single screw, or two screws. Appropriate cephalomedullary fixation ideally deep and central within the femoral head can often be measured with the Tip Apex Distance (TAD) [67]. It should be noted that the original paper describing TAD was done in SHS constructs. Failure of cephalomedullary fixation can be described as either "cut out" or "cut through" and is often related to either quality of reduction or inadequate tip apex distance rather than the implant used [68–70]. A tip apex distance of less than 25 mm will mitigate the chances of screw cutout. This has applied to both cephalomedullary nails as well as SHS constructs [71] (Fig. 28.10a, b).

The use of a helical blade design for fixation has been shown in cadaveric models to resist rotational and translational forces by compaction of cancellous bone [72] (Fig. 28.11a, b). Despite the biomechanical advantage, there is limited clinical data supporting the use of a blade versus a lag screw. Helical blades have been [73]associated with a phenomenon of "cut-through" in which there is medial perforation of the blade. It is recommended that the blade is not fully predrilled and the tip of the blade should be less than 10 mm from the joint surface [74, 75].

Lag screw fixation can consist of either a single or a double lag screw design. Single lag screw fixation while more commonly used is limited by a single point of fixation and can hence be subject to rotational instability [76]. Biomechanically, a dual lag screw design has been shown to have a higher load to failure, decreased varus collapse, and neck rotation [73, 77]. It is important to note that a dual lag screw design can be subject to the Z effect, in which the cephalic screw is subject to more stress under weight-bearing and as a result, the proximal screw advances into the nail while the distal screw toggles and backs out laterally ultimately leading to collapse and penetration proximally [78]. This has also been described in single lag screws as well. To mitigate the risk of the Z-effect while still maintaining rotational control, integrated sliding lag screw designs have been developed. However, a multicenter trial noted no difference in functional mobility, hip function, and patient satisfaction between a SHS

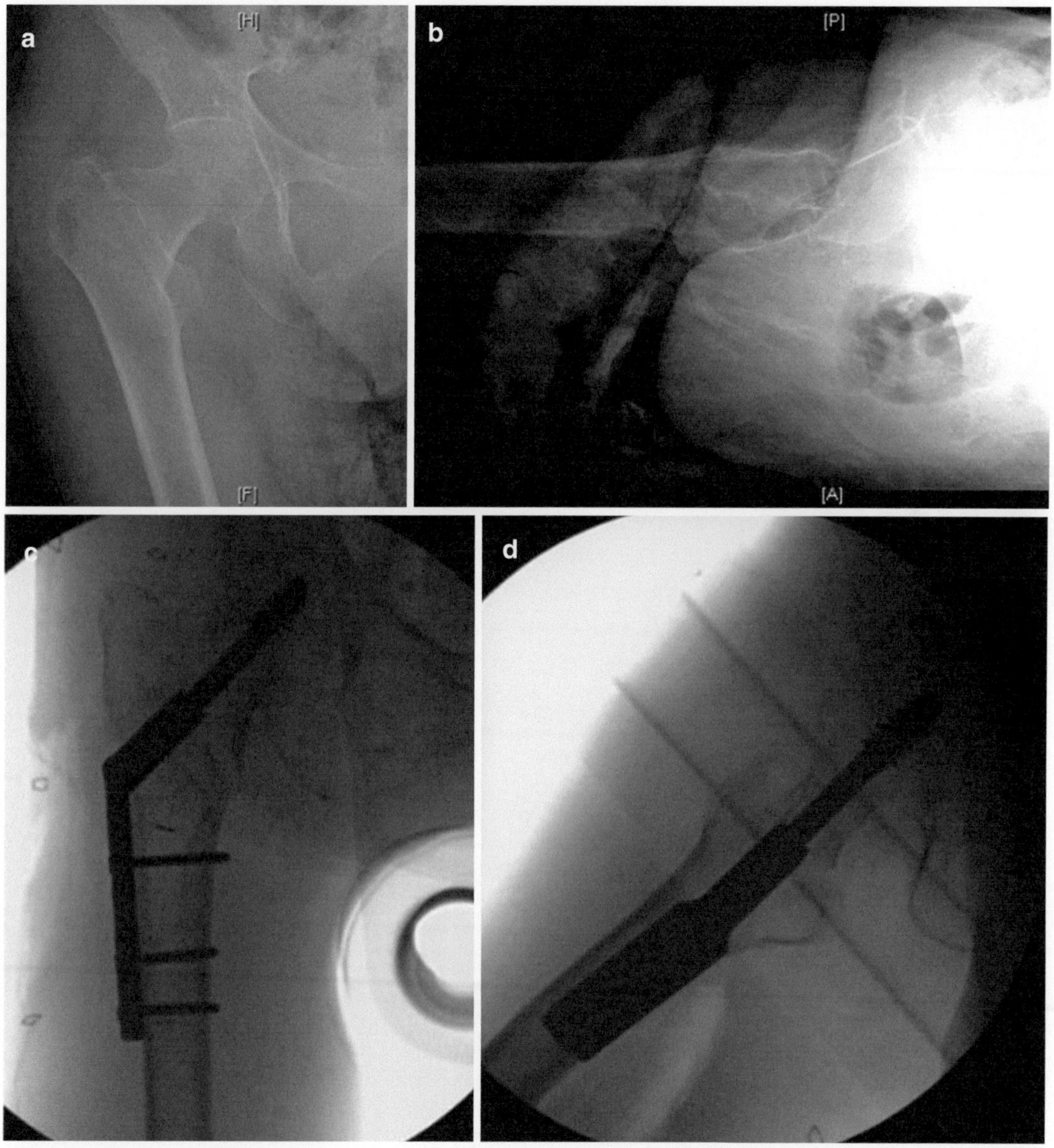

Fig. 28.8 (**a**) AP hip radiograph of a stable intertrochanteric femur fracture. (**b**) Lateral hip radiograph of a stable intertrochanteric femur fracture. (**c**) AP hip radiograph of a stable intertrochanteric femur fracture treated with an SHS. (**d**) Lateral hip radiograph of a stable intertrochanteric femur fracture treated with a SHS

and nailing system with an integrated sliding lag screw [62, 79]. A separate clinical study comparing nailing systems with a single lag screw compared with an integrated sliding lag screw demonstrated increased varus collapse and neck shortening in the single lag screw radiographically at 1 year postoperatively; however, since no patient or clinical outcomes were recorded, the overall effect of these radiographic changes are unknown [80].

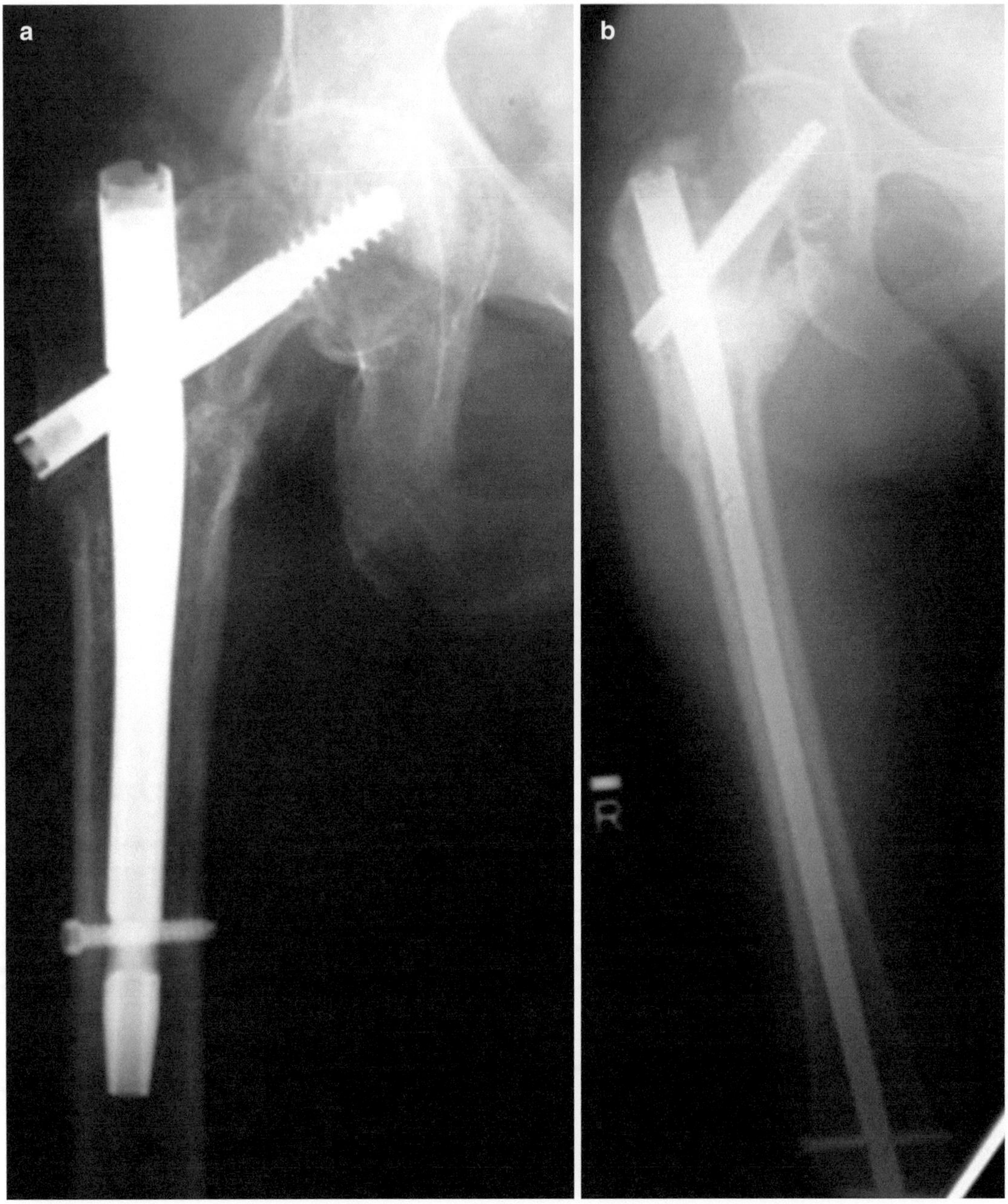

Fig. 28.9 (**a**) Short IMN. (**b**) Long IMN

28.11 Long Versus Short Nail

Currently, both short and long cephalomedullary nails are used in the treatment of intertrochanteric hip fractures. Advantages of using a short CMN include decreased operative time, blood loss, decreased implant cost, and distal locking performed through a targeting jig [76]. However, the theoretical disadvantage is that short nails do not span the entire bone in patients who are prone to falls and are already osteoporotic. The anatomic bow of the femoral shaft needs to be taken into consideration with the use of a long cephalomedullary nail and the radius of curvature (ROC)

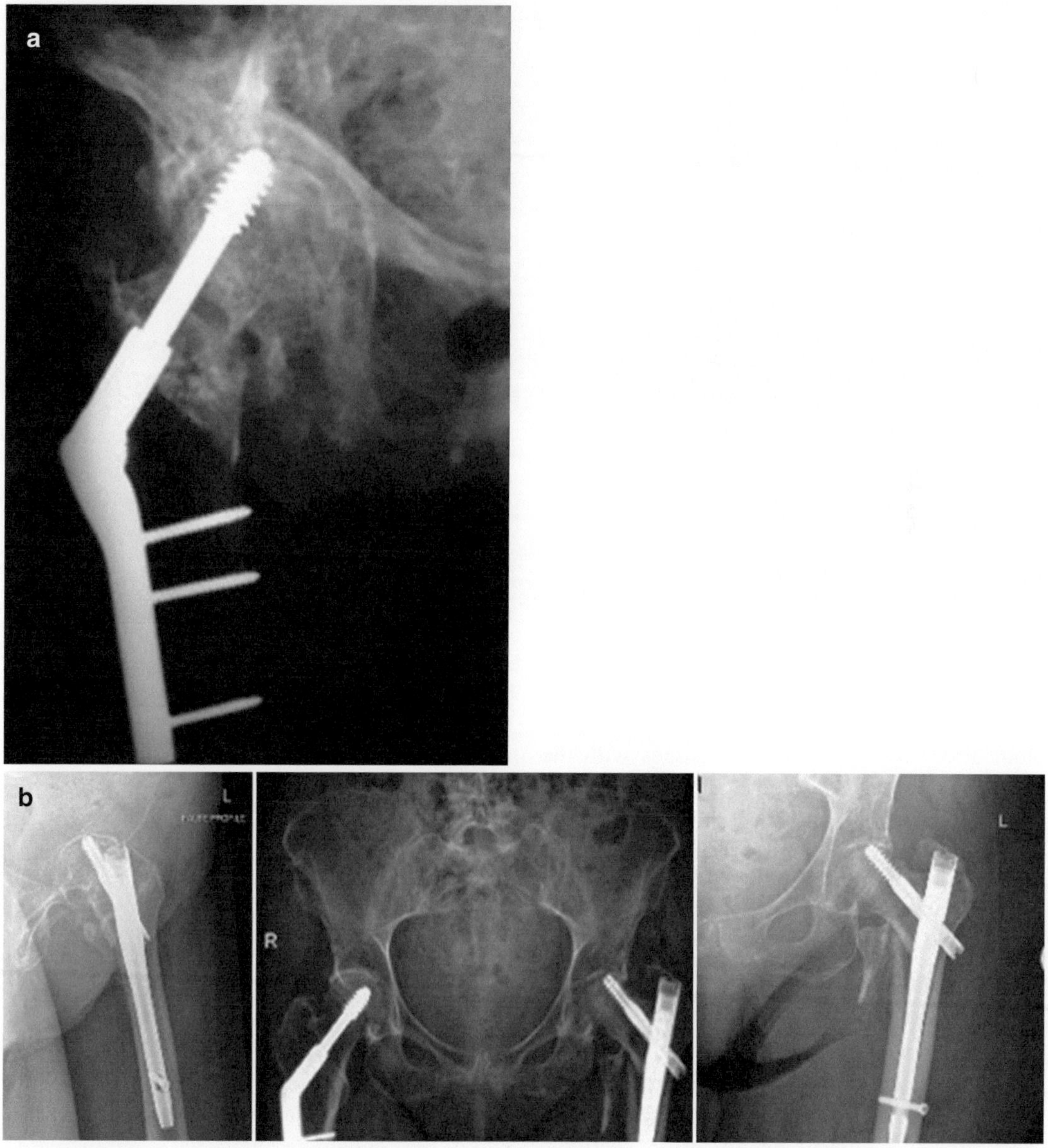

Fig. 28.10 (**a**) AP radiograph demonstrating cutout of a SHS construct. (**b**) AP radiograph demonstrating cutout of a CMN construct

mismatch between the implant and the femur can lead to anterior cortical perforation/impingement [81]. This finding can lead to a significant stress riser in the distal femur in osteoporotic patients. Newer implant designs have focused on improving this design aspect, with more anatomic ROC's.

Regardless of the theoretical risks and benefits of either implant, clinical studies have shown that both are viable options in the treatment of intertrochanteric femur fractures in the absence of subtrochanteric extension. Kleweno et al retrospectively analyzed 559 geriatric patients with intertrochanteric hip fractures treated with either a long or short CMN and noted no difference in the rates of revision surgery; however, the long CMN was associated with statistically significant longer operative time [82]. Hou et al noted higher

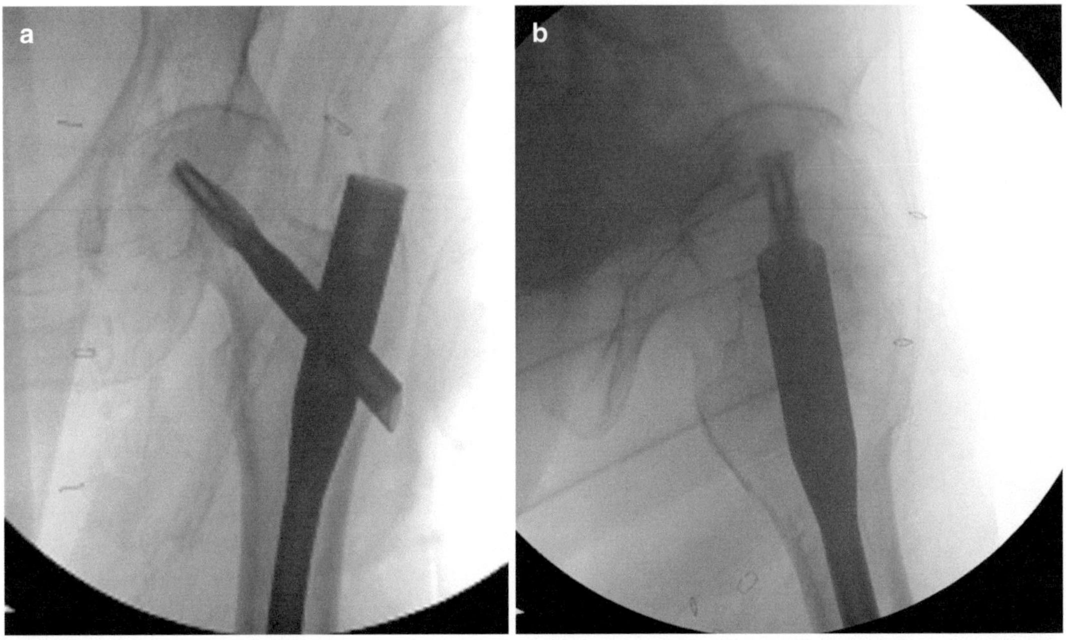

Fig. 28.11 (**a**) AP radiograph demonstrating a helical blade fixation of an intertrochanteric hip fracture. (**b**) Lateral radiograph demonstrating a helical blade fixation of an intertrochanteric hip fracture

blood loss and longer operative times with the use of a long nail. Ultimately, both groups had similar rates of intraoperative and postoperative complications and similar rates of union amongst all fracture types [83].

28.12 Implant-related Complications

Ultimately, two-part stable fractures treated with SHSs have minimal complication rates [84]. However, discussed in prior sections, patients with potentially unstable fractures or grossly unstable fractures can have failure rates of the SHS by over 15% [85]. Excluding improper surgical technique, the failure rates can be as low as 5% [86]. Failure occurs with progressive varus collapse of the femoral head leading to cutting out of the cephalomedullary screw. It important to recognize that the use of the SHS in unstable fractures despite proper surgical technique can have a greater amount of postoperative collapse compared to a cephalomedullary device [86]. While this collapse is not considered a failure of fixation and does not fall into screw "cut out", it may alter hip biomechanics and gait quality most notably when collapse surpasses 2 CM [87].

Cephalomedullary nails due to biomechanical superiority have had an increased trend in usage. Original designs of cephalomedullary nails were fraught with postoperative femoral shaft fracture, which ranged anywhere from 5 to 15% [88–90]. After design modifications made to the proximal end of the cephalomedullary nails and increased surgeon familiarity, the number of peri-implant fractures decreased significantly [91]. In a large retrospective study of cephalomedullary nails for the treatment of intertrochanteric femur fractures, the overall reported rate of postoperative femoral shaft fractures was about 0.6%. Despite the theoretical risks of a short nail ending in a region of a stress riser, a sub-analysis in this cohort did not demonstrate any increased risk of a short versus long nail [92].

28.13 Value-Based Care Algorithm

As mentioned before, the increasing trend in using cephalomedullary fixation has not decreased the perioperative mortality and morbidity of these injuries nor has it demonstrated any superiority in functional outcomes [93, [94]. Intramedullary nail implants can be up to 100% more expensive than the SHSs and its increased use has raised concerns regarding cost [56]. Surgeon comfort with the implant, risk of failure, implant costs, as well as industry influence are the driving variables for implant choice. Swart et al noted by analyzing failure rates, the intramedullary nail was more cost-effective as the risk of SHS failure increased. Hence in the A1 fractures, the SHS was more cost-effective and in A3 fractures the intramedullary nail was more cost-effective. In A2 fractures, the SHS was more cost-effective 70% of the time; however, they noted that fixation failure rate was the major driver of cost [95]. Egol et al implemented an algorithm treating stable intertrochanteric fractures with a SHS, unstable fractures with a short cephalomedullary nail, and fractures with distal extension such as reverse obliquity patterns or subtrochanteric extension with a long cephalomedullary nail. Adherence to this algorithm not only decreased rates of postoperative complications, it also led to significant cost savings [96].

28.14 Subtrochanteric Femur Fractures

Subtrochanteric femur fractures are defined as those occurring within 5 cm of the distal aspect of the lesser trochanter. These fractures have had an increase in incidence in the hip fracture population and are often a result of low-energy trauma in this population [97]. Over two-thirds of all subtrochanteric femur fractures occur in patients over the age of 50 [98]. Due to the presence of osteoporosis in this patient population, a portion of these patients may be on bisphosphonate therapy care must be taken to recognize patients who fall under this category of bisphosphonate-related (atypical) subtrochanteric femur fractures [99]. These fractures may not only occur from ground-level falls, but may also occur spontaneously with or without prodromal pain [99].

These fractures present a challenge as the deforming forces of the proximal femur are an obstacle to overcome. Furthermore, these fractures have a short working length, making manipulation and reduction at times challenging to gain and maintain. The classic deformity of the proximal femur is brought on by its multiple muscle attachments. The Iliopsoas acts as a strong flexor and external rotator, the short external rotators add an additional external rotation moment, and the gluteus medius and minimus abduct the proximal femur [100].

28.15 Atypical Subtrochanteric Femur Fractures

Atypical femur fractures are a relatively recent recognized fracture pattern and fall within the subcategory of subtrochanteric femur fractures. These fractures have increased morbidity and poor healing and have had an association with the long-term use of bisphosphonates. Despite this, there is still much research that is pending to understand the true pathogenesis behind these fracture patterns. What is though is that the use of bisphosphates inhibits osteoclastic function from allowing repair in the area of high tensile and compressive forces leading to microdamage and stress reactions [101]. Furthermore, the collagen cross-linking from bisphosphonates creates more brittle bone. This combination leads to eventual failure in high areas of stress such as the subtrochanteric region. While the awareness of this injury has increased, the overall incidence is still low and is thought to be between 1.5 and 23 cases per 100,000 person years [102].

Upon treating a patient, a thorough history is required to assist in identifying potential risk factors linking them toward having an atypical femur fracture. Patients should be asked if they not only have been on bisphosphonate therapy but also for the duration of time. Furthermore, it is important to understand the mechanism behind the injury and also if there are any prodromal

Table 28.2 Major and minor criteria for atypical bisphosphonate fractures

Major	Minor
The fracture must be associated with minimal to no trauma	Generalized increase in cortical thickening of the femoral diaphysis
The fracture line originates at the lateral cortex and is substantially transverse in its orientation, although it may become more oblique as it progresses medially along the femur	Unilateral or bilateral prodromal symptoms such as dull or aching pain in the groin or thigh
Complete fractures extend through both cortices and may be associated with a medial spike	Bilateral incomplete or complete diaphysis fractures
The fracture is non-comminuted or minimally comminuted	Delayed fracture healing
There is focal periosteal or endosteal thickening of the lateral cortex at the fracture site (beaking for flaring)	

symptoms such as thigh or groin pain [102]. The Task Force of the American Society for Bone and Mineral Research have defined the following major criteria for which the patient must meet four of to have an atypical femur fracture [102]. Minor criteria may be present or not (Table 28.2).

Ultimately, patients should also be questioned about the contralateral extremity as well. In the setting of prodromal symptoms without an obvious fracture, an MRI can demonstrate focal lateral cortical thickening or signs of a fracture line [103].

28.16 Surgical Management of Subtrochanteric Femur Fractures

Generally, all subtrochanteric femur fractures will require surgical treatment, unless the patient is nonambulatory or has medical comorbidities that would preclude surgical treatment. Options for treatment include IM Nails and fixed-angle plate and screw constructs. Specific implants utilized with these fractures include: centromedullary nails, cephalomedullary nails, SHSs, proximal femur locking plates, and a 95-degree blade plate. Nailing can be performed with either a piriformis start point or through a trochanteric entry with equivalent results; however, it is important to understand the geometry of the nail being used as well as proximal locking options [104]. Trochanteric start points have been utilized more frequently for theoretical ease of obtaining a start point on a more subcutaneous portion of the proximal femur. Depending on the manufacturer, each nail will have a various-proximal bend; however, this bend may induce a varus or valgus force on the nail depending on the start point [105]. A lateral start point on the trochanter, even with an adequate reduction, may induce a varus deformity once the nail is finally seated (Fig. 28.12). Due to patient's proximal femur morphology, there is no true ideal starting point for a trochanteric entry nail; however, starting at the tip of the trochanter or slightly medial may avoid a malreduction caused by the proximal bend of the nail [106].

Whether treatment is done on a flat top table or on a fracture table, the deforming forces of the proximal femur make imaging to obtain a starting point challenging. The C-arm will have to come over the top of the patient to account for the external rotation deformity. It is imperative to obtain a proper AP and lateral view of the proximal femur as the nail entry site is crucial for intramedullary nailing. If the deformity is such that reduction is difficult, percutaneous schanz pins or a ball spike pusher can be used to counteract the deforming forces to easier obtain imaging for a start point. A variety of methods exist in obtaining reduction for the proximal femur and should be done by graduated closed reduction methods. Options include a mallet, manual pressure, and use of an intramedullary reduction tool or "finger" [107]. Graduated open techniques can consist of ball spike pushers, schanz pins, and bone hooks which can be used to manipulate the proximal and distal fragments for reduction (Fig. 28.13a–d). Ultimately if unable to close reduce an open reduction is required. Following an open lateral approach to the proximal femur clamp assisted reduction can be performed in a

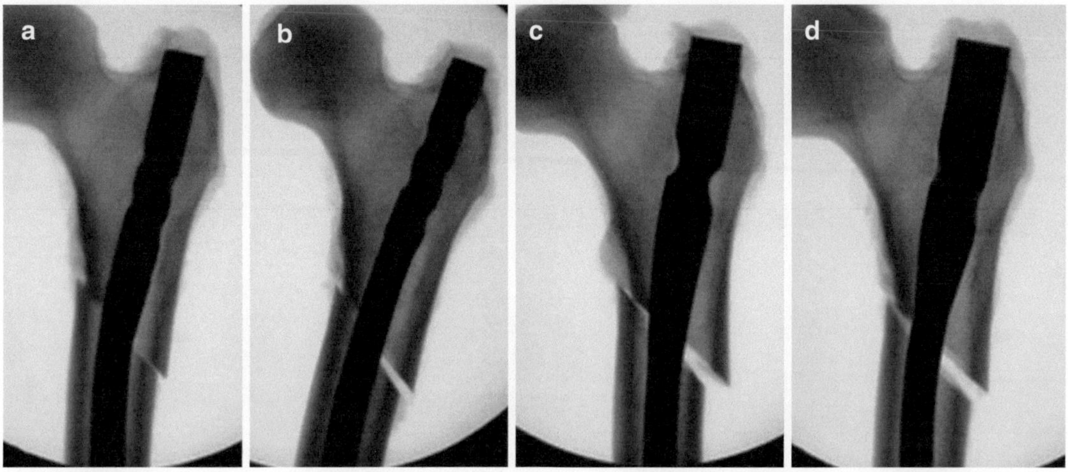

Fig. 28.12 (**a–d**) Demonstrate the effect of a lateral start point for different cephallomedullary nails in a subtrochanteric femur fracture resulting in a varus malunion. Courtesy of Ostrum et al.

biologically friendly manner to obtain and maintain a reduction of the proximal femur for efficient and accurate nailing with good clinical results [108]. Regardless of the technique used, the goals of surgery include spending time obtaining an appropriate start point and maintaining reduction while reaming to avoid malreduction that could occur prior to nail placement. "Push past" reaming can be used as a reduction aid as to not eccentrically ream at the fracture site and allow to nail assist with correction [109]. It must be noted that this technique is not as powerful in the metaphyseal region. In terms of proximal screw orientation, while crossed proximal screws are biomechanically stronger than parallel screws in the femoral head, they are often reserved for more distal or diaphyseal fracture patterns [110]. In geriatric patients, a large diameter cephalomedullary screw is used for increased fixation due to its larger size within the femoral head.

28.17 Surgical Management of Atypical Femur Fractures

While the primary goal for surgical management of these fractures remains the same as non-atypical subtrochanteric femur fractures, atypical femur fractures are pathologic in nature and require special attention [111]. One of the most common complications during intramedullary nailing includes fracture propagation or iatrogenic fracture due to the brittle nature of the bone [112]. Care should be taken to not only measure the canal diameter, but also to scrutinize and locate the size of any bony pedestals. These bony pedestals or areas of lateral intramedullary sclerosis can deflect reamers leading to reaming of the medial cortex [101]. To avoid a translational or angular deformity, this area can be over-reamed after fracture reduction with a larger diameter reamer or ultimately may an open approach and burred down. For patients with MRI/radiographic evidence of stress reaction with prodromal symptoms, Egol et al reported a 100% healing rate with 81% relief of pain following prophylactic treatment [113].

28.18 Managing Complications in Subtrochanteric Femur Fractures

The main causes of malunion are often due to the inability to obtain an adequate reduction intraoperatively or with improper placement of a nail. A lateral start point can be salvaged by eccentrically reaming out the medial bone with

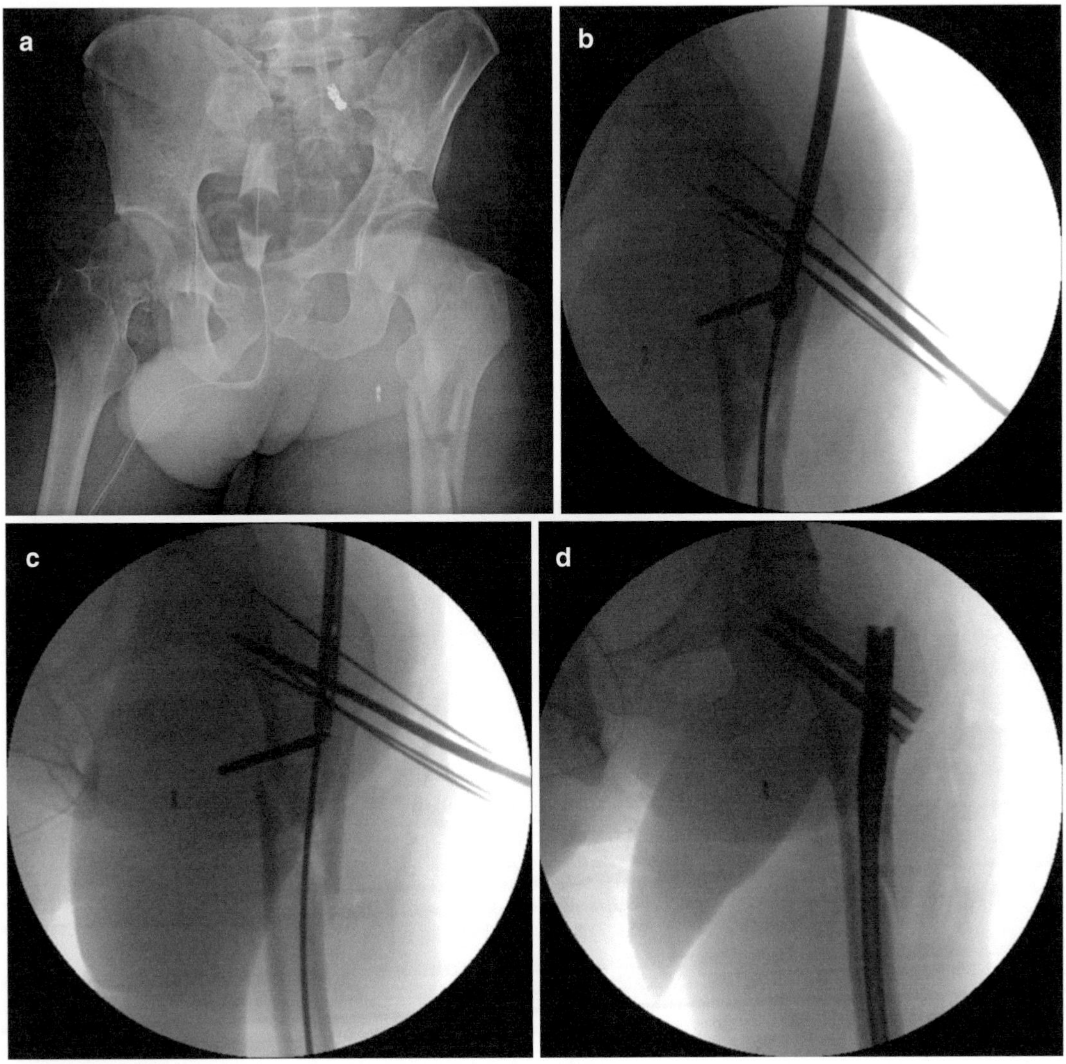

Fig. 28.13 (**a**) AP radiograph demonstrating a comminuted subtrochanteric femur fracture. (**b**) Fluoroscopy demonstrates the use of percutaneous schanz pins to act as blocking drill bits as well as to manipulate the proximal fragment. (**c**) Fluoroscopy demonstrates placement of the nail around the percutaneous schanz pins. (**d**) Final AP demonstrates interval reduction and alignment after nail placement

a large diameter reamer to walk the start point more medial. However, varus mal-reduction and flexion of the proximal segment if not addressed can not only cause failure of the proximal femur fixation but also severely affect hip biomechanics. While there is a dearth of literature on treatment for this, the authors preference is to remove the intramedullary implant, osteotomized the fracture site, and place a blade plate (Fig. 28.14a–c).

Risks of nonunion and malunion are particularly noted to be higher in atypical femoral fractures due to the pathologic nature of the bone as well as varus malalignment [114, 115]. In a large multicenter series, the revision rate for these fractures was noted to be about 12% with a union rate of 5.2 months in those who did not need a reoperation [111]. This could be partly due to the fact that these fractures were able to be identified preoperatively allowing for appropriate surgical planning.

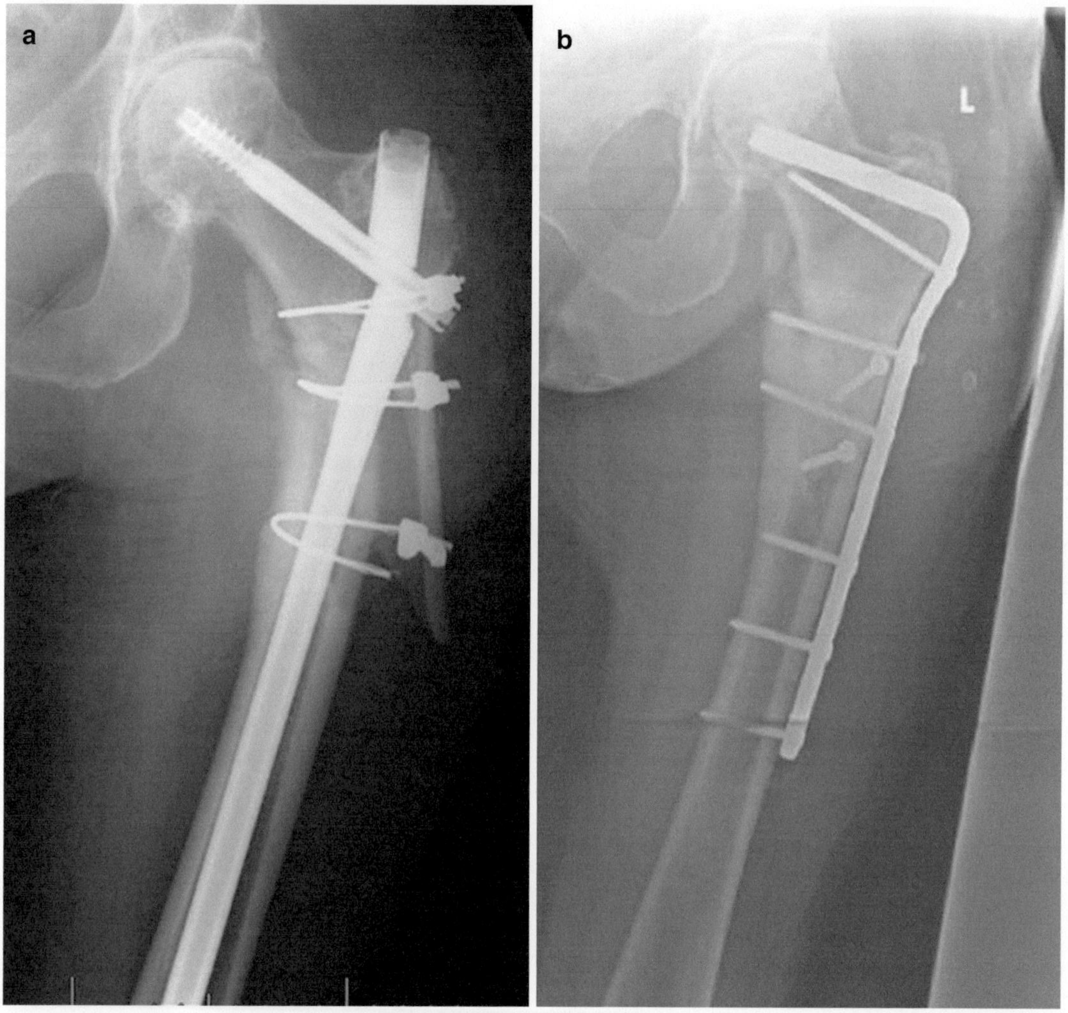

Fig. 28.14 (**a**) AP hip radiograph demonstrating varus failure of a subtrochanteric femur fracture. (**b**) AP hip radiograph postoperative revision of subtrochanteric malunion with blade plate. (**c**) Lateral hip radiograph of postoperative revision of subtrochanteric malunion with blade plate

28.19 Conclusion

Proximal femur fractures whether they are intracapsular or extracapsular in the geriatric population continue to increase in numbers. Treatment of these injuries has a major impact on the health care system and is one of the most expensive diagnoses. While surgical techniques and implants continue to evolve, the rate of mortality after these injuries continues to remain the same. Risk stratification and dedicated geriatric hip fracture services have been utilized to identify patients at risk for increased complications and optimize patients as necessary prior to surgery.

Regardless of injury type, a thorough patient history should be completed and the preoperative radiographs should be scrutinized for appropriate preoperative planning. All current literature points to an anatomic reduction of the proximal femur and technically sound application of the implant to avoid both intraoperative and postoperative pitfalls. Sound evidence-based algorithms have also been developed for the surgical management of proximal femur fractures to optimize outcomes and improve cost.

While the primary goal of surgical intervention is to allow immediate mobilization and to return patients to their pre-injury level of function, poor bone quality, medical comorbidities, and patient frailty can make this difficult.

References

1. Bergstrom U, Jonsson H, Gustafson Y, Pettersson U, Stenlund H, Svensson O. The hip fracture incidence curve is shifting to the right. Acta Orthop. 2009;80(5):520–4.
2. Gullberg B, Johnell O, Kanis JA. World-wide projections for hip fracture. Osteoporos Int. 1997;7(5):407–13.
3. Cooper C, Campion G, Melton LJ 3rd. Hip fractures in the elderly: a world-wide projection. Osteoporos Int. 1992;2(6):285–9.
4. Burge R, Dawson-Hughes B, Solomon DH, Wong JB, King A, Tosteson A. Incidence and economic burden of osteoporosis-related fractures in the United States, 2005-2025. J Bone Miner Res. 2007;22(3):465–75.
5. Hung WW, Egol KA, Zuckerman JD, Siu AL. Hip fracture management: tailoring care for the older patient. JAMA. 2012;307(20):2185–94.
6. Khan MA, Hossain FS, Ahmed I, Muthukumar N, Mohsen A. Predictors of early mortality after hip fracture surgery. Int Orthop. 2013;37(11):2119–24.
7. Tornetta P 3rd, Mostafavi H, Riina J, et al. Morbidity and mortality in elderly trauma patients. J Trauma. 1999;46(4):702–6.
8. Gallagher SF, Williams B, Gomez C, et al. The role of cardiac morbidity in short- and long-term mortality in injured older patients who survive initial resuscitation. Am J Surg. 2003;185(2):131–4.
9. Wilson MS, Konda SR, Seymour RB, Karunakar MA. Carolinas trauma network research G. early predictors of mortality in geriatric patients with trauma. J Orthop Trauma. 2016;30(9):e299–304.
10. Konda SR, Lack WD, Seymour RB, Karunakar MA. Mechanism of injury differentiates risk factors for mortality in geriatric trauma patients. J Orthop Trauma. 2015;29(7):331–6.
11. Merloz P. Optimization of perioperative management of proximal femoral fracture in the elderly. Orthop Traumatol Surg Res. 2018;104(1S):S25–30.
12. Rosell PA, Parker MJ. Functional outcome after hip fracture. A 1-year prospective outcome study of 275 patients. Injury. 2003;34(7):529–32.
13. Koval KJ, Oh CK, Egol KA. Does a traction-internal rotation radiograph help to better evaluate fractures of the proximal femur? Bull NYU Hosp Jt Dis. 2008;66(2):102–6.
14. Bazylewicz DB, Egol KA, Koval KJ. Cortical encroachment after cephalomedullary nailing of the proximal femur: evaluation of a more anatomic radius of curvature. J Orthop Trauma. 2013;27(6):303–7.
15. Sadozai Z, Davies R, Warner J. The sensitivity of CT scans in diagnosing occult femoral neck fractures. Injury. 2016;47(12):2769–71.
16. Pejic A, Hansson S, Rogmark C. Magnetic resonance imaging for verifying hip fracture diagnosis why, when and how? Injury. 2017;48(3):687–91.
17. Heijckmann AC, Huijberts MS, Geusens P, de Vries J, Menheere PP, Wolffenbuttel BH. Hip bone mineral density, bone turnover and risk of fracture in patients on long-term suppressive L-thyroxine therapy for differentiated thyroid carcinoma. Eur J Endocrinol. 2005;153(1):23–9.
18. Heetveld MJ, Raaymakers EL, van Eck-Smit BL, van Walsum AD, Luitse JS. Internal fixation for displaced fractures of the femoral neck. Does bone density affect clinical outcome? J Bone Joint Surg Br. 2005;87(3):367–73.
19. Swiontkowski MF, Harrington RM, Keller TS, Van Patten PK. Torsion and bending analysis of internal fixation techniques for femoral neck fractures: the role of implant design and bone density. J Orthop Res. 1987;5(3):433–44.
20. Zlowodzki M, Bhandari M, Keel M, Hanson BP, Schemitsch E. Perception of Garden's classification for femoral neck fractures: an international survey of 298 orthopaedic trauma surgeons. Arch Orthop Trauma Surg. 2005;125(7):503–5.
21. Kakar S, Tornetta P 3rd, Schemitsch EH, et al. Technical considerations in the operative management of femoral neck fractures in elderly patients: a multinational survey. J Trauma. 2007;63(3):641–6.
22. Panteli M, Rodham P, Giannoudis PV. Biomechanical rationale for implant choices in femoral neck fracture fixation in the non-elderly. Injury. 2015;46(3):445–52.
23. Hoffmann JC, Kellam J, Kumaravel M, Clark K, Routt MLC, Gary JL. Is the cranial and posterior screw of the "inverted triangle" configuration for femoral neck fractures safe? J Orthop Trauma. 2019;33(7):331–4.
24. Wang J, Jiang B, Marshall RJ, Zhang P. Arthroplasty or internal fixation for displaced femoral neck fractures: which is the optimal alternative for elderly patients? A meta-analysis. Int Orthop. 2009;33(5):1179–87.
25. Bray TJ. Femoral neck fracture fixation. Clinical decision making. Clin Orthop Relat Res. 1997;339:20–31.
26. Krastman P, van den Bent RP, Krijnen P, Schipper IB. Two cannulated hip screws for femoral neck fractures: treatment of choice or asking for trouble? Arch Orthop Trauma Surg. 2006;126(5):297–303.
27. Fixation using alternative implants for the treatment of hip fractures I. fracture fixation in the operative management of hip fractures (FAITH): an international, multicentre, randomised controlled trial. Lancet. 2017;389(10078):1519–27.
28. Ort PJ, LaMont J. Treatment of femoral neck fractures with a sliding compression screw and two Knowles pins. Clin Orthop Relat Res. 1984;190:158–62.
29. Parker MJ. Hemiarthroplasty versus internal fixation for displaced intracapsular fractures of the hip in elderly men: a pilot randomised trial. Bone Joint J. 2015;97-B(7):992–6.

30. Parker MJ, Stockton G. Internal fixation implants for intracapsular proximal femoral fractures in adults. Cochrane Database Syst Rev 2001(4):CD001467.
31. Broderick JM, Bruce-Brand R, Stanley E, Mulhall KJ. Osteoporotic hip fractures: the burden of fixation failure. Scientific World Journal. 2013;2013:515197.
32. Parker MJ. Lateral versus posterior approach for insertion of hemiarthroplasties for hip fractures: a randomised trial of 216 patients. Injury. 2015;46(6):1023–7.
33. Yamagata M, Chao EY, Ilstrup DM, Melton LJ 3rd, Coventry MB, Stauffer RN. Fixed-head and bipolar hip endoprostheses. A retrospective clinical and roentgenographic study. J Arthroplast. 1987;2(4):327–41.
34. Kanto K, Sihvonen R, Eskelinen A, Laitinen M. Uni- and bipolar hemiarthroplasty with a modern cemented femoral component provides elderly patients with displaced femoral neck fractures with equal functional outcome and survivorship at medium-term follow-up. Arch Orthop Trauma Surg. 2014;134(9):1251–9.
35. Hedbeck CJ, Blomfeldt R, Lapidus G, Tornkvist H, Ponzer S, Tidermark J. Unipolar hemiarthroplasty versus bipolar hemiarthroplasty in the most elderly patients with displaced femoral neck fractures: a randomised, controlled trial. Int Orthop. 2011;35(11):1703–11.
36. Coleman SH, Bansal M, Cornell CN, Sculco TP. Failure of bipolar hemiarthroplasty: a retrospective review of 31 consecutive bipolar prostheses converted to total hip arthroplasty. Am J Orthop (Belle Mead NJ). 2001;30(4):313–9.
37. Azegami S, Gurusamy KS, Parker MJ. Cemented versus uncemented hemiarthroplasty for hip fractures: a systematic review of randomised controlled trials. Hip Int. 2011;21(5):509–17.
38. Berend ME, Smith A, Meding JB, Ritter MA, Lynch T, Davis K. Long-term outcome and risk factors of proximal femoral fracture in uncemented and cemented total hip arthroplasty in 2551 hips. J Arthroplast. 2006;21(6 Suppl 2):53–9.
39. Ahn J, Man LX, Park S, Sodl JF, Esterhai JL. Systematic review of cemented and uncemented hemiarthroplasty outcomes for femoral neck fractures. Clin Orthop Relat Res. 2008;466(10):2513–8.
40. Tannast M, Mack PW, Klaeser B, Siebenrock KA. Hip dislocation and femoral neck fracture: decision-making for head preservation. Injury. 2009;40(10):1118–24.
41. Macaulay W, Pagnotto MR, Iorio R, Mont MA, Saleh KJ. Displaced femoral neck fractures in the elderly: hemiarthroplasty versus total hip arthroplasty. J Am Acad Orthop Surg. 2006;14(5):287–93.
42. Gregory RJ, Wood DJ, Stevens J. Treatment of displaced subcapital femoral fractures with total hip replacement. Injury. 1992;23(3):168–70.
43. Keating JF, Grant A, Masson M, Scott NW, Forbes JF. Randomized comparison of reduction and fixation, bipolar hemiarthroplasty, and total hip arthroplasty. Treatment of displaced intracapsular hip fractures in healthy older patients. J Bone Joint Surg Am. 2006;88(2):249–60.
44. Mahmoud SS, Pearse EO, Smith TO, Hing CB. Outcomes of total hip arthroplasty, as a salvage procedure, following failed internal fixation of intracapsular fractures of the femoral neck: a systematic review and meta-analysis. Bone Joint J. 2016;98-B(4):452–60.
45. Swart E, Roulette P, Leas D, Bozic KJ, Karunakar M. ORIF or arthroplasty for displaced femoral neck fractures in patients younger than 65 years old: an economic decision analysis. J Bone Joint Surg Am. 2017;99(1):65–75.
46. Slover J, Hoffman MV, Malchau H, Tosteson AN, Koval KJ. A cost-effectiveness analysis of the arthroplasty options for displaced femoral neck fractures in the active, healthy, elderly population. J Arthroplast. 2009;24(6):854–60.
47. Parker MJ, Pryor GA, Anand JK, Lodwick R, Myles JW. A comparison of presenting characteristics of patients with intracapsular and extracapsular proximal femoral fractures. J R Soc Med. 1992;85(3):152–5.
48. Forte ML, Virnig BA, Swiontkowski MF, et al. Ninety-day mortality after intertrochanteric hip fracture: does provider volume matter? J Bone Joint Surg Am. 2010;92(4):799–806.
49. Schipper IB, Steyerberg EW, Castelein RM, van Vugt AB. Reliability of the AO/ASIF classification for pertrochanteric femoral fractures. Acta Orthop Scand. 2001;72(1):36–41.
50. Hsu CE, Shih CM, Wang CC, Huang KC. Lateral femoral wall thickness. A reliable predictor of post-operative lateral wall fracture in intertrochanteric fractures. Bone Joint J. 2013;95-B(8):1134–8.
51. Gotfried Y. The lateral trochanteric wall: a key element in the reconstruction of unstable pertrochanteric hip fractures. Clin Orthop Relat Res. 2004;425:82–6.
52. Parker MJ. Trochanteric hip fractures. Fixation failure commoner with femoral medialization, a comparison of 101 cases. Acta Orthop Scand. 1996;67(4):329–32.
53. Im GI, Shin YW, Song YJ. Potentially unstable intertrochanteric fractures. J Orthop Trauma. 2005;19(1):5–9.
54. Chen F, Wang Z, Bhattacharyya T. Convergence of outcomes for hip fracture fixation by nails and plates. Clin Orthop Relat Res. 2013;471(4):1349–55.
55. Roberts KC, Brox WT, Jevsevar DS, Sevarino K. Management of hip fractures in the elderly. J Am Acad Orthop Surg. 2015;23(2):131–7.
56. Socci AR, Casemyr NE, Leslie MP, Baumgaertner MR. Implant options for the treatment of intertrochanteric fractures of the hip: rationale, evidence, and recommendations. Bone Joint J. 2017;99-B(1):128–33.
57. Leung KS, So WS, Shen WY, Hui PW. Gamma nails and dynamic hip screws for peritrochanteric

fractures. A randomised prospective study in elderly patients. J Bone Joint Surg Br. 1992;74(3):345–51.
58. Adams CI, Robinson CM, Court-Brown CM, McQueen MM. Prospective randomized controlled trial of an intramedullary nail versus dynamic screw and plate for intertrochanteric fractures of the femur. J Orthop Trauma. 2001;15(6):394–400.
59. Curtis MJ, Jinnah RH, Wilson V, Cunningham BW. Proximal femoral fractures: a biomechanical study to compare intramedullary and extramedullary fixation. Injury. 1994;25(2):99–104.
60. Parker MJ, Handoll HH. Gamma and other cephalocondylic intramedullary nails versus extramedullary implants for extracapsular hip fractures in adults. *Cochrane Database Syst Rev* 2010(9):CD000093.
61. Bohl DD, Basques BA, Golinvaux NS, Miller CP, Baumgaertner MR, Grauer JN. Extramedullary compared with intramedullary implants for intertrochanteric hip fractures: thirty-day outcomes of 4432 procedures from the ACS NSQIP database. J Bone Joint Surg Am. 2014;96(22):1871–7.
62. Matre K, Vinje T, Havelin LI, et al. TRIGEN INTERTAN intramedullary nail versus sliding hip screw: a prospective, randomized multicenter study on pain, function, and complications in 684 patients with an intertrochanteric or subtrochanteric fracture and one year of follow-up. J Bone Joint Surg Am. 2013;95(3):200–8.
63. Bretherton CP, Parker MJ. Femoral medialization, fixation failures, and functional outcome in trochanteric hip fractures treated with either a sliding hip screw or an intramedullary nail from within a randomized trial. J Orthop Trauma. 2016;30(12):642–6.
64. Ahrengart L, Tornkvist H, Fornander P, et al. A randomized study of the compression hip screw and gamma nail in 426 fractures. Clin Orthop Relat Res. 2002;401:209–22.
65. Pajarinen J, Lindahl J, Michelsson O, Savolainen V, Hirvensalo E. Pertrochanteric femoral fractures treated with a dynamic hip screw or a proximal femoral nail. A randomised study comparing post-operative rehabilitation. J Bone Joint Surg Br. 2005;87(1):76–81.
66. Reindl R, Harvey EJ, Berry GK, Rahme E. Canadian orthopaedic trauma S. intramedullary versus extramedullary fixation for unstable intertrochanteric fractures: a prospective randomized controlled trial. J Bone Joint Surg Am. 2015;97(23):1905–12.
67. Baumgaertner MR, Curtin SL, Lindskog DM, Keggi JM. The value of the tip-apex distance in predicting failure of fixation of peritrochanteric fractures of the hip. J Bone Joint Surg Am. 1995;77(7):1058–64.
68. Huang X, Leung F, Liu M, Chen L, Xu Z, Xiang Z. Is helical blade superior to screw design in terms of cut-out rate for elderly trochanteric fractures? A meta-analysis of randomized controlled trials. Eur J Orthop Surg Traumatol. 2014;24(8):1461–8.
69. Stern R, Lubbeke A, Suva D, Miozzari H, Hoffmeyer P. Prospective randomised study comparing screw versus helical blade in the treatment of low-energy trochanteric fractures. Int Orthop. 2011;35(12):1855–61.
70. Ibrahim I, Appleton PT, Wixted JJ, DeAngelis JP, Rodriguez EK. Implant cut-out following cephalomedullary nailing of intertrochanteric femur fractures: are helical blades to blame? Injury. 2019;50(4):926–30.
71. Geller JA, Saifi C, Morrison TA, Macaulay W. Tip-apex distance of intramedullary devices as a predictor of cut-out failure in the treatment of peritrochanteric elderly hip fractures. Int Orthop. 2010;34(5):719–22.
72. Goffin JM, Pankaj P, Simpson AH, Seil R, Gerich TG. Does bone compaction around the helical blade of a proximal femoral nail anti-rotation (PFNA) decrease the risk of cut-out?: a subject-specific computational study. Bone Joint Res. 2013;2(5):79–83.
73. Kubiak EN, Bong M, Park SS, Kummer F, Egol K, Koval KJ. Intramedullary fixation of unstable intertrochanteric hip fractures: one or two lag screws. J Orthop Trauma. 2004;18(1):12–7.
74. Frei HC, Hotz T, Cadosch D, Rudin M, Kach K. Central head perforation, or "cut through," caused by the helical blade of the proximal femoral nail antirotation. J Orthop Trauma. 2012;26(8):e102–7.
75. Flores SA, Woolridge A, Caroom C, Jenkins M. The utility of the tip-apex distance in predicting axial migration and Cutout with the trochanteric fixation nail system helical blade. J Orthop Trauma. 2016;30(6):e207–11.
76. Baldwin PC 3rd, Lavender RC, Sanders R, Koval KJ. Controversies in intramedullary fixation for intertrochanteric hip fractures. J Orthop Trauma. 2016;30(12):635–41.
77. Kouvidis GK, Sommers MB, Giannoudis PV, Katonis PG, Bottlang M. Comparison of migration behavior between single and dual lag screw implants for intertrochanteric fracture fixation. J Orthop Surg Res. 2009;4:16.
78. Strauss EJ, Kummer FJ, Koval KJ, Egol KA. The "Z-effect" phenomenon defined: a laboratory study. J Orthop Res. 2007;25(12):1568–73.
79. Santoni BG, Nayak AN, Cooper SA, et al. Comparison of femoral head rotation and Varus collapse between a single lag screw and integrated dual screw intertrochanteric hip fracture fixation device using a cadaveric hemi-pelvis biomechanical model. J Orthop Trauma. 2016;30(4):164–9.
80. Serrano R, Blair JA, Watson DT, et al. Cephalomedullary nail fixation of intertrochanteric femur fractures: are two proximal screws better than one? J Orthop Trauma. 2017;31(11):577–82.
81. Egol KA, Chang EY, Cvitkovic J, Kummer FJ, Koval KJ. Mismatch of current intramedullary nails with the anterior bow of the femur. J Orthop Trauma. 2004;18(7):410–5.
82. Kleweno C, Morgan J, Redshaw J, et al. Short versus long cephalomedullary nails for the treatment of intertrochanteric hip fractures in patients older than 65 years. J Orthop Trauma. 2014;28(7):391–7.

83. Hou Z, Bowen TR, Irgit KS, et al. Treatment of pertrochanteric fractures (OTA 31-A1 and A2): long versus short cephalomedullary nailing. J Orthop Trauma. 2013;27(6):318–24.
84. Harrington P, Nihal A, Singhania AK, Howell FR. Intramedullary hip screw versus sliding hip screw for unstable intertrochanteric femoral fractures in the elderly. Injury. 2002;33(1):23–8.
85. Davis TR, Sher JL, Horsman A, Simpson M, Porter BB, Checketts RG. Intertrochanteric femoral fractures. Mechanical failure after internal fixation. J Bone Joint Surg Br. 1990;72(1):26–31.
86. Whale CS, Hulet DA, Beebe MJ, et al. Cephalomedullary nail versus sliding hip screw for fixation of AO 31 A1/2 intertrochanteric femoral fracture: a 12-year comparison of failure, complications, and mortality. Curr Orthop Pract. 2016;27(6):604–13.
87. Zielinski SM, Keijsers NL, Praet SF, et al. Femoral neck shortening after internal fixation of a femoral neck fracture. Orthopedics. 2013;36(7):e849–58.
88. Bridle SH, Patel AD, Bircher M, Calvert PT. Fixation of intertrochanteric fractures of the femur. A randomised prospective comparison of the gamma nail and the dynamic hip screw. J Bone Joint Surg Br. 1991;73(2):330–4.
89. Radford PJ, Needoff M, Webb JK. A prospective randomised comparison of the dynamic hip screw and the gamma locking nail. J Bone Joint Surg Br. 1993;75(5):789–93.
90. Butt MS, Krikler SJ, Nafie S, Ali MS. Comparison of dynamic hip screw and gamma nail: a prospective, randomized, controlled trial. Injury. 1995;26(9):615–8.
91. Bhandari M, Schemitsch E, Jonsson A, Zlowodzki M, Haidukewych GJ. Gamma nails revisited: gamma nails versus compression hip screws in the management of intertrochanteric fractures of the hip: a meta-analysis. J Orthop Trauma. 2009;23(6):460–4.
92. Bojan AJ, Beimel C, Speitling A, Taglang G, Ekholm C, Jonsson A. 3066 consecutive gamma nails. 12 years experience at a single Centre. BMC Musculoskelet Disord. 2010;11:133.
93. Anglen JO, Weinstein JN. American Board of Orthopaedic Surgery Research C. nail or plate fixation of intertrochanteric hip fractures: changing pattern of practice. A review of the American board of orthopaedic surgery database. J Bone Joint Surg Am. 2008;90(4):700–7.
94. Radcliff TA, Regan E, Cowper Ripley DC, Hutt E. Increased use of intramedullary nails for intertrochanteric proximal femoral fractures in veterans affairs hospitals: a comparative effectiveness study. J Bone Joint Surg Am. 2012;94(9):833–40.
95. Swart E, Makhni EC, Macaulay W, Rosenwasser MP, Bozic KJ. Cost-effectiveness analysis of fixation options for intertrochanteric hip fractures. J Bone Joint Surg Am. 2014;96(19):1612–20.
96. Egol KA, Marcano AI, Lewis L, Tejwani NC, McLaurin TM, Davidovitch RI. Can the use of an evidence-based algorithm for the treatment of intertrochanteric fractures of the hip maintain quality at a reduced cost? Bone Joint J. 2014;96-B(9):1192–7.
97. Sullivan MP, Baldwin KD, Donegan DJ, Mehta S, Ahn J. Geriatric fractures about the hip: divergent patterns in the proximal femur, acetabulum, and pelvis. Orthopedics. 2014;37(3):151–7.
98. Ng AC, Drake MT, Clarke BL, et al. Trends in subtrochanteric, diaphyseal, and distal femur fractures, 1984-2007. Osteoporos Int. 2012;23(6):1721–6.
99. Thompson RN, Phillips JR, McCauley SH, Elliott JR, Moran CG. Atypical femoral fractures and bisphosphonate treatment: experience in two large United Kingdom teaching hospitals. J Bone Joint Surg Br. 2012;94(3):385–90.
100. Jackson C, Tanios M, Ebraheim N. Management of Subtrochanteric Proximal Femur Fractures: a review of recent literature. Adv Orthop. 2018;2018:1326701.
101. Githens M, Garner MR, Firoozabadi R. Surgical Management of Atypical Femur Fractures Associated with Bisphosphonate Therapy. J Am Acad Orthop Surg. 2018;26(24):864–71.
102. Shane E, Burr D, Abrahamsen B, et al. Atypical subtrochanteric and diaphyseal femoral fractures: second report of a task force of the American Society for Bone and Mineral Research. J Bone Miner Res. 2014;29(1):1–23.
103. Black JD, Kancherla VK, De Long WG Jr. A review of atypical femoral fractures from a tertiary care teaching hospital: an alarming trend? J Orthop Trauma. 2016;30(4):182–8.
104. Starr AJ, Hay MT, Reinert CM, Borer DS, Christensen KC. Cephalomedullary nails in the treatment of high-energy proximal femur fractures in young patients: a prospective, randomized comparison of trochanteric versus piriformis fossa entry portal. J Orthop Trauma. 2006;20(4):240–6.
105. Ostrum RF, Marcantonio A, Marburger R. A critical analysis of the eccentric starting point for trochanteric intramedullary femoral nailing. J Orthop Trauma. 2005;19(10):681–6.
106. Streubel PN, Wong AH, Ricci WM, Gardner MJ. Is there a standard trochanteric entry site for nailing of subtrochanteric femur fractures? J Orthop Trauma. 2011;25(4):202–7.
107. Yoon RS, Donegan DJ, Liporace FA. Reducing subtrochanteric femur fractures: tips and tricks, do's and don'ts. J Orthop Trauma. 2015;29(Suppl 4):S28–33.
108. Afsari A, Liporace F, Lindvall E, Infante A Jr, Sagi HC, Haidukewych GJ. Clamp-assisted reduction of high subtrochanteric fractures of the femur: surgical technique. J Bone Joint Surg Am. 2010;92(Suppl 1 Pt 2):217–25.
109. Gary JL, Munz JW, Burgess AR. "push-past" reaming as a reduction aid with intramedullary nailing of metadiaphyseal and diaphyseal femoral shaft fractures. Orthopedics. 2014;37(6):393–6.
110. Grisell M, Moed BR, Bledsoe JG. A biomechanical comparison of trochanteric nail proximal screw

configurations in a subtrochanteric fracture model. J Orthop Trauma. 2010;24(6):359–63.
111. Bogdan Y, Tornetta P 3rd, Einhorn TA, et al. Healing time and complications in operatively treated atypical femur fractures associated with bisphosphonate use: a Multicenter retrospective cohort. J Orthop Trauma. 2016;30(4):177–81.
112. Prasarn ML, Ahn J, Helfet DL, Lane JM, Lorich DG. Bisphosphonate-associated femur fractures have high complication rates with operative fixation. Clin Orthop Relat Res. 2012;470(8):2295–301.
113. Egol KA, Park JH, Rosenberg ZS, Peck V, Tejwani NC. Healing delayed but generally reliable after bisphosphonate-associated complete femur fractures treated with IM nails. Clin Orthop Relat Res. 2014;472(9):2728–34.
114. Favinger JL, Hippe D, Ha AS. Long-term radiographic follow-up of bisphosphonate-associated atypical femur fractures. Skelet Radiol. 2016;45(5):627–33.
115. Schilcher J. High revision rate but good healing capacity of atypical femoral fractures. A comparison with common shaft fractures. Injury. 2015;46(12):2468–73.

29 Specifics of Surgical Management: Pelvis

Chima D. Nwankwo, Edward R. Westrick,
Gregory T. Altman, and Daniel T. Altman

29.1 Introduction

Osteoporosis decreases bone mass and bone quality and directly increases the risk of fracture [1]. Lourie was the first to use the term "spontaneous osteoporotic fracture of the sacrum" [2]. Fragility fractures of the pelvic (FFP) ring are a clinical entity that include disruptions of the bony pelvis due to low-energy mechanisms and atraumatic events. In 2005, pelvic fractures made up 7% of all osteoporotic fractures, and that number is expected to increase by 56% by 2025 in the United States [3]. There has been a marked increase in the incidence of these fractures in Finland, the Netherlands, and Germany [4–6]. This is likely secondary to aging populations, increasing global life expectancy, recognition of fragility fractures of the pelvis as a significant source of pain and disability, and more extensive use of advanced imaging tools such as computed tomography (CT) and magnetic resonance imaging (MRI).

C. D. Nwankwo
Department of Orthopaedic Surgery, New York-Presbyterian Brooklyn Methodist Hospital/Columbia University Medical Center, Brooklyn, NY, USA

E. R. Westrick · G. T. Altman · D. T. Altman (✉)
Department of Orthopaedic Surgery, Allegheny Health Network, Drexel University College of Medicine, Pittsburgh, PA, USA
e-mail: daniel.altman@ahn.org

29.2 Clinical Significance

In comparison to the high-quality research and clinical algorithms that guide management of geriatric hip fractures, the evidence base for management and clinical outcomes of FFP ring is lacking. One study which assessed 63 community-dwelling patients reported that 95% of patients with pubic rami fractures returned to their pre-injury baseline, half required home care at discharge, and there was a 1-year mortality rate of 9.5% [7]. Hill and colleagues reviewed 286 consecutive patients over age 60 with pubic rami fractures and report that most surviving patients return to their original place of residence, but have worse levels of mobility. They report a 1-year mortality rate of 13.3% and significantly worse survival than an age-matched cohort from the general population [8]. In their retrospective series, Taillandier et al. reviewed 60 patients with pelvic insufficiency fractures and reported an inpatient complication rate of 40% and a 1-year mortality of 14.3% [9]. Breuil reports that 52% of individuals hospitalized due to osteoporotic pelvic fractures had inpatient complications including urinary tract infections, pressure ulcers, and pneumonia. They report a 1-year mortality of 22% [10]. In their matched retrospective cohort study of 1154 institutionalized nursing home patients with low-energy pelvic fractures, Rapp showed that excess mortality was found in women (HR 1.83) and men (HR 2.95) 1 month after fracture [11]. In their inquiry

H.-C. Pape et al. (eds.), *Senior Trauma Patients*, https://doi.org/10.1007/978-3-030-91483-7_29

to find clinical predictors of outcome, Marrinan prospectively followed a cohort of patients with osteoporotic pelvic fractures and report an in-patient mortality rate similar to hip fractures and found that the odds of changing from independent to institutionalized accommodation were significantly associated with age and length of hospital stay [12].

It also appears that the severity of initial fracture displacement does not modify the morbidity and mortality of low-energy fractures of the pelvic ring in the elderly. Mears and Berry report that morbidity and mortality rates for non-displaced pubic rami fractures and sacral insufficiency fractures are similar to those for more displaced pelvic fractures [13]. Despite the absence of level 1 data, there is clear evidence from numerous studies that FFP ring are associated with significant morbidity due to inpatient complications, need for institutionalized care upon discharge, loss of independence and functional mobility, and an elevated mortality over age-matched controls.

29.3 Classification

In 1986 in their retrospective analysis of plain radiographs of 142 patients with pelvic ring injuries, Young et al. identified four distinct patterns of injuries that correlated with the direction and location of the traumatizing energy [14]. This formed the basis of the Young-Burgess classification [15–16]. In this scheme, an anterior-posterior compressive force vector applied to the pelvis causes external rotation of the ilium with diastasis of the pubic symphysis or vertical fracture of the pubic rami. A lateral compressive force applied to the pelvis causes internal rotation of the ipsilateral hemipelvis with resultant fractures of the ilium, sacrum, disruption of the sacroiliac joint, and horizontal fractures of the pubic rami. When an axial force is applied to either hemipelvis, a vertical shear injury results with complete disruption of the sacroiliac ligaments or complete vertical pelvic fractures on the injured side.

In the geriatric population, low-energy traumatic events are much more common. These accidents do not typically cause significant injury to intra-pelvic organs, significant neurovascular injury, or damage to the soft tissue envelope [17]. Fragility fractures of the pelvis are typically non- or minimally displaced and are the result of a ground-level fall, or from repetitive stress through pathologic bone. Lateral compression fracture patterns and unilateral, bilateral, and transverse sacral fractures are frequently observed in this population [17]. The distinct patterns of bony injury observed in fragility fractures of the pelvis may be due to different anatomic areas of the pelvis exhibiting varying amounts of bone loss. In a CT study, Wagner and colleagues suggested that bone loss (measured by Hounsfield units) in the para-foraminal lateral region of the sacrum explains why this area is often involved in fragility fractures of the sacrum. They also reported that transverse fractures located between S1 and S2 may occur because of decreased bone mass in the S2 vertebral body [18]. These findings are also supported by Linstrom et al who theorized that the fracture lines in sacral insufficiency fractures follow areas of lowest sacral bone mass and highest strain [19].

Rommens and Hoffman propose that fragility fractures of the pelvis are, in many ways, different from pelvic ring fractures in non-osteoporotic bone and have developed a novel classification scheme [17]. In this arrangement, there are 4 types of FFP ring, with FFP Type-I and Type-II fractures being non-displaced/stable injuries and FFP Type-III and Type-IV being displaced/unstable injuries. FFP Type-I fractures involve only the anterior pelvic ring, Type-II fractures are non-displaced posterior ring fractures, Type-III fractures are displaced unilateral posterior pelvic ring injuries, and Type-IV fractures involve displaced bilateral posterior pelvic ring fractures. Each fracture type is further divided into A, B, and C subcategories (Fig. 29.1). In their series, Type-II lesions accounted for over 50% of the fragility fractures [20]. They recommend surgical stabilization of Type-III and Type-IV lesions.

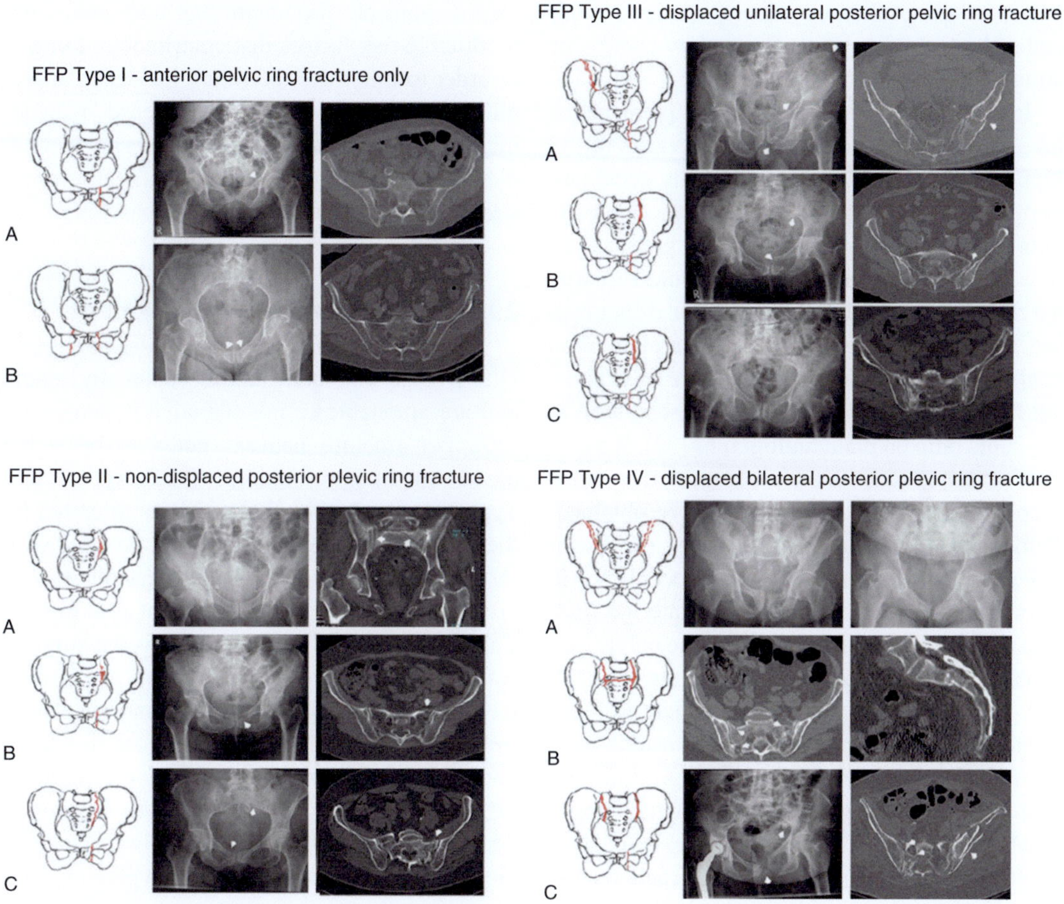

Fig. 29.1 FFP type III displaced unilateral posterior pelvic ring fracture

29.4 Diagnosis

Patients with fragility fractures of the pelvis typically present after a fall. The fall may have been precipitated by an acute neurologic or cardiovascular event, or may be a mechanical fall due to gait instability, lack of an adequate ambulatory aid, or because of an environmental hazard. It is important to note that elderly patients may suffer multiple bony lesions after a fall, so a careful musculoskeletal exam must be conducted. Pelvic fractures that occur without a history of trauma are called insufficiency fractures. These typically occur in the sacrum when the bone fails under physiological loads. These patients usually present with subacute or more chronic symptoms, and sometimes the only presenting sign is pain and progressive loss of mobility. Patients with fragility or insufficiency fractures of the pelvis may present with hip, groin, gluteal, thigh, and lower back pain. Pain with weight-bearing or complete inability to bear weight may be present. Additionally, affected patients might have difficulty with bed mobility, find it painful to lay on the affected hemipelvis, and have pain with transfers. Clinical signs seen in high-energy pelvic traumas such as bruising, groin and gluteal hematomas, limb shortening, and florid hemodynamic instability are often absent. The presence of dementia, communication difficulties, and the absence of direct caretakers or family members, may also complicate the clinical picture. Given these factors, the clinician must maintain a high index of suspicion for fragility fractures of the pelvis when evaluating elderly patients with ambulatory dysfunction after a low-energy or atraumatic mechanism.

Initial imaging should involve a plain radiograph of the pelvis, and orthogonal views of the hips may also be obtained if clinically necessary to rule out a hip fracture. Given low bone density, poor bone mineralization, and the presence of bowel gas, non-displaced fracture lines or cortical disruptions are often obscured or difficult to see, and fractures are often missed on plain films [21]. In the chronic setting, evidence of exuberant healing and callus formation may be seen at the pubic rami on plain radiographs [22]. If a pelvic fracture is seen on the anteroposterior radiograph, inlet and outlet views should be obtained. Some authors recommend obtaining a CT scan when the index of suspicion for an occult pelvic fracture is high, or to further illustrate the fracture type and assess the stability of the pelvic ring when a fracture is seen on plain films [17, 23–25]. They argue that prompt assessment and recognition of posterior pelvic ring lesions may allow for an optimized treatment algorithm that will accurately triage patients into the proper rehabilitative pathway. CT imaging is vital in identifying H-type or U-type sacral fractures that are typically only identified on sagittal CT scans [17]. Conventional CT scans are unable to detect microfractures of cancellous bone, which explains its inferior sensitivity in detecting sacral insufficiency fractures in comparison to MRI. If the origin of pelvic pain remains ambiguous after obtaining plain radiographs and CT imaging, MRI may be given consideration in the diagnostic workup [26].

29.5 Treatment

The management of fragility fractures of the pelvis involves a multidisciplinary approach with input from orthopedic surgeons, geriatric medicine physicians, physical therapists, nursing staff, and social workers. Each member of this team is essential for the efficient diagnosis, optimal management, and timely recovery with minimal inpatient complications from this injury. This team is also responsible for identifying and addressing modifiable risk factors that contribute to fall risk in order to minimize the future incidence of fragility fractures. Osteoporosis disease management should also be initiated [20]. The primary management objective is pain relief, early mobilization, and a return to pre-injury baseline.

29.5.1 Nonoperative Management

Often these fractures are mechanically stable and are amenable to nonoperative management [20]. For fracture patterns noted to be stable based on imaging studies (FFP Type-I and Type-II lesions), weight-bearing as tolerated by the patient is allowed. This should be done with instruction and support from physiotherapists after appropriate pain management is achieved. The patient should be followed by the surgical team while they are hospitalized to ensure that they are continuing to progress, and outpatient follow-up should be continued post discharge until evidence of fracture healing and cessation of symptoms. Surgical intervention is considered in cases of pelvic ring instability, spinopelvic dissociation, and secondarily in patients with stable injuries involving the posterior ring that are unable to ambulate or transfer due to pain. Additionally, there has probably been an underappreciation of instability in these fractures. In fact, recently Rommens et al documented progression in 14% of patients with fragility fracture of the pelvis with female patients being at the highest risk [27].

29.5.2 Surgical Management

In the past decade, there has been an increased emphasis on operative intervention. There is an expectation that the pain relief gained by fixation would support early mobilization, and this benefit outweighs the anesthetic risk and complications posed by surgery. Prior to any surgical procedure in this patient population, preoperative evaluation by the geriatric medicine and anesthesia providers must be conducted. The surgeon must understand the pelvic fracture patterns and the osteology and osseous fixation pathways in detail as described by Bishop and Routt. [28] The conditions for a safe and time-conscious surgery must be optimized in understanding the physiologic reserve in the elderly. This may include giving a bowel regimen to reduce bowel gas and improve visualization when percutaneous fixation is considered, proper communication with the operating room nurse and surgical technician, and working with an experienced fluoroscopy operator. Multiple techniques exist for surgical stabilization of fragility fractures of the pelvis. Most often these techniques are percutaneous and can involve combined posterior and anterior pelvic ring stabilization.

29.5.2.1 Sacroplasty

Sacroplasty is a minimally invasive percutaneous procedure where cement is injected into the sacral alar in order to stabilize a fragility fracture of the sacrum. This technique was introduced by Garant in 2002. [29] Sacroplasty is contraindicated in the setting of local infection, sacral decubitus ulcers, allergy to PMMA cement, and displaced sacral fractures or fractures involving the neural foramen [30].

The technique can be conducted under local anesthesia, conscious sedation, or a general anesthetic. Prone positioning on a radiolucent table is typically utilized. The technique can be done using conventional fluoroscopy or CT guidance. Fluoroscopy is both cost-efficient, widely available, and it can be used for real-time monitoring of cement deposition [31]. Inlet, outlet, and lateral radiographic projections are utilized. In the setting of poor bone density, bowel gas, and soft tissue obstruction, it can be difficult or even impossible to visualize the bony elements of the pelvis. CT guidance does not have these limitations; however, it results in a higher amount of radiation exposure, and it takes longer to perform [32]. There are various cement insertion techniques described, and the approach utilized is determined by the location of the lesion and the patient's anatomy [30]. The injection cannula can be inserted along the short axis of the sacrum (perpendicular to the posterior cortex) and advanced in a posterior-anterior trajectory either medial to or lateral to the sacral foramina.

There are no randomized trials evaluating the utility of sacroplasty; however, there are several case series, retrospective studies, and prospective cohort studies which report pain relief and improved mobility [33–37]. Injuries to nerves and vascular structures from trochar placement and cement extrusion are notable complications of sacroplasty. Cement can extrude into the sacroiliac joint, through the anterior sacral cortex and unto the L5 nerve root, into the disc space, into the local venous plexus, and into the neuroforamina. Bayley and colleagues reported the rate of cement leakage in their series to be 8 out of 108 patients [36].

29.5.2.2 Percutaneous Posterior Pelvic Ring Stabilization

Operative intervention is recommended in displaced/unstable fractures of the posterior pelvic ring. Stabilization historically required open reduction and internal fixation (ORIF) using trans-iliac bars or posterior plating. Open techniques for placement of iliosacral screws were developed in the 1980s [38]. In the ensuing decade, this technique was modified to enable percutaneous placement of implants [39, 40]. Percutaneous internal fixation has resulted in decreased operating time, soft tissue injury, and blood loss compared with open procedures [41]. This is even more important in the elderly patient given their limited physiological reserves, and the need for rapid rehabilitation postoperatively.

Successful and safe percutaneous placement of percutaneous screws into the pelvis requires reduction of the fracture to minimize the risk of neurovascular injury, nonunion, and malunion. FFP ring is usually non- or minimally displaced. Subsequently, maneuvers such as traction application or manipulation of the hemipelvis with Schanz pins or other devices are less likely to be required. A thorough understanding of the three-dimensional pelvic ring anatomy, the fracture pattern, and their representation on plain radiography and CT imaging is fundamental for this technique [41]. The surgeon must also be wary of variations in sacral morphology (sacral dysmorphism) and should modify surgical techniques as necessary to ensure safe screw placement [42].

Percutaneous posterior pelvic ring fixation is usually done under general anesthesia. A supine or prone position can be utilized. A small stack of folded towels or blankets is placed centrally in the lumbosacral region to raise the pelvis from the operating room table to allow for access to the posterior pelvis. The fluoroscope is positioned on the opposite side of the radiolucent table as the surgeon. Based on the preoperative CT sagittal and axial images, the surgeon should determine the approximate C-arm angles needed to obtain an inlet view of the S1 and S2 vertebral bodies, and plan for the trajectories of the intended screws. The surgical technique requires inlet, outlet, and lateral views. The ideal inlet image of the pelvis superimposes the S1 and S2 vertebral bodies. The outlet view superimposes the superior aspect of the symphysis pubis on the S2 vertebral body and should demonstrate the bilateral sacral neuroforamen. The lateral view of the sacrum should superimpose the greater sciatic notches and should show a distinct iliac cortical density (ICD) posterior to the sacral promontory if the posterior ring is adequately reduced.

29.5.2.3 Iliosacral Screw

It is critical to understand that the "vestibule" is the narrowest part of the bony corridor from the lateral ilium to the S1 sacral body and has a different dimension and orientation from person to person. It extends from the roof of the S1 neuroforamen to the alar slope and it is ovoid in shape [43]. The bony corridor of the vestibule extends in an anterior and superior direction. Given that most sacral fragility fractures are vertical, the iliosacral screw should be placed perpendicular to the fracture line. In the setting of a dysmorphic sacrum, in order to prevent anterior perforation and potential injury to the L5 nerve root, the screw path must head across the narrow bony corridor of the vestibule—anterior and superior.

The posterosuperior quadrant of the intersection of a vertical line made from the anterior superior iliac spine down toward the table and the long axis of the femur is the working area. A 0.62 mm is placed percutaneously into the ilium and the trajectory is adjusted based on the preoperative plan. Once the appropriate start point is identified, the wire is driven into the ilium and a stab incision is made around this wire to allow for instrumentation. A cannulated drill is placed over this wire and the outer cortex of the ilium is breached—this creates a pilot hole for the iliosacral screw. A guide wire is then placed into the previously drilled pilot hole, and is directed toward the midline of the S1 body using the inlet and outlet projections (Fig. 29.2). On a lateral projection, the wire tip should be below the ICD and above the interosseous tunnel of the S1 nerve root. A cannulated screw can then be placed safely.

Biomechanical studies have shown that iliosacral screws restore stability of the fractured pelvic ring. Multiple iliosacral screws are more stable than a single screw, long screws that enter the denser bone of the S1 sacral body are more stable than shorter screws, and longer thread screws are preferred due to higher pullout strength compared to shorter screws [44–46]. Given the decreased bone mass and bone quality in elderly patients, cement augmentation of iliosacral screws has been proposed by some authors and has been shown to increase stability [47, 48].

29.5.2.4 Transiliac-transsacral Screw

Transsacral (TS) implants that span the bilateral sacroiliac joints are more mechanically stable than bilateral iliosacral screws in bilateral vertical sacral fractures. Transsacral implants are advantageous because they are longer in length, have longer threads, and rely on fixation into the denser cortical bone of the ilium [49]. This makes them particularly effective in patients with poor bone quality. This technique popularized by Routt can be particularly effective in osteoporostic fractures and injuries with significant posterior pelvic instability. [40]

The technique for placement of a TS screw is similar to that described above for IS screws; however, the transiliac–transsacral screw's starting point and trajectory are much more constrained and must be carefully planned. The inlet and outlet views must be carefully scrutinized during this procedure, and tactile feedback dur-

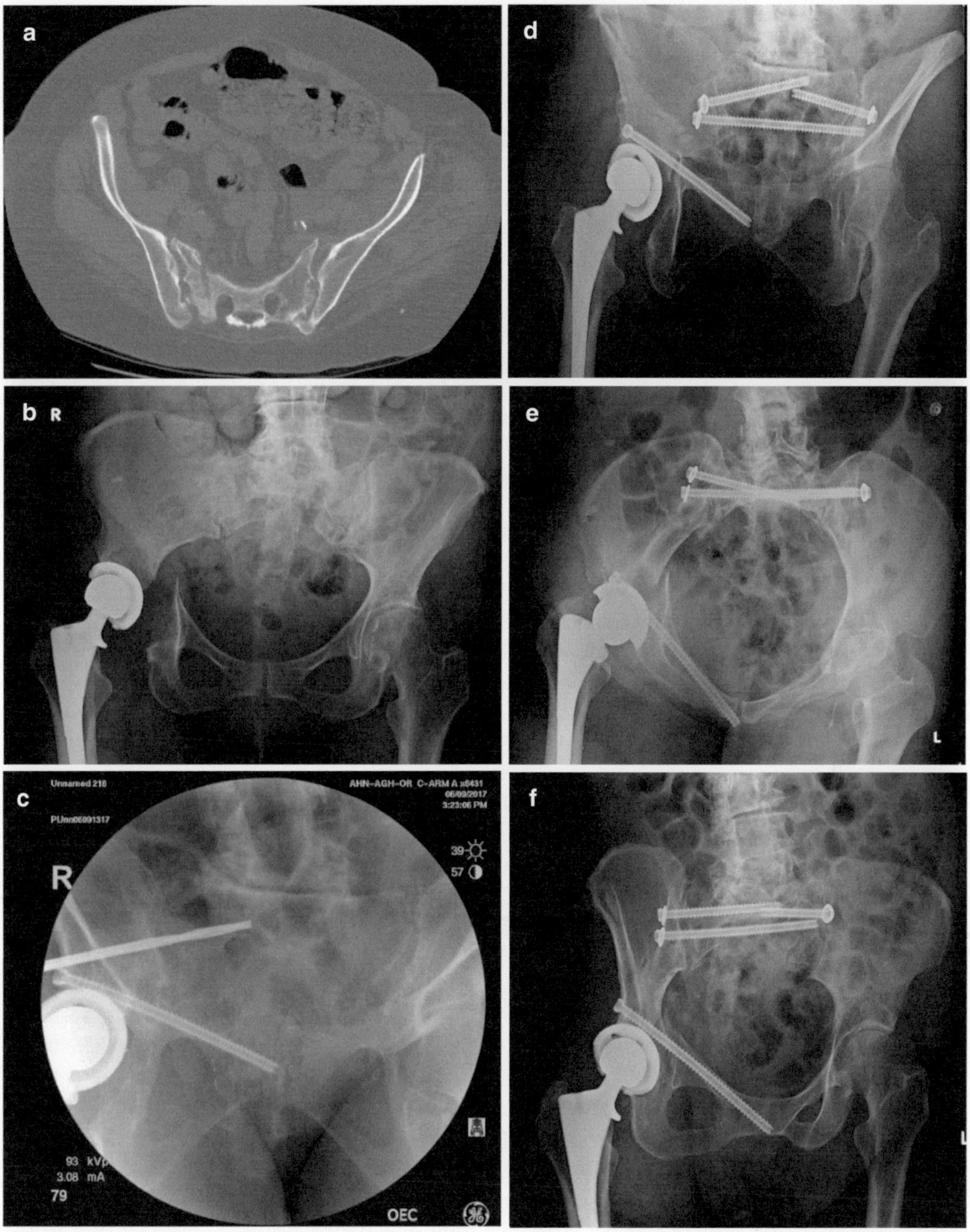

Fig. 29.2 A 72-year-old woman sustained a left periprosthetic transverse acetabular fracture, a right SI joint disruption and a left zone 2 sacral fracture after a ground level fall at home. (**a**) Axial CT scan of the posterior pelvic ring showing a right SI joint disruption and a left zone 2 sacral fracture. (**b**) AP radiograph showing right sacroiliac widening and left displaced transverse acetabular fracture. (**c**) Percutaneous drilling over a guidewire to place a S1 sacroiliac screw. Right antegrade anterior column screw has already been placed to stabilize acetabular fracture. (**d**) Outlet radiograph after placement of left sacroiliac screw at S1 and a transsacral screw at S2. (**e**) Inlet radiograph. (**f**) Obturator oblique radiographs taken at 6 weeks showing healing fractures

ing guidewire placement and drilling is essential. A true lateral sacral view can be obtained prior to crossing the near and far sacral nerve root tunnels to ensure that the tip of the wire is below the ICD and above the interosseous tunnel of the sacral nerve root of the desired segment. A screw measurement should be done prior to exiting the contralateral iliac cortex so that an accurate length assessment can be obtained. Analogous techniques which may offer even greater stability in this setting include a transsacral positioning bar and locked transsacral screws as described by Moed [50–52].

There are no randomized trials evaluating the utility of percutaneous posterior pelvic ring fixation in this patient population; however, there is a growing body of evidence touting these techniques as a way to improve clinical outcomes and decrease morbidity of fragility fracture of the pelvic ring. Hopf and colleagues report on 30 patients with posterior ring fractures and a mean age of 78.4 years treated with percutaneous IS screws. They report a numerical pain reduction from 6.8 to 1.8 [53]. In their series of 11 patients (average age of 67 years) who underwent TS fixation for fragility fractures of the pelvis, Sanders et al report that patients experienced significant improvement in visual analog scale pain scores (9.1 to 3.4) and modified Oswestry Low Back Pain Disability Index during follow-up [54]. Jones retrospectively compared 41 patients with sacral fragility fractures of which 16 were treated operatively and 25 were treated nonoperatively. They report that in patients who failed to ambulate with physical therapy or had significant posterior pelvic pain with ambulation, percutaneous TS screw fixation improved pain, ambulation, and the rate of disposition to home without increasing complications or length of stay [55].

The primary complication seen with percutaneous fixation of the posterior pelvic ring is errant screw placement. In a systematic review and meta-analysis on screw malposition and reviews rates, Zwingmann et al. report a screw malposition rate of 2.6%, although there are individual series that have reported rates as high as 15% [58]. The incidence of neurological injury is reported to be between 0.5 and 7.7% [56]. Recent advancements in imaging including computer navigation and 3D-fluoroscopy are being used clinically with good results and these have significantly reduced the incidence of screw malposition [57, 58]. However, these techniques have not been universally adopted.

29.5.2.5 Anterior Ring Stabilization

Posterior pelvic ring lesions are usually combined with anterior lesions [59]. In a geriatric low-energy mechanism, the fracture typically occurs at the pubic ramus, probably due to the weak cortical and trabecular bone here compared to the stiff symphyseal ligaments [62]. Isolated fractures of the anterior ring (FFP Type-1) should primarily be managed nonoperatively as described earlier in this text. However, Tile et al showed that when the anterior ring was broken, it contributed to a 30% loss in the stability of the pelvic ring [61]. Subsequently, when the posterior pelvic ring is treated surgically, fixation of the anterior part of the pelvis should also be taken into consideration, especially in the bilateral and more unstable settings. Isolated anterior ring stabilization in the setting of concurrent posterior fractures should not be undertaken.

29.5.2.6 Percutaneous Anterior Pelvic Ring Stabilization

In 1995 Routt et al. reported the first results of retrograde transpubic screw placement in 24 patients [62]. Since then, techniques have been described for antegrade pubic rami screw placement as well [63]. Percutaneous fixation is attractive in this patient population because it allows for a minimally invasive surgery that minimizes the significant risk of blood loss, infection, wound complications, ileus, and prolonged postsurgical recuperation from an open approach. This technique utilizes the anterior column corridor of bone that includes the superior pubic rami and passes medially and cranially to the acetabulum. As with all percutaneous fixation techniques in the pelvis, there are significant person-to-person variations and the surgeon must possess a thorough understanding of the relevant osseous and local neurovascular anatomy. Symphyseal disruptions and parasymphyseal fractures cannot be managed with this technique.

29.5.2.7 Retrograde Anterior Column Screw

We use the technique as outlined by Altman and Westrick [64]. Given that the fracture of the superior ramus is usually horizontal or oblique in orientation, and the bone is of such poor quality, we utilize fully threaded screws that effectively function as an internal "splint". A mini-Pfannenstiel incision is made proximal to the pubic symphysis and the cannulated screw guidewire is inserted through the ipsilateral pubic tubercle, aimed posterior and inferior to the anterior inferior iliac spine. The wire is then passed cephalad up the superior pubic ramus. Inlet iliac oblique radiographs are obtained to ensure that the guidewire does not penetrate the inner cortex of the ramus, and outlet obturator oblique radiographs are used to prevent penetration of the hip joint. Following appropriate wire placement, the outer cortex is again drilled and a 6.5 mm or 7.3 mm fully threaded cannulated screw is advanced.

29.5.2.8 Antegrade Anterior Column Screw

For antegrade screws, the authors utilize a starting point is at the junction of a line drawn along the lateral border of the femur through the greater trochanter and a line from the pubic symphysis through the anterior inferior iliac spine. The guidewire is then passed down the superior pubic ramus to the pubic symphysis (Fig. 29.2). Again, frequent inlet iliac oblique and outlet obturator oblique radiographs are obtained before the outer cortex is drilled. An appropriately sized fully threaded screw is inserted [64].

Starr et al report a 15% loss of reduction on follow-up radiographs in a retrospective study of percutaneous fixation of superior rami fractures [65]. They report that an antegrade screw was less likely to lead to fixation failure than retrograde placement, and theorize that this may be because antegrade placement provides screw purchase in the good bone above the acetabulum. They also found that elderly female patients with fractures medial to the visible border of the obturator foramen were at the highest risk of failure. They surmise that in the setting of osteopenic bone, a ramus screw may not provide adequate resistance to recurrence of a lateral compression deformity and this may increase the risk of failure.

29.5.2.9 Anterior Pelvic Ring Plate Fixation

Plate fixation of the anterior pelvic ring is more stable than after retrograde anterior column screw fixation [60]. Plate fixation is preferable in parasymphyseal fractures, when there is significant displacement, and in nonunion cases where there is bone resorption at the ends of the fracture. Plating is relatively contraindicated in the setting of contamination of the surgical field with bowel or bladder contents, in the presence of a transpubic urinary catheter, and in the setting of infection.

Plate fixation can be performed via a midline incision or a Pfannenstiel incision. A longitudinal midline split of the linea alba is made, and the dissection is extended down to the pubic symphysis. The retropubic space is entered gently and the bladder is retracted and protected with a malleable retractor. Dissection is then carried out laterally in subperiosteal fashion. Care is taken to identify and control crossing anastomotic vessels of the corona mortis. 3.5mm curved plates are typically utilized with long cortical screws placed across the pubic body and into the inferior rami. Retroacetabular screws can also be placed to maximize stability [66].

29.5.3 Lumbopelvic Fixation

Lumbopelvic fixation involves fixation from the lumbar spine usually with pedicle screws at L5 and/or L4 to large diameter screws into the posterior ilium which can be inserted open or percutaneously. Lumbopelvic fixation of unstable sacral fractures was introduced by Kach and Trenz and further refined to include triangular osteosynthesis by Schildhauer in the 1990s [67]. The majority of these patients were polytraumatized with high-energy fractures.

Recently lumbopelvic fixation has been further expanded to include osteoporotic fractures,

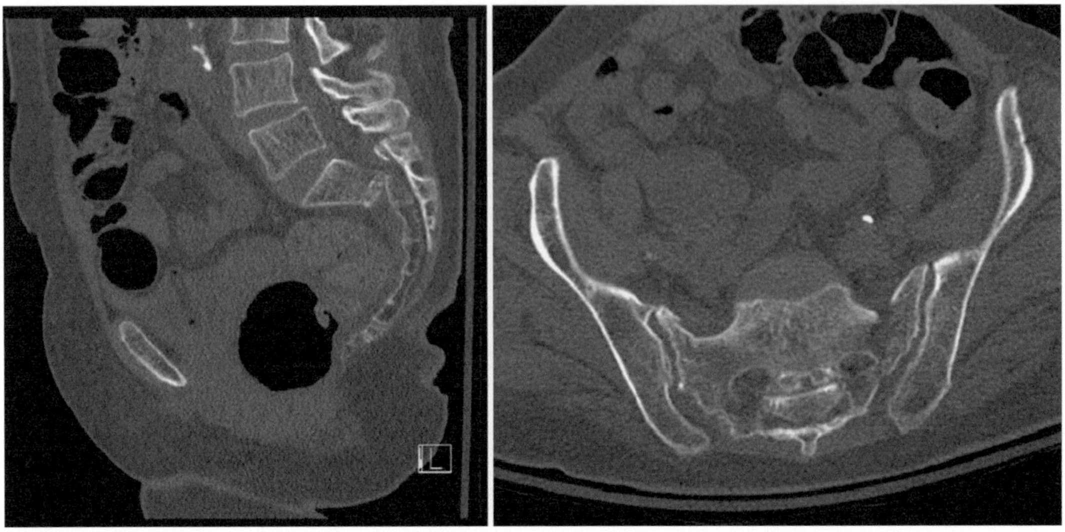

Fig. 29.3 A 65-year-old female fell from standing with delay in diagnosis. Transferred with saddle anesthesia and pelvic pain. Severe displacement transverse component of U type fracture as identified on sagittal CT scan. Not initially identified on Emergency Department AP Pelvic Radiograph

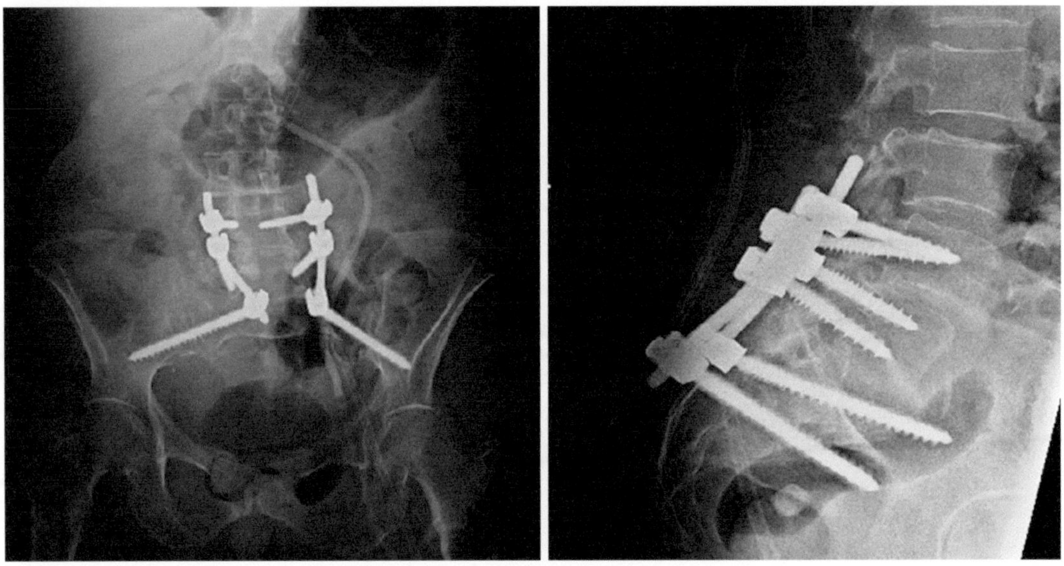

Fig. 29.4 S/P Lumbopelvic fusion with L5-S3 decompression

especially when bilateral and with a transverse sacral component (i.e., U-type and H-type fracture); although there are no long-term follow-up studies or large series (Figs. 29.3 and 29.4). In a recent functional outcome study involving patients treated with percutaneous screw fixation for pelvic fragility fractures, although good functional outcomes were reported on 50 patients, the authors report a revision operation rate of 20% and suggest that trans-sacral screws could probably reduce the reoperation rate [68]. The high rate of screw loosening may indicate the need for anterior rami fixation or additional lumbopelvic fixation.

29.5.4 Pelvic Ring Nonunion

Although the majority of patients who sustain FFP ring typically go on to union without surgical intervention, there is a small subset of patients who develop marked fracture displacement and/or nonunion of the pelvic ring after conservative management or insufficient fixation of the pelvic ring. The actual incidence of pelvic nonunion in the geriatric population is difficult to ascertain. Risk factors for the occurrence of nonunion include prior pelvic radiation, vertical shear pattern, initial nonoperative management, or treatment with only external fixation systems [69, 70]. Pain is the most common symptom described by patients with pelvic nonunion. The pain can be in the anterior or posterior pelvis, activity related, cause sitting discomfort, and even lead to bed confinement in the most severe cases. Neurologic symptoms, gait disturbance, and a sensation of pelvic instability may also be reported. Surgical correction is effective in the treatment of symptomatic pelvic nonunion. Mears reported on a series of 70 patients treated for nonunion of the pelvic ring using standard surgical approaches to debride the nonunion sites, reapproximate the pelvic ring, apply autologous bone graft, and place stable internal fixation. He reported a union rate of over 95% and 79% rate of patient satisfaction. [71] Van den Bosch reported on 11 cases of nonunion of the pelvic ring. Following surgery, improvement in pain and functional status was seen in 82% of patients (82%).

29.6 Summary

There has been an increased incidence and awareness of pelvic ring fractures in the elderly with inherent treatment challenges and resultant disability and associated morbidity and mortality [17, 72]. These fractures are different in multiple aspects from pelvic fractures occurring in younger patients. Physicians and other providers will need to treat the underlying causes associated with these fractures and understand the risk of progression and nonunion. Percutaneous fixation techniques based on sound principles and knowledge of osseous pathways may allow earlier mobilization and improved outcomes.

References

1. NIH Consensus Development Panel on Osteoporosis Prevention, Diagnosis, and Therapy. Osteoporosis prevention, diagnosis, and therapy. JAMA. 2001;285(6):785–95. https://doi.org/10.1001/jama.285.6.785.
2. Lourie H. Spontaneous osteoporotic fracture of the sacrum: an unrecognized syndrome of the elderly. JAMA. 1982;248:715–7.
3. Burge R, Dawson-Hughes B, Solomon DH, Wong JB, King A, Tosteson A. Incidence and economic burden of osteoporosis-related fractures in the United States, 2005–2025. J Bone Miner Res. 2007;22:465–75.
4. Kannus P, Parkkari J, Niemi S, et al. Low-trauma pelvic fractures in elderly Finns in 1970–2013. Calcif Tissue Int. 2015;97:577–80.
5. Nanninga GL, de Leur K, Panneman MJ, et al. Increasing rates of pelvic fractures among older adults: the Netherlands, 1986–2011. Age Ageing. 2014;43:648–53.
6. Andrich S, Haastert B, Neuhaus E, et al. Epidemiology of pelvic fractures in Germany: considerably high incidence rates among older people. PLoS One. 2015;10:e0139078.
7. Koval KJ, Aharonoff GB, Schwartz MC, Alpert S, Cohen G, McShinawy A, et al. Pubic rami fracture: a benign pelvic injury? J Orthop Trauma. 1997 Jan;11(1):7–9.
8. Hill RM, Robinson CM, Keating JF. Fractures of the pubic rami. Epidemiology and five-year survival. J Bone Joint Surg Br. 2001;83(8):1141–4.
9. Taillandier J, Langue F, Alemanni M, et al. Mortality and functional outcomes of pelvic insufficiency fractures in older patients. Joint Bone Spine. 2003;70:287–9.
10. Breuil V, et al. Outcome of osteoporotic pelvic fractures: an underestimated severity. Joint Bone Spine. 2008;75(5):585–6.
11. Rapp K, Cameron ID, Kurrle S, Klenk J, Kleiner A, Heinrich S, Becker C. Excess mortality after pelvic fractures in institutionalized older people. Osteoporos Int. 2010;21(11):1835–9. https://doi.org/10.1007/s00198-009-1154-0.
12. Marrinan S, Pearce MS, Jiang XY, Waters S, Shanshal Y. Admission for osteoporotic pelvic fractures and predictors of length of hospital stay, mortality and loss of independence. Age Ageing. 2014;44(2):258–61. https://doi.org/10.1093/ageing/afu123.
13. Mears SC, Berry DJ. Outcomes of displaced and nondisplaced pelvic and sacral fractures in elderly adults. J Am Geriatr Soc. 2011;59:1309–12.
14. Young JW, Burgess AR, Brumback RJ, Poka A. Pelvic fractures: value of plain radiography in early assessment and management. Radiology. 1986;160:445–51.

15. Dalal SA, Burgess AR, Siegel JH, et al. Pelvic fracture in multiple trauma: classification by mechanism is key to pattern of organ injury, resuscitative requirements, and outcome. J Trauma. 1989;29:981–1000.
16. Burgess AR, Eastridge BJ, Young JW, et al. Pelvic ring disruptions: effective classification system and treatment protocols. J Trauma. 1990;30:848–56.
17. Rommens PM, Wagner D, Hofmann A. Fragility fractures of the pelvis. JBJS Reviews. 2017;5(3):1. https://doi.org/10.2106/jbjs.rvw.16.00057.
18. Wagner D, Kamer L, Sawaguchi T, Richards RG, Noser H, Rommens PM. Sacral bone mass distribution assessed by averaged three dimensional CT models. J Bone Joint Surg Am. 2016;98(7):584–90.
19. Linstrom NJ, Heiserman JE, Kortman KE, Crawford NR, Baek S, Anderson RL, Pitt AM, Karis JP, Ross JS, Lekovic GP, Dean BL. Anatomical and biomechanical analyses of the unique and consistent locations of sacral insufficiency fractures. Spine (Phila Pa 1976). 2009;34(4):309–15.
20. Rommens PM, Ossendorf C, Pairon P, Dietz SO, Wagner D, Hofmann A. Clinical pathways for fragility fractures of the pelvic ring: personal experience and review of the literature. J Orthop Sci. 2015;20(1):1–11.
21. Kirby MW, Spritzer C. Radiographic detection of hip and pelvic fractures in the emergency department. Am J Roentgenol. 2010;194(4):1054–60. https://doi.org/10.2214/ajr.09.3295.
22. Peh WC, Khong PL, Yin Y, Ho WY, Evans NS, Gilula LA, Yeung HW, Davies AM. Imaging of pelvic insufficiency fractures. Radiographics. 1996;16(2):335–48.
23. O'Connor TJ, Cole PA. Pelvic insufficiency fractures. Geriatr Orthop Surg Rehabil. 2014;5:178–90.
24. Lau TW, Leung F. Occult posterior pelvic ring fractures in elderly patients with osteoporotic pubic rami fractures. J Orthop Surg (Hong Kong). 2010;18(2):153–7.
25. Tosounidis G, Wirbel R, Culemann U, et al. Misinterpretation of anterior pelvic ring fractures in the elderly. Unfallchirurg. 2006;109:678–80.
26. Natoli RM, Fogel HA, Holt D, Schiff A, Bernstein M, Summers HD, Lack W. Advanced imaging lacks clinical utility in treating geriatric pelvic ring injuries caused by low-energy trauma. J Orthop Trauma. 2017;31(4):194–9.
27. Rommens PM, Arand C, Hopf JC, Mehling I, Dietz SO, Wagner D. Progress of instability in fragility fractures of the pelvis: an observational study. Injury IntJCare Injured. 2019;50:1966–73.
28. Bishop JA, Routt ML. Osseous fixation pathways in pelvic and acetabular fracture surgery: osteology, radiology and clinical applications. J Trauma Acute Care Surg. 2012;72(6):1502–9.
29. Garant M. Sacroplasty: a new treatment for sacral insufficiency fracture. J Vasc Interv Radiol. 2002;13(12):1265–7.
30. Bastian JD, Keel MJB. Sacroplasty. Fragility Fractures of the Pelvis. 2017;105–117 https://doi.org/10.1007/978-3-319-66572-6_10.
31. Shah RV. Sacral kyphoplasty for the treatment of painful sacral insufficiency fractures and metastases. Spine J. 2012;12(2):113–20.
32. Grossterlinden L, Begemann PG, Lehmann W, Nuechtern J, Schumacher U, Nagel HD, et al. Sacroplasty in a cadaveric trial: comparison of CT and fluoroscopic guidance with and without balloon assistance. Eur Spine J. 2009;18(8):1226–33.
33. Garant M. Sacroplasty: a new treatment for sacral insufficiency fracture. J Vasc Interv Radiol. 2002;13(12):1265–7.
34. Frey ME, Depalma MJ, Cifu DX, Bhagia SM, Carne W, Daitch JS. Percutaneous sacroplasty for osteoporotic sacral insufficiency fractures: a prospective, multicenter, observational pilot study. Spine J. 2008;8(2):367–73.
35. Kortman K, Ortiz O, Miller T, Brook A, Tutton S, Mathis J, et al. Multicenter study to assess the efficacy and safety of sacroplasty in patients with osteoporotic sacral insufficiency fractures or pathologic sacral lesions. J Neurointerv Surg. 2013;5(5):461–6.
36. Bayley E, Srinivas S, Boszczyk BM. Clinical outcomes of sacroplasty in sacral insufficiency fractures: a review of the literature. Eur Spine J. 2009;18(9):1266–71.
37. Butler CL, Given CA 2nd, Michel SJ, et al. Percutaneous sacroplasty for the treatment of sacral insufficiency fractures. AJR. Am J Roentgenol. 2005;184(6):1956–9.
38. Matta J, Saucedo T. Internal fixation of pelvic ring fractures. Clin Orthop. 1989;24283-87
39. Ebraheim N, Rusin J, Coornbs R. Percutaneous computer tomography-stabilization of pelvic fracture: preliminary report. J Orthop Trauma. 1987;1:197–204.
40. Routt ML Jr, Meier M, Kregor P. Percutaneous iliosacral screws with the patient supine technique. Operative Tech Orthop. 1993;3:3545.
41. Routt MLC, Nork SE, Mills WJ. Percutaneous fixation of pelvic ring disruptions. Clin Orthop Relat Res. 2000;375:15–29. https://doi.org/10.1097/00003086-200006000-00004.
42. Miller AN, Routt MLC. Variations in sacral morphology and implications for Iliosacral screw fixation. J Am Acad Orthop Surg. 2011;20(1):8–16. https://doi.org/10.5435/jaaos-20-01-008.
43. Rommens PM, Wagner D, Hofmann A. Iliosacral screw osteosynthesis. Fragility Fractures of the Pelvis. 2017;121–137 https://doi.org/10.1007/978-3-319-66572-6_11.
44. Kraemer W, Hearn T, Tile M, Powell J. The effect of thread length and location and extraction strength of iliosacral lag screws. Injury. 1994;25:5–9.
45. van Zwienen CM, van den Bosch EW, Snijders CJ, Kleinrensink GJ, van Vugt AB. Biomechanical comparison of sacroiliac screw techniques for unstable pelvic ring fractures. J Orthop Trauma. 2004;18:589–95.
46. Mears SC, Sutter EG, Wall SJ, Rose DM, Belkoff SM. Biomechanical comparison of three methods of sacral fracture fixation in osteoporotic bone. Spine. 2010;35(10):E392–5. https://doi.org/10.1097/brs.0b013e3181cb4fcd.

47. Wähnert D, Raschke MJ, Fuchs T. Cement augmentation of the navigated iliosacral screw in the treatment of insufficiency fractures of the sacrum: a new method using modified implants. Int Orthop. 2013;37(6):1147–50.
48. Osterhoff G, Dodd AE, Unno F, Wong A, Amiri S, Lefaivre KA, Guy P. Cement augmentation in sacroiliac screw fixation offers modest biomechanical advantages in a cadaver model. Clin Orthop Relat Res. 2016;474(11):2522–30. https://doi.org/10.1007/s11999-016-4934-9.
49. Gardner MJ, Routt MLC. Transiliac-transsacral screws for posterior pelvic stabilization. J Orthop Trauma. 2011;25(6):378–84.
50. Mehling I, Hessmann MH, Rommens PM. Stabilization of fatigue fractures of the dorsal pelvis with a trans-sacral bar. Operative technique and outcome. Injury. 2012;43(4):446–51. Epub 2011 Sep 1
51. Vanderschot P, Kuppers M, Sermon A, Lateur L. Trans-iliac-sacral-iliac-bar procedure to treat insufficiency fractures of the sacrum. Indian J Orthop. 2009;43(3):245–52.
52. Moed BR, Whiting DR. Locked transsacral screw fixation of bilateral injuries of the posterior pelvic ring: initial clinical series. J Orthop Trauma (United States). 2010;24(10):p616–21.
53. Hopf JC, Krieglstein CF, Müller LP, Koslowsky TC. Percutaneous iliosacral screw fixation after osteoporotic posterior ring fractures of the pelvis reduces pain significantly in elderly patients. Injury. 2015;46(8):1631–6. https://doi.org/10.1016/j.injury.2015.04.036.
54. Sanders D, Fox J, Starr A, et al. Transsacral-Transiliac screw stabilization: veffective for recalcitrant pain due to sacral insufficiency fracture. J Orthop Trauma. 2016;30:469–73.
55. Walker JB, Mitchell SM, Karr SD, Lowe JA, Jones CB. Percutaneous transiliac–transsacral screw fixation of sacral fragility fractures improves pain, ambulation, and rate of disposition to home. J Orthop Trauma. 2018;32(9):452–6. https://doi.org/10.1097/bot.0000000000001243.
56. Zwingmann J, Hauschild O, Bode G, Sudkamp NP, Schmal H. Malposition and revision rates of different imaging modalities for percutaneous iliosacral screw fixation following pelvic fractures: a systematic review and meta-analysis. Arch Orthop Trauma Surg. 2013;133(9):1257–65. https://doi.org/10.1007/s00402-013-1788-4.
57. Zwingmann J, Konrad G, Kotter E, Südkamp NP, Oberst M. Computer-navigated iliosacral screw insertion reduces malposition rate and radiation exposure. Clin Orthop Relat Res. 2009;467:1833–8.
58. Shaw JC, Routt ML, Chip, Gary JL. Intra-operative multi-dimensional fluoroscopy of guidepin placement prior to iliosacral screw fixation for posterior pelvic ring injuries and sacroiliac dislocation: an early case series. Int Orthop. 2017;41(10):2171–7. https://doi.org/10.1007/s00264-017-3447-9.
59. Scheyerer MJ, Osterhoff G, Wehrle S, Wanner GA, Simmen HP, Werner CM. Detection of posterior pelvic injuries in fractures of the pubic rami. Injury. 2012;43(8):1326–9.
60. Acklin YP, Zderic I, Buschbaum J, Varga P, Inzana JA, Grechenig S, Richards RG, Gueorguiev B, Schmitz P. Biomechanical comparison of plate and screw fixation in anterior pelvic ring fractures with low bone mineral density. Injury. 2016;47(7):1456–60. Epub 2016 Apr 22
61. Tile M, Hearn T, Vrahas M. Biomechanics of the pelvic ring. In: Tile M, Helfet D, Kellam J, editors. Chapter 4: Fractures of the pelvis and acetabulum. 3rd ed. Philadelphia: Lippincott Williams and Wilkins; 2003. p. 32–45.
62. Routt M, Simonian P, Grujic L. The retrograde medullary superior pubic ramus screw for the treatment of anterior pelvic ring disruptions: a new technique. J Orthop Trauma. 1995;9:35–40.
63. Starr AJ, Reinert CM, Jones AL. Percutaneous fixation of the columns of the acetabulum: a new technique. J Orthop Trauma. 1998;12:51–5.
64. Altman DT, Westrick ER. Geriatric acetabulum fractures. Geriatric Trauma and Acute Care Surgery. 2017;123–132 https://doi.org/10.1007/978-3-319-57403-5_13.
65. Starr AJ, Nakatani T, Reinert CM, Cederberg K. Superior pubic ramus fractures fixed with percutaneous screws: what predicts fixation failure? J Orthop Trauma. 2008;22(2):81–7. https://doi.org/10.1097/bot.0b013e318162ab6e.
66. Culemann U, Marintschev I, Gras F, Pohlemann T. Infra-acetabular corridor--technical tip for an additional screw placement to increase the fixation strength of acetabular fractures. J Trauma. 2011;70:244–6.
67. Schildhauer TA, Josten C, Muhr G. Triangular osteosynthesis of vertically unstable sacrum fractures: a new concept allowing early weight bearing. JOT. 1998;12(5):307–14.
68. Eckardt H, Egger A, Hasler RM, Zech CJ, Vach W, Suhm N, et al. Good functional outcome in patients suffering fragility fractures of the pelvis treated with percutaneous screw stabilization: assessment of complications and factors influencing failure. Injury Int J Care Injured. 2017;48:2717–23.
69. Mears DC, Velyvis J. In situ fixation of pelvic nonunions following pathologic and insufficiency fractures. J Bone Joint Surg Am. 2002;84(5):721–8.
70. Kanakaris NK, Angoules AG, Nikolaou VS, Kontakis G, Giannoudis PV. Treatment and outcomes of pelvic malunions and nonunions: a systematic review. Clin Orthop Relat Res. 2009;467(8):2112–24. https://doi.org/10.1007/s11999-009-0712-2.
71. Mears DC, Velyvis J. Surgical reconstruction of late pelvic posttraumatic nonunion and malalignment. J Bone Joint Surg Br. 2003;85(1):21–30.
72. Noser J, Dietrich M, Tiziani S, Werner CML, Pape H-C, Osterhoff G. Mid-term follow-up after surgical treatment of fragility fractures of the pelvis. Injury Int J Care Injured. 2018;49:2032–5.

Open Fractures in the Elderly

30

Erin Pichiotino, Dylan Nugent, and Kyle J. Jeray

30.1 Introduction

The global population of the elderly is growing. In the United States, life expectancy has been on the rise for decades, with a 78.6-year life expectancy in 2017 [1], and by the year 2030 one in every five residents will be of retirement age. The Baby Boomer generation, born between 1946 and 1964, was the largest ever born in the United States and has remained the largest segment of the population ever since [1, 2]. As this generation has reached retirement age, and life expectancies have increased, the number of active, elderly individuals has also significantly increased, leading to an increased number of elderly persons sustaining injuries [3]. Many injuries involve the musculoskeletal system, including both low and high-energy traumatic fractures that require the care of orthopedic surgeons. The assumption is that larger numbers of older, active adults would in theory lead to an overall greater number of open fractures even if the incidence remained constant throughout all age groups. However, the incidence is not constant [4], and the mechanisms and locations of open fractures in the elderly are often different than in younger adults [5, 6]. In young adults, road traffic accidents (RTAs) or other high-energy mechanisms are the most frequent cause of open fractures whereas in the elderly a ground-level fall is the most common causative factor [5].

E. Pichiotino · D. Nugent
Department of Orthopedic Surgery, Prisma Health-Upstate, Greenville, SC, USA

K. J. Jeray (✉)
Department of Orthopedic Surgery, Prisma Health-Upstate, Greenville, SC, USA

University of South Carolina School of Medicine Greenville, Greenville, SC, USA
e-mail: Kyle.Jeray@PrismaHealth.org

30.2 Incidence

The incidence of open fractures in the elderly equals or exceeds that of young adult males, with the greatest number of open fractures in the elderly occurring in women [6]. In a study of 2386 open fractures in patients over the age of 15, the incidence of open fractures in the super elderly (patients older than 80 years) was significantly higher than patients under the age of 65. And, the incidence of open fractures in male patients 15–19 years and females >90 years were almost identical, with a progressive increase in the incidence of open fractures in females after the 7th decade of life [5]. The most common open fractures in the elderly involve the distal radius, phalanges of the hand, tibia, and ankle, which are for all intents and purposes, subcutaneous bones [6]. With increased age, the incidence of multiple fractures also increases, and in octogenarians, multiple fractures may be at least four times the incidence of patients younger than sixty-five [6].

H.-C. Pape et al. (eds.), *Senior Trauma Patients*, https://doi.org/10.1007/978-3-030-91483-7_30

The three most common reasons for open fractures in the elderly are simple falls, crush injuries, and RTAs, but falls alone account for more than 50% of all open fractures in patients older than 65 years [5]. A study of 33,704 ankle fractures using Medicare data found that the rate of all ankle fractures (closed or open) was highest in white women (5.8 per 1000) and lowest in white males (1.5 per 1000) [7]. There is a steady decline in the incidence of open fractures in men after the age of 60, while the incidence sharply rises in women of the same age [5]. Reasons for this include the soft tissue and bone changes associated with menopause leading to increased susceptibility in women. Further exacerbating the risk is that women have a longer life expectancy than men. The shorter life expectancy in men may lead to fewer men surviving to an age where low-energy open fractures would become common. Additionally, the overall health condition may be worse, and the activity level decreased, in age-matched elderly men compared to women leading to fewer open injuries [6, 8].

30.3 Evaluation

Multiply injured elderly patients requiring orthopedic trauma care are not uncommon due to high early survival rates as a result of well-established prehospital care protocols such as Basic Life Support (BLS)®, Advanced Trauma Life Support (ATLS)®, and timely resuscitation in trauma centers. As in younger individuals, care for the multiply injured elderly patient should be provided by skilled multidisciplinary teams that can help manage medical comorbidities, polypharmacy concerns, and the delicate resuscitation efforts required to control fluid shifts and metabolic imbalances that may be exacerbated by a more vulnerable physiologic state.

The initial evaluation of an elderly patient with an open fracture should begin with a thorough history of the event leading to the injury as well as pertinent medical history that could impact treatment, rehabilitation, and outcomes. Important facets of the history include mechanism of injury such as low-energy falls versus high-energy trauma such as motor vehicle collisions or pedestrian versus auto injuries. Preexisting medical conditions and baseline functional status should be investigated to help guide treatment and postoperative rehabilitation goals. It is important to obtain an accurate list of medications for resuscitative and perioperative guidance.

It is crucial to understand if the injury occurred because of an underlying medical process such as a myocardial infarction, stroke, hypoglycemia, hypotension, or neurological derangement. Additionally, it is important to consider if the injury could be complicated by associated injuries such as intracranial hemorrhage due to anticoagulant use or renal failure and rhabdomyolysis due to immobility and delayed presentation, both more commonly seen in the elderly. A 2017 study by Wongrakpanich et al found that a fall was the most frequent cause of rhabdomyolysis in a cohort of patients over 65 years with creatinine kinase levels in excess of five times the normal limits [9]. They demonstrated that acute kidney injury (AKI), peak decline in glomerular filtration rate (GFR), and greater than eight preadmission medications were all independent prognostic predictors of lower overall survival after rhabdomyolysis in the elderly [9]. Another study found that elderly patients in critical care settings had a 20% higher rate of AKI compared to younger patients [10]. With the increased risk of kidney dysfunction and potential for rhabdomyolysis in elderly patients even after a fall from standing, early involvement of hospitalist and geriatric teams with a thorough medical workup and resuscitation plan is prudent.

30.3.1 Patient Factors and Comorbidities

With age comes increasing comorbidities, many of which are linked to increased mortality and morbidity. For example, diabetes mellitus (DM) is increasing worldwide and subsequent micro- and macro-vascular changes, chronic inflammation, and hyperglycemia can effect both bony and soft-tissue healing. Both type 1 and type 2 DM have been found to have negative effects of bone turnover, strength, and density [11–13] and have been seen as significant risk factors for postoperative infections after open fractures [14, 15]. Diabetes treatment can also be problematic, with medications such as thiazolidinediones causing decreased osteoblast formation and subsequent increased bone loss. In contrast, insulin is thought to be anabolic in bone, though implications on fracture healing are limited at this point [11]. Ultimately, elderly patients with diabetes are at increased risk of infection, delayed bony healing and nonunion, and skin and soft-tissue problems after open fractures. The goal for the healthcare team is tight glycemic control, consideration of additional fixation constructs, and longer clinical monitoring after open fractures to help minimize complications.

Hormonal changes have been linked to skin aging and fragility of the soft tissues [5, 16–18]. It is believed that the thinning of the subcutaneous tissue, disordered collagen, and altered water content associated with menopause is the reason why open fractures continue to be more common in elderly women. One study showed that skin thickness was actually an independent predictor of osteoporosis due to the decline in collagen with age in both skin and bone [19]. An example of the fragility of skin on the medial ankle after a ground-level fall can be seen in Fig. 30.1. Ultimately, both aging and menopausal effects are associated with collagen atrophy and the consequential decrease in elasticity, putting elderly patients at increased risk of open fractures.

It is well established that bone density decreases while fracture risk increases with age, particularly in postmenopausal women. Many patients are first diagnosed with osteoporosis after they sustain a fragility fracture, which can complicate treatment management and outcomes [20, 21]. Major risk factors for osteoporosis development and fragility fractures include nutritional deficiencies including insufficient calcium and Vitamin D. Fragility fractures also have a higher risk of complications such as infection, fixation failure, and increased morbidity and mortality rates [20–22].

Obesity is another important factor to consider. There is some evidence that obesity is not a risk factor for the occurrence of open fractures.

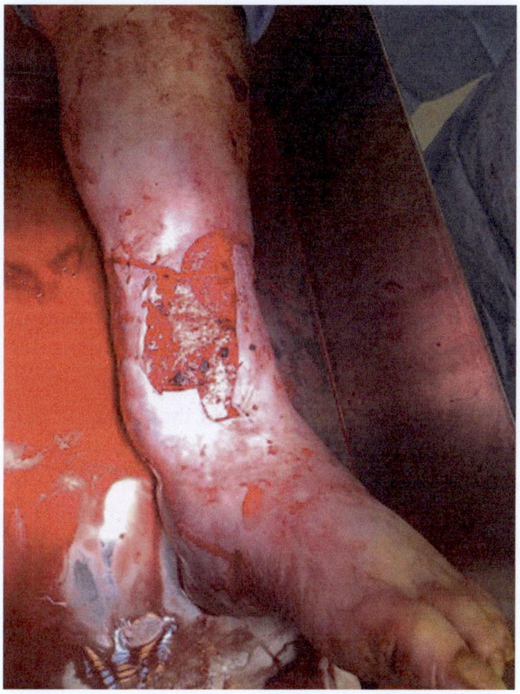

Fig. 30.1 Extensive skin degloving in a 79-year old female after a fall from standing resulting in a Gustillo Anderson Type IIIA open trimalleolar ankle fracture-dislocation

Court-Brown et al found the prevalence of fractures in general decreases after age 50 in obese females and 60 years in obese males, and there was no association between the prevalence of open or multiple fractures and obesity in all ages [25]. However, obesity has generally shown to increase the rate of complications following open fractures (Yarboro also has an article in Injury in 2016 on obesity increasing complications in tibia fxs). Obesity is associated with chronic inflammation due to elevated inflammatory markers and cytokines, which can contribute to insulin resistance, cardiac disease, metabolic syndrome, and endothelial dysfunction [23–26]. These physiologic changes in obese patients of all ages increase the risk of complications such as infection, fracture fixation due to increased stress, cardiovascular compromise, and even mortality in some studies [23, 26]. However, a recent study looking at open ankle fractures found an overall increased risk of complications in obese patients. However, in a subgroup analysis, while obese patients younger than 60 versus exhibited a significant risk of complications over nonobese patients, interestingly, obese patients older than 60 did not exhibit the same increased risk [24]. Regardless of the effect of obesity on postoperative complications, body habitus may be prohibitive for certain operative set-ups including bed weight limits and/or implant guide sizes. Obese patients should be carefully evaluated pre- and postoperatively by anesthesia and medicine teams. Obesity needs to be taken into consideration for all per-operative decision-making by the orthopedic surgery team, even though its impact on elderly open fractures is still in question. Future studies are needed to better delineate the effects of obesity specifically in elderly patients with open fractures.

Smoking has established risks on both bony and soft-tissue healing [14, 27–29]. An early study by Hollenbach et al. found reduced hip bone mineral density in both men and women over 60 years who were smokers and a dose-response relationship between change in smoking status and hip bone density, supporting that smoking cessation was beneficial to reducing bone density loss later in life [27]. A prospective, observational population-based study followed over one thousand women and found that both former and current smokers had increased risk for any fracture and osteoporotic fractures compared to nonsmokers. Smoking cessation showed a decreased risk for vertebral fractures, but did not significantly change risk of other types of fractures in this cohort [28]. A 2012 systematic review and meta-analysis across surgical specialties found significantly more postoperative healing complications in smokers compared to nonsmokers and smoking cessation was found to reduce surgical site infections (SSIs), but not other complications such as wound necrosis or complication or decreased bone healing [29]. Due to these potentially modifiable risks, it is our recommendation that smoking cessation begins on presentation for open fracture patients.

Other pharmacologic agents can effect bony and soft-tissue healing, both in a positive or negative manner. Drugs including cytostatics (i.e., chemotherapy/cytotoxic drugs) in oncologic treatment, fluoroquinolone antibiotics, corticosteroids, and cox inhibitors (NSAIDS) are thought to inhibit fracture healing [30]. Antiepileptic drugs (AEDS) and antidepressants have also been shown to have a negative effect on bone health and may require more aggressive osteoporosis management in these patients [31]. Others such as bone-morphogenetic proteins (BMP), parathyroid hormone (PTH), and selective prostaglandin agonists can stimulate bony healing [30] Thus, it is important to carefully examine a patient's history and medical list when considering treatment and outcomes of open fractures, particularly in the elderly.

Preexisting use of anticoagulation is common in elderly patients, and in most cases should not delay initial management of open fractures needing formal debridement, irrigation, and stabilization. Consultation with medical or cardiology specialists may be necessary to determine the best plan for managing anticoagulation in the perioperative period to minimize the risks of both embolic complications related to holding anticoagulation as well as the bleeding and wound healing complications associated with "operating through" anticoagulation. Dineen et al reported the safety of continuing aspirin in nearly all orthopedic procedures. There is evidence, however, that withdrawing antiplatelet therapy, such as clopidogrel, can be problematic due to the acute-phase reaction and systemic inflammatory response that increases platelet adhesiveness and reduces fibrinolysis after trauma [32]. While no significant evidence exists that stopping clopidogrel for primary prevention of cardiovascular disease is harmful, it is recommended to restart it within 24 h of surgery if hemostasis is adequate [32, 33]. To extrapolate from hip fracture data for a similar demographic cohort, a recent meta-analysis on clopidogrel use in hip fractures found there was no clinically significant bleeding risk when surgery was done on the hip fracture, but there was increased risk of cardiovascular events if stopped [34]. These studies support the safety in continuing aspirin and clopidogrel for urgent surgical procedures. If for some reason antiplatelet therapy is stopped, it should be restarted within 24 h to decrease the risk for postoperative cardiovascular events.

30.3.2 Examination

A thorough examination is necessary in any patient with an apparent open fracture. The potentially dramatic appearance of wounds and/or deformities associated with open fractures can serve as distractors to both patients and health care providers. In the elderly, simple falls or other low-energy mechanisms may result in other injuries. So careful examination should be diligently performed in a systematic fashion so that other injuries are not overlooked. Again, underlying medical conditions and medications should be elucidated for the reasons discussed.

30.3.3 Imaging

Standard plain radiographs in orthogonal planes of all joints and extremities with obvious or suspected injuries should be obtained as part of the initial workup of an elderly patient with an open fracture. Advanced imaging may be obtained of specific, complex injuries such as those around the elbow, knee, or ankle to assist with preoperative and intra-operative decision-making. Additionally, imaging of the head and/or c-spine should be considered for any patient presenting with signs of head or facial trauma, confusion, or neck pain because even a low-energy fall may cause significant injury to the more rigid spine.

It is essential to keep in mind that often the poor soft tissue around the fractures may mask the true extent of the injury. Stress views may be helpful to elucidate a higher-grade injury. Sometimes they are performed in the emergency room, but most often in the operating room. An example of poor soft-tissue quality leading to instability in an ankle fracture-dislocation can be seen in Fig. 30.2.

30.3.4 Classification

The Gustilo-Anderson classification is still broadly used for open fracture classification and may be used in elderly patients with the caveat that soft-tissue wounds in the elderly may appear more severe than the underlying bone injury or mechanism of trauma would otherwise suggest [35]. It is prudent to go beyond simply classifying the open fracture and to describe the soft-tissue injury in detail for the benefit of others who may be involved in serial debridement or definitive coverage when necessary. The Orthopaedic Trauma Association (OTA) has developed a new classification system for open fractures to address these potential discrepancies, which includes specification of injury to five subcategories: skin, muscle, arterial, contamination, and bone loss [36].

Examples of characteristic, open ankle fractures in the elderly can be seen in Fig. 30.3a–e. These transverse lacerations, which fail in tension, are the most common soft-tissue pattern in elderly ankle fractures.

30.4 Management

The initial management of open fractures in the elderly is similar to that in young patients, but with special consideration given to potential comorbidities, polypharmacy effects, and poor physiologic reserve. As discussed previously, comorbidities and frailty increase with age, which can make the assessment and treatment of open fractures challenging. The ultimate goals for managing open fractures include preventing infection, facilitating soft-tissue healing, bone healing, and early mobilization to restore patient function [37].

30.4.1 Systemic Antibiotic Therapy

Elderly patients should receive early, broad-spectrum, systemic antibiotics ideally within 3 h from injury, as recommended by the current

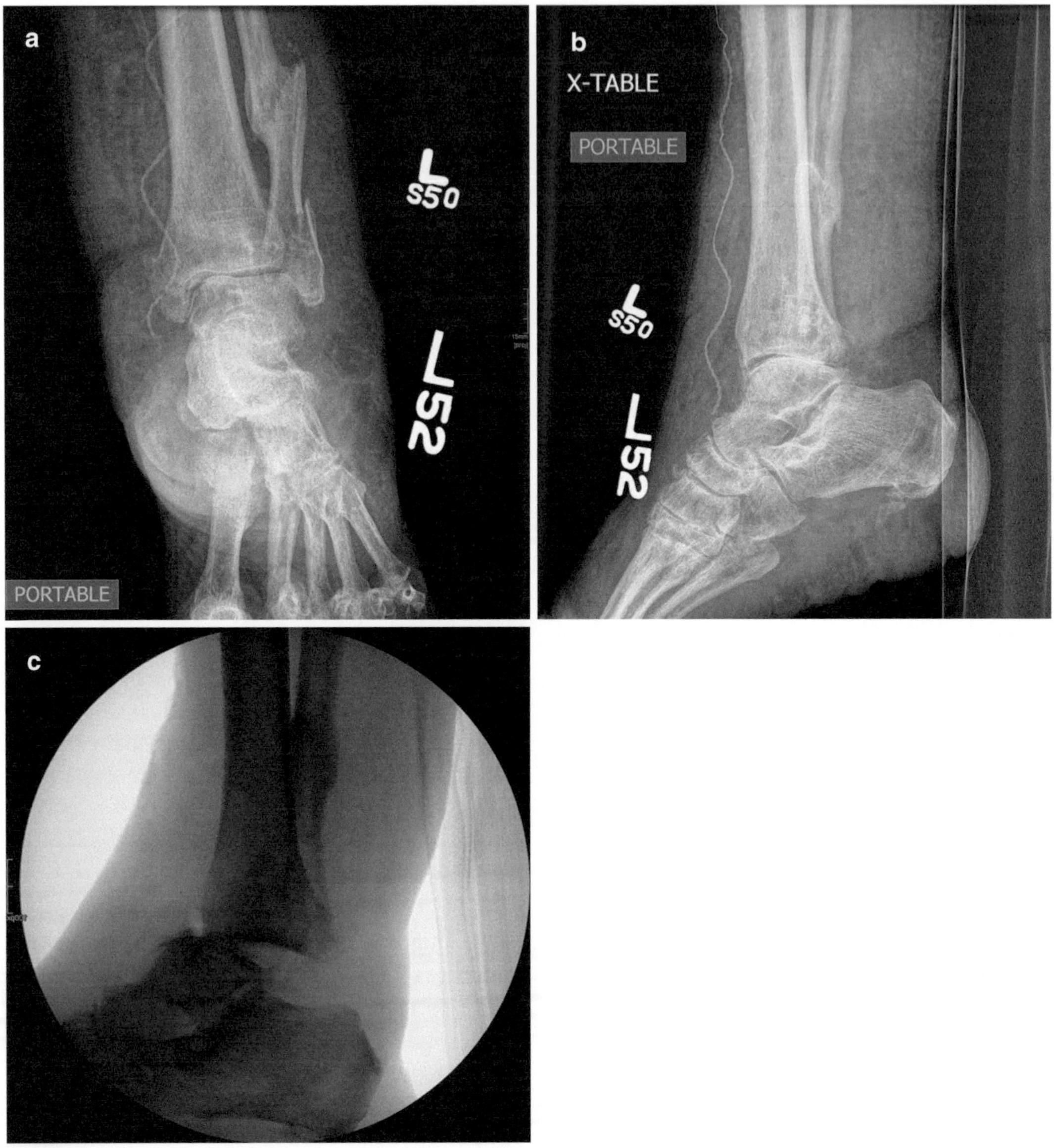

Fig. 30.2 (**a**) Antero-posterior (AP) and (**b**) lateral injury films of a 79-year old female after a fall from standing resulting in a type IIIa open ankle fracture-dislocation. Images (**a–b**) show what appears to be a simple bimalleolar ankle fracture pattern in the setting of a prior fibular mal-union, however, (**c**) intraoperative fluoroscopy showed this injury to be a trimalleolar ankle fracture-dislocation

Eastern Association for the Surgery of Trauma (EAST) guidelines [38], as studies show a significant reduction in infection with antibiotic coverage after open fractures [39–41, 50]. Gram-positive coverage, such as with first-generation cephalosporins (i.e., cefazolin), should be given for uncontaminated or clean appearing wounds, and gram-negative coverage, such as aminoglycosides (i.e., gentamicin) or fourth-generation cephalosporins (i.e., cefepime), should be added for contaminated wounds and Gustilo type III fractures. Literature also supports using penicillin or ampicillin for concerns of anaerobic infection for wounds contaminated with feces and/or soil [39, 42]. Varying antibiotic protocols exist for highly contaminated wounds using combina-

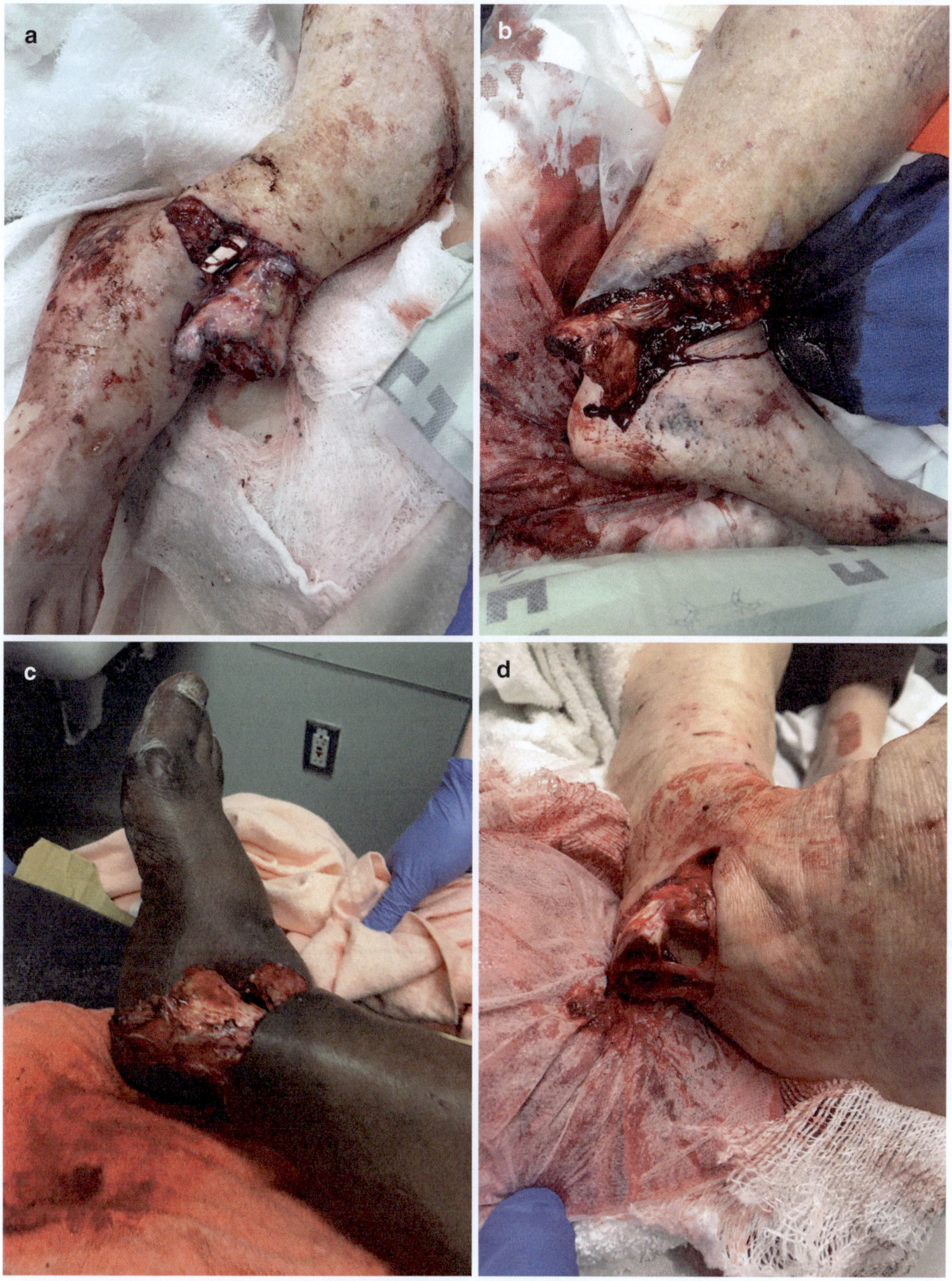

Fig. 30.3 (**a**) Extruded distal tibia plafond with classic transverse medial ankle wound in an elderly female after a ground-level fall resulting in a type IIIa open, trimalleolar ankle fracture-dislocation. (**b**) type IIIa open fracture-dislocation after a ground-level fall in an 89-year old female with obvious necrosis of the skin edges (**c**) type IIIb open ankle fracture-dislocation after a fall from height in an elderly male and (**d, e**) transverse lateral ankle wound with an ankle fracture-dislocation in an elderly female patient after a ground-level fall resulting in a type IIIA open injury

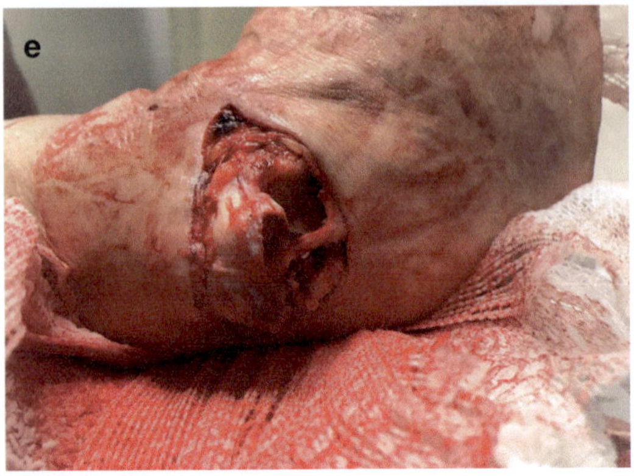

Fig. 30.3 (continued)

tions of other agents including ciprofloxacin, piperacillin-tazobactam, and clindamycin. However, scarce literature exists to compare these in terms of efficacy or safety profiles [38, 39, 42]. And, with the rising community and hospital prevalence of methicillin-resistant staphylococcus aureus (MRSA) as a feared pathogen in open fractures, some protocols include MRSA coverage (i.e., vancomycin), however, guidelines are still lacking in this area [43]. However, a pilot randomized trial by Saveli et al compared cefazolin to cefazolin plus vancomycin in 140 open fracture patients of all ages and found no significant difference in SSI rates between groups [44]. Routine use of vancomycin for open fractures should be approached with caution especially in the elderly as there are potential complications associated with the use of vancomycin.

Nephrotoxicity, drug-drug interactions, or other potentially serious adverse effects should be accounted for when considering the use of any systemic antibiotics, which may necessitate monitoring of serum creatinine and drug levels. And, higher risk for acute kidney injury is seen in patients with hypotension and higher injury severity scores (ISS) on presentation [45], making elderly patients with open fractures at very high risk. There is an increased risk of nephrotoxicity specifically with aminoglycoside administration with greater patient age, longer duration of therapy, higher dosing, and concurrent use with other nephrotoxic agents [46]. Because of this, routine use of gentamicin should be avoided, if possible, in elderly patients with open fractures due to their high risk of kidney injury and our institution has removed gentamicin from routine use even in younger patients.

Duration of antibiotic treatment has also been heavily investigated. The EAST guidelines recommend a maximum of 72 h from the time of injury, but not more than 24 hours after soft-tissue coverage as a Level II recommendation [38]. The British Orthopaedic Association recommends no longer than 24–48 h for Gustilo Type I fractures and a maximum of 72 h or until definitive soft-tissue closure, whichever is shorter for type II and III fractures [47]. Similarly, a recent meta-analysis of 32 studies on antibiotic treatment duration in open fractures in all ages could not support any benefits of using prophylactic antibiotics past 72 h, regardless of the severity of injury or time to soft-tissue coverage [42]. The newest review article from the American Academy of Orthopaedic Surgeons also did not find evidence to support antibiotics beyond 24 h after definitive coverage or debridement and sterile dressing placement [43].

While there remains some uncertainty in the optimal antibiotics used, duration of treatment, and subsequent risk profile of prophylactic antibiotics, our institutional policy is to administer 2 grams of IV Cefazolin every 8 h for Gustilo Type I and II fractures for 24 h and 2 g Ceftriaxone every 24 h for Type III fractures for a total duration of 72 h or 24 h after wound closure, whatever is shorter. Clindamycin 900 mg every eight hours is administered for those with penicillin allergies in type I and II fractures and Aztreonam 2 g every 8 h is added for type III injuries. Decisions for safe antibiotic prophylaxis should be discussed with pharmacologic, medicine, and/or geriatrics teams for appropriate monitoring, if indicated.

30.4.2 Local Antibiotic Therapy

There has been increasing interest in local antibiotic therapy for use in open fractures in recent years. Local administration in bone cement or powder forms rarely causes systemic side effects, but can produce high concentrations in the nearby tissues [39, 49]. One study by Moehring et al compared local and systemic therapies for Gustilo type II, IIIA, and IIIB fractures and found similar infection rates using systemic first-generation cephalosporins versus local therapy with tobramycin-eluting beads. However, the study was underpowered due to the small sample size, so no definitive conclusions could be determined [50]. A more recent systematic review and meta-analysis showed a risk reduction in subsequent fracture-related infections of 11% with the addition of prophylactic local antibiotics given for open limb fractures compared to systemic therapy alone, however, the authors themselves caution against the interpretation of these results secondary to heterogeneity, bias, and limited quality studies included in analysis [51].

Important factors to consider with local antibiotic use include mechanism of injury, extent of soft tissue and bone involvement and contamination, surgical factors including planned return procedures, and patient factors. At this point, use of local therapy should be used on a case-by-case basis using clinical judgment.

30.4.3 Debridement and Irrigation

Thorough debridement and irrigation are essential to help prevent infection. Provisional irrigation and debridement of gross contamination should be completed upon presentation to the emergency room. Formal debridement should be completed ideally within 24 h, if possible. The ultimate goal of surgical debridement is to maintain a clean wound bed with viable tissues and to remove devitalized bone fragments to prevent infection [37]. Along with debridement, irrigation is performed with a variety of options. The FLOW study investigation suggested that reoperation rates were similar regardless of irrigation pressures and that saline had lower reoperation rates than castile soap solutions in the treatment of open fractures [52]. With this, it is our opinion that normal saline at low pressures is adequate irrigation fluid after appropriate debridement. Per Anglen et al., 3 l of saline for type I fractures, 6 l for type II fractures, and 9 l for type III fractures is common practice [53] It is our practice to perform debridement and irrigation as soon as possible (within 24 h at the latest) with gravity flow sterile saline using a minimum of 3, 6, and up to 9 l for Gustilo type I, II, and III, respectively.

30.5 Provisional Fixation

In addition to urgent surgical irrigation and debridement, fracture stabilization should be planned to allow for optimal wound care, minimize additional soft-tissue injury, and enable patient mobilization and rehabilitation. The stabilization strategy should be dictated by the patient's overall health and medical conditions, other injuries, and the condition of the soft-tissue envelope which may be much more tenuous in the elderly than in younger patients.

Temporary stabilization with splinting, external fixation, or provisional internal fixation are all valid options for the elderly patient. The choice of immobilization should take into account definitive surgical plans, the need for ongoing wound care or soft-tissue assessment, and the potential risks of further compromise to the bone or soft tissues. Plaster immobilization may be restrictive to soft-tissue swelling, decrease access to wounds, cause thermal injury at the time of application, and/or cause additional soft-tissue injury or pressure ulceration if not applied with the utmost care.

External fixation can also play a role in provisional fixation of elderly open fractures as it can allow access for early soft-tissue stabilization. However, it is associated with pin tract infections that can be superficial or deep and lead to greater morbidity. External fixation may also lead to fewer options for definitive fixation by limiting screw placement at the time of definitive plating. Although rare, another difficulty with external fixation may include inability to obtain sufficient stability, even temporarily given the soft-tissue or fracture locations.

30.6 Definitive Fixation

Definitive care should be provided as soon as medically appropriate and surgically prudent. A key consideration in treating open elderly fractures is bone quality and density as this can impact the ability to maintain fixation. This is compounded by the difficulty in treating fractures with associated soft-tissue injuries and the potential complications associated with an extended healing period. Wagner et al found the delay in fracture healing with age to be partially attributed to a decrease in both number and function of mesenchymal stem cells that assist with bone regeneration and direction of angiogenesis by endothelial progenitor cells [54]. In addition, when managing elderly patients who may be frail and unable to comply with limited weight-bearing, every effort should be made to provide a fixation construct that will allow for the greatest amount of early mobility and weight-bearing or activities of daily living when possible. At times, this may require creatively adapting fixation constructs in poor bone to meet the needs of the elderly and frail patient.

Strategies that may be beneficial include definitive fixation at the time of initial debridement to minimize the risks of multiple anesthetics, blood loss, and soft-tissue injury, and making every effort to minimize the length of procedures. There is evidence to suggest that early definitive care may decrease subsequent procedures, infection rates, and possibly expedite rehabilitation and bony union compared to delayed fixation/closure [55–58]. In a small series of 21 open distal radius fractures, the authors found a low rate of complications with only one deep infection and adequate functional results in elderly patients treated with a single definitive procedure [55]. A 2020 retrospective case-control study of 88 open ankle fractures of all ages compared immediate internal fixation with primary closure to temporary fixation with delayed definitive fixation and wound closure. While they found no significant difference between infection rates, the early cohort had significantly fewer reoperations and shorter hospital stays with similar clinical outcomes to the staged cohort [57]. Similarly, a 2017 review showed that definitive internal fixation and wound closure/coverage was associated with lower mortality rates and better functional outcomes compared to external fixation or wound healing by secondary intent in elderly patients with low-energy open ankle fractures [58].

Creative fixation strategies have been explored for the treatment of open fractures, specifically in elderly or frail patients. For example, Armstrong et al. reported on the use of tibiocalcaneal nails and early soft-tissue coverage for the initial management of type IIIB open ankle fractures in a frail population to allow for stable fixation and early mobilization and weight-bearing. They demonstrated a low rate of complications and no reoperations with timely return to ambulation [59]. Other novel techniques include distal fibulectomy, tibial shortening, and subsequent tibiotalar arthrodesis as a salvage procedure after open ankle fractures in the elderly, which may be indicated in patients with extensive soft-tissue injuries and comorbidities that preclude flap coverage or in cases of a failed free flap, as described by Crespo et al [60]. An example of early, definitive fixation with percutaneous medial malleolus and calcaneo-tibial fixation can be seen in Fig. 30.4.

In a severely debilitated patient who is minimally ambulatory or has limited independent functional capabilities, an amputation may be a reasonable definitive surgical option to minimize the risks of repeated surgeries and anesthetics. However, an amputation in an elderly person may be much more limiting in terms of postoperative rehab and independence. Thus, the decision for surgical fixation versus amputation should be made on an individual basis after carefully weighing the risks and benefits as described above.

Overall, early definitive fracture fixation and wound coverage with early mobilization improve overall functional outcomes in open fractures in the elderly [55].

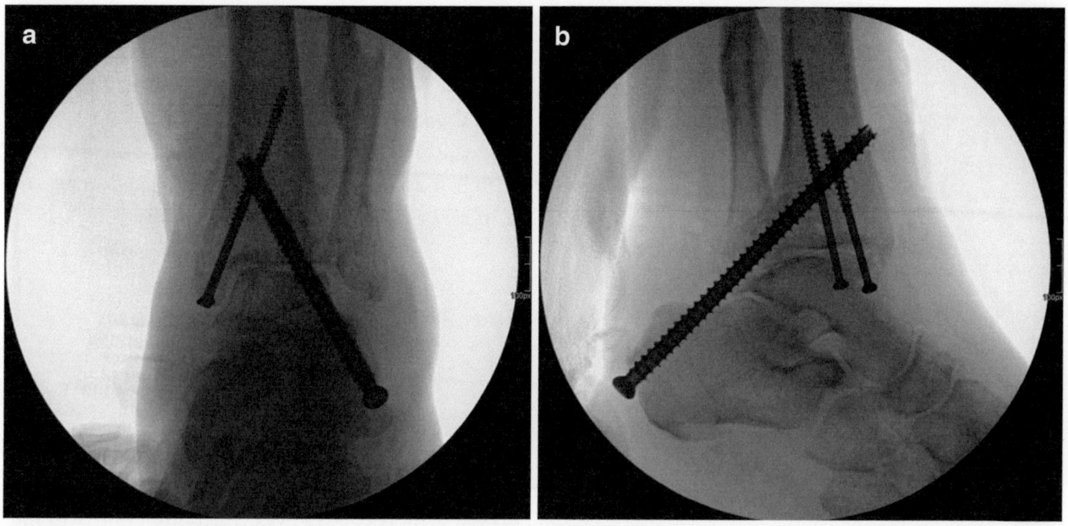

Fig. 30.4 The patient referenced in Figs. 30.1 and 30.2 was treated with provisional irrigation and debridement and definitive, percutaneous medial malleolus and calcaneo-tibial fixation with non-pressure wound therapy until definitive coverage was completed with split-thickness skin grafting (STSG) by our plastic surgery colleagues (Fig. 30.5) as seen in both the (**a**) AP and (**b**) lateral intraoperative fluoroscopy

30.6.1 Wound Coverage

Careful soft-tissue management should be a priority in all stages of open fracture management in elderly patients. The optimal timing for wound closure or soft-tissue reconstruction remains controversial, however, studies do support increased risks with delayed closure. A 2016 study by Ovaska et al., found a 16% wound necrosis rate after primary wound closure in patients of all ages after surgical fixation of open ankle fractures, with independent risk factors including Gustilo grade III open injuries, ASA>=2, and use of pulsatile lavage. There was no statistical difference in wound necrosis rates, however, when stratified in patients older than 65 years of age. Despite this, it was the authors' conclusion that grade III ankle fracture wounds should not be closed primarily even in elderly patients [61]. A propensity-matched cohort study by Jenkinson et al found a 4.1% deep infection rate with immediate primary closure of lower-grade open fractures versus 17.8% in delayed primary closure, though this study was not stratified by age [62]. At our institution, we advocate for primary closure when possible. However, in cases that are grossly contaminated or have high-grade soft-tissue injuries, the surgeon may elect to delay closure.

Unfortunately, high-grade soft-tissue injuries are difficult to treat, specifically with exposed bone, which can be compounded in elderly patients due to their poor soft tissue and aging skin. In the elderly, the viability of local soft-tissue flaps is a concern because of baseline fragility of the skin, underlying vascular disease, and medical and physiologic factors that may impair healing [59, 63, 64]. Furthermore, specifically as it relates to ankle fractures, local flap coverage or the use of STSG can be difficult or impossible as the vasculature required for the local flaps or the soft-tissue beds for STSGs are often involved in the zone of injury [60]. An example of a successful STSG in an elderly patient with an open ankle fracture can be found in Fig. 30.5.

While free flaps are considered, the treatment of choice when there is low possibility of local flaps working, some authors have argued that age, comorbidities, and patient factors including DM, peripheral vascular disease, and coronary artery disease are relative contraindications [60, 65–67]. Other authors have argued that age is not a contraindication to rotational and free-tissue

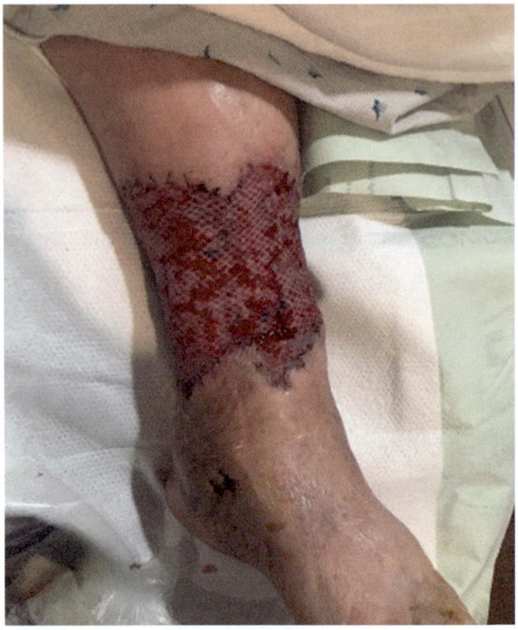

Fig. 30.5 Healing split-thickness skin grafting of the patient referenced in Fig. 30.1 after multiple surgical debridements and subsequent internal fixation

transfers and such "aggressive" soft-tissue coverage options may be the best way to minimize infection risks and time of wound healing [59, 63, 67]. An early retrospective review of 100 patients older than 65 who had free-flap reconstruction—ten of which had lower extremity traumatic wounds—by Serletti et al found an overall success rate of 97% for free flaps, supporting similar success rates in elderly patients compared to the general population [65]. Qian et al performed a systematic review and meta-analysis of 17 studies (453 free-style flaps) and found no statistically significant difference in complications after free flaps in patients over 60 years old [68]. In contrast, a 2019 study of 77 patients undergoing free flaps found a statistically significant relationship between flap loss and age (correlation coefficient 0.3, p = 0.006) [66]. While the majority of these studies included oncologic reconstructions in various anatomic areas, they do provide insight into flap coverage in the elderly population, which may be applicable to open fracture management. So, free flaps should be considered in the elderly but one must perform an adequate patient evaluation and workup, including angiography and/or nutritional status when indicated [69]. Early conversations with plastic surgery and/or orthopedic colleagues with experience in flap coverage should be had to discuss appropriate soft-tissue management, which may ultimately change surgical decisions if there is no adequate coverage option.

30.6.2 Negative Pressure Wound Therapy

Use of negative pressure wound therapy (NPWT) has become widely used for open fracture wounds over the past 20 years. Literature to support the efficacy of use, however, remains controversial. And, to our knowledge, there are no studies stratified by age.

A retrospective cohort study by Blum et al of open tibial fractures comparing NPWT to conventional dressings found a decreased rate of deep infection in the NPWT group (8.4% v 20.6%, p = 0.01). This study was not stratified by age—the average age was 40.3 in the NPWT group and 36.8 in the conventional group—and there was a greater proportion of type IIIB injuries in the NPWT group (50% vs. 25%, p = 0.001). In addition, free flaps were used more frequently in NPWT group versus the conventional group (28% v 14%). However, there was no difference in the rate of primary closure, skin grafting, or local flaps between groups. Use of NPWT, Gustilo type, associated major trauma, transfusion rates, time to initial debridement, and time to definitive fracture fixation were independent univariate predictors of deep infection in this study [70]. Similarly, a 2020 review selected 10 studies for meta-analysis and found a significantly decreased rate of deep infection in the NPWT group (OR 0.43, $p < 0.0001$). Flap failure was also significantly reduced in the NPWT group (OR 0.37, p = 0.04). But, there was no statistical difference between groups in regards to amputation, fracture union, flap frequency, ICU stay, or hospital stay in subgroup analysis [71].

The WOLLF Randomized Clinical Trial compared NPWT versus standard wound management after the first surgical debridement in open fractures of the lower limbs. While patients were younger, with an average age of 45.3 years and 74% were male, there were no statistically significant differences in patients' Disability Rating Index scores at 12 months, number of deep SSIs, or in quality of life. Additionally, there was a low probability of cost-effectiveness in this study [72]. Similarly, a 2018 Cochrane Database Systematic Review included seven randomized controlled trials (1377 participants) and found moderate-certainty evidence that there was no clear difference between standard care and NPWT at 6 weeks for open fractures and moderate-certainty evidence that NPWT is not cost-effective for open fracture wound treatment [73].

Deep infection is a feared complication after open fractures. Contradictory evidence exists in the literature and uncertainty remains as to whether NPWT affects the rate of wound infections, adverse events, time to closure or patient-reported outcomes based on this review. Despite the questionable benefit, it is the author's opinion that NPWT should be considered for elderly open fractures in light of the bony and soft-tissue susceptibilities as mentioned earlier in this chapter.

30.6.3 Venous Thromboembolic Prophylaxis (VTE)

Elderly patients with open fractures are at increased risk for postoperative venous thromboembolic prophylaxis (VTE) in the first 5–7 days postoperatively during which a potential deep vein thrombosis (DVT) remains in the early, acute phase. Virchow's triad is activated—from use of a tourniquet and/or decreased mobilization postoperatively causing venous stasis, fracture and/or surgical manipulations causing endothelial vascular damage, and increased hypercoagulability as the body's response to trauma—which puts orthopedic patients at especially high risk [33]. The incidence of symptomatic DVT has been reported to be in the range from 40 to 60% after major orthopedic surgery [74]. Thus, postoperative venous thromboembolism (VTE) prophylaxis is recommended. While various guidelines exist, it is our practice that patients receive low-molecular-weight heparin (LMWH) and/or novel Xa inhibitors with mechanical prophylaxis while inpatient and for a minimum of 10–14 days per the American College of Chest Surgeons (CHEST) guidelines [75]. Patients can then be transitioned to a maintenance VTE prophylaxis—including aspirin—for up to 35 days or at least until the patient is adequately mobilizing [74, 75]. While the CHEST guidelines do not suggest thromboprophylaxis for isolated lower extremities injuries—even if they require immobilization—it is our departmental policy to prescribe it if there are concerns for mobility issues.-And as the medications and comorbidities in the elderly patients can be complex, decisions for VTE prophylaxis should be discussed with the hospitalists and/or geriatric medical teams.

30.6.4 Mobilization and Weight-bearing

Early mobilization and weight-bearing are a priority in the elderly population to minimize complications and prevent further injuries. Older patients may be unable to comply with limited weight-bearing restrictions due to debility, balance, and gait disturbances at baseline, or from dementia or cognitive impairment. Every effort should be made to provide a stable enough construct to allow immediate weight-bearing when possible and to provide appropriate resources for assistive devices and adaptive equipment when activities must be restricted.

When mobility and/or weight-bearing must be limited, extra assistance may be required from inpatient and outpatient rehabilitation specialists, home-health nursing, and family or other caregivers to ensure basic hygiene needs, daily mobilization and repositioning, and postoperative wound care are met.

30.6.5 Bone Health

Osteoporosis-related fragility fractures are an epidemic worldwide, and various resources exist to enable providers to evaluate and treat these patients. A coordinated postfracture education and treatment program are essential and should be considered for all elderly open fracture patients [76]. As previously mentioned, calcium and vitamin D supplementation is indicated in patients with deficiencies and/or osteoporosis to help prevent bone loss following fracture, as well as an attempt to reduce secondary fracture risk [21].

Part of the workup includes assessing the quality of bone and then where indicted beginning treatment. Osteoporotic treatment medications are separated into anabolic agents, including PTH analogues, and anti-resorptive medications, including bisphosphonates, denosumab, calcitonin, and estrogen receptor modular [20]. It is now widely accepted that secondary prevention can be safely implemented as a preventive measure as soon as possible after a fragility fracture, and prefracture treatment does not need to be delayed or paused, as the benefits of treatment outweigh the potential risks of delayed fracture healing [20]. And although not definitive in the literature, there may be a role for treatment with an anabolic drug to aid in the healing of elderly fractures. For example, a 2011 study by Peichl et al found a decreased time to healing after pelvic ring fractures in osteoporosis patients who were treated with daily, subcutaneous PTH compared to those who were not [77].

30.7 Outcomes and Complications

When an efficient, multidisciplinary approach is carried out, good outcomes can be achieved even in elderly patients with open fractures. However, age and preexisting comorbidities can pose challenges often leading to increased risk of infection, nonunion, and mortality.

30.7.1 Infection and Wound Complications

Despite improvements in antimicrobial coverage, prompt irrigation and debridement, and delicate soft-tissue management, infection is a feared consequence of open injuries and can be complicated by comorbidities in the elderly and/or iatrogenic from surgical intervention and implants [78]. Infection rates for even closed injuries show less favorable results in older versus younger cohorts. Pagliaro et al. found an 8% rate of deep infection out of a cohort of 23 patients with both open and closed fractures [79]. In a series of 237 geriatric ankle fractures, Aigner et al. found that increased operative time was the only independent risk factor associated with development of complications, and surgical time and presence of an open fracture were risk factors for requiring a revision surgery [15]. A study of 21 grade IIIB open, unstable ankle fractures treated with tibiocalcaneal nail fixation and soft-tissue coverage found six superficial wound infections (28%) [59]. Another retrospective analysis by Khadim et al. of 99 elderly patients with type IIIB open lower limb fractures—with the majority treated with locoregional flaps more than free flaps secondary to low-energy injuries—found a 1% flap failure rate and 1% deep infection rate [63]. A study by White et all retrospectively reviewed 13 open ankle fractures in adult patients of all ages with diabetes and found a 64% rate of wound complication, 36% of which developed deep infection, and 42% of which ultimately required amputation. And, only 21% of these patients archived bony union without complication [80]. Clinical and radiographic examples of lateral incision wound breakdown after open reduction internal fixation and primary closure of an open ankle fracture in an elderly patient can be found in Fig. 30.6.

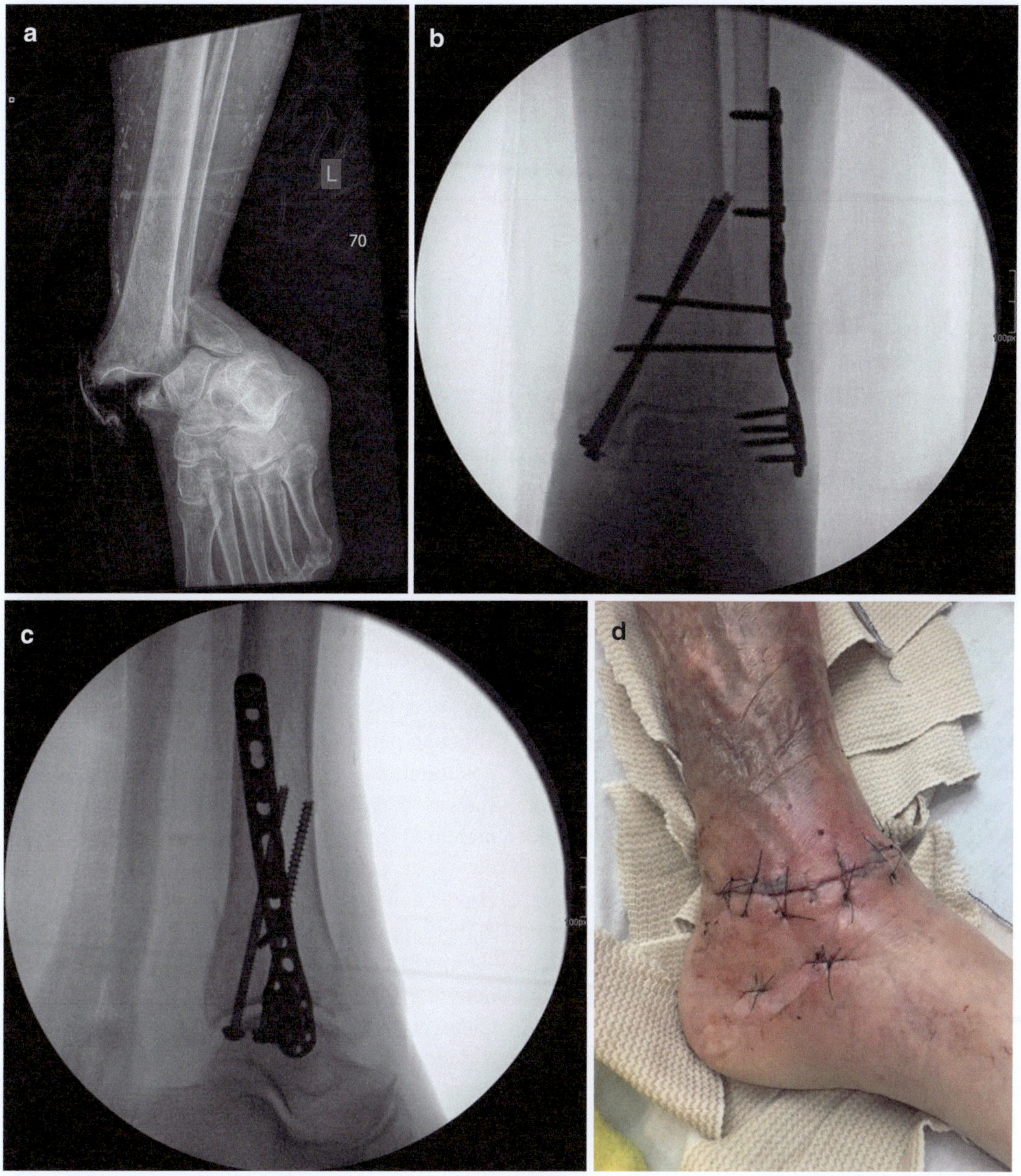

Fig. 30.6 (**a**) Injury and (**b, c**) intra-operative fixation radiographs for the elderly female with an open ankle fracture-dislocation with clinical photos as seen in Fig. 30.4. (**d**) Open, medial injury wound that was primarily closed, and (**e**) surgical incision with wound breakdown and exposed plate on the lateral side

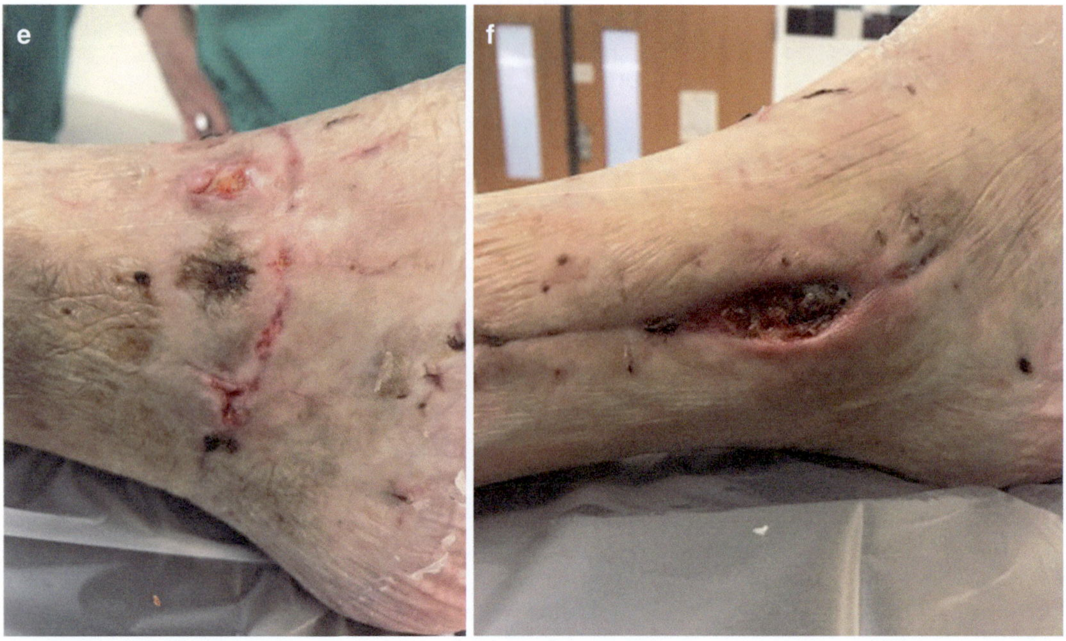

Fig. 30.6 (continued)

Based on the studies presented above, infections after open fracture vary widely and are influenced by many factors other than age alone, and can be estimated between 1 and 36% for deep infection [63, 80] with up to a 64% wound complication rate in patients with diabetes [80]. Evaluating patient risk factors including diabetes, obesity, home medicines, skin and soft-tissue quality, and nutrition status are essential to help to attempt to stratify risks preoperatively. Furthermore, intraoperative considerations such as adequate debridement and irrigation, delicate soft-tissue handling, and shorter operative times may help decrease risks. And, as mentioned above, arguably the most important, early administration of broad-spectrum antibiotics significantly reduces the incidence of wound infections [38–45, 51].

30.7.2 Nonunion

Nonunion is an established complication with any fracture that can negatively affect patient outcomes. There is evidence supporting increasing age as a factor for fracture healing inhibition, although patient comorbidities also play a role in nonunion risk. For example, clinical studies have shown diabetic patients not only have an increased fracture risk but also have a higher incidence of delayed union or nonunion and an almost doubled time to healing compared to non-diabetic patients [13, 81].

Age has also been shown to be a risk factor for nonunion after both closed and open fractures. Clement et al found that frailer, elderly patients had more substantial injuries, an increased risk of open fractures, and a higher rate of nonunion compared to their younger counterparts [82]. Zura et al. found that nonunion after all fractures in Medicare beneficiaries was more likely to occur in people with certain comorbidities, including smoking, obesity, type I and II diabetes, osteoarthritis and rheumatoid arthritis, open fractures, osteoporosis, and alcoholism. Interestingly, in this study patients that were older than 75 were less likely to go on to nonunion compared to patients under 75 years old [83]. While the literature on the effect of age on bone healing is still inconclusive, it is important to identify that the risks of nonunion are multifactorial with both injury- and patient-related factors. Modifiable risk factors such as smoking, bone health, and nutrition should be addressed with the patient as soon as possible in attempts to reduce the nonunion risk.

30.7.3 Mortality

Mortality rates after open fractures in elderly patients have been shown to be higher compared to closed fractures and higher in elderly patients compared to their younger counterparts—even after closed fractures [83–87]. A 2013 review of both closed and open tibial diaphysis fractures in patients >65 years found a 17% overall 120-day mortality rate. When breaking this down by 65–80 years of age, the 120-day mortality was 9%, and the mortality rate for those >80 years of age was 30%. This study also found a 33% 120-day mortality rate in all patients over 65 years of age patients with open fractures [82]. A Swedish study of 3777 open tibial fractures found an increased risk of adjusted 90-day mortality in elderly patients (25.7%)—comparable to mortality rates in hip fracture patients—with increased risk of cardiovascular and respiratory failure [86]. Another study by Toole et al found a 27% mortality rate after open ankle fractures in the elderly at a mean of 2.67 ± 2.02 months from injury, and a staggering 81% of these patients were found to have >=3 comorbidities [87]. A smaller study of only 21 grade IIIB open, unstable ankle fractures treated with tibiocalcaneal nail fixation and soft-tissue coverage found a 15% three-month mortality rate [59].

The literature supports increased mortality rates after open fractures in elderly patients. Closed fracture mortality rates in elderly patients ranged from 4.9 to 9% [83–85] but open fracture mortality rates in elderly patients were even higher, ranging from 15 to 33% in these studies [59, 82, 86, 87]. Thus, patients and their families should be adequately counseled on the long-term risks, including higher mortality rates, after sustaining open fractures.

30.8 Summary of Recommendations

Open fractures in the elderly are becoming more common and remain difficult to treat for a myriad of age-specific concerns including poor bone quality and quantity, aging skin, delay in wound and bone healing, and overall extended recovery periods with difficulty mobilizing postoperatively.

While there is limited literature published specifically on open fractures in the elderly, our recommended mainstays of treatment include:

- Multidisciplinary care teams including geriatric and/or hospitalist-based medicine to ensure patients are well resuscitated and to avoid poly-pharmacy or drug-drug interactions.
- Early administration of broad-spectrum systemic antibiotic prophylaxis on presentation with Cefazolin in Gustilo type I and II fractures for 24 h and Ceftriaxone for type III fractures, to minimize nephrotoxicity of aminoglycoside use, for 72 h or 24 h after wound coverage, whichever is shorter.
- Local antibiotic therapy should be used on a case-by-case basis, specifically for extensive soft-tissue wounds or contaminated fractures.
- Urgent debridement, irrigation, and provisional fixation as necessary with splinting, external fixation, or provisional internal fixation until definitive fixation can be completed when soft tissue allows.
- The emphasis for fixation is on stability considering poor-quality and/or low-density bone with the goal of weight-bearing through the injured extremity whenever possible.
- Early involvement of plastic surgery or flap proficient orthopedic surgery colleagues for soft-tissue coverage as indicated.
- Low-molecular-weight heparin (LMWH), novel Xa inhibitors, and/or aspirin and mechanical VTE prophylaxis for a minimum of 10–14 days, but ideally for 35 days, per CHEST guidelines [75]
- Early mobilization with trained geriatric therapists.

- Close postoperative follow-up including radiographs to monitor bony healing.
- Early involvement of osteoporosis management and/or treatment, if indicated.

References

1. Arias, E., Xu, J. United States Life Tables, 2017. National Vital Statistics Reports. Volume 68, Number 7. US Department of Health and Human Services Center for Disease control and Prevention. https://www.cdc.gov/nchs/data/nvsr/nvsr68/nvsr68_07-508.pdf (2019) Accessed 30 Mar 2020
2. United States Census Bureau. 2017 National population projections tables: main series. https://www.census.gov/data/tables/2017/demo/popproj/2017-summary-tables.html (2017). Accessed 13 Apr 2020.
3. Court-Brown CM, Duckworth AD, Clement ND, McQueen MM. Fractures in older adults. A view of the future? Injury. 2018;49(12):2161–6.
4. Bugler KE, Clement ND, Duckworth AD, White TO, McQueen MM. Open ankle fractures: who gets them and why? Arch Orthop Trauma Surg. 2015;135(3):297–303.
5. Court-Brown CM, Biant LC, Clement ND, Bugler KE, Duckworth AD, McQueen MM. Open fractures in the elderly. The importance of skin ageing. Injury. 2015;46(2):189–94.
6. McQueen MM. Global forum: fractures in the elderly. J Bone Joint Surg Am. 2016;98(9):e36.
7. Koval KJ, Lurie J, Zhou W, Sparks MB, Cantu RV, Sporer SM, Weinstein J. Ankle fractures in the elderly: what you get depends on where you live and who you see. J Orthop Trauma. 2005;19(9):635–9.
8. Court-Brown CM, Clement ND, Duckworth AD, Aitken S, Biant LC, McQueen MM. The spectrum of fractures in the elderly. Bone Joint J. 2014;96(3):366–72.
9. Wongrakpanich S, Kallis C, Prasad P, Rangaswami J, Rosenzweig A. The study of rhabdomyolysis in the elderly: an epidemiological study and single center experience. Aging Dis. 2018;9(1):1.
10. Hain D, Paixao R. The perfect storm: older adults and acute kidney injury. Crit Care Nurs Q. 2015;38(3):271–9.
11. Elamir Y, Gianakos AL, Lane JM, Sharma A, Grist WP, Liporace FA, Yoon RS. The effects of diabetes and diabetic medications on bone health. J Orthop Trauma. 2020;34(3):e102–8.
12. Ferrari SL, Abrahamsen B, Napoli N, Akesson K, Chandran M, Eastell R, Fuleihan GE, Josse R, Kendler DL, Kraenzlin M, Suzuki A. Diagnosis and management of bone fragility in diabetes: an emerging challenge. Osteoporos Int. 2018;29(12):2585–96.
13. Jiao H, Xiao E, Graves DT. Diabetes and its effect on bone and fracture healing. Curr Osteoporos Rep. 2015;13(5):327–35.
14. Kortram K, Bezstarosti H, Metsemakers WJ, Raschke MJ, Van Lieshout EM, Verhofstad MH. Risk factors for infectious complications after open fractures; a systematic review and meta-analysis. Int Orthop. 2017;41(10):1965–82.
15. Aigner R, Salomia C, Lechler P, Pahl R, Frink M. Relationship of prolonged operative time and comorbidities with complications after geriatric ankle fractures. Foot Ankle Int. 2017;38(1):41–8.
16. Bonifant H, Holloway S. A review of the effects of ageing on skin integrity and wound healing. Br J Community Nurs. 2019;24(Suppl. 3):S28–33.
17. Gist S, Tio-Matos I, Falzgraf S, Cameron S, Beebe M. Wound care in the geriatric client. Clin Interv Aging. 2009;4:269.
18. Reus TL, Brohem CA, Schuck DC, Lorencini M. Revisiting the effects of menopause on the skin: functional changes, clinical studies, in vitro models and therapeutic alternatives. Mech Ageing Dev. 2019;4:111193.
19. Yoneda PD, Biancolin SE, Gomes MS, Miot HA. Association between skin thickness and bone density in adult women. An Bras Dermatol. 2011;86(5):878–84.
20. Hak DJ. The biology of fracture healing in osteoporosis and in the presence of anti-osteoporotic drugs. Injury. 2018;49(8):1461–5.
21. Fischer V, Haffner-Luntzer M, Amling M, Ignatius A. Calcium and vitamin D in bone fracture healing and post-traumatic bone turnover. Eur Cell Mater. 2018;22(35):365–85.
22. Von Rüden C, Augat P. Failure of fracture fixation in osteoporotic bone. Injury. 2016;1(47):S3–10.
23. Spitler CA, Hulick RM, Graves ML, Russell GV, Bergin PF. Obesity in the polytrauma patient. Orthop Clin North Am. 2018;49(3):307–15.
24. Gil JA, Durand W, Johnson JP, Goodman AD, Daniels AH. Effect of obesity on perioperative complications, hospital costs, and length of stay in patients with open ankle fractures. J Am Acad Orthop Surg. 2019;27(11):e529–34.
25. Court-Brown CM, Duckworth AD, Ralston S, McQueen MM. The relationship between obesity and fractures. Injury. 2019;50(8):1423–8.
26. Hoffmann M, Lefering R, Gruber-Rathmann M, Rueger JM, Lehmann W. Trauma registry of the German Society for Trauma Surgery. The impact of BMI on polytrauma outcome. Injury. 2012;43(2):184–8.
27. Hollenbach KA, Barrett-Connor E, Edelstein SL, Holbrook T. Cigarette smoking and bone mineral density in older men and women. Am J Public Health. 1993;83(9):1265–70.
28. Thorin MH, Wihlborg A, Åkesson K, Gerdhem P. Smoking, smoking cessation, and fracture risk in

elderly women followed for 10 years. Osteoporos Int. 2016;27(1):249–55.
29. Sørensen LT. Wound healing and infection in surgery: the clinical impact of smoking and smoking cessation: a systematic review and meta-analysis. Arch Surg. 2012;147(4):373–83.
30. Aspenberg P. Drugs and fracture repair. Acta Orthop. 2005;76(6):741–8.
31. Miziak B, Chrościńska-Krawczyk M, Czuczwar SJ. An update on the problem of osteoporosis in people with epilepsy taking antiepileptic drugs. Expert Opin Drug Saf. 2019;18(8):679–89.
32. Dineen PF, Curtin RJ, Harty JA. A review of the use of common antiplatelet agents in orthopaedic practice. J Bone Joint Surg Br. 2010;92(9):1186–91.
33. Flevas DA, Megaloikonomos PD, Dimopoulos L, Mitsiokapa E, Koulouvaris P, Mavrogenis AF. Thromboembolism prophylaxis in orthopaedics: an update. EFORT Open Rev. 2018;3(4):136–48.
34. Soo CG, Della Torre PK, Yolland TJ, Shatwell MA. Clopidogrel and hip fractures, is it safe? A systematic review and meta-analysis. BMC Musculoskelet Disord. 2016;17(1):136.
35. Gustilo RB, Mendoza RM, Williams DN. Problems in the management of type III (severe) open fractures: a new classification of type III open fractures. J Trauma. 1984;24(8):742–6.
36. Orthopaedic trauma association: open fracture study group. A new classification scheme for open fractures. J Orthop Trauma. 2010;24(8):457–64.
37. Zalavras CG, Patzakis MJ, Holtom PD, Sherman R. Management of open fractures. Infect Dis Clin N Am. 2005;19(4):915–29.
38. Hoff WS, Bonadies JA, Cachecho R, Dorlac WC. East practice management guidelines work group: update to practice management guidelines for prophylactic antibiotic use in open fractures. J Trauma Acute Care Surg. 2011;70(3):751–4.
39. Griffin M, Malahias M, Khan W, Hindocha S. Update on the Management of Open Lower Limb Fractures. Open Orthop J. 2012;6:571.
40. Gosselin RA, Roberts I, Gillespie WJ. Antibiotics for preventing infection in open limb fractures. Cochrane Database Syst Rev. 2004;1
41. Obremskey W, Molina C, Collinge C, Nana A, Tornetta P III, Sagi C, Schmidt A, Probe R, Ahn J, Browner BD. Current practice in the management of open fractures among orthopaedic trauma surgeons. Part a: initial management. A survey of orthopaedic trauma surgeons. J Orthop Trauma. 2014;28(8):e198–202.
42. Messner J, Papakostidis C, Giannoudis PV, Kanakaris NK. Duration of administration of antibiotic agents for open fractures: meta-analysis of the existing evidence. Surg Infect. 2017;18(8):854–67.
43. Garner MR, Sethuraman SA, Schade MA, Boateng H. Antibiotic prophylaxis in open fractures: evidence, evolving issues, and recommendations. J Am Acad Orthop Surg. 2020;28(8):309–15.
44. Saveli CC, Belknap RW, Morgan SJ, Price CS. The role of prophylactic antibiotics in open fractures in an era of community-acquired methicillin-resistant Staphylococcus aureus. Orthopedics. 2011;34(8):611–6.
45. Saveli CC, Morgan SJ, Belknap RW, Ross E, Stahel PF, Chaus GW, Hak DJ, Biffl WL, Knepper B, Price CS. Prophylactic antibiotics in open fractures: a pilot randomized clinical safety study. J Orthop Trauma. 2013;27(10):552–7.
46. Tessier JM, Moore B, Putty B, Gandhi RR, Duane TM. Prophylactic gentamicin is not associated with acute kidney injury in patients with open fractures. Surg Infect (Larchmt). 2016;17(6):720–3.
47. Paterson DL, Robson JM, Wagener MM. Risk factors for toxicity in elderly patients given aminoglycosides once daily. J Gen Intern Med. 1998;13(11):735–9.
48. Nanchahal J, Nayagam S, Khan U, Moran C, Barrett S, Sanderson F, Pallister I. Standards for the management of open fractures of the lower limb. British Association of Plastic, Reconstructive and Asthetic Surgeons. Royal Society of Medicine Press Ltd.. http://www.bapras.org.uk/professionals/clinical-guidance/open-fractures-of-the-lower-limb Accessed 13 Apr 20
49. Eckman JJ, Henry SL, Mangino PD, Seligson DA. Wound and serum levels of tobramycin with the prophylactic use of tobramycin-impregnated polymethylmethacrylate beads in compound fractures. Clin Orthop Relat Res. 1988;237:213–5.
50. Moehring HD, Gravel C, Chapman MW, Olson SA. Comparison of antibiotic beads and intravenous antibiotics in open fractures. Clin Orthop Relat Res. 2000;372:254–61.
51. Morgenstern M, Vallejo A, McNally MA, Moriarty TF, Ferguson JY, Nijs S, Metsemakers WJ. The effect of local antibiotic prophylaxis when treating open limb fractures: a systematic review and meta-analysis. Bone Joint Res. 2018;7(7):447–56.
52. Investigators F. A trial of wound irrigation in the initial management of open fracture wounds. N Engl J Med. 2015;373(27):2629–41.
53. Anglen JO. Wound irrigation in musculoskeletal injury. J Am Acad Orthop Surg. 2001;9(4):219–26.
54. Wagner DR, Karnik S, Gunderson ZJ, Nielsen JJ, Fennimore A, Promer HJ, Lowery JW, Loghmani MT, Low PS, McKinley TO, Kacena MA. Dysfunctional stem and progenitor cells impair fracture healing with age. World J Stem Cells. 2019;11(6):281.
55. Kaufman AM, Pensy RA, O'Toole RV, Eglseder WA. Safety of immediate open reduction and internal fixation of geriatric open fractures of the distal radius. Injury. 2014;45(3):534–9.
56. DeLong WG, Born CT, Wei SY, Petrik ME, Ponzio R, Schwab CW. Aggressive treatment of 119 open fracture wounds. J Trauma Acute Care Surg. 1999;46(6):1049–54.

57. Peterson DL, Schuurman M, Geamanu A, Padela MT, Kennedy CJ, Wilkinson J, Vaidya R. Early definitive care is as effective as staged treatment protocols for open ankle fractures caused by rotational mechanisms: a retrospective case control study. J Orthop Trauma. 2020; https://doi.org/10.1097/BOT.0000000000001734.
58. Wijendra A, Alwe R, Lamyman M, Grammatopoulos GA, Kambouroglou G. Low energy open ankle fractures in the elderly: outcome and treatment algorithm. Injury. 2017;48(3):763–9.
59. Armstrong L, Jackson J, Riddick A. Tibiotalocalcaneal nail fixation and soft tissue coverage of Gustilo–Anderson grade 3B open unstable ankle fractures in a frail population; a case series in a major trauma centre. Foot Ankle Surg. 2018;24(4):347–52.
60. Crespo AM, Rautenberg AF, Siev N, Saadeh P, Egol KA. Fibulectomy, tibial shortening, and ankle arthrodesis as an alternative treatment of nonhealing wounds following open ankle fracture in compromised elderly adults. Foot Ankle Int. 2015;36(1):103–7.
61. Ovaska MT, Madanat R, Mäkinen TJ. Predictors of postoperative wound necrosis following primary wound closure of open ankle fractures. Foot Ankle Int. 2016;37(4):401–6.
62. Jenkinson RJ, Kiss A, Johnson S, Stephen DJ, Kreder HJ. Delayed wound closure increases deep-infection rate associated with lower-grade open fractures: a propensity-matched cohort study. J Bone Joint Surg Am. 2014;96(5):380–6.
63. Khadim MF, Emam A, Wright TC, Chapman TW, Khan U. A comparison between the major trauma Centre management of complex open lower limb fractures in children and the elderly. Injury. 2019;50(7):1376–81.
64. Noblet TM, Jackson PC, Foster P, Taylor DM, Harwood PJ, Wiper JD. Managing soft tissues in severe lower limb trauma in an ageing population. Injury. 2018;49(6):1197–202.
65. Serletti JM, Higgins JP, Moran S, Orlando GS. Factors affecting outcome in free-tissue transfer in the elderly. Plast Reconstr Surg. 2000;106(1):66–70.
66. Ekin Y, Günüşen İ, Özdemir ÖY, Tiftikçioğlu YÖ. Effect of coagulation status and co-morbidity on flap success and complications in patients with reconstructed free flap. Turk J Anaesthesiol Reanim. 2019;47(2):98.
67. Xiong L, Gazyakan E, Kremer T, Hernekamp FJ, Harhaus L, Saint-Cyr M, Kneser U, Hirche C. Free flaps for reconstruction of soft tissue defects in lower extremity: a meta-analysis on microsurgical outcome and safety. Microsurgery. 2016;36(6):511–24.
68. Qian Y, Li G, Zang H, Cao S, Liu Y, Yang K, Mu L. A systematic review and meta-analysis of free-style flaps: risk analysis of complications. Plast Reconstr Surg Glob Open. 2018;6(2)
69. Jordan DJ, Malahias M, Hindocha S, Juma A. Suppl 2: M5: flap decisions and options in soft tissue coverage of the lower limb. Open Orthop J. 2014;8:423.
70. Blum ML, Esser M, Richardson M, Paul E, Rosenfeldt FL. Negative pressure wound therapy reduces deep infection rate in open tibial fractures. J Orthop Trauma. 2012;26(9):499–505.
71. Grant-Freemantle MC, Ryan ÉJ, Flynn SO, Moloney DP, Kelly MA, Coveney EI, O'Daly BJ, Quinlan JF. The effectiveness of negative pressure wound therapy versus conventional dressing in the treatment of open fractures: a systematic review and meta-analysis. J Orthop Trauma. 2020;34(5):223–30.
72. Costa ML, Achten J, Bruce J, Davis S, Hennings S, Willett K, Petrou S, Jeffery S, Griffin D, Parker B, Masters J. Negative-pressure wound therapy versus standard dressings for adults with an open lower limb fracture: the WOLLF RCT. Health Technol Assess. 2018;22(73):1.
73. Newton K, Dumville JC, Costa ML, Norman G, Bruce J, Iheozor-Ejiofor Z. Negative pressure wound therapy for open traumatic wounds. Cochrane Database Syst Rev. 2018;2018(7)
74. Geerts WH, Bergqvist D, Pineo GF, Heit JA, Samama CM, Lassen MR, Colwell CW. Prevention of venous thromboembolism: American College of Chest Physicians evidence-based clinical practice guidelines. Chest. 2008;133(6):381S–453S.
75. Falck-Ytter Y, Francis CW, Johanson NA, Curley C, Dahl OE, Schulman S, Ortel TL, Pauker SG, Colwell CW Jr. Prevention of VTE in orthopedic surgery patients: antithrombotic therapy and prevention of thrombosis: American College of Chest Physicians evidence-based clinical practice guidelines. Chest. 2012;141(2):e278S–325S.
76. Fojas MC, Southerland LT, Phieffer LS, Stephens JA, Srivastava T, Ing SW. Compliance to the joint commission proposed Core measure set on osteoporosis-associated fracture: review of different secondary fracture prevention programs in an open medical system from 2010 to 2015. Arch Osteoporos. 2017;12(1):16.
77. Peichl P, Holzer LA, Maier R, Holzer G. Parathyroid hormone 1-84 accelerates fracture-healing in pubic bones of elderly osteoporotic women. J Bone Joint Surg Am. 2011;93(17):1583–7.
78. Elniel AR, Giannoudis PV. Open fractures of the lower extremity: current management and clinical outcomes. EFORT Open. 2018;3(5):316–25.
79. Pagliaro AJ, Michelson JD, Mizel MS. Results of operative fixation of unstable ankle fractures in geriatric patients. Foot Ankle Int. 2001;22(5):399–402.
80. White CB, Turner NS, Lee GC, Haidukewych GJ. Open ankle fractures in patients with diabetes mellitus. Clin Orthop Relat Res. 2003;1(414):37–44.
81. Cozen L. Does diabetes delay fracture healing? Clin Orthop Relat Res. 1972;1(82):134–40.
82. Clement ND, Beauchamp NJ, Duckworth AD, McQueen MM, Court-Brown CM. The outcome of tibial diaphyseal fractures in the elderly. Bone Joint J. 2013;95(9):1255–62.
83. Zura R, Braid-Forbes MJ, Jeray K, Mehta S, Einhorn TA, Watson JT, Della Rocca GJ, Forbes K, Steen

RG. Bone fracture nonunion rate decreases with increasing age: a prospective inception cohort study. Bone. 2017;1(95):26–32.
84. SooHoo NF, Krenek L, Eagan MJ, Gurbani B, Ko CY, Zingmond DS. Complication rates following open reduction and internal fixation of ankle fractures. J Bone Joint Surg Am. 2009;91(5):1042–9.
85. Moran CG, Wenn RT, Sikand M, Taylor AM. Early mortality after hip fracture: is delay before surgery important? J Bone Joint Surg Am. 2005;87(3):483–9.
86. Tampe U, Widmer LW, Weiss RJ, Jansson KÅ. Mortality, risk factors and causes of death in Swedish patients with open tibial fractures-a nationwide study of 3, 777 patients. Scand J Trauma Resusc Emerg Med. 2018;26(1):62.
87. Toole WP, Elliott M, Hankins D, Rosenbaum C, Harris A, Perkins C. Are low-energy open ankle fractures in the elderly the new geriatric hip fracture? J Foot Ankle Surg. 2015;54(2):203–6.

Obesity and the Senior Trauma Patient

31

Douglas Lundy, Sydney E. Burke, and Jennifer L. Bruggers

31.1 Introduction

It is well understood that increased age is a known risk factor in the survival and outcome of trauma patients, and the addition of obesity as a comorbidity certainly complicates the scenario. Even so, studies concerning obesity and trauma provide results that may not be necessarily intuitive, and obesity may ironically be protective to the patient in certain situations. The World Health Organization has defined the various degrees of obesity as follows: not obese (BMI 18.5–29.9 kg/m^2), mild obesity (BMI 30.0–34.9 kg/m^2), moderate obesity (BMI 35.0–39.9 kg/m^2), and severe obesity (BMI $\geq$ 40.0 kg/m^2). Trauma surgeons must understand the impact of obesity on the outcome of their elderly patients, and strategies to mitigate these issues should be deployed.

31.2 Obesity and Trauma

Much has been written regarding the effect of obesity on the injured patient, and obese patients are at greater risk of injury than normal-weight patients. Joseph et al. [1] studied the effect of obesity in patients injured in motor vehicle collisions. They found that patients with morbid obesity were 1.52 times more likely to die in a motor vehicle collision than normal-weight occupants. This effect was identified regardless of whether the patient was restrained or whether the airbags were deployed. Hartka et al. [2] found that due to body habitus, seatbelt restraints tend to displace anteriorly in obese patients. This horizontal, but not vertical positioning of the seat belt, may produce different injury patterns than in normal-weight individuals. Dubois et al. [3] reported interesting findings regarding extremes of body mass index (BMI) and death resulting from motor vehicle collisions. They found that elderly patients (over 85 years of age) with very low BMI (less than 18) as well as those with very high BMI (greater than 42.5) had a significantly increased chance of dying from injuries resulting from a motor vehicle collision compared with a cohort of similar weight individuals who were less than 25 years of age. Ironically, a moderate BMI of 27.5 seemed to have a protective effect for elderly patients compared to their younger counterparts. These studies show that obese patients are at greater risk than normal-weight individuals during motor vehicle collisions, but the manifestations of this influence are variable.

31.3 Obesity and the Elderly Trauma Patient

Obesity seems to have a direct correlation in falls in elderly patients. Several studies examining large databases have demonstrated this connec-

D. Lundy (✉) · S. E. Burke · J. L. Bruggers
St. Luke's University Health Network, Bethlehem, PA, United States
e-mail: douglas.lundy@sluhn.org; jennifer.bruggers@wellstar.org

H.-C. Pape et al. (eds.), *Senior Trauma Patients*, https://doi.org/10.1007/978-3-030-91483-7_31

tion. Neri et al. [4] performed a meta-analysis of 31 manuscripts comprising 1.7 million patients. They found a relative risk of 1.16 that obese older adults would sustain a fall compared to their normal-weight equivalents, and that obese patients were also far more likely to report multiple falls. Interestingly, although the obese patients were at increased risk of falling, there was not a reported concomitant increase in reported injuries from falls in the obese subgroup. Handrigan et al. [5] found a similar correlation, and they studied the rate of falls in different weight subclasses. They found that both underweight (BMI less than 18.5) and obese (BMI more than 30) older Canadians were more likely to fall than their normal and overweight counterparts, and this effect was noted in men more than women. They also identified that only obese men were at more risk in sustaining a fall-related injury compared to their female counterparts. Barry et al. [6] queried the database from the Global Burden of Disease and determined that blunt trauma due to falls was related to an increase in injury in elderly patients, and the blunt trauma sustained from these falls caused an increase in mortality in the elderly population. They did not find an increase in mortality in the obese group compared to the normal-weight group, and they attributed this lack of difference to the high percentage of comorbidities found in both cohorts. These varied findings are frequently seen in studies regarding the effect of obesity in elderly patients, and the intuitive conclusion that obese patients always have poor outcomes is not always supported.

Several studies have also demonstrated the incidence of injury in older patients relative to BMI. Kim et al. [7] screened 300,000 Koreans between the age of 50 and 80 regarding the incidence of a proximal femoral fracture. They found that overweight individuals (men with a BMI between 27.5 and 29.9 and women with a BMI between 25 and 27.4) had the lowest incidence of proximal femoral fracture compared with other subgroups. They found that not only did obese persons have a higher risk of fracture, but underweight patients were at increased risk of fracture as well. Conversely, Zhang et al. [8] reported that underweight nursing home residents were more likely to sustain a proximal femoral fracture than residents who were mildly and moderately-to-severely obese. The literature in general seems to agree that extremely underweight and severely obese patients are at risk for proximal femoral fracture relative to patients with more moderate BMI.

Obesity does affect outcome after an elderly patient sustains an injury. The effect of obesity has been examined in elderly patients who have sustained a proximal femoral fracture. Kosar et al. [9] found that both length of stay after surgery and likelihood of readmission to the hospital were increased in obese patients with a proximal femoral fracture compared to the normal-weight cohort. In fact, they found that as the degree of obesity increased (from mild to moderate to severe), the patients were more likely to be readmitted and have an increased length of stay. Kempegowda et al. [10] found a similar effect in patients who had sustained an intertrochanteric femoral fracture. In their study, obese patients (BMI between 30 and 39.9) were statistically more likely to have post-operative complications including respiratory and electrolyte issues and even sepsis. This effect was magnified in patients with a BMI greater than 40. They also found that the duration of surgery and length of stay was also significantly increased in obese patients. Zajonz and coauthors [11] found obese patients were more likely to develop a perioperative infection after hemiarthroplasty in the treatment of patients with a femoral neck fracture. These studies all agree that obese patients should anticipate longer length of stay, more complications, and higher rates of readmission than their nonobese counterparts.

Obesity affects injured patients in other ways as well. Ssentongo et al. [12] reported a significant degree of hyperglycemia in their geriatric trauma patients. They recognized that hyperglycemia in this elderly obese cohort directly increased the rate of infections, length of stay, and death. Mauck et al. [13] reported that obese patients were more likely to develop chronic pain after a motor vehicle collision than normal-weight patients. They found this effect to be especially true in patients with morbid obesity. In patients sustaining severe traumatic brain injury, Czorlich et al. [14] found that patients with a BMI greater than 35 were statistically more likely to die from their injury, and if they did survive, they were far more likely to have a poor neurological outcome.

31.4 Sarcopenic Obesity

A subset of obesity is defined by sarcopenia which is the relative decrease of muscle mass and strength. Not surprisingly, sarcopenic patients can expect worse outcomes after injury. Follis et al. [15] found that women with sarcopenic obesity had a higher risk of falls, and that this risk was greatest in Hispanic women. Chang and coauthors [16] found that sarcopenia magnified the effect of obesity in terms of outcome in their study of elderly patients. Patients with low paraspinal muscle density and low skeletal muscle index were statistically more likely to have increased hospital length of stay after fracture. They also found that these patients had higher transfusion demands than normal patients. Liao et al. [17] found that augmenting resistance training with protein supplementation effectively increased function in older adults with sarcopenia. In the meta-analysis including 17 randomized controlled trials, they found that the addition of protein supplementation to resistance exercise was more beneficial in obese sarcopenic patients than in those with normal-weight sarcopenia.

31.5 Obesity Paradox

Ironically, the presence of obesity does not always predict poor outcomes in patients with injury, and studies have failed to show a difference in some variables compared with normal-weight cohorts. Childs et al. [18] examined the effect of obesity in their series of patients with fractures. Although obese patients were more likely to suffer acute renal failure, infections, and longer periods in intensive care, they did not find any difference in terms of mortality, pulmonary issues, or the presence of multiple organ failure compared with normal-weight individuals. Rock and coauthors [19] examined the trauma hospital admissions in Detroit over a 9-year period. They found that although obese patients had a longer length of stay, their mortality was no higher than the normal-weight patients. Chen et al. [20] found no difference in the rate of hepatic or splenic injuries between obese and normal-weight patients in their study of solid organ injury in adult patients who sustained blunt trauma.

In terms of a specific injury, other studies have failed to demonstrate a difference between the obese population and normal-weight patients. Thorud et al. [21] found no difference in bone healing between different BMI groups in their study of foot and ankle fractures. Specifically, obese and morbidly obese patients were able to heal their fractures just as well as their normal-weight counterparts. Likewise, Acosta-Olivio et al. [22] examined the effect of obesity on the severity of patients presenting with a distal radial fracture. Their study failed to demonstrate any difference in severity between normal-weight individuals and those with obesity. So, although obesity complicates recovery after injury and increases the likelihood of proximal femoral fractures in the elderly, surgeons cannot always assume that obesity predisposes patients to more severe injuries and complications.

In 2003, Kalantar-Zadeh and coauthors [23] described the "protective" effect of obesity against cardiovascular disease and mortality in their series of dialysis patients. They dubbed this effect as the "obesity paradox", and many other studies have noted that obesity may have a positive influence in certain situations. Modiq et al. [24] found that comorbidity-matched obese patients had a lower mortality rate than other patients in their series of proximal femoral fractures. As noted in previous studies, they found that patients with very low BMI were at higher risk of mortality and failing to return home after fracture if they did survive. Rios-Diaz and coauthors [25] also noted a protective effect of obesity in their series of patients with severe soft tissue infections. They found that obese individuals had a lower mortality rate than normal-weight patients with this disease.

Conversely, Zhang et al. [26] believe that the obesity paradox seen in patients with proximal femoral fractures should be attributed to patient selection rather than a true protective effect. They compared the population of patients with proximal femoral fracture who underwent more urgent surgery with elective hip surgery patients in a nonurgent setting. Regression models demonstrated that although the "obesity paradox" existed in the fractured patients, there was no such protective finding in obese patients undergoing elective hip surgery, and they found that obese patients had a statistical increase in wound infections compared to normal-weight patients. They attributed the phenomenon of the obesity paradox to selection criteria in that surgeons tended to operate on only the healthiest obese patients whereas they would operate on sicker normal-weight patients.

31.6 Best Practices in the Treatment of Injured Elderly Patients with Obesity

Regardless of the conflicting literature regarding obesity in the elderly trauma patient, there is ample evidence that obesity compromises the ability of this already compromised group to recover. Surgeons should strongly consider these strategies to optimize recovery from injury in obese elderly patients:

1. Modified venous thromboembolism (VTE) prophylaxis (modified medications and dosing techniques).
2. Modified oxygenation procedures, adjusted positioning during intubation, and preoperative obstructive sleep apnea (OSA) assessment.
3. Consideration of hypocaloric high-protein diet after critical illness/surgery.
4. Adjustments to avoid surgical site infections and wound complications.

Obesity is a known risk factor in the development of VTE, and these patients present to the trauma center in the "prothrombic" state [27]. This condition is presumed due to enhanced platelet activity, impaired fibrinolysis, and activation of endothelial cells. Because of the decrease in vascularity in adipose tissue, fixed-dose regimens of anticoagulants may be insufficient in this patient group, and weight-based prophylactic treatment may be more effective in preventing VTE. Mechanical prophylaxis should be used in conjunction with chemical prophylaxis, and mechanical methods should not be used alone.

Patients with obesity are well known for presenting with difficult airways and OSA [28]. These patients often desaturate prior to intubation, and their airway can be difficult to manage when they are supine. The patient's end-expiratory volume may be reduced up to 69% after induction due to the decrease in functional reserve capacity [29]. Obese patients often present with OSA, and this condition is often undiagnosed in 10–20% of patients with a BMI greater than 35 [30]. Effective treatment of OSA may decrease pain resulting in lower doses of opioids which can lead to further respiratory failure. Recommendations for treating elderly obese patients include:

- Positioning the patient before intubation in a 30° reverse Trendelenburg position or 25° head-up position can improve preoxygenation.
- Maintaining positive end-expiratory pressure (PEEP) of 10 cm H_2O during preoxygenation increases time of apnea without hypoxemia by average time of 1 min.
- Pre-oxygenate obese patients with high-flow nasal cannula to increase oxygen delivery during apneic period.
- Maintain low tidal volume ventilation after intubation.
- Evaluate patients for OSA by using these screening tools:
  - Snoring, tiredness, observed apnea, high blood pressure (STOP).
  - Body mass index, age, neck circumference, and gender (Bang).

- Avoid postoperative complications and maximize recovery by assessing for OSA before surgery.
- Mitigate OSA in patients with CPAP, BiPAP, or an oral appliance.

Obese patients are disadvantaged from a nutritional standpoint, and they should be optimized to encourage healing. Surgeons should consider a hypocaloric, high-protein diet after surgery to maximize healing. Obese patients lose protein at accelerated rate during critical illness as they consume muscle as fuel source [29]. Clinical outcomes are at least equivalent, if not improved, in patients consuming high-protein hypocaloric feeding than those consuming high-protein eucaloric feeding [30].

Lastly, as noted previously, obese patients are more likely to have wound complications than normal-weight patients. Surgeons should consider weight-based dosing of perioperative antibiotics to ensure adequate coverage. Minimally invasive techniques should be used whenever possible, since tensions on the edges of the wound edges are often increased in obese patients thus causing decreased oxygen supply to the surgical site [28].

References

1. Joseph B, Hadeed S, Haider AA, et al. Obesity and trauma mortality: sizing up the risks in motor vehicle crashes. Obes Res Clin Pract. 2017;11:72–8.
2. Hartka TR, Carr HM, Smith BR, et al. Does obesity affect the position of seat belt loading in occupants involved in real-world motor vehicle collisions? Traffic Inj Prev. 2018;28(Suppl 1):S70–5.
3. Dubois S, Mushquash AR, Weaver R, et al. Age modifies the association between driver's body mass index and death following motor vehicle crashes. Traffic Inj Prev. 2018;19:728–33.
4. Neri SGR, Oliverira JS, Dario AB, et al. Does obesity increase the risk and severity of falls in people aged 60 years and older? A systematic review and meta-analysis of observational studies. J Gerontol A Biol Sci Med Sci. 2020;75:952–60.
5. Handrigan GA, Maltais N, Gagné M, et al. Sex-specific association between obesity and self-reported falls and injuries among community-dwelling Canadians aged 65 and older. Osteoporos Int. 2017;28:483–94.
6. Barry R, Modaressi M, Duran R, et al. The impact of obesity on outcomes in geriatric blunt trauma. Am Surg. 2019;85:188–95.
7. Kim SH, Yi SW, Yi JJ, et al. Association between body mass index and the risk of hip fracture by sex and age: a prospective study. J Bone Miner Res. 2018;33:1603–11.
8. Zhang N, Lu SF, Zhou Y, et al. Body mass index, falls, and hip fractures among nursing home residents. J Gerontol A Biol Sci Med Sci. 2018a;73:1403–9.
9. Kosar CM, Thomas KS, Gozalo PL, et al. Effect of obesity on postacute outcomes of skilled nursing facility residents with hip fracture. J Am Geriatr Soc. 2018;66:1108–14.
10. Kempegowda H, Richard R, Borade A, et al. Obesity is associated with high perioperative complications among surgically treated intertrochanteric fracture of the femur. J Orthop Trauma. 2017;31:352–7.
11. Zajonz D, Brand A, Lycke C. Risk factors for early infection following hemiarthroplasty in elderly patients with a femoral neck fracture. Eur J Trauma Emerg Surg. 2019;45:207–12.
12. Ssentongo A, Ssentongo P, Armen S, et al. Central obesity is a predictor of stress hyperglycemia in critically ill geriatric trauma patients. Curr Dev Nutr. 2019;13(Suppl 1)
13. Mauck MC, Hu J, Sefton C, et al. Obesity increases the risk of chronic pain development after motor vehicle collision. Pain. 2019;160:670–5.
14. Czorlich P, Dreimann M, Emami P. Body mass index >35 as independent predictor of mortality in severe traumatic brain injury. World Neurosurg. 2017;107:515–21.
15. Follis S, Cook A, Bea JW, et al. Association between sarcopenic obesity and falls in multiethnic cohort of postmenopausal women. J Am Geriatr Soc. 2018;66:2314–20.
16. Chang CD, Wu JS, Mhuicheartaigh JN, et al. Effect of sarcopenia on clinical and surgical outcome in elderly patients with proximal femur fracture. Skelet Radiol. 2017;47:771–7.
17. Liao CD, Tsauo JY, Wu YT, et al. Effects of protein supplementation combined with resistance exercise on body composition and physical function in older adults: a systematic review and meta-analysis. Am J Clin Nutr. 2017;106:1078–91.
18. Childs BR, Nahm NJ, Dolenc AJ, Vallier HA. Obesity is associated with more complications and longer hospital stays after orthopaedic trauma. J Orthop Trauma. 2015;29:504–9.
19. Rock K, Hayward RD, Edhavan E. Obesity and hospital outcomes following traumatic injury: associations in 9 years of patient data from a single metropolitan area. Clin Obes. 2019;9(2):e12293.
20. Chen AK, Jeffcoach D, Stivers JC, et al. The impact of obesity on severity of solid organ injury in the adult population at a level I trauma center. Trauma Surg Acute Care Open. 2019;12(1):e000318.

21. Thorud JC, Mortensen S, Thoroud JL, et al. Effect of obesity on bone healing after foot and ankle long bone fractures. J Foot Ankle Surg. 2017;56:258–62.
22. Acosta-Olivo C, Gonzalez-Saldivar JC, Villarreal-Villarreal G, et al. Correlation between obesity and severity of distal radius fractures. Orthop Traumatol Surg Res. 2017;103:199–202.
23. Kalantar-Zadeh K, Block G, Humphreys MH, Kopple JD. Reverse epidemiology of cardiovascular risk factors in maintenance dialysis patients. Kindey Int. 2003;63:793–808.
24. Modiq K, Erdelfelt A, Mellner C, et al. "Obesity paradox" holds true for patients with hip fracture: a registry-based cohort study. J Bone Joint Surg Am. 2019;101:888–95.
25. Rios-Diaz AJ, Lin E, Williams K, et al. The obesity paradox in patients with severe soft tissue infections. Am J Surg. 2017;214:385–9.
26. Zhang JC, Matelski J, Gandhi R, et al. Can patient selection explain the obesity paradox in orthopaedic hip surgery? An analysis of the ACS-NSQIP registry. Clin Orthop Relat Res. 2018b;476:964–73.
27. Freeman AL, Pendleton RC, Rondina MT. Prevention of venous thromboembolism in obesity. Expert Rev Cardiovasc Ther. 2010;8:1711–21.
28. Lang LH, Parekh K, Tsui BYK, Maze M. Perioperative management of the obese surgical patient. Br Med Bull. 2017;124:135–55.
29. Gray S, Dieudonne B. Optimizing care for trauma patients with obesity. Cureus. 2018;10:e3021.
30. Choban P, Dickerson R, Malone A, et al. A.S.P.E.N. clinical guidelines: nutrition support of hospitalized adult patients with obesity. J Parenter Enteral Nut. 2013;37:714–44.

Spinal Fracture in the Elderly

32

Paul A. Anderson

32.1 Introduction

Osteoporosis is the loss of bone mineral density and degraded bone microarchitecture resulting in increased fracture risk. Fractures occur in both the axial and appendicular skeleton with the latter usually associated with falls while the former may be atraumatic. The increased prevalence of osteoporosis in the aging population results in a greater number of elderly patients having fragile spinal fractures, the most common type of fracture. Many injuries are the results of low-energy trauma, although atraumatic fractures and nonclinical fractures are common. Morbidity and mortality of these fractures are similar to that of hip fracture with corresponding cost of treatment and utilization of hospital resources. To maximize outcomes and avoid complications in this frail population spinal fractures in the elderly should be treated with a comprehensive care pathway.

Geriatric spine fractures are distinguished from those in younger patients as they usually result from low-energy trauma such as a ground-level fall or coughing. The fracture patterns are compressive in nature and are stable injuries without neurologic involvement. Neurologic injury occurs when spinal stenosis is preexisting or from retropulsion of bone fragments into the spinal canal. Unlike younger patients, retropulsion can occur late as the fracture collapses over time. Spinal cord injury, although rare, is associated with poor outcome and death in the majority of elderly patients. Osteoporosis is usually a significant causative factor in the development of the fracture and requires assessment and secondary treatment to prevent further fracture in elderly patients.

The purpose of this chapter is to review the epidemiology of geriatric cervical and thoracolumbar fractures. Further, the classification and treatment of the elderly patients with these fractures will be reviewed. Finally, the role of secondary fracture prevention will be emphasized.

32.2 Epidemiology of Osteoporotic Spinal Injuries

In 2015, fragility fractures occur in an estimated 2.3 million people annually in the United States with hip and spine being most prevalent at 14 and 23% respectively [1]. It is estimated that the incidence will increase to 3.2 million over the next two decades [2]. In patients greater than 50 years of age, the 10-year fracture risk of the hip is 0.9% while all fractures are 6.9%, increasing with age and in women [1]. However, spine fractures are underreported as more than half are nonclinical

P. A. Anderson (✉)
Department of Orthopedics Surgery and Rehabilitation, University of Wisconsin UWMF Centennial Bldg, Madison, WI, USA
e-mail: anderson@ortho.wisc.edu

H.-C. Pape et al. (eds.), *Senior Trauma Patients*, https://doi.org/10.1007/978-3-030-91483-7_32

(asymptomatic) and the cervical spine is not included in many analyses. In 2018, Lewicki calculated annual cost of caring for osteoporotics as $57 billion [2].

Secondary fractures are common after an initial osteoporotic fracture. The overall incidence in the Medicare population in the first year is 15% for all initial fracture sites with new fractures occurring most commonly in the hip and spine [1]. For patients with an initial spine fracture, additional fractures occurred in the spine in 6% and elsewhere 9% of cases [1].

32.3 Assessment of the Spine in Geriatric Patients

Geriatric patients require the same comprehensive evaluation protocols as other patients. The geriatric patient presents challenges from preexisting cognitive changes, comorbidities, higher pain tolerance, and degenerative changes that may mimic injury. In addition, fractures may be evident but their acuity may be difficult to discern.

Protocols for the evaluation of the cervical spine in geriatric patients have been established, although in general are not as sensitive as in younger adults [3, 4]. Patients may not have pain but when it is present should prompt radiologic evaluation. Patients with evidence of craniofacial trauma need careful evaluation to rule out cervical spine injury. Palpation of the entire spinal column is performed to determine tenderness, kyphosis and gibbous deformity, or any bruising. Spinal tenderness is an important finding to aid in identification of acuity and is used to determine candidacy for vertebral augmentation. A complete neurologic examination is performed including cranial nerve, motor sensory, and reflexes per the ASIA guidelines [5]. Ambulatory patients should have their height measured using a floor-mounted stadiometer. A loss of 2 cm of height from the last measurement or 4 cm from maximum height suggests osteoporosis and vertebral fracture and is an indication for spinal imaging [6].

Patients with pain, tenderness, evidence of craniofacial trauma, or neurologic deficits require radiographic imaging. To evaluate the cervical spine, CT is recommended. Patients with central cord syndrome or other spinal cord injuries should have MRI. Either biplanar radiographs or CT scan can be used to evaluate thoracolumbar injuries. If a thoracolumbar fracture is present then further evaluation to determine severity and acuity is needed and is best performed by MRI. On MRI, increased signal intensity on T2-weighted or fat-suppressed images should be correlated to the level of pain. However, in some patients, fractures at the thoracolumbar junction may have pain localized in the lower lumbar spine.

In the geriatric patient, assessment of bone quality is important. If CT is available, then opportunistic CT can be used where a region of interest (ROI) is drawn in a vertebral body (L1 if possible) and the mean Hounsfield Unit (HU) measured from the PACS elliptical tool [7]. The mean HU provides an estimate of the bone mineral density. Thresholds have been established that rule in osteoporosis at L1 (HU < 100); and rule out (HU > 150) [7]. Other findings are preexisting erosive changes at C2 that predispose to dens fractures, spinal canal narrowing in the cervical spine (less than 10 mm) confirming spinal stenosis, and healing status to determine fracture acuity. Patients at risk of vertebral artery injury such as vertebral displacement or fractures in proximity to the vertebral arteries are assessed using CT angiography.

32.4 Cervical Spine Fractures in the Elderly

The incidence of cervical spine fractures in geriatric patients is increasing 3.5 times faster than the population in general [8]. In geriatric patients, cervical spine injuries have a 1-year mortality of 24% and in those with spinal cord injuries a mortality of up to 44% [9]. Further, geriatric patients returned home after injury in one-third of cases [10].

Falls are the most common mechanism of cervical spine injuries in older patients, occurring in up to 75% of cases. Because of kyphotic posture and the head tilting forward, the face and forehead often hit the ground first creating a hypertension injury to the cervical spine. The hyperextension is often focused at C2 resulting in an odontoid fracture or Hangman's type fracture, the most common injury types. Also, hyperextension can transiently result in spinal cord compression due to a pincer mechanism between infolded ligamentum flava and bulging disc annulus or osteophyte. This becomes critical due to preexisting spinal canal narrowing from degenerative changes and clinically can result in a central cord injury. This spinal cord injury is characterized by more profound weakness of upper extremities than the lower extremities.

Although geriatric patients can have cervical spine injuries typical of other adults, this review will focus on those particular to the older population. The most common cervical spine injuries are of C2 and, in particular, odontoid fractures. In over 50% of patients, there are preexisting erosive changes from degeneration that predispose to fractures, Fig. 32.1a–c [11]. In some cases, the age of the fracture will be difficult to discern. These fractures are unstable, although spinal cord injury is uncommon. Displacement will usually be posterior which is also increased when the patient lies supine due to thoracic kyphosis and the head alignment forward creates a large gap between the occiput and bed/pillow.

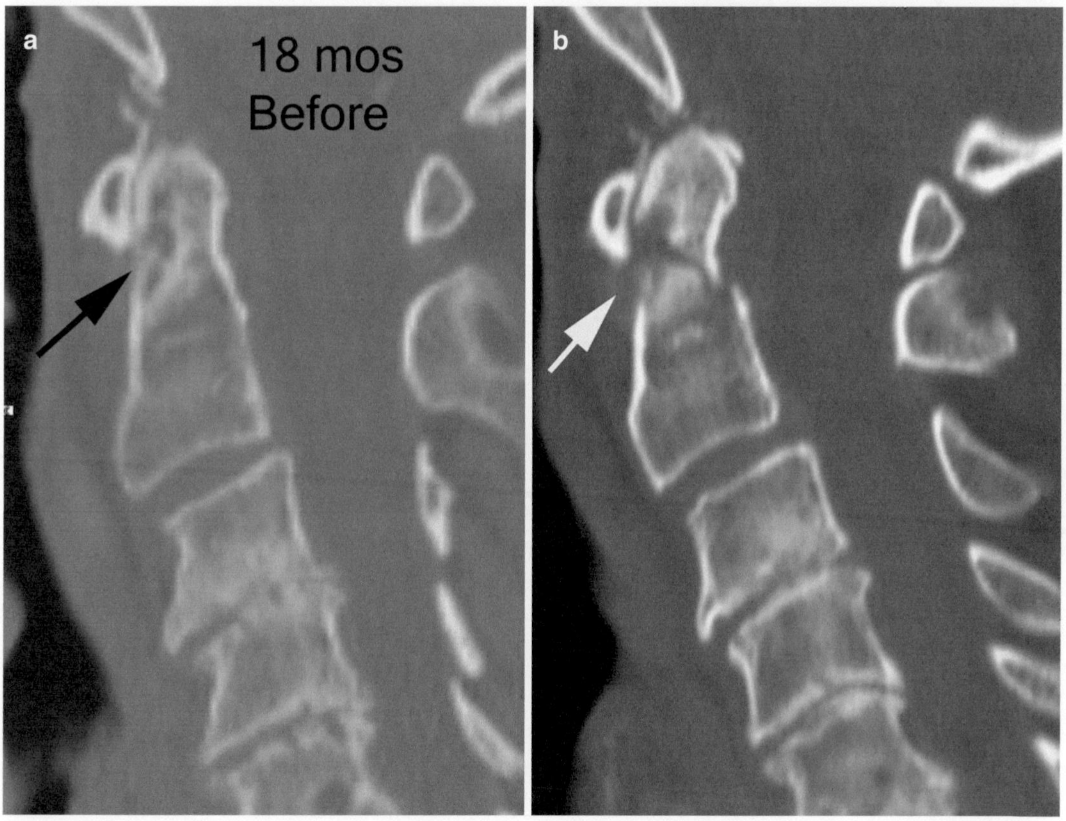

Fig. 32.1 (**a**) A 79-year-old male with significant cognitive changes following stroke who had CT angiogram 18 months before sustaining a fall. The odontoid process is intact but there is significant cystic erosion anteriorly (arrow). (**b**) He presented to emergency room after a fall complaining of neck pain. CT shows and a Type 2 posterior angulated odontoid process fracture (arrow). He was treated nonoperatively in soft collar. (**c**) One year later, he had a head CT to evaluate cognitive changes that shows an odontoid fracture nonunion (arrow). He had no neck pain and no neurologic findings that were felt to be from the odontoid fracture. No treatment for his C2 fracture was recommended

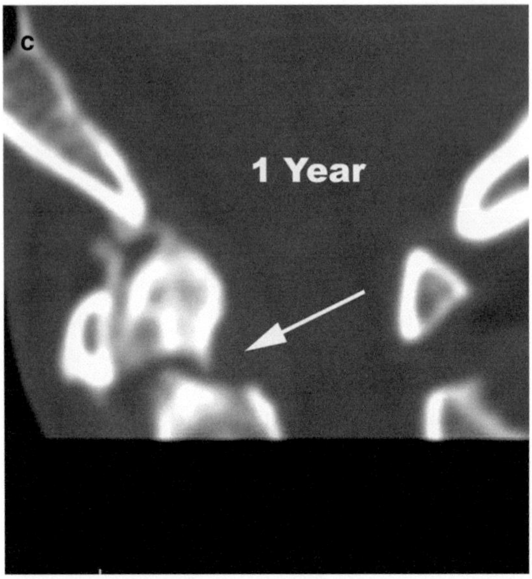

Fig. 32.1 (continued)

32.4.1 Odontoid Fractures

Odontoid fractures are classified as: Type 1 located at the dens tip and associated with alar ligament disruption; Type 2 through the odontoid waist rostral to the atlantoaxial articulation; and Type 3 that extend into the body. These may be associated with other cervical injuries, most commonly a posterior arch fracture of the atlas.

The treatment of Type 1 odontoid fractures is conservative with a collar unless associated with craniocervical disassociation which is treated by occipital cervical fusion [12]. The Type 3 fracture has a good prognosis being in trabecular bone and is also initially treated nonoperatively in a collar [12]. After patient mobilization, an upright radiograph is checked to assure maintenance of alignment. If proven to be unstable then posterior C1-2 fusion can be considered.

The treatment of geriatric Type 2 odontoid fractures remains controversial. A multicenter observational study evaluated 322 geriatric patients with odontoid fracture found a 14% morality rate at 30 days, 18% at 12 months, and by 2 years 44% had died [13]. Surgical treatment was associated with a lower mortality but selection bias may have been present. In the 50 patients treated initially nonoperatively, 22% developed nonunion of whom two-thirds subsequently had surgery [14]. However, no patient treated nonoperatively had late neurologic deterioration. Functional outcomes were better in the operatively compared to nonoperatively treated patients [15].

For geriatric patients with Type 2 odontoid fractures, the author recommends nonoperative treatment for those with severe cognitive disorders, non-displaced fractures, and age indeterminate fractures, Fig. 32.1a–c. The treatment goals should be rapid mobilization and avoidance of complications related to treatment, not necessarily to obtain fracture healing. Decubitus ulcers are prevented by careful fitting of orthosis, proper education, or the use of soft collar instead of any more rigid orthosis altogether. Cognitively-impaired individuals are at greatest risk for skin breakdown. Aspiration is common due to immobilization in an orthosis, retropharyngeal swelling from the fracture, poor gag reflex, and the use of opioid medications. We recommend a swallow evaluation for these patients before allowing feeding. The use of a halo-vest should be avoided in the geriatric patient [16].

Geriatric patients with Type 2 odontoid fractures who are active and have displacement are considered surgical candidates. The authors recommend a posterior C1-2 fusion with rigid instrumentation such as C1-2 transarticular screws or C1 lateral mass-C2 pedicle screws constructs. Careful evaluation of the location of the vertebral artery is recommended when planning surgery to avoid iatrogenic injury. Postoperatively, patients should be rapidly mobilized with as little immobilization as practicable. Odontoid screw fixation is contraindicated as this is associated with greater mortality and potential loss of fixation.

32.4.2 Central Cord Syndrome

Older patients develop loss of disc height, osteophyte formation, and thickening and infolding of the ligamentum flava which all reduce the cros-sectional area of the spinal canal. Transient hyperextension can then cause a pincer force on the cord causing a spinal cord injury. The most common manifestation is a central cord syndrome where the more central aspect of the cord containing the gray matter and the more centrally located white matter tracts to the upper extremities are affected to a greater degree than the lower extremity tracts [17]. Clinically, patients have worse upper extremity than lower extremity function although the clinical deficits can vary considerably. The prognosis of these injuries is generally thought to be good with the return of walking ability in over 85% of cases although hand function may remain poor [17]. However, older patients improve less than younger patients.

CT may not show any evidence of injury although degenerative changes and narrowing of the spinal canal may be present, Fig. 32.2a. The midsagittal diameter between the disc space and ligamentum flavum when <10 mm indicates spinal stenosis. Fractures to the posterior elements such as lamina, lateral mass, and spinous process can be present, as well as avulsion fractures of the anterior vertebral bodies. Displacement is less common but is usually a retrolisthesis consistent with hyperextension mechanism. An MRI is indicated and will show spinal stenosis at one or multiple levels, swelling of the spinal cord, and spinal cord signal changes consistent with contusion or edema, Fig. 32.2b.

The initial treatment of central cord syndrome in geriatric patients should be resuscitation and in particular, maintaining a high oxygen saturation and mean arterial pressure to minimum 85 mmHg [18]. This is continued for 7 days and may require pressor and intensive care unit admission. The

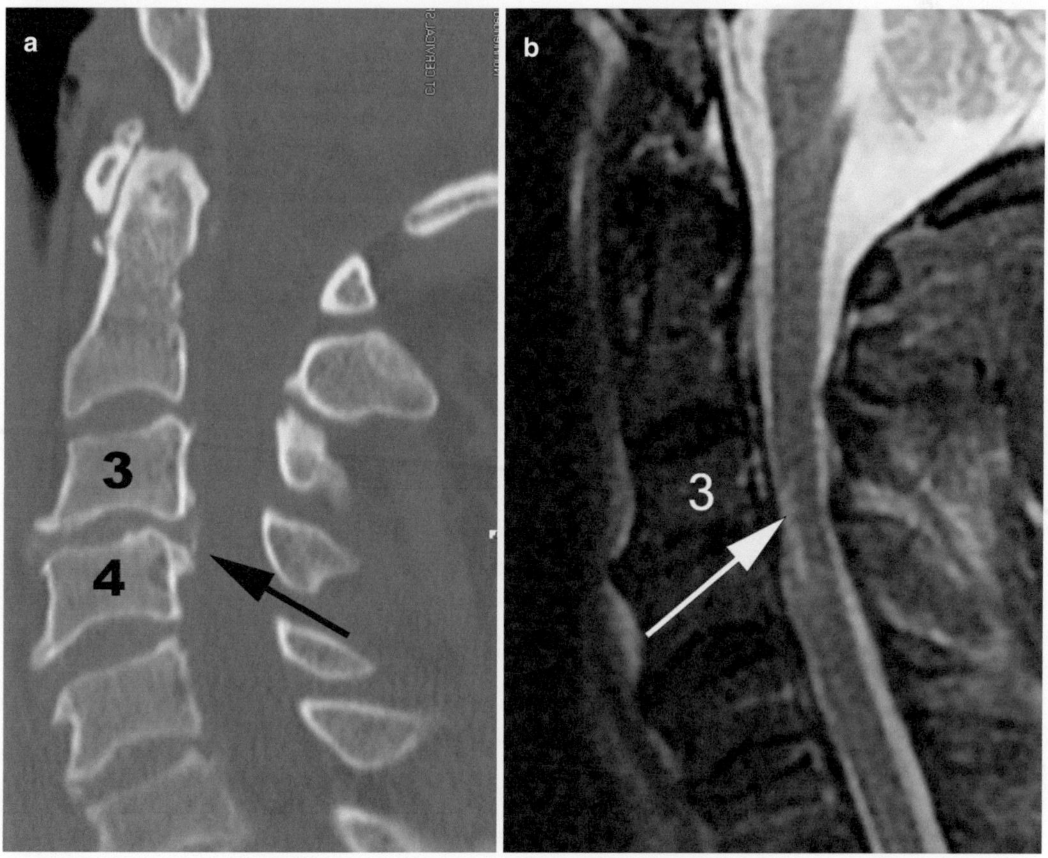

Fig. 32.2 (**a**) A 67-year-old female had a ground-level fall and presented with a central cord syndrome. Her lower extremities had Grade 3-4 motor function, there was no hand function and Grade 2 motor function in deltoid and biceps muscles. The sagittal CT shows no fracture or subluxation. There is ossification of the posterior longitudinal ligament at C3-4 (arrow)and a narrow spinal canal. (**b**) T2 fat-suppressed MRI demonstrates spinal stenosis with increased signal at C3-4 in the anterior aspect of the cord. (**c**) Postoperative lateral radiograph after laminoplasty C3-C6 and reconstruction with plates. (**d**) T2 MRI one year after injury showing bright cord signal changes at C3-4 but resolution of spinal stenosis. She had made significant neurologic recovery except in hands but is living independently

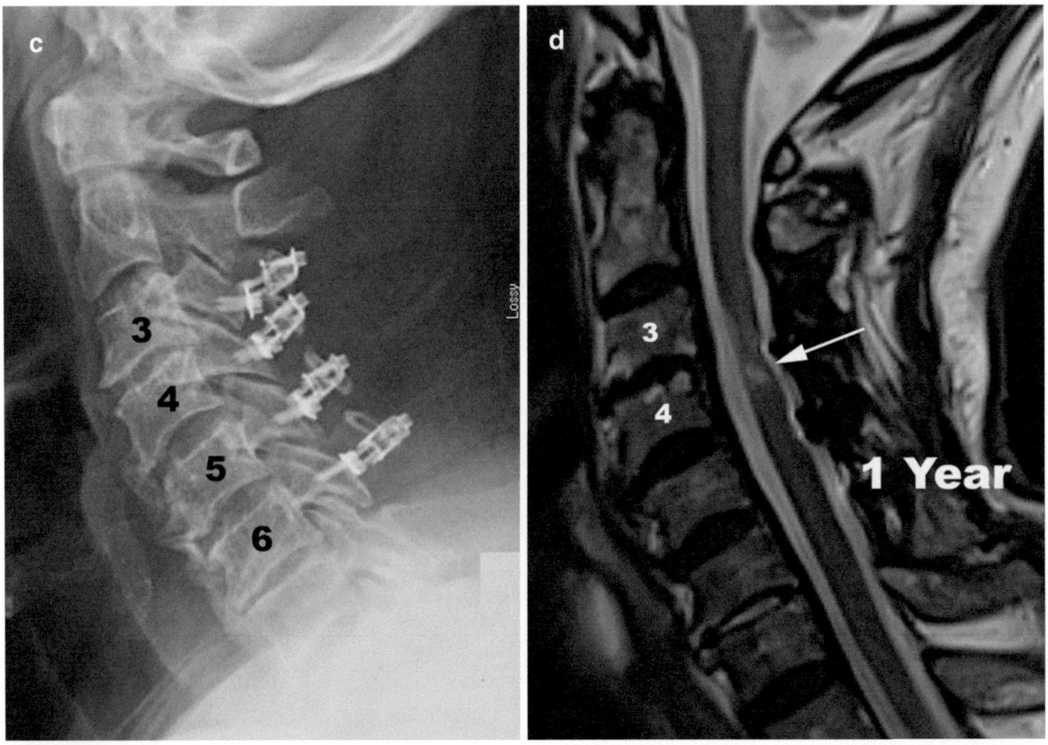

Fig. 32.2 (continued)

role of methylprednisolone in geriatric patients and spinal cord injury remains controversial. Methylprednisolone increases mortality risk in geriatric patients and efficacy has been shown to be only minimal and therefore should be used with caution and only in individuals without other injures or comorbidities [18].

The role of surgery remains controversial. Initially, the prognosis was felt to be excellent and that surgery was not likely to improve outcomes and could be harmful. However, more recently, excellent outcomes in central cord syndrome have been reported with surgical treatment [17–19]. Clear indications for surgery are unstable and/or displaced injuries. Further, patients making rapid recovery and those without ongoing spinal cord compression are best treated initially nonoperatively. Patients with significant deficits and ongoing compression appear to benefit from surgical decompression, Fig. 32.2c, d. The surgical approach varies depending upon pathology, number of levels involved, and presence of any fractures or ligamentous injuries. The authors recommend patients with 1–2 segments of ventral compression undergo an anterior decompression and fusion. In the more common situation of multilevel stenosis, a laminoplasty can be performed. There is no consensus regarding the timing of surgery in the management of central cord syndromes. In a recent narrative review, Divi noted that while strong evidence is insufficient they recommend surgery be performed within 24 h in patients with ongoing cord compression [19].

32.5 Thoracolumbar Fractures

The most common osteoporotic fracture occurs in the thoracolumbar spine, only one-third of which are clinically evident. The consequences of a clinical thoracolumbar fracture are similar to hip fracture with mortality rates up to 25% at 1 year and only 30% of Medicare patients surviving at 5 years [1]. Chen also reported that thoracolumbar compression fractures were associated with a diminution of independent living with fewer than half of patients living at home [20]. In addition, at 6 months pain was still significant and fear of further pain and loss of independence became dominant [21].

Unlike cervical and other fragility fractures, thoracolumbar spine fractures may occur spontaneously without an injury or from lifting, coughing, or Valsalva. The resultant forces cause anterior compression and fracture. The fractures are usually described as compression fractures, which imply loss of vertebral body height and wedging of the vertebrae. Less common is a burst fracture where the posterior vertebral body wall is retropulsed into the spinal canal causing spinal stenosis, Fig. 32.3a. This can occur over time as the vertebral body collapses. Other fracture variants are the pincer fracture where the cranial caudal disc herniated into the intervening vertebral body splitting it into two pieces. Occasionally, clefts will develop likely from the disc or nonunion. Stability, the ability to withstand physiologic loads, is most often maintained after compression fractures although should be assessed by upright radiographs [22]. If significant collapse or kyphotic deformity develops, then the fracture is unstable and may be a candidate for an intervention. Genant has provided a classification based on severity of fracture that is useful for epidemiologic purposes but does not aid in clinical care [6].

32.6 Treatment of Thoracolumbar Osteoporotic Vertebral Fractures

32.6.1 Nonoperative Treatment of Vertebral Fractures

The majority of patients with thoracolumbar osteoporotic compression fractures can be treated nonoperatively (Table 32.1). In fact, two-thirds of

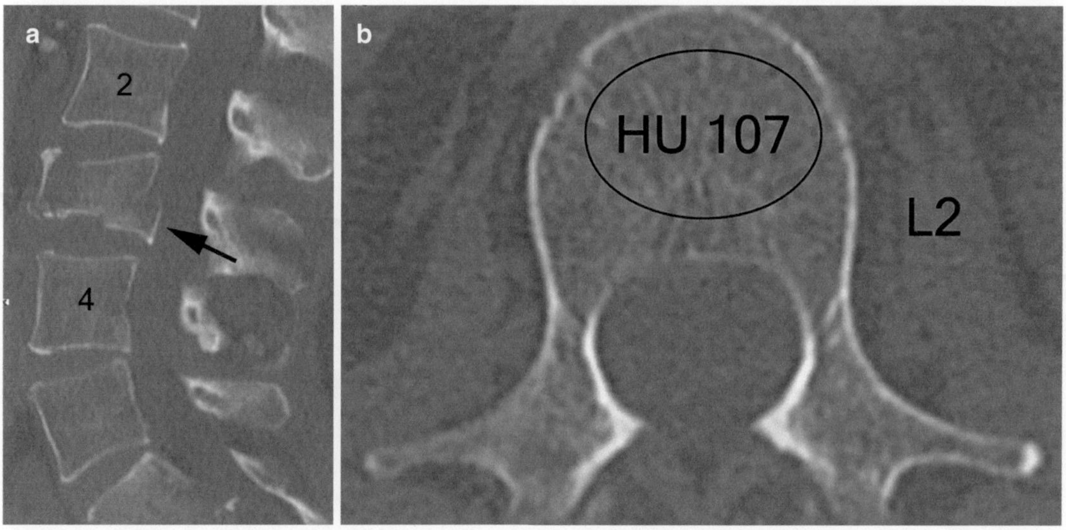

Fig. 32.3 (**a**) A Sagittal CT of 68 year-old female showing L3 burst fracture following a fall. She has history of steroid use and osteopenia. The arrow indicates retropulsed bone from posterior inferior body of L3. (**b**) Axial CT at L2 above her fracture. The mean Hounsfield Unit (HU) in the region of interest (Oval) was 107 indicating likely osteoporosis. (**c**) At 3 months follow-up, she is doing poorly with increasing back and leg pain. Lateral radiograph shows further collapse and increased retropulsion of bone into spinal canal at L3. (**d**) Sagittal T2 MRI at 3 months confirming retropulsion of bone into spinal canal at L3 (arrow). (**e**) Lateral radiograph 1 year after minimally invasive corpectomy L3 and reconstruction with expandable cage from L2 to L4 and second-stage posterior pedicle screw instrumentation. The pedicle screws were augmented with bone cement. (**f**) Anterior posterior radiography one year after surgery

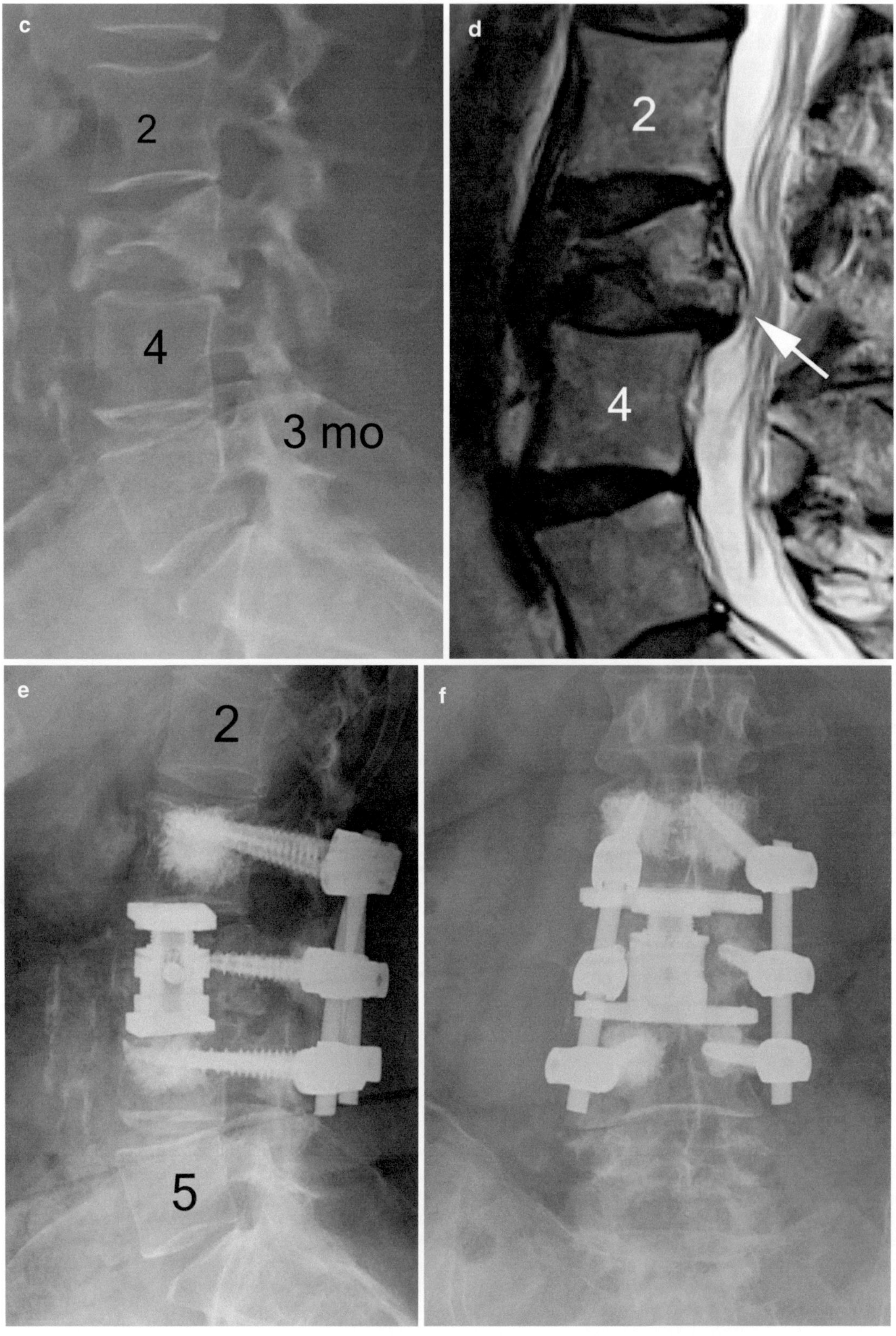

Fig. 32.3 (continued)

Table 32.1 Management options for elderly patients with spinal fractures

Treatment	Method	Alternative method
Observation	Serial radiographs	No further imaging
Pain control	Minimize use of opioids	Consider advanced pain control methods
Physical therapy	Short-term mobilization, body mechanics, extension exercises	Long-term strength, impact loading, fall prevention
Orthotic management	Limited benefit Poor tolerance	Avoidance or surgery
Advance pain management	Facet blocks/epidural injections	Rhizotomy
Cement augmentation	Vertebroplasty	Kyphoplasty
Surgical treatment	Stabilization/instrumentation	Decompression and stabilization
Secondary fracture prevention	Fracture liaison services such as own the bone	Primary care

fractures are not even clinically evident although their presence indicates a likelihood of osteoporosis. The goal of treatment is to allow immediate mobilization, improve body mechanics (avoid flexion as much as possible), reduce fall risk, and manage pain. In addition, secondary fracture prevention should be provided.

The authors recommend that stability be assessed in acute fractures by simply obtaining an upright radiograph and measuring angular deformity of the injured segment and comparing to supine images such as CT or MRI if available [22]. This will provide an index of how much instability is present. Patients with minimal collapse are excellent candidates for nonoperative treatment. In hospitalized patients, physical and occupational therapy should be consulted to aid patient mobilization, educate regarding protective body mechanics, assess fall risk, and instruct patients in activities of daily living. A home physical therapy visit after discharge should be considered to assess safety. Exercise is important after osteoporotic vertebral fracture. In a systematic review, Ebling found that exercise had positive effects on mobility, balance, back extensor strength, and may improve pain [23]. No recommendations can be made on a specific type of exercise and will likely be dependent upon individual patient preferences and needs.

Pain control is often a major patient concern. It is best to use multimodal pain management. Opioids should be used judiciously to avoid complications, addiction, and mental status changes. Further, opioids significantly increase the likelihood of future falls.

Bracing is often utilized, although efficacy for management of thoracolumbar compression fractures is lacking. In a randomized control trial comparing no brace, a soft brace, and a rigid orthosis, Kim found no difference in pain, function, and radiographic findings [24]. Similarly, Li found no differences between a custom TLSO and lumbosacral corset [25]. This is consistent with the findings of Bailey that found no differences in any outcome parameter from orthotic treatment of burst fractures (more severe injury) between orthosis and no orthosis [26]. However, Merraciello found that the Spinomed dynamic brace had greater improvement in pain and function than a rigid 3-point brace [27]. Bracing is, in general, poorly tolerated in geriatric patients, reduces mobilization, and has poor compliance and satisfaction. Given questionable efficacy, the author does not routinely use this modality.

32.6.2 Cement Augmentation

Cement augmentation is the installation of a biomaterial, most commonly polymethylmethacrylate (PMMA), to stiffen the fractured vertebrae. Two methods are available vertebroplasty and kyphoplasty. In vertebroplasty, the patient is positioned prone thereby obtaining some postural reduction, and a 12–14-gauge needle is placed transpedicular into the vertebral body and cement is inserted. Kyphoplasty uses a larger cannula placed transpedicular and then reduction is obtained positionally by use of an expandable balloon and cement is then inserted. Both procedures can be done under local anesthesia. In both cases cement polymerizes quickly and there is often rapid improvement and no specific postoperative care or bracing is required.

Controversy exists over the effectiveness of cement augmentation. Multiple randomized clinical trials have been performed comparing outcomes of cement augmentation to nonoperative treatment or sham surgery; however, they report conflicting results [23]. Most of the conflicts reflect differences in control arms with sham-controlled trials showing no or less benefit from cement augmentation. A recent guideline based on a meta-analysis using the sham control studies thus recommended against using vertebroplasty [23]. However, the methodology used to formulate this guideline has been contraindicated [28]. The sham control was a local anesthetic injection down to the periosteum which itself has been shown to be an active treatment. Further numerous flaws in the selected studies were present such as investigator bias, inadequate sample size, lack of consistency of diagnosis, long enrollment periods (averaging over 4 years), enrollment greater than 6 months after fracture, and crossover when sham patients obtain vertebroplasty but for statistical purposes remain in the sham group [29]. In another meta-analysis, Beall reported the opposite results [30]. Balloon kyphoplasty and vertebroplasty had greater pain and functional improvement than nonsurgical management. Although both techniques were associated with higher secondary fracture rate, this was not statistically significant.

A multidisciplinary panel of experts utilized the RAND method to develop a clinical care pathway for the use of cement augmentation based on best available evidence [31]. The panel identified common signs and symptoms and recommended use of advanced imaging such as MRI. Cement augmentation was recommended in patients with persistent symptoms who had two to four unfavorable findings: progression of height loss, severe impact on function, kyphotic deformity, and >25% vertebral height reduction. In addition, the panel recommended all patients receive secondary fracture prevention.

32.6.3 Indications for Cement Augmentation

The indications for cement augmentation are persistent severe pain, unable to mobilize or care for oneself, progressive collapse, spinal instability between supine images and upright radiographs, or a nonunion or cleft in the vertebral body. The timing of intervention in relation to the onset of symptoms or fracture remains controversial. In general, a short period (2–3 weeks) of nonoperative treatment should be attempted if the patient can be mobilized and be cared for at home. However, in hospitalized patients or patients who are failing to care for themselves at home, cement augmentation has been shown to be highly effective with rapid improvement and early discharge.

32.6.4 Technique

Both procedures are done in the prone position either on special tables (Jackson) or by rolls and pillows. Traditionally the procedure can be done under local anesthesia, although in some patients, conscious sedation may be required. Achieving spine extension by judicious use of pillows and rolls can aid fracture reduction and improve alignment. For lumbar vertebrae, a transpedicular approach is used. For thoracic spine, depending on the pedicle size, a transpedicular or paraspinal approach is used [32]. Under biplanar fluoroscopic imaging the starting point for needle placement is identified and local anesthesia down to the periosteum is placed. An 11-gauge Jamshidi needle is then placed onto the lateral edge of the pedicle on the anteroposterior image at its midpoint vertically. The needle is advanced to the posterior vertebral body checking both anteroposterior and lateral images. When the needle is just entering the body the tip should be within or just at the medial edge of the pedicle. Depending on where the fracture is located the needle can be advanced either caudally or cranially into the anterior third of the vertebral body. In most cases bilateral approaches will be used; however, some practitioners may use only a unilateral approach. A recent meta-analysis showed no differences between unilateral and bilateral approaches if at least 4 cc of cement was injected [33]. Liquid PMMA cement is instilled under biplanar fluoroscopic control carefully assessing vertebral body fill and watching for extravasation. The most common sites of extravasation are into the intervertebral disc or into veins and subsequently the vena cava. Most important is to stop cement installation if the cement is tracking posteriorly toward the spinal canal. Best results are obtained when 3–4 cc are used per side and the cement interdigitates into native bone.

In kyphoplasty, a balloon (or more recently other devices) is inserted into the vertebral body which is expanded, thus reducing height loss and correcting kyphosis. The procedure uses a larger cannula than vertebroplasty and is more expensive. Once the vertebra is expanded a cavity has been created that is filled with cement. Because of the use of a larger cannula and creation of a cavity, more viscous cement can be placed with less tendency for extravasation. Clinical results are equal or better than vertebroplasty [34]. Overall small improvements in kyphotic alignments and vertebral body expansion are achieved, although the clinical significance is unknown.

32.6.5 Complications of Cement Augmentation

Complications from cement augmentation are rare with few reported cases of neurologic deficits. In fact, in the ASBMR clinical review, the only case of paraplegia was in an untreated patient [23]. Extravasation can be seen in up to 40% of cases but is rarely clinically significant except when it occurs intradiscally and may be associated with junctional fracture of the next vertebrae [35, 36]. Overall, new fractures occur slightly more frequently but not statistically significantly after cement augmentation.

32.6.6 Surgical Treatment of Osteoporotic Thoracolumbar Fractures

Most patients with osteoporotic fractures do not require surgery since neurologic compromise is rare, and bone quality with patient frailty precludes major spine reconstructions. Thus, only case series involving selected patients with specific indications are reported. The surgical indications are neurologic deficits with spinal canal narrowing, progressive spinal deformity localized to a few segments, and correction of sagittal plane imbalance. Prior to surgery unless an emergency condition, patients should undergo medical and bone health optimization. The latter is similar to the program for secondary fracture prevention includes diagnostic testing, screening for secondary causes of osteoporosis, correction of nutritional deficiencies, and if warranted anti-osteoporotic medication [37]. The authors prefer an anabolic agent for this purpose. Correction of osteoporosis unless dictated by urgency should be for 3–4 months or longer for more complex surgeries such multilevel osteotomies. Insufficient treatment of the osteoporosis will likely lead to further failure and revision surgery.

Thoracolumbar osteoporotic burst fractures can be treated with anterior corpectomy, insertion of cage, and supplemental posterior fixation. Less invasive techniques that use transpsoas approach to the vertebral body and percutaneous screws are appealing in this frail population, Fig. 32.3a–f. Alternatives are posterior instrumentation and decompression, or balloon kyphoplasty combined with posterior instrumentation [38, 39]. In addition cement augmentation of pedicle screws can be used. Sudo reported excellent neurologic recovery and maintenance of alignment in 21 patients treated with posterior decompression and fusion [39]. Marco noted improvement in all patients with neurologic deficits who were treated with balloon kyphoplasty and posterior instrumentation [38]. In patients with multilevel compression fractures with progressive deformity the authors have performed percutaneous posterior instrumentation without fusion successfully. An additional surgery to remove the hardware is required 6–12 months later.

The treatment of osteoporotic-related spinal deformity is complex and associated with significant morbidity and mortality [40]. Usually one or more osteotomies will be required along with multiterminal fixation [41]. Unfortunately fractures at either end of construct in up to 80% of cases [42]. Suh compared two-stage anterior posterior instrumentation to closing wedge posterior osteotomy and found better results with the latter technique although this was technically demanding [43].

32.7 Secondary Fracture Prevention

The goal of secondary fracture prevention is to prevent further fracture that can result in greater morbidity and mortality. The 12-month incidence of a secondary fracture after an initial spine fracture is 15%, with few patients receiving secondary fracture prevention. Barton found that in vertebral fracture patients presenting to the emergency room only 2% had a DXA 2 years before or within 1 year after fracture. Anti-osteoporotic therapy was started in only 7% of patients while the refracture rate was 36% within 2 years.

The initial fracture provides a teaching or sentinel event so that changes can occur to prevent further fracture. This program is called Secondary fracture prevention or fracture liaison service (FLS) [44]. The FLS is a comprehensive program that identifies patients with fragility fractures, provides education, and communication with other providers. Most importantly patients are evaluated for bone status usually with a DXA, screened for secondary cause of osteoporosis, recommended to eliminate toxins such as excessive alcohol intake and smoking, assess fall risk and suggest exercise programs for increase loading and improve muscle strength and reduce fall risk. Nutritional deficits are corrected. Medications if indicated by current guidelines are offered [6, 45]. The American Orthopedic association has developed a comprehensive program that can be adopted that encourages practitioners to take ownership of osteoporosis after fracture and that assures patients receive secondary fracture care [46].

Secondary fracture programs are highly effective and significantly reduce the cost of caring for additional fractures [1]. Wasfie compared refracture rate after spinal fracture before and after instituting a FLS [47]. Refracture at 24 months was reduced from 56% to 37%. Bawa utilized a Medicare database and found that only 10.6% of beneficiaries received anti-osteoporotic medication after fracture; however, this reduced secondary fracture risk by 40% [48]. Beall has shown that teriparatide administration significantly reduces secondary fractures after cement augmentation [49].

32.8 Conclusion

Elderly patients with spinal fractures have similar outcomes to those with hip fracture, including risk of mortality, loss of independence, and destitution. Further, patients become fearful of reoccurrence and lose social interactions. Two cervical injury patterns are seen frequently: odontoid fractures and central cord syndrome. Controversies regarding treatment remain despite large observational trials. Thoracolumbar fragility fractures indicate that patients have osteoporosis and are usually initially treated nonoperatively. Cement augmentation appears useful but is controversial for those who are suffering pain and disability. Surgical treatment is needed rarely and requires preoperative medical and bone optimization as complications are frequent. Finally, all geriatric patients with spinal fractures should receive secondary fracture prevention.

References

1. Hansen D, Bazell C, Pellzzari P, Pyenson B. Milliman Research Report. Medicare cost of osteoporotic fractures. The clinical and cost burden of an important consequence of osteoporosis 2019;2019.
2. Lewiecki EM, Wright NC, Curtis JR, et al. Hip fracture trends in the United States, 2002 to 2015. Osteoporosis Int. 2018;29:717–22.
3. Schoenfeld AJ, Beck AW, Harris MB, Anderson PA. Evaluating the cervical spine in the blunt trauma patient. J Am Acad Orthop Surg. 2019;27:633–41.
4. Goode T, Young A, Wilson SP, Katzen J, Wolfe LG, Duane TM. Evaluation of cervical spine fracture in the elderly: can we trust our physical examination? Am Surg. 2014;80:182–4.
5. Kirshblum SC, Waring W, Biering-Sorensen F, et al. Reference for the 2011 revision of the international standards for neurological classification of spinal cord injury. J Spinal Cord Med. 2011;34:547–54.
6. Cosman F, de Beur SJ, LeBoff MS, et al. Clinician's guide to prevention and treatment of osteoporosis. Osteoporos Int. 2014;25:2359–81.
7. Anderson PA, Polly DW, Binkley NC, Pickhardt PJ. Clinical use of opportunistic computed tomography screening for osteoporosis. J Bone Joint Surg Am. 2018;100:2073–81.
8. Zusman NL, Ching AC, Hart RA, Yoo JU. Incidence of second cervical vertebral fractures far surpassed the rate predicted by the changing age distribution and growth among elderly persons in the United States (2005–2008). Spine. 2013;38:752–6.
9. Keller JM, Sciadini MF, Sinclair E, O'Toole RV. Geriatric trauma: demographics, injuries, and mortality. J Orthop Trauma. 2012;26:e161–5.
10. Damadi AA, Saxe AW, Fath JJ, Apelgren KN. Cervical spine fractures in patients 65 years or older: a 3-year experience at a level I trauma center. J Trauma. 2008;64:745–8.
11. Shinseki MS, Zusman NL, Hiratzka J, Marshall LM, Yoo JU. Association between advanced degenerative changes of the atlanto-dens joint and presence of dens fracture. J Bone Joint Surg Am. 2014;96:712–7.
12. Ryken TC, Hadley MN, Aarabi B, et al. Management of isolated fractures of the axis in adults. Neurosurgery. 2013;72(Suppl. 2):132–50.
13. Chapman J, Smith JS, Kopjar B, et al. The AOSpine North America geriatric odontoid fracture mortality study: a retrospective review of mortality outcomes for operative versus nonoperative treatment of 322 patients with long-term follow-up. Spine. 2013;38:1098–104.
14. Smith JS, Kepler CK, Kopjar B, et al. Effect of type II odontoid fracture nonunion on outcome among elderly patients treated without surgery: based on the AO Spine North America geriatric odontoid fracture study. Spine. 2013;38:2240–6.
15. Vaccaro AR, Kepler CK, Kopjar B, et al. Functional and quality-of-life outcomes in geriatric patients with type-II dens fracture. J Bone Joint Surg Am. 2013;95:729–35.
16. Harrop JS, Hart R, Anderson PA. Optimal treatment for odontoid fractures in the elderly. Spine. 2010;35:S219–27.
17. Brooks NP. Central cord syndrome. Neurosurg Clin N Am. 2017;28:41–7.
18. Fehlings MG, Tetreault LA, Wilson JR, et al. A clinical practice guideline for the Management of Patients with Acute Spinal Cord Injury and Central Cord Syndrome: recommendations on the timing (≤24 hours versus >24 hours) of decompressive surgery. Global Spine J. 2017;7:195s–202s.
19. Divi SN, Schroeder GD, Mangan JJ, et al. Management of Acute Traumatic Central Cord Syndrome: a narrative review. Global Spine J. 2019;9:89s–97s.
20. Chen AT, Cohen DB, Skolasky RL. Impact of nonoperative treatment, vertebroplasty, and kyphoplasty on survival and morbidity after vertebral compression fracture in the medicare population. J Bone Joint Surg Am. 2013;95:1729–36.
21. Svensson HK, Olofsson EH, Karlsson J, Hansson T, Olsson LE. A painful, never ending story: older women's experiences of living with an osteoporotic vertebral compression fracture. Osteoporos Int. 2016;27:1729–36.
22. Chen YJ, Lo DF, Chang CH, Chen HT, Hsu HC. The value of dynamic radiographs in diagnosing painful vertebrae in osteoporotic compression fractures. AJNR Am J Neuroradiol. 2011;32:121–4.
23. Ebeling PR, Akesson K, Bauer DC, et al. The efficacy and safety of vertebral augmentation: a second ASBMR task force report. J Bone Miner Res. 2019;34:3–21.
24. Kim HJ, Yi JM, Cho HG, et al. Comparative study of the treatment outcomes of osteoporotic compression fractures without neurologic injury using a rigid brace, a soft brace, and no brace: a prospective randomized controlled non-inferiority trial. J Bone Joint Surg Am. 2014;96:1959–66.
25. Li M, Law SW, Cheng J, Kee HM, Wong MS. A comparison study on the efficacy of SpinoMed(R) and soft lumbar orthosis for osteoporotic vertebral fracture. Prosthetics Orthot Int. 2015;39:270–6.
26. Bailey CS, Urquhart JC, Dvorak MF, et al. Orthosis versus no orthosis for the treatment of thoracolumbar burst fractures without neurologic injury: a multicenter prospective randomized equivalence trial. Spine J. 2014;14:2557–64.
27. Meccariello L, Muzii VF, Falzarano G, et al. Dynamic corset versus three-point brace in the treatment of osteoporotic compression fractures of the thoracic and lumbar spine: a prospective, comparative study. Aging Clin Exp Res. 2017;29:443–9.
28. Beall DP. Response to: randomized controlled trial of vertebroplasty versus kyphoplasty in the treatment of

vertebral compression fractures. J Neurointerv Surg. 2016;8:763–4.
29. Beall DP, Tutton SM, Murphy K, Olan W, Warner C, Test JB. Analysis of reporting bias in vertebral augmentation. Pain Physician. 2017;20:E1081–e90.
30. Beall D, Lorio MP, Yun BM, Runa MJ, Ong KL, Warner CB. Review of vertebral augmentation: an updated meta-analysis of the effectiveness. Int J Spine Surg. 2018;12:295–321.
31. Hirsch JA, Beall DP, Chambers MR, et al. Management of vertebral fragility fractures: a clinical care pathway developed by a multispecialty panel using the RAND/UCLA appropriateness method. Spine J. 2018;18:2152–61.
32. Beall DP, Parsons B, Burner S. Technical strategies and anatomic considerations for an Extrapedicular modified inferior endplate access to thoracic and lumbar vertebral bodies. Pain Physician. 2016;19:593–601.
33. Chen YC, Zhang L, Li EN, et al. Unilateral versus bilateral percutaneous vertebroplasty for osteoporotic vertebral compression fractures in elderly patients: a meta-analysis. Medicine. 2019;98:e14317.
34. Wang B, Zhao CP, Song LX, Zhu L. Balloon kyphoplasty versus percutaneous vertebroplasty for osteoporotic vertebral compression fracture: a meta-analysis and systematic review. J Orthop Surg Res. 2018;13:264.
35. Khosla A, Diehn FE, Rad AE, Kallmes DF. Neither subendplate cement deposition nor cement leakage into the disk space during vertebroplasty significantly affects patient outcomes. Radiology. 2012;264:180–6.
36. Matouk CC, Krings T, Ter Brugge KG, Smith R. Cement embolization of a segmental artery after percutaneous vertebroplasty: a potentially catastrophic vascular complication. Interv Neuroradiol. 2012;18:358–62.
37. Kadri A, Binkley N, Hare KJ, Anderson PA. Bone health optimization in orthopaedic surgery. J Bone Joint Surg Am. 2020;
38. Marco RA, Kushwaha VP. Thoracolumbar burst fractures treated with posterior decompression and pedicle screw instrumentation supplemented with balloon-assisted vertebroplasty and calcium phosphate reconstruction. J Bone Joint Surg Am. 2009;91:20–8.
39. Sudo H, Ito M, Kaneda K, et al. Anterior decompression and strut graft versus posterior decompression and pedicle screw fixation with vertebroplasty for osteoporotic thoracolumbar vertebral collapse with neurologic deficits. Spine J. 2013;13:1726–32.
40. Kim WJ, Lee ES, Jeon SH, Yalug I. Correction of osteoporotic fracture deformities with global sagittal imbalance. Clin Orthop Relat Res. 2006;443:75–93.
41. Suk SI, Kim JH, Lee SM, Chung ER, Lee JH. Anterior-posterior surgery versus posterior closing wedge osteotomy in posttraumatic kyphosis with neurologic compromised osteoporotic fracture. Spine. 2003;28:2170–5.
42. Okuda S, Oda T, Yamasaki R, Haku T, Maeno T, Iwasaki M. Surgical outcomes of osteoporotic vertebral collapse: a retrospective study of anterior spinal fusion and pedicle subtraction osteotomy. Global Spine J. 2012;2:221–6.
43. Cho HM, Lee K, Min W, et al. Survival and functional outcomes after hip fracture among nursing home residents. J Korean Med Sci. 2016;31:89–97.
44. Bunta AD, Edwards BJ, Macaulay WB Jr, et al. Own the bone, a system-based intervention, improves osteoporosis care after fragility fractures. J Bone Joint Surg Am. 2016;98:e109.
45. Camacho PM, Petak SM, Binkley N, et al. American association of clinical endocrinologists and American college of endocrinology clinical practice guidelines for the diagnosis and treatment of postmenopausal osteoporosis – 2016. Endocr Pract. 2016;22:1–42.
46. Edwards BJ, Bunta AD, Anderson J, et al. Development of an electronic medical record based intervention to improve medical care of osteoporosis. Osteoporos Int. 2012;23:2489–98.
47. Wasfie T, Jackson A, Brock C, Galovska S, McCullough JR, Burgess JA. Does a fracture liaison service program minimize recurrent fragility fractures in the elderly with osteoporotic vertebral compression fractures? Am J Surg. 2019;217:557–60.
48. Bawa HS, Weick J, Dirschl DR. Anti-osteoporotic therapy after fragility fracture lowers rate of subsequent fracture: analysis of a large population sample. J Bone Joint Surg Am. 2015;97:1555–62.
49. Beall DP, Feldman RG, Gordon ML, et al. Patients with prior vertebral or hip fractures treated with teriparatide in the direct assessment of nonvertebral fractures in community experience (DANCE) observational study. Osteoporos Int. 2016;27:1191–8.

Part VII

Intensive Care Management of the Geriatric Patient

Standard Operating Procedures in Geriatric Polytrauma

33

F. Ziegenhain, H. Teuber, and K. O. Jensen

33.1 Background

33.1.1 Trauma Mechanism

Trauma in younger patients is primarily characterized by high-energy mechanisms such as traffic accidents. In geriatric patients, serious injuries can occur even in low-energy trauma mechanisms. Studies have shown that elderly polytraumatized patients most commonly sustain their injuries in falls from a height of less than 3 m [1, 2]. A significant number of these falls occur at home from standing height. Therefore, geriatric polytrauma injuries seem to constitute a different entity of injuries than the injuries found in young polytraumatized patients [3–6].

33.1.2 SOPs: General Aspects

SOPs are commonly used in many different fields, for example, to introduce a new product or in the military. Further, SOPs play an increasing role in everyday medical decision-making. For common diseases and standard situations in hospitals, SOPs have been developed to ensure a high quality of care. In minor injuries (e.g. femoral neck fracture, osteoporotic spine injuries) or inpatient treatment protocols (e.g. delirium prophylaxis, osteoporosis therapy, nutrition, etc.) SOPs are well established. They provide a guide for medical staff on how best to move forward in specific clinical constellations. To generate a SOP, outcomes of existing processes must be critically evaluated. Based on that, standardized recommendations are formulated. Several studies have shown significantly improved patient outcomes in trauma care after the introduction of standard operating procedures [7, 8].

33.1.3 Injury Severity

Injury mechanisms in elderly patients differ from those in younger patients. Low-energy trauma mechanisms are common, and do not usually suggest a severely injured patient. Studies, however, show a different reality. Geriatric patients often suffer severe injuries from minor trauma [9]. A younger patient who stumbles and falls will most likely not sustain severe injuries. Due to comorbidities and slower protective reflexes, geriatric patients may for example sustain a hip fracture or severe traumatic brain injury after a same-level fall [10].

F. Ziegenhain · H. Teuber · K. O. Jensen (✉)
Department of Trauma, University Hospital Zurich, Zurich, Switzerland
e-mail: franziska.ziegenhain@usz.ch; kaioliver.jensen@usz.ch

H.-C. Pape et al. (eds.), *Senior Trauma Patients*, https://doi.org/10.1007/978-3-030-91483-7_33

33.1.4 Frailty/Biological Age

Frailty and biological age are commonly used expressions in the setting of the elderly patient [11, 12]. Frailty refers to the physiological vulnerability of an individual to acute stressors due to preexisting conditions. Frailty increases late in life, and patients with increased comorbidities are considered biologically older as a result of increased frailty. Several authors have developed scores to estimate the frailty of elderly individuals [12–14]. Studies have shown that patients with high frailty scores are more likely to have an adverse outcome [15, 16].

Most frailty scores include similar parameters such as weight loss and an increasing loss of independence. However, while frailty plays a critical role in patient outcomes, it is a difficult entity to quantify [11, 16–19].

33.1.5 Comorbidities

Comorbidities of the geriatric patient require treating physicians to take many more factors into consideration before making therapeutic decisions. In trauma, for example, the ability to estimate trauma severity and blood loss by assessing basic vital parameters may be more difficult since many elderly patients take beta-blockers and other antihypertensive medication. This blunts the physiological response to stress and blood loss and a reactive tachycardia may be fully absent [10, 20].

While the prevalence of common comorbidities varies between countries, the most frequently found diseases are very similar and are listed in Table 33.1 [21–23].

Table 33.1 Most frequent comorbidities in geriatric trauma patients

Most frequent comorbidities [21–23]
• Cardiovascular diseases • Hypertension • Diabetes mellitus • Neurodegenerative diseases • Cancer • Arthritis • Chronic pulmonary diseases

33.2 SOP for Geriatric Polytrauma

33.2.1 General Considerations

Studies addressing standardized trauma care in all severely injured patients especially showed significant benefits in geriatric trauma patients [24]. Different challenges are confronted when treating the severely injured elderly patient, and some general considerations should be taken into account early. For example, due to the high probability of adverse outcomes, an ICU admission with maximum medical care in a severely injured, frail, and unwilling geriatric patient may be ethically contraindicated. This underlines the need for specialized SOPs dedicated to geriatric trauma patients.

However, many critically injured elderly patients benefit from intensive care and this option should not be ruled out based on patient age alone. We, therefore, recommend initiating intensive care when indicated, while closely defining and then frequently reevaluating what therapeutic option is best for the patient. Whenever possible, these options should be discussed with the patient directly. If this is not possible due to the patient's condition, the medical team should act according to the patient's health care directive if available. Family members are also an important resource to help determine the presumed will of the patient. If none of these options are available, the medical team must reach a consensus on the treatment objective. For these reasons, the development of an SOP for assessing ICU admission and intensive care treatment in elderly polytraumatized patients would in our opinion be of tremendous help in every institution. In summary, before treatment can be initiated in critically injured patients, an assessment should be made if it would benefit the patient.

33.2.2 Development of Consensus Group and Future Direction

The goal is to develop evidence-based SOPs for the trauma care of critically ill elderly patients in the ICU. An interdisciplinary international consensus group comprised of traumatologists,

Table 33.2 Participating subspecialties of the interdisciplinary international consensus group

Participating subspecialties
Traumatology
Orthopedic surgery
Anesthesiology
Intensive care medicine
Geriatric medicine
Medical ethics

orthopedic surgeons, intensivists, anesthesiologists, medical ethics experts, and geriatricians experienced in the treatment of severely injured geriatric patients, and with previous experience in SOP/guideline development was therefore created (Table 33.2). This task force of the German trauma association section for geronto-traumatology (Sektion Alterstraumatologie der DGU®) has now begun the development of a SOP for severely injured geriatric patients.

33.2.2.1 Literature Search

A literature search was conducted to identify SOPs that have already been developed or suggested. Furthermore, a review of national and local guidelines as well as expert opinions was carried out. When using the term "Standard operating procedures geriatric trauma" in a literature search, about 250 results were found. Most of the national and local guidelines contain clear information on fracture treatment and general considerations such as fall and delirium prophylaxis. For the treatment of severely injured geriatric patients in the intensive care unit, no specific SOPs were found. Therefore, the initial focus turned towards the development of a new guideline to clarify the indications for ICU admission of severely injured geriatric patients after initial management in the emergency department or trauma bay.

33.2.2.2 Inclusion Criteria

A flowchart to evaluate which patients meet the criteria for the geriatric trauma SOP was developed and agreed upon in a consensus meeting. Included were all trauma patients aged 65 years or older. Relevant baseline characteristics (injuries, age, preexisting conditions) are collected in a list of criteria.

33.2.2.3 Exclusion Criteria

Patients under 65 years old, intubated patients due to the definite need for ICU treatment, and those patients who died during initial trauma management in the trauma bay were excluded.

33.2.2.4 Discussion

This initial list was discussed in two Delphi rounds during two separate consensus conferences. In another consensus meeting, a simple point-based triage scoring sheet was developed and the scoring system as well as the included parameters were extensively discussed.

The entire process of discussion and voting was highly standardized and well documented, and resulted in a flowchart and a score chart. A small registry of geriatric trauma patients was utilized to validate the initially developed triage score. A validation study with a bigger sample size is in progress.

At the same time, the DGU consensus group started to generate a SOP for the treatment of severely injured geriatric patients in the ICU. In order to create a guideline that is easy to follow and understand, the group decided to organize the SOP into organ-based rather than problem-based chapters (Table 33.3). Since ethics play an especially important role in geriatric care, ethical considerations with different therapeutic options based on those considerations form a substantial component of the SOP.

33.2.3 Therapeutic Options

Therapeutic decisions are based on the patient's desired therapeutic goals and the burdens and risks of potential treatment options. Advanced care planning, designed to ensure that patients receive their desired emergency care in the event of a life-threatening crisis, has been further developed in recent years. In Germany, a one-paged sheet with detailed patient wishes in the setting of acute illness or injury, referred to as Physician Orders for Life-Sustaining Treatment (POLST or ÄNo, in German), can be added to an advanced directive [25]. Based on these choices, three treatment options exist:

Table 33.3 SOP chapters for the treatment of severely injured geriatric patients in the ICU

SOP chapters	
CNS	Delirium Reduced brain volume
Cardiovascular system	Volume management Transfusions Catecholamines Cardiovascular diseases
Coagulation	
Pulmonary system	Ventilator-associated pneumonia Thoracic trauma Tracheotomy Pulmonary diseases
Nephrology	Dialysis
Liver	
Pharmacology and medication	
Infectiology/immunologic system	
Gastrointestinal tract	Nutrition Digestion
Musculoskeletal system	Frailty/preexisting condition Physiotherapy/Ergotherapy
Skin	Decubitus
Externa	Pacemakers Catheter
Ethical problems	Therapy limitations Reanimation Comfort therapy

33.2.3.1 Option A

Option A is a treatment plan with the goal of maintaining life with all necessary medical interventions. This is the standard treatment option if the patient has no known advance directive. This option includes initial mechanical resuscitation and intubation, but also extends to any therapeutic escalation that may be necessary, or treatment of complications associated with resuscitation that may occur. Patients under this treatment option should receive maximum care, including institutional, surgical, and conservative therapies. [25]

33.2.3.2 Option B

Option B is a limited version of the first option. This is an individualized approach to maximizing care with certain restrictions or limitations depending on the patient's particular situation, wishes, and/or physical limitations. This may for example state that resuscitation should be limited to drug resuscitation and prohibit mechanical resuscitation. Further, certain limited surgical interventions may be a good treatment option, while high-risk or high-morbidity surgeries should not be performed. In general, the patient can choose to exclude up to four major therapeutic options including cardiopulmonary resuscitation, invasive ventilation, and ICU admission. As a last step, the patient can also exclude any hospital treatment at all. [25]

33.2.3.3 Option C

Option C describes a palliative situation with a care plan designed to maximize comfort and quality of life without attempting to extend the life of the patient. Admission to the ICU may still be an option to ensure best supportive care. This option can either be medically indicated or the wish of the patient [25].

33.3 Summary

The first important steps towards realizing standardized treatment of polytraumatized geriatric patients in the ICU have been taken, but much work remains. Apart from validating a new triage score to assess the indication for ICU admission, SOPs for intensive care of elderly patients after severe trauma are in development. It should be the aim in the coming years to establish these evidence-based SOPs to attain the best possible care for geriatric patients after trauma.

References

1. Wutzler S, Lefering R, Laurer HL, Walcher F, Wyen H, Marzi I. Veränderungen in der Alterstraumatologie. Unfallchirurg [Internet]. 2008; 111(8):592–8. Verfügbar unter:. https://doi.org/10.1007/s00113-008-1448-2.
2. Spering C, Lefering R, Bouillon B, Lehmann W, von Eckardstein K, Dresing K. It is time for a change in the management of elderly severely injured patients! An analysis of 126,015 patients from the TraumaRegister DGU®. Eur J Trauma Emerg Surg [Internet]. 2019.; Verfügbar unter:; https://doi.org/10.1007/s00068-019-01229-8.
3. Sterling DA, O'Connor JA, Bonadies J. Geriatric falls: injury severity is high and disproportionate to mechanism. J Trauma Acute Care Surg [Internet]. 2001;50(1) Verfügbar unter: https://journals.lww.com/jtrauma/Fulltext/2001/01000/Geriatric_Falls__Injury_Severity_Is_High_and.21.aspx
4. Brown CVR, Rix K, Klein AL, Ford B, Teixeira PGR, Aydelotte J. A comprehensive investigation of comorbidities, mechanisms, injury patterns, and outcomes in geriatric blunt trauma patients. Am Surg. 2016;82(11):1055–62.
5. Kocuvan S, Brilej D, Stropnik D, Lefering R, Komadina R. Evaluation of major trauma in elderly patients -- a single trauma center analysis. Wien Klin Wochenschr [Internet]. 2016;128(7):535–42. Verfügbar unter:. https://doi.org/10.1007/s00508-016-1140-4.
6. Ziegenhain F, Scherer J, Kalbas Y, Neuhaus V, Lefering R, Teuben M, Sprengel K, Pape H-C, Jensen KO, The TraumaRegister DGU. Age-Dependent Patient and Trauma Characteristics and Hospital Resource Requirements—Can Improvement Be Made? An Analysis from the German Trauma Registry. Medicina. 2021;57(4):330. https://doi.org/10.3390/medicina57040330.
7. Schoeneberg C, Schilling M, Burggraf M, Fochtmann U, Lendemans S. Reduction in mortality in severely injured patients following the introduction of the treatment of patients with severe and multiple injuries guideline of the German society of trauma surgery a retrospective analysis of a level 1. Injury [Internet]. 2014;45(3):635–8. Verfügbar unter:. https://doi.org/10.1016/j.injury.2013.11.024.
8. Grimshaw JM, Russell IT. Effect of clinical guidelines on medical practice: A systematic review of rigorous evaluations. Obstet Gynecol Surv. 1994;49(7):469–70.
9. Fröhlich M, Caspers M, Lefering R, Driessen A, Bouillon B, Maegele M. Do elderly trauma patients receive the required treatment? Epidemiology and outcome of geriatric trauma patients treated at different levels of trauma care. Eur J Trauma Emerg Surg [Internet]. 2019.; Verfügbar unter:; https://doi.org/10.1007/s00068-019-01285-0.
10. Luchette FA, Yelon JA. Geriatric trauma and critical care: second edition. In: Geriatric trauma and critical care. 2; 2017. p. 1–464.
11. Clegg A, Young J, Iliffe S, Rikkert MO, Rockwood K. Frailty in elderly people. Lancet. 2013;381(9868):752–62.
12. Pijpers E, Ferreira I, Stehouwer CDA, Nieuwenhuijzen Kruseman AC. The frailty dilemma. Review of the predictive accuracy of major frailty scores. Eur J Intern Med [Internet]. 2012;23(2):118–23. Verfügbar unter:. https://doi.org/10.1016/j.ejim.2011.09.003.
13. Juma S, Taabazuing M-M, Montero-Odasso M. Clinical frailty scale in an acute medicine unit: a simple tool that predicts length of stay. Can Geriatr J [Internet]. 2016;19(2):34–9. Verfügbar unter: https://www.ncbi.nlm.nih.gov/pubmed/27403211
14. de Vries NM, Staal JB, van Ravensberg CD, Hobbelen JSM, Olde Rikkert MGM, der Sanden MWG N-v. Outcome instruments to measure frailty: a systematic review. Ageing Res Rev [Internet]. 2011;10(1):104–14. Verfügbar unter:. https://doi.org/10.1016/j.arr.2010.09.001.
15. Chen C-L, Chen C-M, Wang C-Y, Ko P-W, Chen C-H, Hsieh C-P. Frailty is associated with an increased risk of major adverse outcomes in elderly patients following surgical treatment of hip fracture. Sci Rep [Internet]. 2019;9(1):19135. Verfügbar unter: https://www.ncbi.nlm.nih.gov/pubmed/31836751
16. Flaatten H, De Lange DW, Morandi A, Andersen FH, Artigas A, Bertolini G. The impact of frailty on ICU and 30-day mortality and the level of care in very elderly patients (≥ 80 years). Intensive Care Med. 2017;43(12):1820–8.
17. Bischoff HA, Staehelin HB, Willett WC. The effect of undernutrition in the development of frailty in older persons. J Gerontol Ser A. 2006;61(6):585–9.
18. Brooks SE. Evidence – based C are of geriatric trauma patients. 2017;97:1157–74.
19. Kim S, Han H-S, Jung H, Kim K, Hwang DW, Kang S-B. Multidimensional frailty score for the prediction of postoperative mortality risk. JAMA Surg [Internet]. 2014;149(7):633–40. Verfügbar unter:. https://doi.org/10.1001/jamasurg.2014.241.
20. Peck KA, Calvo RY, Schechter MS, Sise CB, Kahl JE, Shackford MC, u. a. The impact of preinjury anticoagulants and prescription antiplatelet agents on outcomes in older patients with traumatic brain injury. J Trauma Acute Care Surg [Internet]. 2014;76(2)

Verfügbar unter: https://journals.lww.com/jtrauma/Fulltext/2014/02000/The_impact_of_preinjury_anticoagulants_and.25.aspx
21. NCDC 2030. NCD Countdown 2030: worldwide trends in non-communicable disease mortality and progress towards Sustainable Development Goal target 3.4. Lancet (London, England) [Internet]. 2018;392(10152):1072–88. Verfügbar unter: https://www.ncbi.nlm.nih.gov/pubmed/30264707
22. GBD. 2016 D and II and P. Global, regional, and national incidence, prevalence, and years lived with disability for 328 diseases and injuries for 195 countries, 1990–2016: a systematic analysis for the Global Burden of Disease Study 2016. Lancet (London, England) [Internet]. 2017;390(10100):1211–59. Verfügbar unter: https://www.ncbi.nlm.nih.gov/pubmed/28919117
23. Jaul E, Barron J. Age-related diseases and clinical and public health implications for the 85 years old and over population. Front Public Heal [Internet]. 2017;5:335. Verfügbar unter: https://www.ncbi.nlm.nih.gov/pubmed/29312916
24. Peterer L, Ossendorf C, Jensen KO, Osterhoff G, Mica L, Seifert B. Implementation of new standard operating procedures for geriatric trauma patients with multiple injuries: a single level I trauma centre study. BMC Geriatr [Internet]. 2019;19(1):359. Verfügbar unter:. https://doi.org/10.1186/s12877-019-1380-z.
25. Bvp Z Von. Behandlung im Voraus planen – Bedeutung für die Intensiv- und Notfallmedizin Einleitung Befähigung als konstitutives Element von Patientenselbstbestimmung Ein neues Konzept: Behandlung im Voraus planen (Advance Care Planning). Ungelöste Herausforderunge. 2018:62–70.

34 Specifics of Surgical Management: Patient in Critical Condition

Sascha Halvachizadeh and Hans-Christoph Pape

34.1 Introduction

The constant increase of life expectancy leads to a constant increase of elderly patients, especially of the western population [1]. In 2060, approximately one-third of the European population will be 65 years and older; the proportion of octogenarians is estimated to increase from 6% in 2015 to 11% in 2040 [2]. Similarly, in the US an estimated 1 in 5 residents will be elderly by the year 2050 [3]. The past two decades showed a substantial increase in the elderly population in critical conditions that require intensive care management [4, 5]. Constant improvements in managing chronic diseases have resulted in more active lifestyles in the elderly, leading to an increase in incidences of injuries [6]. Currently, traumatic injuries are the fifth leading cause of death in elderly patients [7]. In 2017 more than 1 in 4 patients included in the German Trauma Registry (DGU®) were 70 years and older [2]. The median age of patients in critical condition approaches 65 years in many countries, and the proportion of critically ill octogenarians will increase faster compared to any other cohort in the intensive care unit (ICU) [8]. Aging alters the physiologic capacity to respond to injury [9, 10]. In 1984 Harborview Medical Center published a review of 100 trauma patients older than 70 years that reported a 85% survival rate but noted that 88% did not return to their previous level of independence [11]. The article stated: "... with impact preexisting disease has on survival following injury has not been adequately studied" [12]. In the early 1990s, Scalea et al [13] recognized that blunt traumata in geriatric patients is a very different disease process compared to the young patient. Further, they stated that elderly trauma patients sustaining multiple blunt trauma to be at considerably higher risk compared to younger patients [13]. Several studies have shown, that geriatric trauma patients sustain an injury severity score (ISS) of 16 points or greater after considerably low-energy trauma compared to the high-energy trauma that is required for young patients to sustain a similar severity of injuries [14, 15]. Polytraumatized geriatric patients show substantial differences in injury distribution and injury management compared to young patients [16] (Table 34.1).

In geriatric patients, low-energy trauma mechanism leads to ISS of 16 points or greater. One of the most important steps towards improving surgical management of geriatric patients in critical condition is to acknowledge the outcome differences in geriatric injured patients and connecting those outcomes to differences in physiology and physiologic responses to injuries.

S. Halvachizadeh · H.-C. Pape (✉)
Department of Trauma, University Zurich,
Universitäts Spital Zürich, Zurich, Switzerland
e-mail: hans-christoph.pape@usz.ch

H.-C. Pape et al. (eds.), *Senior Trauma Patients*, https://doi.org/10.1007/978-3-030-91483-7_34

Table 34.1 Three most common blunt injuries with Abbreviated Injury Scale (AIS) ≥3 in different age groups

18–59 years	60–69 years	70–79 years	≥80 years
Thoracic (52.8%)	Head/neck (53.8%)	Head/neck (57.4%)	Head/neck (58.9%)
Head/neck (46.2%)	Thoracic (49.1%)	Thoracic (43.0%)	Extremities (36.0%)
Extremities (42.6%)	Extremities (32.2%)	Extremities (43.0%)	Thoracic (32.5%)

34.2 Comorbidities and Changes of Organ Systems Associated with Aging

With age, the number of comorbidities per patient increases. The mean number of comorbidities per patient is 2.6 (SD 2.2) in patients aged between 65–84 years, and increases to a mean of 3.6 (SD 2.3) in patients aged 85 years or over [17]. Comorbidities are associated with increased mortality [18]. Amongst the most common comorbidities are hypertension, diabetes, chronic obstructive pulmonary disease, cardiac failure, cancer, and cognitive impairment [17, 19]. The patient with comorbidities in critical condition is associated with higher in-hospital and long-term mortality rates [20–22]. In the past decades, physiological changes that decrease reserve capacities in aging patients have been extensively studied (Table 34.2) [23–26].

Impairment of the central nervous system increases the rate of agitation and delirium in geriatric trauma patients [28]. The cardiac function declines by 50% between the ages 20 and 80 years and the patients experience 30% of all myocardial infarctions, and 60% of all cardiovascular associated deaths in this age group [29, 30]. A review of more than 4000 trauma patients found a significant increase in mortality in geriatric patients whose heart rates were greater than 90 beats per minute (bpm), an association not seen until a heart rate of 130 bpm in younger patients [31]. They further found a marked increase of mortality in geriatric trauma patients with a systolic blood pressure less than 110 mmHg, but not until a systolic blood pressure of less than 95 mmHg in young patients [31]. Vital signs are less predictive of mortality in geriatric trauma patients [32]. The cardiovascular responses to trauma in geriatric patients are not comparable to the physiologic responses in young patients. Heart rates greater than 90 bpm or systolic blood pressure less than 110 mmHg should increase awareness in the trauma surgeon.

34.3 Treatment of Geriatric Trauma Patients

One of the most important factors in treating TBIs is the treatment of the underlying coagulatory pathology. With increased prescription of anticoagulants, the rate of intracranial hemorrhage (ICH) increased substantially [33]. Patients that need regular anticoagulation or antiplatelet therapy have been shown to suffer from delayed ICH, thus lowering the threshold for repeated cCT scans after initial negative cCT [34]. Further, routine neurologic observation is mandatory and a repeated cCT if the Glasgow Coma Scale (GCS) drops by 2 points or more (Table 34.3).

Pulmonary contusions are the most common blunt thoracic trauma injuries and occur in up to 75% of patients [35]. Cases with more than three fractured ribs are associated with 31% risk of pneumonia in geriatric patients compared to 17% in younger patients; mortality increases to 33% [36]. Further, rib fractures in geriatric patients are associated with an increased risk of splenic injury (OR 1.7) or liver injury (OR 1.4). Treatment should include optimal, multimodal analgesia with consequent physiotherapeutic guided breathing training to minimize the risk of respiratory failure and ensuing ventilator support [37]. In cases with failed conventional analgesic regime, consider epidural analgesia [38]. Consider open reduction internal fixation (ORIF) of rib fractures in selected patients [39–42].

In the treatment of abdominal injuries, consider the altered physiologic response to trauma in geriatric patients. A matched cohort study

Table 34.2 Changes in specific organ systems that are associated with aging [27]

Organ system	Pathology	Result
Central nervous	Cortical atrophy Plaque build-up in c.-v. vessels Decreased cerebellar function Polypharmacy	5 sensations ↓ Cognitive decline ↓ Balance ↓ and falls ↑ Agitation and delirium ↑
Cardiovascular	Muscle/conductive pathways replaced with fat and fibrous tissue Stiffness ↑ Beta-blocker medication	Arrhythmia ↑ Cardiac output ↓ Systemic vascular resistance ↑ Compensatory tachycardia ↓ (masks hypovolemia)
Respiratory	Kyphosis, intervertebral space ↓ Rigid chest wall Muscle mass ↓ Lung elasticity ↓ Alveolar surface ↓ Cough reflex ↓ Muco-cilliary function ↓ Microorganism ↑	Intercostal space ↓ Concentration of inhalative agents ↓ Air trapping Hyperinflammation Effectiveness pulm.System ↓↓ Residual volume ↑ FEVs and FVC ↓ Postoperative complications ↑↑ (ARDS)
Renal	Glomerulosclerosis Intimal thickening of vessels Renovascular reflex ↓↓	Cortical glomeruli ↓ Renovascular dysautonomy Preserving function in hypo-/hypertension ↓↓ Acute kidney injuries
Gastro-intestinal	Malnutrition	Postoperative morbidity ↑ Perioperativ mortality ↑ Length of stay ↑ Quality of life ↓

Table 34.3 Treating injuries

Traumatic Brain Injuries (TBI)	Low threshold to perform Head CT (cCT) scan Treat coagulopathy Manage anticoagulants -> increase rate of delayed intracerebral haemorrhage (ICH) Correction of INR
Blunt trauma to the chest	Consider pulmonary contusions (75% of cases) Fractures of more than 3–4 ribs increases risk of pneumonia Consider splenic injuries and liver injuries Adequate pain management Ventilation support and oxygenation Aggressive physiotherapy Consider open reduction and internal fixation of rib fractures in selected patients Chest tubes
Abdominal injuries	Diagnostics with whole body CT decreases mortality Conservative treatment in hemodynamically stable patients Angioembolization in selected cases Do not trust the "normal" vital signs (might be masked)
Extremities	Adequate soft tissue management Aim for early mobilization to reduce immobilization associated complications Address osteoporosis Physiotherapeutic guided movement

showed, that half of the geriatric patients that died after penetrating trauma had normal vital signs [43].

34.4 Critical Care

An adequate triage of geriatric trauma patients in the intensive care unit (ICU) might be a crucial step in improving morbidity and mortality. It has been shown that geriatric patients had significantly lower ICU admission rates compared with younger patients with similar injury severity [44]. Yet, several studies described improved outcomes after early trauma team activation and intensive monitoring in the geriatric [13, 45].

The initial management of the trauma patient should be based on the Advance Trauma and Life Support (ATLS) system, independent of age [46]. However, it has been shown that the injury severity in elderly patients is often underestimated and under-triaged [15]. The rate of under-triaged elderly ranges from 15% to 49% resulting in inadequate care [47] that results in increased overall mortality [48]. Early aggressive diagnostics and treatment, and the threshold to admit elderly trauma patients to the ICU should be low. The continuous thoughtful invasive monitoring is beneficial and the interdisciplinary treatment is indispensable in addressing associated comorbidities for the pot-acute care [50]. When taking the changed physiologic response to trauma into account, performing adequate and early appropriate diagnostics, and accounting for the patient's age and comorbidities, studies have shown that the rate of under-triage might be significantly reduced [49]. Geriatric consultation helps to identify additional diagnoses and improve outcome with decreased 30-day mortality [49].

34.5 Conclusion

The critical care of trauma patients depends only to a certain degree on age. Comorbidities, patient`s will, and the interdisciplinary approach are crucial elements in triatic the geriatric patient in critical condition. It is of high importance to recognize the changed physiological responses in geriatric patients to certain conditions and to lower the threshold for diagnostics.

References

1. Sampalis JS, Nathanson R, Vaillancourt J, Nikolis A, Liberman M, Angelopoulos J, et al. Assessment of mortality in older trauma patients sustaining injuries from falls or motor vehicle collisions treated in regional level I trauma Centers. Ann Surg. 2009;249(3):488–95.
2. Gather A, Gruetzner PA, Muenzberg M. Polytrauma in old age-knowledge from the TraumaRegister DGU (R). Chirurg. 2019;90(10):791–4.
3. Moore L, Turgeon AF, Sirois M-J, Lavoie A. Trauma Centre outcome performance: a comparison of young adults and geriatric patients in an inclusive trauma system. Injury-Int J Care Injured. 2012;43(9):1580–5.
4. Flaatten H. Intensive care in the very old: are we prepared? Acta Anaesthesiol Scand. 2007;51(5):519–21.
5. Laake JH, Dybwik K, Flaatten HK, Fonneland IL, Kvale R, Strand K. Impact of the post-world war II generation on intensive care needs in Norway. Acta Anaesthesiol Scand. 2010;54(4):479–84.
6. Jacobs DG. Special considerations in geriatric injury. Curr Opin Crit Care. 2003;9(6):535–9.
7. Aschkenasy MT, Rothenhaus TC. Trauma and falls in the elderly. Emerg Med Clin North Am. 2006;24(2):413.
8. de Flaatten H, et al. The status of intensive care medicine research and a future agenda for very old patients in the ICU. Intensive Care Med. 2017;43(9):1319–28.
9. Broos PLO, Dhoore A, Vanderschot P, Rommens PM, Stappaerts KH. Multiple trauma in elderly patients – factors influencing outcome - importance of aggressive care. Injury-Int J Care Injured. 1993;24(6):365–8.
10. Morris JA, Mackenzie EJ, Damiano AM, Bass SM. Mortality in trauma patients – the interaction between host factors and severity. J Trauma-Injury Infect Crit Care. 1990;30(12):1476–82.
11. Brooks SE, Peetz AB. Evidence-based Care of Geriatric Trauma Patients. Surg Clin North Am. 2017;97(5):1157–74.
12. Oreskovich MR, Howard JD, Copass MK, Carrico CJ. Geriatric trauma - injury patterns and outcome. J Trauma-Injury Infect Crit Care. 1984;24(7):565–72.
13. Scalea TM, Simon HM, Duncan AO, Atweh NA, Sclafani SJA, Phillips TF, et al. Geriatric blunt multiple trauma – improved survival with early invasive monitoring. J Trauma-Injury Infect Crit Care. 1990;30(2):129–36.
14. Switzer JA, Gammon SR. High-energy skeletal trauma in the elderly. J Bone Joint Surg-Am Vol. 2012;94A(23):2195–204.

15. Soles GLS, Tornetta PI. Multiple trauma in the elderly: new management perspectives. 2011;25:S61–5.
16. Wutzler S, Lefering R, Laurer HL, Walcher F, Wyen H, Marzi I, et al. Changes in geriatric traumatology. An analysis of 14,869 patients from the German trauma registry. Unfallchirurg. 2008;111(8):592–8.
17. Barnett K, Mercer SW, Norbury M, Watt G, Wyke S, Guthrie B. Epidemiology of multimorbidity and implications for health care, research, and medical education: a cross-sectional study. Lancet. 2012;380(9836):37–43.
18. Menotti A, Mulder I, Nissinen A, Giampaoli S, Feskens EJM, Kromhout D. Prevalence of morbidity and multimorbidity in elderly male populations and their impact on 10-year all-cause mortality: the FINE study (Finland, Italy, Netherlands, elderly). J Clin Epidemiol. 2001;54(7):680–6.
19. Salive ME. Multimorbidity in older adults. Epidemiol Rev. 2013;35:75–83.
20. Bagshaw SM, Webb SAR, Delaney A, George C, Pilcher D, Hart GK, et al. Very old patients admitted to intensive care in Australia and New Zealand: a multi-Centre cohort analysis. Crit Care. 2009;13(2)
21. Zampieri FG, Colombari F. The impact of performance status and comorbidities on the short-term prognosis of very elderly patients admitted to the ICU. BMC Anesthesiol. 2014;14
22. Stavem K, Hoel H, Skjaker SA, Haagensen R. Charlson comorbidity index derived from chart review or administrative data: agreement and prediction of mortality in intensive care patients. Clin Epidemiol. 2017;9:311–20.
23. Zeleznik J. Normative aging of the respiratory system. Clin Geriatr Med. 2003;19(1):1.
24. Hughes VA, Frontera WR, Roubenoff R, Evans WJ, Singh MAF. Longitudinal changes in body composition in older men and women: role of body weight change and physical activity. Am J Clin Nutr. 2002;76(2):473–81.
25. Guidet B, Vallet H, Boddaert J, De Lange DW, Morandi A, Leblanc G, et al. Caring for the critically ill patients over 80: a narrative review. Ann Intensive Care. 2018;8
26. Marzetti E, Leeuwenburgh C. Skeletal muscle apoptosis, sarcopenia and frailty at old age. Exp Gerontol. 2006;41(12):1234–8.
27. Brooks SE, Peetz AB. Evidence-based care of geriatric trauma patients. Surg Clin N Am 2017;97(5):1157-+.
28. Barr J, Fraser GL, Puntillo K, Ely EW, Gelinas C, Dasta JF, et al. Clinical practice guidelines for the management of pain, agitation, and delirium in adult patients in the intensive care unit. Crit Care Med. 2013;41(1):263–306.
29. Martin MJ, Perez-Alonso AJ, Asensio JA. Vascular complications and special problems in vascular trauma. Eur J Trauma Emerg Surg. 2013;39(6):569–89.
30. Martin RS, Farrah JP, Chang MC. Effect of aging on cardiac function plus monitoring and support. Surg Clin N Am. 2015;95(1):23.
31. Heffernan DS, Thakkar RK, Monaghan SF, Ravindran R, Adams CA Jr, Kozloff MS, et al. Normal presenting vital signs are unreliable in geriatric blunt trauma victims. J Trauma-Injury Infect Crit Care. 2010;69(4):813–8.
32. Martin JT, Alkhoury F, O'Connor JA, Kyriakides TC, Bonadies JA. 'Normal' vital signs belie occult hypoperfusion in geriatric trauma patients. Am Surg. 2010;76(1):65–9.
33. Bechtel BF, Nunez TC, Lyon JA, Cotton BA, Barrett TW. Treatments for reversing warfarin anticoagulation in patients with acute intracranial hemorrhage: a structured literature review. Int J Emerg Med. 2011;4
34. Docimo S Jr, Demin A, Vinces F. Patients with blunt head trauma on anticoagulation and antiplatelet medications: can they be safely discharged after a Normal initial cranial computed tomography scan? Am Surg. 2014;80(6):610–3.
35. Simon B, Ebert J, Bokhari F, Capella J, Emhoff T, Hayward T, et al. Management of pulmonary contusion and flail chest: an eastern Association for the Surgery of trauma practice management guideline. J Trauma Acute Care Surg. 2012;73:S351–S61.
36. Bulger EM, Arneson MA, Mock CN, Jurkovich GJ. Rib fractures in the elderly. J Trauma-Injury Infect Crit Care. 2000;48(6):1040–6.
37. Scales DC, Fischer HD, Li P, Bierman AS, Fernandes O, Mamdani M, et al. Unintentional continuation of medications intended for acute illness after hospital discharge: a population-based cohort study. J Gen Intern Med. 2016;31(2):196–202.
38. Bulger EM, Edwards T, Klotz P, Jurkovich GJ. Epidural analgesia improves outcome after multiple rib fractures. Surgery. 2004;136(2):426–30.
39. Nirula R, Allen B, Layman R, Falimirski ME, Somberg LB. Rib fracture stabilization in patients sustaining blunt chest injury. Am Surg. 2006;72(4):307–9.
40. Slobogean GP, MacPherson CA, Sun T, Pelletier M-E, Hameed SM. Surgical fixation vs nonoperative Management of Flail Chest: a meta-analysis. J Am Coll Surg. 2013;216(2):302.
41. Pieracci FM, Rodil M, Stovall RT, Johnson JL, Biffl WL, Mauffrey C, et al. Surgical stabilization of severe rib fractures. J Trauma Acute Care Surg. 2015;78(4):883–7.
42. Majercik S, Vijayakumar S, Olsen G, Wilson E, Gardner S, Granger SR, et al. Surgical stabilization of severe rib fractures decreases incidence of retained hemothorax and empyema. Am J Surg. 2015;210(6):1112–6.
43. Roth BJ, Velmahos GC, Oder DB, Vassiliu P, Tatevossian R, Demetriades D, et al. Penetrating trauma in patients older than 55 years: a case-control study. Injury-Int J Care Injured. 2001;32(7):551–4.
44. Taylor MD, Tracy JK, Meyer W, Pasquale M, Napolitano LM. Trauma in the elderly: intensive care unit resource use and outcome. J Trauma-Injury Infect Crit Care. 2002;53(3):407–14.
45. Demetriades D, Karaiskakis M, Velmahos G, Alo K, Newton E, Murray J, et al. Effect on outcome of early

intensive management of geriatric trauma patients. Br J Surg. 2002;89(10):1319–22.
46. Brasel KJ, Atls S, American College of Surgeons' Committee on Trauma; International ATLS Working Group. Advanced trauma life support (ATLS (R)): the ninth edition. J Trauma Acute Care Surg. 2013;74(5):1363–6.
47. Meldon SW, Reilly M, Drew BL, Mancuso C, Fallon W. Trauma in the very elderly: a community-based study of outcomes at trauma and non-trauma centers. J Trauma-Injury Infect Crit Care. 2002;52(1):79–84.
48. Chang DC, Bass RR, Cornwell EE, MacKenzie EJ. Undertriage of elderly trauma patients to state-designated trauma centers. Arch Surg. 2008;143(8):776–81.
49. Kristensen PK, Thillemann TM, Soballe K, Johnsen SP. Can improved quality of care explain the success of orthogeriatric units? A population-based cohort study. Age Ageing. 2016;45(1):66–71.
50. Smithson L, Morrell J, Kowalik U, Flynn W, Guo WA. Injury in the aged: geriatric trauma care at the crossroads. J Trauma Acute Care Surg. 2015;78(6):1162–7.

Plastic Surgery: Hand and Soft Tissue Trauma in the Elderly Patient

35

Jan A. Plock, Flavien Mauler, Andreas Weber, and Christian Tschumi

35.1 Introduction

The aging population worldwide is exhibiting an increase in chronic disease prevalence. Regarding trauma, this has been attributed to sarcopenia and osteoporosis, both associated with frailty.

As bone, muscle, and soft tissues interact functionally and metabolically, it is no surprise that plastic surgery and hand surgery play an important role in the elderly patient. While frailty and fracture risk have been discussed elsewhere, this chapter is intending to provide more insight into the specifics of hand fractures and blunt hand trauma as well as nerve injury, acute and chronic soft tissue trauma exhibiting special needs of treatment in the elderly population.

35.2 Hand Trauma

Geriatric patients account for about 25% of trauma admissions [1–3]. This number is going to increase, considering that the population older than 65 years is expected to reach 16% of the population by 2050 [4]. On one hand, the incidence of osteoporotic fractures due to low-energy trauma is increasing constantly in the elderly population [5]. On the other hand, more people are getting older but stay in good physical health for longer, living more actively, doing sport and leisure activities, and therefore being exposed to more injuries [6].

J. A. Plock (✉) · F. Mauler · A. Weber · C. Tschumi
Division of Plastic Surgery and Hand Surgery, Kantonsspital Aarau, Aarau, Switzerland
e-mail: jan.plock@ksa.ch

35.2.1 Fractures

35.2.1.1 Distal Radius

The distal radius fracture is the second most frequent fracture in people >65 years old where it occurs at a disproportionately higher rate compared to the younger population. Collectively, this group of fracture types accounts for 18% of all fractures in the older population and represents the most common open fracture type in women [7].

In the initial physical examination in patients with distal radius fractures, the evaluating clinician should pay close attention to skin tearing, which increases with age. Additionally, vascular status must be assessed, as well as careful neurological examination to rule out an acute carpal tunnel syndrome, which has been reported in 5.4–8.6% of all patients presenting with a distal radius fracture [8].

The radiological evaluation of distal radius fractures includes anteroposterior, lateral, and sometimes oblique views. In the case of a complex intra-articular fracture, the use of computed tomography (CT) may help in treatment planning regardless of whether or not surgery is indicated.

H.-C. Pape et al. (eds.), *Senior Trauma Patients*, https://doi.org/10.1007/978-3-030-91483-7_35

There is no consensus on whether to treat a distal radius fracture surgically or not in elderly patients [9]. Non-displaced or minimally displaced fractures are usually treated with splinting, although some patients may benefit from an internal fixation, allowing for earlier mobilization, and reducing the risk of secondary dislocation if a "walker" has to be used. The indication for closed reduction with a manual traction technique or with the finger-trap traction is still debated. Surgical treatments include closed reduction and Kirschner wire fixation, open reduction and volar or dorsal plate fixation, internal distraction plate, and arthroplasty.

Lutz et al. showed in their case-control study a significantly higher complication rate in operated patients. Although they found a greater number of malunions in the nonsurgically treated group. There was no significant difference in pain and disability at 1-year post-trauma between surgically and nonsurgically treated patients [10]. However, it should be noted that improvement in radiographic alignment may not lead to a better clinical outcome in this population [9].

35.2.1.2 Hand and Finger Fractures

Metacarpal and phalangeal fractures are among the most common fractures in patients >65 years old [7]. Non-displaced or minimally displaced fractures can be treated nonsurgically. Displaced fractures may be reduced under local anesthesia and protected by splinting or stabilized with percutaneously introduced K-wires. Our preferred duration for splinting or K-wire stabilization is 4 weeks with X-ray control before removal and starting progressive overload. If a stable internal fixation would allow for early mobilization, then this approach should be considered. In a study with 198 patients, Wollstein et al. showed that age was not associated with fracture healing time in adult patients. Particularly patients above 75 years with metacarpal fracture were not associated with longer healing time [11].

35.2.2 Activated Osteoarthritis

Osteoarthritis of the hand is a common condition in older patients. Importantly, the extent of radiologic joint damage in osteoarthritis does not necessarily correlate with pain perception. Acute blunt trauma can however activate an inflammatory response leading to massively increased pain levels [12]. First-line treatment is mostly nonsurgical. Splinting of the joint for a couple of days during the acute inflammatory response may be beneficial in reducing pain-related periarticular stiffness or muscle deconditioning [13]. The addition of hand rehabilitation and occupational therapy can benefit patients through minimizing disability and retaining muscle function and proprioception. Topical NSAIDs are an alternative to oral medication. They can be effective in alleviating pain associated with osteoarthritis while minimizing potential complications associated with long-term use [13, 14]. Intra-articular injections of corticosteroids or hyaluronic acid derivatives (HA) are commonly in use to treat painful degenerative joints. Corticosteroids may have an earlier onset of action, but a longer duration of pain relief has been described for HA. Eventually, surgical procedures ranging from denervation, joint resection, with or without tendon interposition, to joint replacement arthroplasty or arthrodesis may be indicated for persisting pain and functional impairment.

35.2.3 Nerve Injuries

The incidence of nerve injuries in the elderly has increased over the last 30 years [3]. Peripheral nerve lesions in the elderly should be treated the same way as in younger individuals. However, Verdú et al. demonstrated that age is associated with a delay in Wallerian degeneration and a slower rate of regeneration [15]. Furthermore, there is a slower rate of axonal regeneration, with a decreased density of regenerating axons. Other studies also demonstrated impaired terminal sprouting of regenerated axons and collateral sprouting of intact adjacent axons, which may be limiting factors for target reinnervation and functional recovery [16].

In a study with 161 patients >60 years, who underwent digital replantation—over 90% of the fingers survived at the 1-year follow-up point. Notably, though, patients aged 70 years or older had an increased risk of replantation failure. Overall functional outcome was inferior in the older patients, which may have been due to decreased sensory recovery [17]. The indication for thumb and finger replantation in the older patient therefore should be individualized depending on the type of injury, the general state of health, functional demands, and rehabilitative potential. Age alone should not be an absolute contraindication to finger replantation today as good outcomes can be achieved [18].

35.2.4 Hand Rehabilitation

Hand function declines gradually with age. After age 65, individuals demonstrate diminished hand and finger range-of-motion (ROM), strength, ability to control submaximal pinch posture, manual speed, and hand sensation [19]. These age-related changes are often accompanied by underlying pathologies such as osteopenia/osteoporosis, osteoarthritis, rheumatoid arthritis, and Parkinson's disease [20]. Hand trauma and the need for immobilization may aggravate functional deterioration associated with these conditions and promote joint stiffness. Therefore, early hand therapy is crucial in elderly patients after hand trauma. To provide adequate and appropriate hand rehabilitation without causing further damage or overexertion, clinicians and therapists must understand the dynamics of age-related functional deterioration [20]. Unfortunately, there is still a paucity of data on optimal hand rehabilitation for this vulnerable patient group.

35.3 Soft Tissue Trauma

Wound healing is normally a well-defined sequence over time. Changes in the soft tissue and skin of elderly patients have diverse intrinsic and extrinsic effects [21], resulting in reduced protection against mechanical and physical trauma. Impaired wound-healing capacity and consequential development of chronic nonhealing wounds have tremendous impact on the individual quality of life and socioeconomic cost. Well-known reasons to vary wound healing are age, nutritional status, hormonal factors, medications such as immunosuppressives, anti-inflammatory agents, and anticoagulants, local wound conditions, underlying disease states [22] all frequently present and alternated in the elderly population. Soft tissue trauma is therefore a threat to the older patient, that needs early and thorough attention to avoid serious consequences.

35.3.1 Bruising

The tendency for bruising is proportional to the physiological changes in aging soft tissue. Aging skin undergoes a process of dermal, subcutaneous tissue loss and epidermal thinning. Among other reasons vascular changes such as delayed angiogenesis, increased capillary fragility in body mass, and increased vascular lesions are responsible for common bruising in elderly people [23, 24]. The use of anticoagulants is a significant risk factor for senile purpura, ecchymoma and hematoma [21]. Extensive ecchymosis and hematoma can cause chronic anemia if occurring repeatedly. Mainly though the bleeding into tissues increases significantly the risk of acquiring skin tears [25].

The medical treatment of bruising includes adequate skin care with proper lubrication and sufficient analgesia. Topical ointments contending nonsteroidal anti-inflammatory drugs optionally with heparin may serve the purpose. Finally, prevention of bruising should be the first priority for patients, caregivers, and healthcare providers.

35.3.2 Skin Tears

Payne and Martin [25–27] published a definition of skin tear in 1990 and revised it in 1993: "a skin tear is a traumatic injury occurring principally on the extremities of older adults as a result of shearing or friction forces which separate the epidermis from the dermis (partial-thickness wound) or which separate the epidermis and the

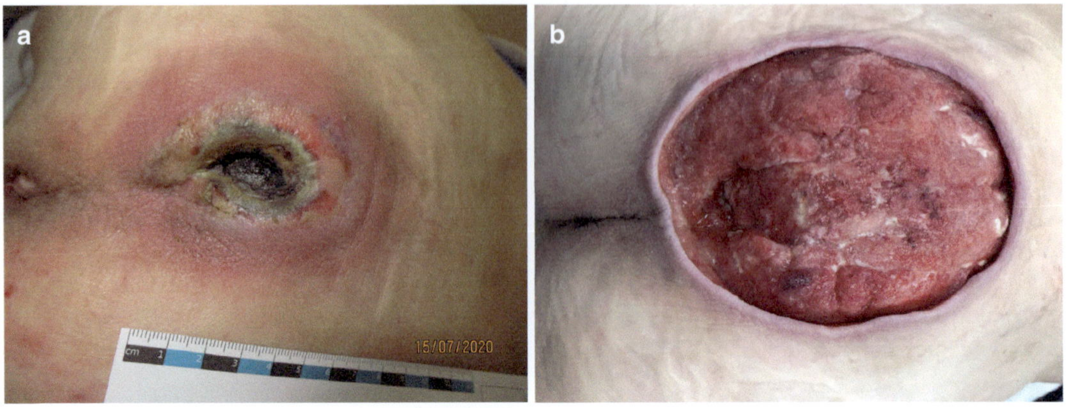

Fig. 35.1 Unstageable pressure injury before (**a**) and after surgical debridement and wound temporization (**b**). The extent of tissue injury can only be suspected in (**a**). Proper expert wound care is required to achieve wound temporization and inhibit deterioration of the wound

dermis from underlying structures (full-thickness wound)". This definition was later included by Carville et al. as part of the Skin Tear Audit Research (STAR) classification system (Fig. 35.1) [25].

Lacerations usually occur in very old, critically ill or medically compromised patients, and in individuals requiring assistance with personal care [21, 25]. Essential characteristics of tears in these patients are that they are very common with the highest incidence in long-term care facilities. The cause is often a minimal mechanic trauma during daily activities or caregiving. Furthermore, skin tears have a high potential risk of evolving into complex chronic wounds [28].

Wound healing is slower in the elderly and may be affected by concomitant conditions, such as diabetes mellitus or vascular disease. Additionally, as already discussed, intrinsic and extrinsic factors such as malnutrition, dehydration, venous insufficiency or smoking may also reduce the healing potential in skin injuries [29].

The same principles used to manage other wounds should be applied when treating skin lacerations [30]. Wound assessment including skin flap or pedicle type using a validated documentation system [25, 27] should be performed before any treatment. Wound cleansing and removal of any necrotic tissue follow the assessment and is essential. Moist wound healing in healable wounds has a high-level evidence support and is an integral part in any wound management [21, 22]. Although skin lacerations are acute wounds with the potential to be closed by primary suture, the fragility and thinness of the elderly skin requires a different approach.

The skin flap should be approximated as far as possible without using any suturing or adhesive strips. Application of a hydrogel, alginate, lipidocolloid based mesh and foam dressing, soft silicone, foam, or non-adherent dressing depending on the type of wound [21].

Conditioned defects with granulation tissue can be treated with a split skin graft to accelerate wound epithelization and complete healing.

Adequate scar and skin care are mandatory to prevent future skin tears and should remain the primary focus.

35.3.3 Facial Trauma

Caused by well-known reasons the risk of stumbling and falling is increased in geriatric patients and is the most common cause of head and neck injury among the elderly [31]. In aging skin, dermal thickness can be reduced by as much as 20%, a contributing factor in the paper-thin appearance of skin of the face. The skin's elasticity and tensile strength decreases, which increases the skin's vulnerability to trauma [21]. In combination with comorbidities and medications facial trauma in elderly patients can be extensive and demand often a damage-control approach to surgical interventions. Extended diagnostic to rule out concomitant injuries is advisable. Measures to monitor and control coagulation should be initiated promptly. Local adherence to a multidisciplinary, evidence-based treatment protocol is recommanded [32]. The attending physician should be competent in diagnosing and retrieving foreign body objects and surgical treatment and reconstruction of complex injuries of the nose, ear, oral cavity, nerves, and eyelid.

35.3.4 Decollement

Decollement injuries are a result of shearing or friction forces which separate and damage the subcutaneous tissue from underlying structures. The initial evaluation and management of these injuries affects their outcome. Factors contributing to this include diagnostic challenges faced by healthcare providers unfamiliar with this injury type and the lack of clear decision-making strategies. This frequently results in underestimation of underlying tissue damage and delay in definitive wound management increasing the risk of infection [33]. Compared with the previously discussed skin laceration injuries, decollement injuries are caused by higher trauma energy and create significant wound surface and associated injuries with high mortality rates. Any extremity with an associated injury is associated with an increased risk of amputation, particularly an extremity decollement with an underlying bone fracture [34]. Although literature data on this topic is limited, this injuries pattern is comparable to burn injuries. Decollement injuries in elderly patients require a damage-control approach to surgical interventions and an implementation of protocolized modern care. These injuries require usually several operations including complex reconstruction with a high complication rate, most of which are secondary to infections [34].

35.3.5 Burn Injury

With a demographic shift and prolonged independent living more people with decreased vision, age-related alteration of judgment and coordination, reduced mobility, and slower response to danger are prone to burn injuries [35]. The elderly population constitute a vulnerable and often challenging group for specialized burn care [36]. Despite improvement in burn care, age is still among the most significant predictors of mortality after burns [36]. The scores used to predict the outcome of burn injuries should not only include the biological age of the patient but rather the aging progression and functionality of a patient. Treating clinicians must be aware that in the elderly, a burn injury of over 30% total body surface area, the risk of mortality is at least 50% [37].

Although several studies have shown a significant reduction of mortality in the elderly in recent decades [18], others have emphasized that older patients still lag behind on mortality and other outcomes compared to younger patients [35]. Mainly due to significant physiological differences like atrophic skin [21] with initially deeper burns [38], impaired healing, extensive comorbidity and associated medication [39], less physiological reserve and malnutrition [40].

The improvement in overall mortality of elderly burn patients appears to be related to improvements in surgical, anesthetics, and critical care and local infrastructure [36]. There is a trend toward earlier burn debridement, which may have contributed to these improved results but further research is needed to make any conclusion in this special age group [36].

35.4 Secondary Infections

Infections in the older patient are generally more frequent and severe than those in younger adults [41]. The factors responsible for the decreased ability of older individuals to protect against infections are related to the gradual deterioration of the immune system, increased fragility/reduced integrity of the tissue structures, and wasting of soft tissue structures.

Once adults reach the sixth decade of life, their immune system undergoes substantial age-related changes (often referred to as "immunosenescence") [42]. These age-related changes induce decreases in both cellular immunity and humoral immunity. Additionally, multiple comorbidities can contribute to a diminution of immune function.

Age-related changes also affect soft tissue structures. For example, dermal-epidermal junctions are flattened, and dermal-epidermal adhesion is reduced [43]. In patients with dermatoporosis, the loss of the hyalurosome in epidermal keratinocytes becomes attenuated, causing a loss of proliferative capacity, and a decline in volume. A consequence of this weakened state is a reduction in the skin's ability to resist (and recover from) mechanical trauma. Other mechanisms known to compromise skin integrity can be seen in patients with vascular diseases. For example, in patients with peripheral vascular disease - a diminished blood supply allows the tissues to become more susceptible to disease severity and progression.

35.4.1 Soft Tissue Infections

The prevalence of soft tissue (and specifically skin) infections increases with age [43]. As such, even minor mechanical trauma can cause breaks in the epidermis. Unfortunately, once this breakdown occurs, the primary mechanism of immune defense is impaired, and infections often follow. Pathogens can spread in the lower dermis and subcutaneous soft tissue. As such, cellulitis becomes much more common with age [43].

35.4.2 Joint Infection

Joints may become infected by direct inoculation, by hematogenous seeding, or by invasion from a neighboring infection [44–45]. Bacteremia is more likely to colonize in a particular joint with preexisting arthritis. This is particularly true if the arthritic joint also is associated with synovitis [44]. Further, given that severe osteoarthritis is more likely to present in older patients - procedures used to treat infected joints (such as debridement) can be more complicated and likely to fail. This phenomenon is due to cartilage loss where the associated osteophytes create cracks and crevices that allow bacteria to evade complete removal [45].

The particular pathogens involved in joint infections are directly related to the cause of the underlying infection. The most common pathogen in septic arthritis is S. aureus, while Streptococci and other gram-positive bacteria can also be potential causes of septic arthritis. Polymicrobial infection is uncommon but is found more often in patients with small joint septic arthritis. In contrast, gram-negative bacilli are more commonly found in patients where the infection is caused by direct inoculation (such as trauma or intravenous drug use) [46].

35.4.3 Bone Infection

Hematogenous osteomyelitis is more likely to occur in pediatric patients who have a more vigorous blood supply to the bones [45]. Whereas acute non-hematogenous osteomyelitis is more likely in the older patient and occurs due to contiguous spread of infection to the bone from adjacent soft tissues and joints (for example, in patients with decubitus ulcers). Usually, acute osteomyelitis can be cured with antimicrobial therapy alone.

Older patients are more likely to have chronic osteomyelitis from previous injuries, wounds, or diabetic infections [45]. Chronic osteomyelitis may be caused by S. aureus but is often due to gram-negative organisms [47]. The organism of chronic osteomyelitis is identified by the culture of bone biopsy. Because of bone sequestra without blood supply, cure of chronic osteomyelitis with antibiotic therapy alone is rarely, if ever, effective. Therefore, surgical debridement is indicated for chronic osteomyelitis, and a cure is impossible without removing all of the infected bone [47].

35.5 Pressure Injury and Chronic Wounds

Elderly patients are prone to a progressive reduction of homeostatic capacity and vascular compensatory mechanisms on the arterial and venous levels. Microcirculation is significantly impaired. Moreover, pathologies affecting systemic organ systems affect the self-healing processes. Comorbidities and frailty, therefore, make older patients susceptible to soft tissue issues. Instability of soft tissues and chronic deterioration of an acute problem is therefore frequently seen in old and multimorbid patients. Prolonged pressure in the presence of reduced sensitivity turning into pressure injury or acute skin laceration turning into chronic and expanding wounds are observed. Ferris and Harding [48] postulated that chronic wounds may be associated with frailty itself. Evidence is scarce, as multiple confounders in the population make it unlikely to clarify this point. Yet a remarkable association has to be acknowledged.

Pressure injury itself frequently starts as a superficial soreness. However, the real damage is developing under the surface. When the superficial pressure is distributed to the deeper tissues, local ischemia and tissue necrosis are resulting with only the tip of the iceberg visible on the skin level. If the skin is finally ulcerating, the deeper tissues may have already progressed to necrosis and are lacking healing capacity from stage III on (Table 35.1). If the necrotic tissue becomes infected, the wound is getting deeper and fascia, muscle, and bone may become affected in addition. While early stages can be treated conservatively, stages III and IV require surgical debridement.

Treating pressure sores and chronic wounds requires special knowledge and care. The situation in the older patient is challenging with regard to healing capacity, compliance, dynamic changes of frailty, and high risk of further decline in independence and mobility (Table 35.2).

Table 35.1 Skin tear classifications systems describe the type of tear with reference to the loss of tissue and the viability of skin flaps detached from the wound bed. The STAR (Skin Tear Research Audit) classification is assessing swelling, bruising and hematoma in addition to tearing and tissue deficiency, which is the main focus of the ISTAP (International Skin Tear Advisory Panel) classification [49, 50]

STAR skin tear classification system				
Category 1a	Category 1b	Category 2a	Category 2b	Category 3
A skin tear where the edges can be realigned to the normal anatomical position (without undue stretching) and the skin or flap colour **is not** pale, dusky or darkened	A skin tear where the edges can be realigned to the normal anatomical position (without undue stretching) and the skin or flap colour **is** pale, dusky or darkened	A skin tear where the edges **cannot** be realigned to the normal anatomical position and the skin or flap colour **is not** pale, dusky or darkened	A skin tear where the edges **cannot** be realigned to the normal anatomical position and the skin or flap colour **is** pale, dusky or darkened	A skin tear where the skin flap is completely absent

ISTAP skin tear classification		
Type 1	Type 2	Type 3
No skin loss	Partial skin flap loss	Total skin flap loss
Linear tear or flap, which can be repositioned to fully cover the wound bed	Flap, which does not fully cover the wound bed	Tear with total wound bed exposure

Table 35.2 Pressure injury staging is assessing the depth of tissue injury and damage, as well as exposure of subdermal structures. Usually pressure injury occurs over bony prominences or pressure points, e.g. heel, malleolus, trochanter, sacrum, scapula, elbows, back of head

Stage 1	Stage 2	Stage 3	Stage 4	Unstageable
Redness or discolouration of intact skin	Blister or partial loss of dermis	Full thickness loss of skin, exposure of fat	Full thickness loss of tissue, exposure of bone, tendon, muscle	Full thickness loss of tissue, with slough of eschar covering the wound bed

35.6 Treatment Principles

The key factor to healing pressure injury not only in the older patient, but especially in the elderly, is mobilization. As long as the patient is bed-bound or resistant to pressure relief, only restricted treatment with wound care, positioning, pressure relieving mattresses, and in case of additional infection, antibiotic treatment is advisable. Yet wound healing is more effective if pressure changes through mobilization lead to an increase of systemic blood pressure and microcirculation of the wound bed. If physiotherapy is capable of mobilizing the patient, further surgical steps can be planned.

Correcting malnutrition is an additional prerequisite, that is mandatory to address. Loss of lean body mass through immobilization should be limited. Enteral or parenteral feeding are measures that affect patients drastically, but addressing protein intake, vitamins, trace minerals, and electrolytes is compulsive if further deterioration is to be avoided.

Debridement should be as minimal as possible. Only third- and fourth-degree pressure injuries should be treated surgically. First necrotic tissue is to be removed and conditioning of the wound bed is advised. Different concepts from moist wound care with hydrogels, alginate, or negative wound pressure therapy have shown value. If healing capacity is sufficient secondary wound healing can be attempted. If progress is slow or the wound is large and deep flap surgery may accelerate the process and gain valuable time for the patient. Flaps should be planned in such a fashion that sufficient tissue is available for upholstering bony protuberances, if these cannot be removed. Patients should again be mobilized as early as possible for pneumonia prophylaxis, but especially for gluteal and sacral flaps sitting should be avoided for a couple of weeks.

References

1. Gioffre-Florio M, Murabito LM, Visalli C, Pergolizzi FP, Fama F. Trauma in elderly patients: a study of prevalence, comorbidities and gender differences. G Chir. 2018;39(1):35–40.
2. Keller JM, Sciadini MF, Sinclair E, O'Toole RV. Geriatric trauma: demographics, injuries, and mortality. J Orthop Trauma. 2012;26(9):e161–5.
3. Rosberg HE, Dahlin LB. An increasing number of hand injuries in an elderly population - a retrospective study over a 30-year period. BMC Geriatr. 2018;18(1):68.
4. United Nations. Available from: https://www.un.org/en/sections/issues-depth/ageing.
5. Kanis JA, Oden A, Johnell O, Jonsson B, de Laet C, Dawson A. The burden of osteoporotic fractures: a method for setting intervention thresholds. Osteoporos Int. 2001;12(5):417–27.
6. Schwab CW, Kauder DR. Trauma in the geriatric patient. Arch Surg. 1992;127(6):701–6.
7. Court-Brown CM, Biant LC, Clement ND, Bugler KE, Duckworth AD, McQueen MM. Open fractures in the elderly. The importance of skin ageing. Injury. 2015;46(2):189–94.
8. Niver GE, Ilyas AM. Carpal tunnel syndrome after distal radius fracture. Orthop Clin North Am. 2012;43(4):521–7.
9. Levin LS, Rozell JC, Pulos N. Distal radius fractures in the elderly. J Am Acad Orthop Surg. 2017;25(3):179–87.
10. Lutz K, Yeoh KM, MacDermid JC, Symonette C, Grewal R. Complications associated with operative versus nonsurgical treatment of distal radius fractures in patients aged 65 years and older. J Hand Surg Am. 2014;39(7):1280–6.
11. Wollstein R, Trouw A, Carlson L, Staff I, Mastella DJ, Ashmead D. The effect of age on fracture healing time in metacarpal fractures. Hand (N Y). 2020;15(4):542–6.
12. Goldring MB, Otero M. Inflammation in osteoarthritis. Curr Opin Rheumatol. 2011;23(5):471–8.
13. Mushtaq S, Choudhary R, Scanzello CR. Non-surgical treatment of osteoarthritis-related pain in the elderly. Curr Rev Musculoskelet Med. 2011;4(3):113–22.
14. Altman R, Barkin RL. Topical therapy for osteoarthritis: clinical and pharmacologic perspectives. Postgrad Med. 2009;121(2):139–47.
15. Verdu E, Ceballos D, Vilches JJ, Navarro X. Influence of aging on peripheral nerve function and regeneration. J Peripher Nerv Syst. 2000;5(4):191–208.
16. Kovacic U, Sketelj J, Bajrovic FF. Chapter 26: age-related differences in the reinnervation after peripheral nerve injury. Int Rev Neurobiol. 2009;87:465–82.
17. Kwon GD, Ahn BM, Lee JS, Park YG, Chang GW, Ha YC. The effect of patient age on the success rate of digital replantation. Plast Reconstr Surg. 2017;139(2):420–6.
18. Barzin A, Hernandez-Boussard T, Lee GK, Curtin C. Adverse events following digital replantation in the elderly. J Hand Surg Am. 2011;36(5):870–4.
19. Ranganathan VK, Siemionow V, Sahgal V, Yue GH. Effects of aging on hand function. J Am Geriatr Soc. 2001;49(11):1478–84.
20. Carmeli E, Patish H, Coleman R. The aging hand. J Gerontol A Biol Sci Med Sci. 2003;58(2):146–52.
21. LeBlanc K, Baranoski S. Skin tear consensus panel M. Skin tears: state of the science: consensus statements for the prevention, prediction, assessment, and treatment of skin tears(c). Adv Skin Wound Care. 2011;24(9 Suppl):2–15.

22. Sibbald RG, Orsted HL, Coutts PM, Keast DH. Best practice recommendations for preparing the wound bed: update 2006. Adv Skin Wound Care. 2007;20(7):390–405. quiz 6-7
23. Leblanc K, Baranoski S. Prevention and management of skin tears. Adv Skin Wound Care. 2009;22(7):325–32. quiz 33-4
24. Ratliff CR, Fletcher KR. Skin tears: a review of the evidence to support prevention and treatment. Ostomy Wound Manage. 2007;53(3):32–34, 6, 8–40 passim.
25. Carville K, Lewin G, Newall N, Haslehurst P, Michael R, Santamaria N, et al. A consensus for skin tear classification. Primary Intension. 2007;15(1):18–28.
26. Payne RL, Martin ML. The epidemiology and management of skin tears in older adults. Ostomy Wound Manage. 1990;26:26–37.
27. Payne RL, Martin ML. Defining and classifying skin tears: need for a common language. Ostomy Wound Manage 1993;39(5):16–20, 2–4, 6.
28. Leblanc K, Christensen D, Cook J, Culhane B, Gutierrez O. Prevalence of skin tears in a long-term care facility. J Wound Ostomy Continence Nurs. 2013;40(6):580–4.
29. Gosain A, DiPietro LA. Aging and wound healing. World J Surg. 2004;28(3):321–6.
30. Baranoski S. How to prevent and manage skin tears. Adv Skin Wound Care. 2003;16(5):268–70.
31. Sethi RK, Kozin ED, Fagenholz PJ, Lee DJ, Shrime MG, Gray ST. Epidemiological survey of head and neck injuries and trauma in the United States. Otolaryngol Head Neck Surg. 2014;151(5):776–84.
32. Spahn DR, Bouillon B, Cerny V, Duranteau J, Filipescu D, Hunt BJ, et al. The European guideline on management of major bleeding and coagulopathy following trauma: fifth edition. Crit Care. 2019;23(1):98.
33. Hakim S, Ahmed K, El-Menyar A, Jabbour G, Peralta R, Nabir S, et al. Patterns and management of degloving injuries: a single national level 1 trauma center experience. World J Emerg Surg. 2016;11:35.
34. Velazquez C, Whitaker L, Pestana IA. Degloving soft tissue injuries of the extremity: characterization, categorization, outcomes, and management. Plast Reconstr Surg Glob Open. 2020;8(11):e3277.
35. World Health Organization [Available from: https://www.who.int/news-room/fact-sheets/detail/ageing-and-health.
36. Wearn C, Hardwicke J, Kitsios A, Siddons V, Nightingale P, Moiemen N. Outcomes of burns in the elderly: revised estimates from the Birmingham burn Centre. Burns. 2015;41(6):1161–8.
37. Jeschke MG, Pinto R, Costford SR, Amini-Nik S. Threshold age and burn size associated with poor outcomes in the elderly after burn injury. Burns. 2016;42(2):276–81.
38. Albornoz CR, Villegas J, Sylvester M, Pena V, Bravo I. Burns are more aggressive in the elderly: proportion of deep burn area/total burn area might have a role in mortality. Burns. 2011;37(6):1058–61.
39. Pereira CT, Barrow RE, Sterns AM, Hawkins HK, Kimbrough CW, Jeschke MG, et al. Age-dependent differences in survival after severe burns: a unicentric review of 1,674 patients and 179 autopsies over 15 years. J Am Coll Surg. 2006;202(3):536–48.
40. Sheridan R. Burns at the extremes of age. J Burn Care Res. 2007;28(4):580–5.
41. Gavazzi G, Krause KH. Ageing and infection. Lancet Infect Dis. 2002;2(11):659–66.
42. Listi F, Candore G, Modica MA, Russo M, Di Lorenzo G, Esposito-Pellitteri M, et al. A study of serum immunoglobulin levels in elderly persons that provides new insights into B cell immunosenescence. Ann N Y Acad Sci. 2006;1089:487–95.
43. Laube S. Skin infections and ageing. Ageing Res Rev. 2004;3(1):69–89.
44. McBride S, Mowbray J, Caughey W, Wong E, Luey C, Siddiqui A, et al. Epidemiology, management, and outcomes of large and small native joint septic arthritis in adults. Clin Infect Dis. 2020;70(2):271–9.
45. Mears SC, Edwards PK. Bone and joint infections in older adults. Clin Geriatr Med. 2016;32(3):555–70.
46. Dubost JJ, Couderc M, Tatar Z, Tournadre A, Lopez J, Mathieu S, et al. Three-decade trends in the distribution of organisms causing septic arthritis in native joints: single-center study of 374 cases. Joint Bone Spine. 2014;81(5):438–40.
47. Cunha BA. Osteomyelitis in elderly patients. Clin Infect Dis. 2002;35(3):287–93.
48. Ferris AE, Harding KG. Are chronic wounds a feature of frailty? Br J Gen Pract. 2020;70(694):256–7.
49. Carville K, Lewin G, Newall N, Haslehurst P, Michael R, Santamaria N, et al. A consensus for skin tear classification. Primary Intension. 2007;15(1):18–28.
50. Van Tiggelen H, LeBlanc K, Campbell K, Woo K, Baranoski S, Chang YY, et al. Standardizing the classification of skin tears: validity and reliability testing of the International Skin Tear Advisory Panel Classification System in in 44 countries. Br J Dermatol. 2020;183(1):146–54.

Part VIII

Rehabilitation and Outcomes

Geriatric Rehabilitation

36

Theiler Robert, Freystaetter Gregor, Simmen Hans-Peter, Pothmann Carina Eva Maria, and Neuhaus Valentin

36.1 Background

Geriatric Medicine is the specialty of medicine, which focuses on physical, mental, functional, and social conditions in acute, chronic, rehabilitative, preventive, and end-of-life care in older patients [1]. Geriatric care requires a different approach, especially diagnostic and therapeutic processes need to take the consequences of each intervention including possible adverse events and the patient's wishes into consideration. The conceptional orientation of geriatric care has to ensure the sensitive perception of the special needs of senior patients, the age-appropriate diagnostics and therapy as well as the full utilization of the current individual rehabilitation potentials [1, 2].

36.2 Geriatric Patients

The human organism ordinarily changes with increasing age. As a consequence, we see adapting functional abilities and preferences of aging seniors. Polymorbidity or multiple comorbidities are typically present and functional deficits increase. These issues cause an accumulation of specific medical and nursing problems, the "age-related diseases" as: degenerative bone and joint diseases, hearing deficits and visual disturbances (e.g., macular degeneration, cataract), neurologic diseases (e.g., Alzheimer disease, Parkinson), and sleeping disorders just to mention a few. The risk of acute and chronic cardiovascular diseases, myocardial infarction, stroke, hypertension, cancer, and other chronic diseases like diabetes mellitus steadily increases with aging. People with these diseases require more frequent medical treatment.

According to the guidelines of the medical societies, geriatric patients are characterized by [1, 3]:

- older age, usually 70+ years
- geriatric multimorbidity: presence of various coexisting diseases with the need for treatment;

or by:

- age 80+ years
- age-specific higher vulnerability for complications and secondary events
- danger of manifestation of a chronic state
- and increased risk of loss of autonomy

T. Robert · F. Gregor
Department of Geriatrics, University Hospital of Zurich, Zurich, Switzerland
e-mail: Gregor.Freystaetter@usz.ch

S. Hans-Peter (✉) · P. C. E. Maria · N. Valentin
Department of Trauma Surgery, University Hospital of Zurich, Zurich, Switzerland
e-mail: Hanspeter.Simmen@usz.ch; Carina.Pothmann@usz.ch; Valentin.Neuhaus@usz.ch

H.-C. Pape et al. (eds.), *Senior Trauma Patients*, https://doi.org/10.1007/978-3-030-91483-7_36

In geriatric patients, serious, often chronic, diseases come together with common age-related alterations [1].

Elderly patients with an acute disease often experience and present with atypical symptoms. They are extremely prone to complications and must be seen as a highly vulnerable group. Geriatric multimorbidity is often the result of impaired physiological functions and decreased activities of daily living, in various combinations, in the sense of a "geriatric syndrome". Consequences of geriatric multimorbidity are immobility, dizziness, falls, cognitive deficits, incontinence, decubital ulcer, malnutrition, depression, anxiety, chronic pain, hearing and vision problems, and finally frailty. These geriatric syndromes are prone to complications and loss of independence. Diagnosis and therapy of geriatric syndromes are complex, often challenging requiring expertise and a multi-professional team. Patient's response to treatment is frequently delayed and often social support is required. The main goal of geriatric treatment is to optimize the functional status of the elderly patient and to improve or at least preserve his/her quality of life and autonomy. Geriatric medicine is not set to a specific age range but rather concentrates on individual functional deficits.

Acute events are often successfully treated with geriatric expertise. Due to comorbidities as well as social isolation, an acute medical event may lead to the loss of autonomy and the need for nursing care. The main goal of geriatric medicine is to preserve autonomy and to prevent long-term care placement of this vulnerable patient group. This requires an individualized treatment plan with a distinct medical, preventive, restorative, social, and ethical assessment.

Patients suffering from dementia can be very challenging, as the conditions described above are also often present and are causing problems. Cognitively impaired people are frequently not able to describe their symptoms adequately. Dementia compromises independence of seniors significantly. The prevalence of dementia increases with age from approximately 1.5% at the age of 65 years up to 30% in people over 90 [4]. Dementia quadruples the risk for nursing care. Only 14% of men and 6% of women with dementia did not need care at the time of their death. Patients with the need for nursing care present with longer and more complex courses and often suffer complications like delirium, infections, falls, etc., and as a consequence require higher nursing care levels, higher use of medical services, and also higher use of health insurance benefits.

If dementia is diagnosed and treated at an early stage, the decline can be slowed down and skills are preserved longer [4]. However, early detection of dementia is difficult in people with severe cognitive impairments. Geriatric skills for general practitioners and specialists in hospitals and facilities for disabled people are therefore highly recommended.

36.2.1 Holistic Geriatric Treatment Approach

Geriatric patients often suffer from serious, frequently chronic diseases, that combine with the usual age-related changes. Geriatric care structures and treatment processes must take these special concerns of the elderly patients into account. They must be designed as an overall therapeutic-rehabilitative concept, considering physical, psychological, functional, and social aspects of this patient group. The main goal of the treatment is to optimize the functional status of the patients, improve the quality of life and autonomy, and promote participation.

36.3 Principles of Geriatric Rehabilitation

One of the essential pillars in geriatric rehabilitation is ensuring the quality of life of our elderly patients. Geriatric rehabilitation is mandatory for ethical and economic reasons if there is a risk of lasting impairment of everyday activities and participation in social life, independent of the diseases. The focus in the rehabilitation process lies on the treatment of the consequences of the disease, the impairment of activities, and participation. If necessary, the cause of the disease is

Table 36.1 Type of postacute medical treatment

		Type of post-acute medical treatment		
	Type	Aim	Health professional	Location
(1)	Postacute care	Functional recovery	Monodisciplinary	Outpatient
		Independence		Ambulatory
(2)	Postacute rehabilitation	Functional recovery	Multidisciplinary	In and outpatient
		Independence		
(3)	Palliative care	Symptomatic treatment	Multidisciplinary	In and outpatient

treated in addition to the rehabilitation. Geriatric inpatient and outpatient rehabilitation is carried out close to the place of residence in order to involve relatives and friends in the rehabilitation process. It is the best treatment package for patients over 70 years suffering from several diseases at the same time.

A basic methodological principle of geriatric rehabilitation is the comprehensive geriatric assessment, carried out in an acute care setting, Table 36.1. It is a multi-dimensional assessment of an older person's medical, psychosocial, functional, and environmental resources and problems, and it creates an overall plan for treatment [5]. Based on this, assessments of patients are categorized in three functional categories: robust, prefrail, and frail. Certain domains of this assessment like mobility or quality of life are not only carried out in acute care, but also during the rehabilitation process and in the outpatient setting, in order to monitor the treatment progress.

Special consideration regarding procedures following surgery has to be taken [6]. Following trauma, for example, fractures or hip prosthesis, special guidelines should be followed [7–9]. Malnutrition may be a serious concern [10].

36.4 The Interdisciplinary Rehabilitation Team

Geriatric rehabilitation is characterized by a multi-professional team, as seen in acute care settings namely somatic departments. It includes the following professions:

- physician, physician-assistant, advanced nurse-practitioner
- nursing staff
- physiotherapy/movement therapy
- occupational therapy
- logopedic
- psychologists
- social worker
- dietitian

In acute care, the geriatric team, which often functions as a mobile geriatric triage unit, decides how the future rehabilitation process will be guided, see Fig. 36.1.

Geriatric rehabilitation is guided by the functional status of the individual patients.

36.4.1 Need for Rehabilitation

The need for rehabilitation assumes a physical, mental, or emotional disease to be present and to affect activity limitation and participation in domestic and nondomestic life according to the ICF terminology [11].

The necessity for post-acute rehabilitation is further characterized by the lack of treatment options in acute care. The required conditions are met in a post-acute rehabilitation center, where adequate therapy is carried out by several professions working in a team under medical surveillance in suitable spatial and equipped rooms. There are different types and healthcare professionals during post-acute care, see Table 36.1.

The rehabilitation pathway is guided by the comprehensive geriatric assessment and the classification in robust, prefrail and frail functional status, see Fig. 36.1. There is uncertainty if frail patients have still a potential for successful geriatric rehabilitation [12].

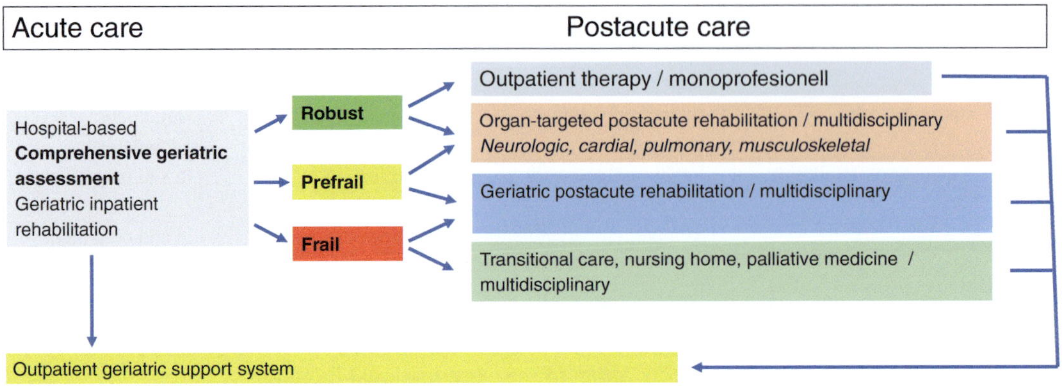

Fig. 36.1 Geriatric rehabilitation pathways

36.4.2 Rehabilitation Potential

Patient must be able to actively participate in the rehabilitation treatment. Therefore, he or she must be in adequate physical and mental condition and necessary resilience. Patients have to agree to the treatment and be motivated for it.

36.4.3 Rehabilitation Goals

Rehabilitation is always carried out in consideration of a rehabilitation goal. In general, this is regaining, improving, or maintaining independency in everyday life performances, in order to return to the previous living environment. The rehabilitation goal can also be to gain back the ability to walk up the stairs to a patient's apartment, which increases her or his independence. The goal for a bedridden patient can be to transfer out of bed for a couple of hours per day.

36.4.4 Positive Rehabilitation Prognosis

Before a rehabilitation is approved by the insurance company the treating doctor evaluates whether the rehabilitation goals are realistically achievable in the period planned for the rehabilitation (positive rehabilitation prognosis). For this, the stage of the disease and the functional deficits, the previous disease progression as well as the ability of its regression have to be recognized under consideration of the personal life circumstances of the person.

References

1. UEMS. Definition of geriatrics. 2008.
2. Geriatriekonzept Baden-Württemberg 2014. 2014.
3. DGGG. Definition Geriatrischer Patienten. 2007. Available from: https://www.ekweende.de/fileadmin/user_upload/abteilungen/geriatrie/info_geriatr_patient.pdf.
4. Dementia UK: Update Second Edition report produced by King's College London and the London School of Economics for the Alzheimer's Society. 2014.
5. Stuck AE, Iliffe S. Comprehensive geriatric assessment for older adults. BMJ. 2011;343:d6799.
6. Stürmer K. Leitlinien Unfallchirurgie der DGU stand, vol. 2018; 2018.
7. Theiler R. Targeted training therapy for secondary prevention of falls and hip fractures praxis. 2017;106(13):701–4.
8. Biggi S, et al. The value of a standardized and reproducible surgical technique in treatment of Vancouver B2 periprosthetic fractures: our experience. Eur J Trauma Emerg Surg. 2019;45(6):1031–8.
9. Liener, U., C. Becker, and K. Rapp, Weissbuch alterstraumatologie. 2018.
10. Renerts K, et al. Effects of a simple home exercise program and vitamin D supplementation on health-related quality of life after a hip fracture: a randomized controlled trial. Qual Life Res. 2019;28(5):1377–86.
11. World Health Organization (WHO). The international classification of functioning, disability and health. Geneva: WHO; 2001.
12. Cameron ID, Kurrle SE. Frailty and rehabilitation. Interdiscip Top Gerontol Geriatr. 2015;41:137–50.

Functional Recovery After Hip Fracture

37

Mohammad Auais, Katie Sheehan, Jay Magaziner, and Lauren Beaupre

37.1 Introduction

Hip fracture is a global public health concern. It is one of the most devastating but preventable injuries among individuals 65 years and older, and one of the most common. Optimal rehabilitation starts at the acute hospital immediately after surgical repair and continues after discharge. When patients are medically stable, they are returned directly to their prior living place (home/long-term care) or sent to an in-patient institution for intensive rehabilitation before being sent home. Hereafter, we will use the term long-term care facility (LTC), also known as a nursing home or extended care facility, to refer to institutions that provide continuous medical and social services for patients with chronic health problems who can no longer remain independent at home. This chapter provides an overview of known consequences of hip fracture and burden on healthcare systems currently and in the future, approaches to defining recovery including the patient's and other stakeholders perspective, and opportunities to improve recovery in different care settings based on emerging evidence, starting with acute care hospital and continuing to different post-acute settings.

This book chapter was submitted for publication in September 2019 and was accepted in Jan 2020.

M. Auais
Department of Physical Therapy, School of Rehabilitation Therapy, Faculty of Health Sciences, Queen's University, Kingston, ON, Canada

K. Sheehan
Department of Population Health Sciences, School of Life Course and Population Sciences, Faculty of Life Sciences and Medicine, Kings College London, London, UK

J. Magaziner (✉)
Department of Epidemiology and Public Health, School of Medicine, University of Maryland, Baltimore, MD, USA
e-mail: JMAGAZIN@som.umaryland.edu

L. Beaupre
Department of Physical Therapy, Faculty of Rehabilitation Medicine, University of Alberta, Edmonton, AB, Canada

37.1.1 Consequences of Hip Fracture

Despite the success of surgical repair in the majority of cases, the short- and long-term outcomes of hip fracture are discouraging. Hip fractures rank among the top ten debilitating disabilities worldwide and result in more mortality and morbidity than all other osteoporotic fractures combined.

The reported mortality rate in the first 12 months after a fracture has in some studies exceeded 30% [1]. Additionally, across studies and regions, men have higher mortality rates, despite them being younger at the time of fracture. While some studies have attributed the excess mortality in men to cardiovascular disease, pneumonia, and sepsis [2, 3], others did not find similar evidence and suggested that it could

H.-C. Pape et al. (eds.), *Senior Trauma Patients*, https://doi.org/10.1007/978-3-030-91483-7_37

be attributed to acute complications after the fracture [4]. This topic requires further investigation [4, 5].

For survivors, 40–78% have not fully recovered 1 year after a fracture [6]. Review of outcomes after hip fracture estimated that on average, 35% of hip fracture survivors were incapable of independent walking a year or more after the injury [7], and 20–60% required assistance with various tasks 2 years after fracture [6]. Immobility after the fracture contributes to the deterioration of balance and muscle strength, which consequently increases the likelihood of subsequent falls, leading to recurrent fractures and further disability.

In the immediate future, the burden on healthcare systems and the resources required to care for patients with hip fractures and its consequences (especially in the community) are expected to increase. Recent research has shown a continuous increase in the absolute number of people with hip fractures, due partly to increased life expectancy [8, 9]. Evidence shows that despite patients with hip fractures getting sicker over time, their in-hospital mortality rates are declining, and direct discharges to home and LTCs are becoming more common [9]. Furthermore, length of stay in acute hospitals is declining, so patients are being discharged to the community earlier, with significant needs. These trends suggest that the economic and societal costs associated with the consequences of hip fracture are likely to increase substantially over the coming decades and that the demand for available resources in the community will also increase.

37.2 Defining Functional Recovery

The conventional goals of management for hip fracture survivors include achieving functional autonomy, return to pre-fracture levels of independence, and the prevention of subsequent fractures; however, a high percentage of patients fail to achieve these goals [6, 10]. The assessment of recovery in individuals surviving hip fracture is important for both research and clinical practice, yet the best method for characterizing recovery following hip fracture remains elusive and may have implications for the delivery of care designed to maximize post-fracture outcomes.

Two conceptually different approaches to defining functional recovery are most used. The first requires that the patient returns to a preexisting level of physical capacity, with an inherent assumption that the pre-functional level is the "normal state". While this approach is common, it is dependent on knowing the patient's pre-fracture status, which can be assessed at a global level (e.g., able to walk without any assistance). Furthermore, using this definition to compare recovery among patients demands accounting for the heterogeneity in pre-fracture functional status. Using this definition as a goal of rehabilitation also assumes that recovery to this point is sufficient, when it is quite possible that patients can improve further. A second approach to defining recovery entails achieving a prespecified functional target that is considered sufficient to declare recovery (e.g., walking a specific distance or autonomy in activities of daily living). The target could include being able to independently carry out a daily activity that is reflective of functional reserves and associated with independence in mobility and everyday life activities. The degree of functional recovery after hip fracture varies on the basis of the definition used. In a previous study comparing these two definitions of recovery, the second definition was better associated with health-related quality of life than the first [11].

A key message is that careful consideration of the definition of recovery used in research or clinical practice is vital, as this can impact clinical decision-making for endorsing a specific intervention or even discharging a patient from rehabilitation.

37.2.1 Patient Perspective on Recovery

Healthcare professionals often adopt a traditional biomedical model to define recovery as the attainment of pre-fracture physical dimensions of

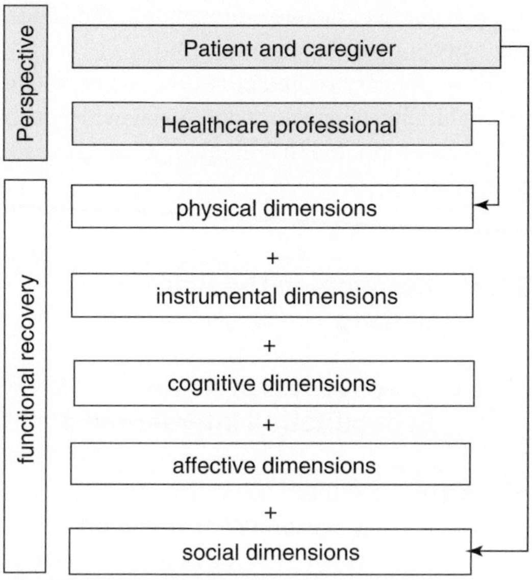

Fig. 37.1 Recovery from the healthcare professional, patient, and caregiver perspective. Reprinted from Sheehan et al. [12]; with permission from Oxford University Press

function. However, patients and caregivers often adopt a more personal definition, which incorporates the patients' perspectives on the importance of functioning well physically, instrumentally, cognitively, affectively, and socially (Fig. 37.1) [12]. This is consistent with the World Health Organization (WHO) approach to healthy aging as having the functional ability to be or to do what the individual has reason to value [13].

In the last 10 years, a series of qualitative studies suggested that uncertainty regarding the most effective rehabilitation is due in part to a lack of understanding of the patient perspective of recovery and rehabilitation after hip fracture. Most of these studies focused on patient perspective in the early post-discharge period (<4 months) [14–16] or at longer-term follow-up (4 months – 8 years post-fracture [16, 17]. Themes related to loss, adaptation to a new functional level, increasing dependence, as well as engagement with resources for recovery (including reliance on professional feedback for motivation and reassurance), need for physical activity and goal setting, and a need for self-determination were reported across studies.

37.2.2 Timing of Recovery

An important consideration in recovery is that time required to achieve recovery is specific to the area of function [18]. This may partly explain why findings vary widely across studies based on the area of function assessed.

Some researchers have argued that there is a time limit for recovery, and that the possibility of patients with hip fractures making further functional gains after this limit (e.g., 4 or 6 months after fracture) is very small [19]. This argument was reinforced by a number of studies showing an overall continuous improvement in many functional tasks up to a specific period of time following fracture, after which functional recovery plateaus. For instance, a 2013 study evaluated a cohort of patients with hip fractures at 1, 3, and 12 months after fracture, and found most recovery occurred during the first 3 months, with a non-clinically significant improvement afterward [20].

However, emerging evidence shows that significant functional improvement can be gained later in the recovery process than previously believed, as long as there is proper rehabilitation provided across the continuum of recovery [21, 22]. This evidence suggests there may be no 'plateau' associated with patients' capacity, but rather implying that any observed plateau may be a consequence of less intensive therapy [11, 23–25]. If health services received by patients end prematurely during the recovery process, the patients subsequently appear to settle into a sedentary lifestyle and gradually start losing functional gains made during rehabilitation in the early months after surgery [11].

37.3 Guidelines for Rehabilitation in the Acute and Subacute Settings

Rehabilitation assists *"individuals who experience disability to achieve and maintain optimal functioning in interaction with their environment"* [26]. Several countries established guidelines and standards for rehabilitation after hip fracture. For example, the National Institute for Health and Care Excellence (NICE) Guideline (updated May 2017) for acute rehabilitation after hip fracture is limited to (1) offering patients a physiotherapy assessment and, unless medically or surgically contraindicated, mobilization on the day after surgery; (2) offering patients mobilization at least once a day and ensuring regular physiotherapy review; and (3) early identification of individual goals for multidisciplinary rehabilitation to recover mobility and independence, and to facilitate return to pre-fracture residence and long-term wellbeing [27]. This led to the Chartered Society of Physiotherapy commissioning the first international audit of rehabilitation after hip fracture [28]. The audit reported marked variation across the country in the extent, quality, and duration of acute rehabilitation after hip fracture. Following publication, they developed a series of standards to align with the current NICE guideline.

Earlier guidelines include the 2015 guidelines for treatment and rehabilitation after hip fracture by the American Academy of Orthopaedic Surgeons. These recommended interdisciplinary care to manage Deep Vein Thrombosis (DVT), prevention and management of delirium, multimodal perioperative pain management, interdisciplinary management of recovery at rehabilitation and LTC facilities, home care therapy after discharge, and osteoporosis assessment and management [29]. In 2011, Bone and Joint Canada published the National Hip Fracture Toolkit detailing evidence for rehabilitation after hip fracture in 2011. The Toolkit promoted early mobility, adequate pain management, and early and continuous transition planning in the acute phase. While the Toolkit acknowledged the challenges of different subacute rehabilitation settings, it also highlighted the need for ongoing intensive rehabilitation irrespective of the rehabilitation setting. In the longer term, the Toolkit suggested community-based exercise programs to optimize physical conditioning and reduce future falls risk. This report noted the shift from a medical model of care in the initial postoperative period to a functional model of care to improve recovery and finally a preventative model of care to avoid further fractures through fall prevention and osteoporosis management [30].

This summary of guidelines is not exhaustive but highlights the need for additional evidence to inform appropriate rehabilitation across the care continuum.

37.4 Recovery in the Acute Setting

37.4.1 Effectiveness of Acute Rehabilitation Interventions

A series of randomized controlled trials explored interventions for rehabilitation after hip fracture in the acute hospital setting (Table 37.1). These interventions were broadly classified as weight-bearing, exercises, increased physiotherapy/occupational therapy, mobility training, balance training, resistance training, electrical stimulation, and/or multidisciplinary care. Most interventions within these classifications adopted different intervention protocols and different primary study outcomes making comparison across studies difficult. Moreover, the evidence for several of these trials was deemed to be of low quality by a number of systematic reviews [31–33].

There is low-quality evidence in favor of early mobilization after hip fracture surgery which has been adopted by clinical guidelines internationally. Proponents of early mobilization argue that delays affect recovery through loss of muscle mass and strength induced by bed rest. Further, a longer time to mobilization may lead to potentially fatal complications such as pulmonary embolism or pneumonia.

The evidence for physiotherapy and/or occupational therapy interventions favors a comprehensive approach with more frequent and longer duration interventions for beneficial effects on promoting independence in activities, general health, and reducing fatigue, as well as falls risk. The benefit of more frequent and longer duration interventions for mobility and function is less clear and may be due in part to specificity of the intervention components. Interventions that target mobility rehabilitation, balance

Table 37.1 Randomized controlled trials of acute rehabilitation interventions after hip fracture

Author year	Sample size	Country	Intervention/control	Primary outcome	Intervention effective
Weight-bearing					
Moseley 2009	160	Australia	I: Twice daily for 60-minutes weight-bearing for 16 weeks (start in acute) C: Usual care	Physical performance and mobility exam	No
Oldmeadow 2006	60	Australia	I: Early weight-bearing C: Delayed weight-bearing	Walking distance	Yes
Sherrington 2004	80	Australia	I: Weight-bearing C: Non-weight-bearing	Physical performance and mobility exam	No
Sherrington 2003	120	Australia	I: Weight-bearing or non-weight-bearing C: Usual care	6-m walk time	No
Increased physiotherapy/occupational therapy					
Bischoff-Ferrari 2010	173	Germany	I: 60 min/day supervised physiotherapy, unsupervised home exercise program C: 30 min/day supervised physiotherapy	Falls	Yes
Karumo 1977	100	Finland	I: Twice daily physiotherapy C: Once daily physiotherapy	Mobility aid use	No
Kimmel 2016	92	Australia	I: 3 times/day supervised physiotherapy sessions C: Usual care	Iowa level of assistance	Yes
Lauridsen 2002	88	Denmark	I: High intensity supervised physiotherapy C: Usual care	Function	No
Martin-Martin 2014	122	Spain	I: Usual care and occupational therapy C: Usual care	GHQ-28, perceived fatigue	Yes
Resnick 2007	155	USA	I: Supervised exercise program C: Usual care	Self-efficacy for walking exercise scale	No
Mobility rehabilitation					
Baker 1991	40	Australia	I: Treadmill gait retraining C: Over-ground gait retraining	Regain pre-fracture mobility	No
Salpakoski 2014	81	Finland	I: Mobility rehabilitation programme C: Usual care	Ability to negotiate stairs	Yes
Balance training					
Monticone 2018	52	Italy	I: 3 weeks of 90 min supervised balance task-specific training 5 times/week C: 3 weeks of 90 min usual care 5 times/week	WOMAC	Yes

(continued)

Table 37.1 (continued)

Author year	Sample size	Country	Intervention/control	Primary outcome	Intervention effective
Resistance training					
Kronborg 2017	90	Denmark	I: Daily physiotherapy with progressive knee-extension strength training C: Usual care	Max isometric knee-extension strength	No
Mendelsohn 2008	20	Canada	I: 4 weeks of 5 physiotherapy and occupational therapy sessions and arm crank ergometer 3 times/week C: 4 weeks of 5 physiotherapy and occupational therapy sessions	V02 peak	Yes
Miller 2006	75	Australia	I: Resistance training/resistance and nutrition C: Education	Gait speed	No
Mitchell 2001	80	UK	I: 6-week quadriceps strength training C: Usual care	Elderly mobility scale	Yes
Electrical stimulation					
Braid 2008	26	UK	I: 6 weeks of electrical stimulation C: Usual care	Elderly mobility scale	No
Gorodetskyi 2007	60	Russia	I: Electrical stimulation C: Placebo stimulation	Pain on walking	Yes
Lamb 2002	27	UK	I: 6 weeks of electrical stimulation C: Placebo stimulation	Regain pre-fracture mobility	Yes

I: intrevention group, C: control group, GHQ-28: General Health Questionnaire – 28, WOMAC: the Western Ontario and McMaster Universities Osteoarthritis Index training, and/or resistance training all show promise for improvements in functional outcomes. Electrical stimulation has conflicting evidence for mobility gains. This may be due in part to insufficient power in the underlying evidence to determine the effectiveness of the intervention on functional outcomes A recent systematic review could not find conclusive evidence on the effect of electrical stimulation on muscle strength and called for further research on this topic [34].

37.4.2 Multidisciplinary Rehabilitation

A Cochrane Systematic Review identified 11 randomized controlled trials of multidisciplinary rehabilitation in the inpatient setting. Pooled estimates for mortality and change in residential status at 1-year follow-up showed no difference between multidisciplinary rehabilitation and usual care. Benefits appeared to be short term and for activities of daily living and mobility outcomes. There is also limited evidence to support the design of effective models of multidisciplinary care for older adults with dementia who fracture their hip [35].

37.4.3 Prognostic Factors of Functional Outcome on Discharge from Acute Care

Uncertainty over the most effective rehabilitation after hip fracture may be due to the heterogenous nature of the underlying population. For example, patients who present with multiple morbidities from a LTC facility may have a differing risk of poor outcome than those who present without multiple morbidities from the community [36]. An understanding of these factors may inform clinical prioritization by identifying those at high risk of poor outcome to target for more intensive rehabilitation.

A recent systematic review identified 33 observational studies of 25 prognostic factors related to functional outcome on discharge [37]. Factors were broadly classified as related to demographics (age, sex, pre-fracture residence), injury (fracture type), comorbidities (Charlson Comorbidity Index, anemia on admission, cognitive function, Parkinson's Disease, pre-fracture function, diabetes, atrial fibrillation, polypharmacy, Vitamin D level), body composition (body mass index, malnutrition), complications (pain, elevated blood urea, perioperative urinary retention, pressure ulcers, delirium, emotional distress, new onset depression), and acute care processes (time to surgery, time to mobilization, length of stay). However, most factors were reported by studies with lower methodological quality.

Two factors from studies with higher quality were associated with functional outcome at discharge—cognitive function and anemia. Systematic review evidence reported a positive effect of rehabilitation after hip fracture on functional outcome for older adults with cognitive impairment [38]. Despite this evidence, cognitively impaired patients are often excluded from trials of new interventions [32]. This may be overcome by tackling the misconception of 'poor potential for recovery' through targeted intensive rehabilitation for patients with cognitive impairment. In addition, clinicians may target patients with cognitive impairment for medication review, for interventions to reduce complications such as delirium, and for early transfer from bed as these were reported barriers to successful rehabilitation. For anemia, randomized controlled trial evidence suggests a more liberal blood transfusion policy does not lead to better recovery of activities of daily living than a more restrictive blood transfusion policy [39]. It may therefore be appropriate to consider the proposed mechanism of action for anemia on functional outcome—frailty and weakness (a feature of frailty). Alone, a more liberal transfusion policy may be insufficient to target both anemia and frailty. A multidisciplinary approach which considers transfusion strategy and more intensive rehabilitation may warrant further study.

37.5 Recovery in People Living in Long-Term Residential Settings

A systematic review of 35 trials of rehabilitation after hip fracture published between 2008 and 2018 indicated 17.2% of potential participants were excluded based on residency in a LTC facility or cognitive impairment [32]. This is important when considering the strength of the available evidence to inform individual patient care and healthcare reform.

People living in long-term residential facilities have a higher risk of hip fracture due to an increased propensity to fall. Further, as cognitive impairment is common in this patient group, access to rehabilitation is limited and evidence is sparse regarding best practices for rehabilitation after hospital discharge [32]. Systematic reviews assessing the impact of cognitive impairment on rehabilitation outcomes have consistently suggested that those with cognitive impairment benefit from rehabilitation, but many of the studies only included those with mild to moderate cognitive impairment who were still residing in the community [38, 40]. Most programs directed at patients with cognitive impairment use a functionally oriented approach, with activities that the patients are likely to value (i.e., walking) that is more likely to engage patients to participate [38].

Two recent controlled trials of LTC residents performed within the nursing home setting following hospital discharge produced conflicting results; a large (n = 240) randomized trial of a 4-week outreach rehabilitation trial showed small benefits in mobility at 4 weeks relative to usual care that were not sustained at 12 months post-fracture [41]. The intervention was not found to be cost-effective. In contrast, a small non-randomized trial (n = 77) reported small sustained benefit in mobility up to 12 months post-fracture after a 10-week outreach rehabilitation program [42]. These results would suggest that more research is warranted in these settings with consideration for duration and intensity of the rehabilitation program.

37.6 Recovery After Discharge from Hospital to the Community

37.6.1 Continuing the Recovery Process in the Community

After patients are discharged home, they usually receive additional healthcare, mainly rehabilitation by community health services. Since the demand for community health services by patients with hip fractures is expected to increase, community health agencies will need to prepare to accommodate this increase and may need to consider innovative solutions to bridge anticipated gaps. Policymakers will need to ensure adequate resources are available, including adequate number of skilled professionals, to cover the expected increase in demand on available resources.

To offset the predicted burden of care for patients with hip fracture, there is an urgent need to establish comprehensive medical and rehabilitation management programs that ensure satisfactory recovery after hip fracture, minimize functional limitations, and prevent subsequent fractures. Currently, any potential benefits derived from interventions during patients' hospital stay may be threatened by the lack of comprehensive post-hospitalization care. An integrated, multidisciplinary, evidence-based hip fracture program spanning the continuum of recovery is a promising solution to help organize patients' care after discharge and promote smooth transitions to facilitate patients' return to normal living. Two main approaches are emerging to help achieve this goal: extended rehabilitation programs that cover the continuum of recovery and integrated approaches that consider the influence of all factors that impact recovery, both physical and nonphysical.

37.6.2 Extended Rehabilitation Over the Continuum of Recovery

Current rehabilitation programs offered post-hip fracture have been shown to be helpful but not sufficient to restore a patient's pre-fracture functional level; consequently, an extended exercise program has been proposed as a promising strategy to improve patients' functional capacities [21, 25]. The aim of these extended programs is to maintain the improvement gained during rehabilitation and continue an upward functional improvement trajectory. Even modest gains in mobility and balance may translate to substantial cost savings if a second hip fracture is prevented or admission to LTC is delayed.

A series of randomized controlled trials tested extended community rehabilitation programs

Table 37.2 Sample randomized controlled trials of extended exercise programs after hip fracture

Author year	Sample size	Country	Intervention/control	Exercise parameters	Outcomes
Home-based programs					
Sherrington and Lord 1997 [90]	42	Australia	I: Unidimensional weight-bearing exercises C: Usual care	Weekly frequency: daily Session duration: NR Intensity: patient's body weight repetitions: 5–50 Sets/session: NR	Muscle strength, postural control, and mobility tests
Sherrington et al. 2004 [91]	90	Australia	I: Group 1--weight-bearing exercises program reflected the way muscles work during daily activities, AND walking; Group 2—Non-weight-bearing group did the same exercises but in non-weight-bearing position C: Usual care	Weekly frequency: daily Session duration: NR Intensity: patient's body weight Repetitions: based on patient performance Sets/session: NR	Muscle strength, physical performance, postural control, and mobility tests
Mangione et al. 2005 [92]	33	United States	I: Group 1--resistance leg training OR group 2-- aerobic training C: Biweekly mailings on a variety of non-exercise topics	Weekly frequency: 1–2 Session duration: 30–40 Intensity: 80% 1RM Repetitions: 8 Sets/session: 3	Muscle strength, physical performance, and mobility tests
Tsauo et al. 2005 [93]	25	Taiwan	I: Strengthening, ROM exercises, functional training, and balance C: Instructed to practice the exercise program given before discharge	Weekly frequency: daily Session duration: NR Intensity: 1 kg Repetitions: 10 Sets/session: 3	Muscle strength, pain, health-related quality of life
Yu-Yahiro et al. 2009 [94]	180	United States	I: Strengthening exercises, functional exercises, and aerobic exercises C: No exercise	Weekly frequency: 5 Session duration: 30 min Intensity: NR Repetitions: 10 Sets/session: 3	Physical activity; energy and program feasibility
Bischoff-Ferrari et al. 2010 [44]	173	Switzerland	I: Strengthening, balance, and functional training C: Vitamin D, no extra exercise after acute care	Weekly frequency: daily Session duration: 30 min Intensity: NR Repetitions: Not reported Sets/session: Not reported	Falls, hospital readmission, muscle strength, and physical performance

(continued)

Table 37.2 (continued)

Author year	Sample size	Country	Intervention/control	Exercise parameters	Outcomes
Mangione et al. 2010 [95]	26	United States	I: Strengthening exercises for both limbs using machines C: Conventional (TENS) + guided imagery	Weekly frequency: 2 Session duration: 30–40 min intensity: 80% Repetitions: 8 Sets/session: 3	Muscle strength, physical performance, and mobility tests
Ziden et al. 2010 [96]	102	Sweden	I: Individualized home rehab program for 3 weeks with a focus on outdoor ambulation C: Standard care	NR	Outdoor ambulation, functional performance, mobility, balance, health-related quality of life, depression
Orwig et al. 2011 [97]	180	United States	I: Stretching exercises, strengthening exercises for upper and lower limbs using Thera-band products and aerobic exercises, including stepping C: Usual care	Weekly frequency: 1–3 Session duration: 30 min/ part Intensity: NR Repetitions: 10 Sets/session: 3	Physical activity, BMD Functional performance, mobility tests, balance health-related quality of life, pain
Latham et al. 2014 [22]	232	United States	I: Functional exercises led by PT to be later performed at home independently. Monthly follow-up calls provided for program modifications if needed C: In home and phones calls, cardiovascular education	Weekly frequency:3 Session duration: 3 min/ part intensity: 3 levels of resistance using bands Repetitions: NR Sets/session: NR	Functional performance, mobility, muscle strength, adverse events, balance, self-efficacy
Edgren et al. 2015 [98]	81	United States	I: Strengthening exercises, balance exercises, functional exercises C: Received exercises to do at home, at hospital prior to discharge same as intervention group.	Weekly frequency: 3–5 Session duration: 30 min Intensity: NR Repetitions: NR Sets/session: NR	Physical performance

Community-based programs					
Hauer et al. 2002 [99]	28	Germany	I: Session started with warm-up, then high-intensity progressive resistance training and progressive functional balance training C: Met 3 times a week for 1 h, practiced motor placebo activities not supposed to be relevant to study purposes	Weekly frequency: 3 Session duration: 1.5 h resistance + 45 min balance Intensity: 70–90% Repetitions: 10–15 Sets/session: 2–3	Muscle strength, postural control, physical performance, and mobility tests
Binder et al. 2004 [21]	90	United States	I: Two 3-mo-long phases of exercising: Phase 1: Flexibility, balance, coordination, movement speed Phase 2: Progressive resistance training was added to the first phase C: A low-intensity exercise program that would mimic standard care after surgery and a weekly phone call	Weekly frequency: 3 Session duration: 45–90 min intensity: 65%–100% repetitions: 8–12 Sets/session: 3	Functional performance and assistive devices use
Peterson et al. 2004 [48]	70	United States	I: High-intensity strengthening circuit exercise training, balance, gait training program C: Usual care	Weekly frequency: 2 session duration: 60 min Intensity: 60% 1RM Repetitions: NR Sets/session: NR	Muscle strength and mobility tests
Portegijs et al. 2008 [100]	46	Finland	I: Resistance strengthening program to reduce asymmetric deficit and to increase strength and power of the lower limb C: Usual care	Weekly frequency: 2 session duration: 1–1.5 h Intensity: 40%–80% 1RM repetitions: 8–12 Sets/session: 2–4	Muscle strength, physical performance, balance, and mobility tests
Sylliaas et al. 2011 [23]	150	Norway	I: Started with warm-up, then strengthening exercises: Standing knee flexion, lunge, sitting knee extension, and leg extension C: Usual care	Weekly frequency: 3^c session duration: 45–60 min Intensity: 70%–80% 1RM repetitions: 8–15 Sets/session: 3	Balance, physical performance, mobility tests, health-related quality of life
Singh et al. 2012 [101]	124	Australia	I: High-intensity progressive resistance training of upper and lower body muscle strength and balance training C: Usual care	Weekly frequency: 2 session duration: NR intensity: 80% 1RM Repetitions: 8 Sets/session: 3	Mortality, institutionalization, functional performance, use of assistive devices

I: intrevention group, C: control group,. NR: not reported; ROM: range of motion; 1RM: one repetition maximum, BMd: bone mineral density after hip fracture (Table 37.2). In summary, these interventions show that weight-bearing exercises seemed to have a larger effect on lower extremity strength and increasing function compared to non-weight-bearing exercises. The most effective way of delivering a hip fracture recovery program seemed to be with a combination of supervised exercise training with some form of an instructional component (e.g., a booklet or a DVD) [43]. The exercise programs frequency varied from daily exercises to twice per week. The most common frequency of exercise was three times a week. The research studies that had patients exercise more frequently per week seemed to have more positive results. The most common strengthening exercises were hip abduction, hip flexion, knee flexion, and extension as well as ankle plantar flexion. Stepping exercises, stair training and sit-to-stand exercises were also very common. The combination of strengthening, functional, and balance exercises seemed to significantly reduce participants' rate of falls [44]. The most recent literature emphasizes functional exercises in extended programs [22].

An identified gap in available studies is the lack of pain management. Pain is a common symptom that older adults experience during their hip fracture recovery. According to Williams et al., there is a strong relationship between pain and delayed recovery from a hip fracture [45]. Pain can be debilitating and can interfere with one's activities of daily living including one's ability to exercise. Pain is a modifiable factor in one's recovery and, therefore, an important component to address in future community exercise programs.

There are two settings in which to offer extended rehabilitation programs: home-based and community-based. In a systematic review and meta-analysis of extended rehabilitation programs, those offered in both settings were found to be effective in improving health outcomes, but a sensitivity analysis showed that pooled effects for the community-based were larger and more likely to be statistically significant [25]. Larger effects in the community-based studies could be explained because exercise tends to be of higher intensity in community settings, and more sophisticated equipment is available. Another explanation might be that the group setting encourages social interaction among people sharing the same condition (which may increase participation in more intensive programs), reduces cost because one session is offered to a group of patients, and enhances motor learning for participants [46, 47]. Nevertheless, such community-based interventions might result in lack of compliance with the study and a decrease in the number of patients willing to participate [48, 49].

37.6.3 Managing Nonphysical Factors in Rehabilitation Programs

The effects of traditional rehabilitation may vary significantly among patients, and many fail to recover after hip fracture, suggesting there are factors beyond surgery and physical rehabilitation contributing to outcomes. Numerous factors have been shown to influence recovery after a hip fracture, including age, sex, and pre-fracture functional level among many others [50]. In addition, nonphysical factors, such as social and psycho-cognitive influences, could play an important role in recovery [51–56]. Current medical management after hip fracture focuses mainly on physical rehabilitation with nonphysical factors not commonly considered [24, 53]. However, emerging evidence suggests incorporating these additional factors into rehabilitative care models could improve recovery outcomes, reducing mortality and economic burden, and ensuring an improved quality of life for the growing population of older adults with hip fractures [52, 54–56]. Furthermore, patients' definition of recovery usually incorporates the importance of having good physical functioning, and also social, cognitive, and affective good functioning (see Fig. 37.1) [12].

Two main groups of nonphysical factors, social and psycho-cognitive factors, are believed to considerably influence recovery from hip fracture.

37.6.3.1 Social Factors and Recovery

A 2019 review of the role of social factors in recovery after hip fracture found that high levels of social support and higher socioeconomic status were associated with an increase in functional recovery, a decrease in mortality, and positive change in other health outcomes, such as length of hospital stay and quality of life after fracture [57]. One possible mechanism to explain this relationship is the positive effect of social support on self-efficacy (i.e., beliefs in one's ability to perform tasks) [49]. Self-efficacy has the potential to act as a protective factor, and low self-efficacy, potentially as a result of the injury and its consequences, may cause a patient to restrict functioning and negate rehabilitation gains [53]. Through social interaction, patients may receive encouragement, leading to better psychosocial health and higher confidence and self-efficacy, which could increase compliance with physical rehabilitation programs and prevent future falls [49, 58]. Social contact may also help alleviate feelings of depression or anxiety, which could be a barrier to patients increasing functional capacity [59]. However, the importance of social factors in recovery from hip fracture is currently under-researched, lacking rigorously designed studies and interventions, and should be further investigated.

37.6.3.2 Psycho-cognitive Factors and Recovery

Recent literature also suggests that there is a significant relationship between several psycho-cognitive factors and recovery after hip fracture. The presence of psycho-cognitive disorders predicts worse health outcomes, specifically mortality and delayed functional recovery.

To date, the main psycho-cognitive disorders investigated include overall cognitive impairment, delirium, depression, and dementia. Numerous studies report a significant association between overall cognitive impairment and poor physical outcomes [24, 60–71]. For example, Kos et al. found that patients with moderate and severe cognitive impairment showed a poorer recovery of mobility at 3 months after surgery than did patients with mild or no impairment [60].

Another important factor after fracture is delirium. Several studies have demonstrated that delirium is associated with increased mortality and poor outcomes after hip fracture [72, 73]. Ruggerio et al. found that delirium resulted in a two-fold increase in the risk of mortality within 1-year after hip fracture [74]. Presence of postoperative delirium was a predictor of 1- [75, 76], 6- [77–79], and 12-month mortality [80] after hip fracture. Also, delirium is a risk factor for contralateral hip fractures [81] and longer hospital stay [76, 79].

Depression was found in several studies to be significantly associated with poor recovery and mortality, especially when co-occurring with cognitive impairments [82] or with other mood disorders [68]. Nightingale and colleagues found that a diagnosis of depression soon after hip fracture greatly increased risk of death in the following 2 years [72]. Some studies that did not find statistically significant relationship between depression and recovery commented on the clinical importance of the results [79].

There appear to be a cumulative effect of psycho-cognitive disorders on recovery post-hip fracture. Givens et al. showed that one mood disorder, such as depression, or one cognitive disorder, at 1-month post-fracture, was associated with one or more adverse outcomes, and when considered together, each additional disorder (whether mood or cognitive) was associated with greater odds of 1-month adverse outcomes [68, 76].

37.6.3.3 Clinical Implications

This growing body of literature indicating that nonphysical factors can significantly affect recovery after hip fracture has substantial implications for clinicians and policymakers, particularly given that many of these factors are modifiable. Recovery programs for patients after hip fractures should not focus solely on the physical aspects of recovery. In terms of incorporating social factors, it is important to encourage patients to return to the community, where they should have adequate services available and strategies to promote social inclusion [83].

Clinicians and health authorities need to implement early screening to recognize psycho-cognitive disorders and prevent them from leading to sub-optimal recovery and increased mortality after hip fractures. Several authors have also proposed the development and use of a simple but thorough bedside test to recognize changes in cognition [74, 84].

Efforts should be also focused on preventable and treatable issues like delirium. The diagnosis of postoperative delirium remains mostly clinical. Clinical features of delirium can be summarized as impairment of awareness, thinking, memory, perception, psychomotor behavior, and emotion [85]. Education of healthcare professionals on these features and on principles of deferential diagnosis can increase the recognition of delirium, which is the first step of effective interventions. Patients are at high risk of developing delirium during the postoperative period; however, delirium occurring at this period is specifically amenable to management [85]. Organized approaches to detect and manage delirium, which involve providing preoperative psychological support and careful postoperative management, is superior to traditional reactive care and can reduce the occurrence of delirium [85].

In addition to delirium, Rathbun et al. emphasize the need for better depression screening and management for a full year after hip fracture, especially in individuals with a history of depressive symptoms [86, 87]. Identifying mental health issues such as depression and implementing treatment can have a positive effect on recovery, and can support staff when planning rehabilitation and discharge destination [88].

Further studies with robust research designs (e.g., RCTs) are required to understand the role of social and psycho-cognitive factors in recovery from hip fracture, and to provide specific clinical direction on how to account for these nonphysical factors in the rehabilitation process [89]. See Figs. 37.2 and 37.3 for the top five priorities in studying social and psycho-cognitive factors, respectively, from a global survey of clinicians and researchers with experience in hip fracture.

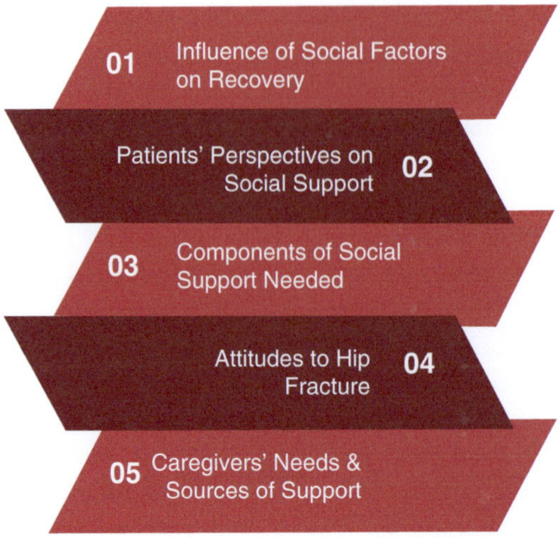
01 Influence of Social Factors on Recovery
Patients' Perspectives on Social Support 02
03 Components of Social Support Needed
Attitudes to Hip Fracture 04
05 Caregivers' Needs & Sources of Support

Fig. 37.2 Top five priorities in studying social factors. Reprinted from Auais et al. [88]; with permission from Elsevier

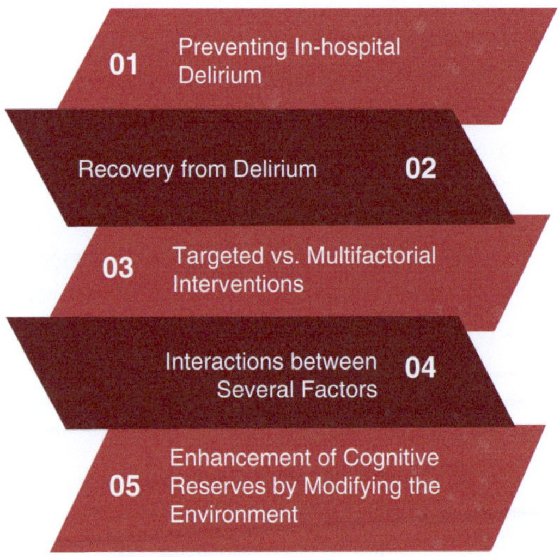

Fig. 37.3 Top five priorities in studying psycho-cognitive factors. Reprinted from Auais et al. [88]; with permission from Elsevier

37.7 Next Steps for Rehabilitation Research

There are several meaningful steps that could improve rehabilitation after hip fracture. First, evidence is lacking to inform the most appropriate rehabilitation after hip fracture for vulnerable proportions of the population including those from supported facility-based care. Future research should consider evaluation of rehabilitation extending across the care continuum, care contexts, and for the entire patient population experiencing hip fracture. Second, there is a need for future trials to identify core outcomes/outcome measures for use in rehabilitation interventions after hip fracture that incorporate not only physical function, but also instrumental, cognitive, affective, and social outcomes to better reflect patient, carer, and clinical definitions of recovery after hip fracture. Finally, national audit data collection that led to the defined best practice tariffs for surgical and medical care after hip fracture reduced mortality and length of stay after hip fracture. Rehabilitation should also capitalize on this evidenced success through a collection of rehabilitation process and structure measures in international audits to inform future rehabilitation best practice tariffs and quality improvement initiatives.

37.8 Summary

As life expectancy increases worldwide, hip fractures are projected to become an even greater global health problem in the near future. The care process of patients with hip fracture starts in the acute settings where patients typically undergo a surgical procedure to repair the fracture and continue in both inpatient and outpatient settings to promote patient recovery post-fracture. In the acute setting, guidelines for rehabilitation after hip fracture recommend interdisciplinary care to manage possible complications such as delirium, pain, and circulatory system problems. Further, these recent guidelines support a shift from the traditional medical model of care in the early period after surgery to a more holistic, functional model of care to improve recovery, regardless of treatment setting. Several factors have been identified as relevant to recovery in the acute setting, including demographics, fracture type, comorbidities, body composition, complications in the hospital (pain, perioperative urinary retention, delirium, new onset depression), and timely care (time to surgery, time to mobilization).

Additional healthcare from community health services should continue when patients are discharged home. The demand for community health services by patients with hip fractures is expected to continue to rise; community health agencies will need to prepare for this increased demand and consider innovative solutions to bridge gaps. Therefore, current care models require review and revision to ensure adequate resource provision, especially in the community to balance the expected increase in demand and meet the needs of older, frail adults who survive their hip fracture to improve their outcomes.

The rehabilitation services offered in hospitals, rehabilitation institutions, and early health services after discharge in the community usually improve patients' functional outcomes, including mobility and activities of self-care. However, initial improvement may not blossom into full recovery or to complete independent living. Potential benefits derived during the hospital stay and provision of rehabilitation services may be threatened through lack of comprehensive and sufficient post-hospitalization care. Comprehensive programs, extending far beyond the acute setting and usual care are needed to ensure adequate recovery and prevention of subsequent fractures, and to minimize the functional limitations associated with hip fractures. Additionally, these programs should cover recovery from physical impairments while addressing other nonphysical challenges and disorders, such as lack of social support and psycho-cognitive disorders. Recent studies suggest that social factors (e.g., social support) and psycho-cognitive factors (e.g., delirium and depression) can play critical roles in recovery, but these factors are not currently common targets for evaluation and/or management in hip fracture rehabilitation programs or research. Incorporating these factors into rehabilitation programs for patients with hip fractures will enhance their recovery and reduce the burden on care providers, healthcare systems, and society.

Acknowledgement The authors would like to aknowledge the support and contribution of the Fragility Fracture Network.

References

1. Abrahamsen B, van Staa T, Ariely R, Olson M, Cooper C. Excess mortality following hip fracture: a systematic epidemiological review. Osteoporos Int. 2009;20(10):1633–50.
2. Fransen M, Woodward M, Norton R, Robinson E, Butler M, Campbell AJ. Excess mortality or institutionalization after hip fracture: men are at greater risk than women. J Am Geriatr Soc. 2002;50(4):685–90.
3. Sterling RS. Gender and race/ethnicity differences in hip fracture incidence, morbidity, mortality, and function. Clin Orthop Rel Res. 2011;469(7):1913–8.
4. Kannegaard PN, van der Mark S, Eiken P, Abrahamsen B. Excess mortality in men compared with women following a hip fracture. National analysis of comedications, comorbidity and survival. Age Ageing. 2010;39(2):203–9.
5. Sterling RS. Gender and race/ethnicity differences in hip fracture incidence, morbidity, mortality, and function. Clin Orthop Relat Res. 2011;469(7):1913–8.
6. Dyer SM, Crotty M, Fairhall N, Magaziner J, Beaupre LA, Cameron ID, et al. A critical review of the long-term disability outcomes following hip fracture. BMC Geriatr. 2016;16(1):158.
7. Bertram M, Norman R, Kemp L, Vos T. Review of the long-term disability associated with hip fractures. Inj Prev. 2011;17(6):365–70.
8. Chen IJ, Chiang CY, Li YH, Chang CH, Hu CC, Chen DW, et al. Nationwide cohort study of hip fractures: time trends in the incidence rates and projections up to 2035. Osteoporosis international: a journal established as result of cooperation between the European Foundation for Osteoporosis and the National Osteoporosis Foundation of the USA. 2015;26(2):681–8.
9. Auais M, Morin S, Nadeau L, Finch L, Mayo N. Changes in frailty-related characteristics of the hip fracture population and their implications for healthcare services: evidence from Quebec. Canada Osteoporosis Int. 2013;24(10):2713–24.
10. Siris ES. Patients with hip fracture: what can be improved? Bone. 2006;38(2 Suppl 2):S8–12.
11. Auais M, Morin SN, Finch L, Ahmed S, Mayo N. Toward a meaningful definition of recovery after hip fracture: comparing two definitions for community-dwelling older adults. Arch Phys Med Rehabil. 2018;99(6):1108–15.
12. Sheehan KJ, Smith TO, Martin FC, Johansen A, Drummond A, Beaupre L, et al. Conceptual framework for an episode of rehabilitative care after surgical repair of hip fracture. Phys Ther. 2019;99(3):276–85.
13. Organization WH. World report on ageing and health. Luxembourg; 2015.
14. Langford D, Edwards N, Gray SM, Fleig L, Ashe MC. "Life Goes On". Everyday tasks, coping self-efficacy, and independence: exploring older adults' recovery from hip fracture. Qual Health Res 2018:1049732318755675.
15. Sims-Gould J, Stott-Eveneshen S, Fleig L, McAllister M, Ashe MC. Patient perspectives on engagement in recovery after hip fracture: a qualitative study. J Aging Res. 2017;2017:2171865.
16. Bruun-Olsen V, Bergland A, Heiberg KE. "I struggle to count my blessings": recovery after hip fracture from the patients' perspective. BMC Geriatr. 2018;18(1):18.
17. Pol M, Peek S, van Nes F, van Hartingsveldt M, Buurman B, Krose B. Everyday life after a hip fracture: what community-living older adults perceive as most beneficial for their recovery. Age Ageing. 2019;48(3):440–7.
18. Magaziner J, Hawkes W, Hebel JR, Zimmerman SI, Fox KM, Dolan M, et al. Recovery from hip fracture in eight areas of function. J Gerontol A Biol Sci Med Sci. 2000;55(9):M498–507.
19. Koot VCM, Peeters PHM, De Jong JR, Clevers GJ, Van Der Werken C. Functional results after treatment of hip fracture: a multicentre, prospective study in 215 patients. Eur J Surg. 2000;166(6):480–5.
20. Young Y, Xiong K, Pruzek RM, Brant LJ. Examining heterogeneity of functional recovery among older adults with hip fractures. J Am Med Dir Assoc. 2010;11(2):132–9.
21. Binder EF, Brown M, Sinacore DR, Steger-May K, Yarasheski KE, Schechtman KB. Effects of extended outpatient rehabilitation after hip fracture: a randomized controlled trial. JAMA. J Am Med Assoc. 2004;292(7):837–46.
22. Latham NK, Harris BA, Bean JF, Heeren T, Goodyear C, Zawacki S, et al. Effect of a home-based exercise program on functional recovery following rehabilitation after hip fracture: a randomized clinical trial. JAMA. 2014;311(7):700–8.
23. Sylliaas H, Brovold T, Wyller TB, Bergland A. Progressive strength training in older patients after hip fracture: a randomised controlled trial. Age Ageing. 2011;40(2):221–7.
24. Sylliaas H, Thingstad P, Wyller TB, Helbostad J, Sletvold O, Bergland A. Prognostic factors for self-rated function and perceived health in patient living at home three months after a hip fracture. DisabilRehabil Int Multidisciplinary J. 2012;34(14):1225–31.
25. Auais MA, Eilayyan O, Mayo NE. Extended exercise rehabilitation after hip fracture improves Patients' physical function: a systematic review and meta-analysis. Phys Ther. 2012;92(11):1437–51.
26. World Health Organization. World report on disability. Geneva; 2011. Available from https://www.who.int/disabilities/world_report/2011/report/en/

27. National Institute for Health and Clinical Excellence (NICE). Hip fracture management: clinical guideline. Updated: May 2017. Available from https://www.nice.org.uk/guidance/cg124.
28. The Chartered Society of Physiotherapy. Hip fracture rehabilitation in physiotherapy practice. 2018.; available from https://www.csp.org.uk/publications/hip-fracture-rehabilitation-physiotherapy-practice 2019.
29. The American Academy of Orthopaedic Surgeons. Appropriate use criteria for postoperative rehabilitation of low energy hip fractures in the elderly. 2015.
30. Bone and Joint Canada. National Hip Fracture Toolkit. 2011. Available from: http://boneandjointcanada.com/wp-content/uploads/2014/05/National-hip-fracture-toolkit-June-2011.pdf31.
31. Handoll HH, Sherrington C, Mak JC. Interventions for improving mobility after hip fracture surgery in adults. Cochrane Database Syst Rev. 2011;(3):CD001704.
32. Sheehan KJ, Fitzgerald L, Hatherley S, Potter C, Ayis S, Martin FC, et al. Equity in rehabilitation interventions after hip fracture surgery: a systematic review. Age Ageing, 10.1093/ageing/afz031. 2019;48, 4:489–97.
33. Diong J, Allen N, Sherrington C. Structured exercise improves mobility after hip fracture: a meta-analysis with meta-regression. Br J Sports Med. 2016;50(6):346–55.
34. Davison Rianne P, Jordan W, Auais MM. A systematic review of using electrical stimulation to improve clinical outcomes after hip fractures. Physiotherapy Theory and Practice. 1–19. https://doi.org/10.1080/09593985.2021.1894620.
35. Smith TO, Hameed YA, Cross JL, Henderson C, Sahota O, Fox C. Enhanced rehabilitation and care models for adults with dementia following hip fracture surgery. Cochrane Database Syst Rev. 2015, CD010569;6
36. Sheehan KJ, Sobolev B, Chudyk A, Stephens T, Guy P. Patient and system factors of mortality after hip fracture: a scoping review. BMC Musculoskelet Disord. 2016;17(1):166.
37. Sheehan K, Williamson L, Alexander J, Filliter C, Sobolev B, Guy P, et al. Prognostic factors of functional outcome after hip fracture surgery: a systematic review. Age Ageing. 2018;47(5):661–70.
38. Resnick B, Beaupre L, McGilton KS, Galik E, Liu W, Neuman MD, et al. Rehabilitation interventions for older individuals with cognitive impairment post-hip fracture: a systematic review. J Am Med Dir Assoc. 2016;17(3):200–5.
39. Gregersen M, Borris LC, Damsgaard EM. Postoperative blood transfusion strategy in frail, anemic elderly patients with hip fracture: the TRIFE randomized controlled trial. Acta Orthop. 2015;86(3):363–72.
40. Muir SW, Yohannes AM. The impact of cognitive impairment on rehabilitation outcomes in elderly patients admitted with a femoral neck fracture: a systematic review. J Geriatr Phys Ther (2001). 2009;32(1):24-32.
41. Crotty M, Killington M, Liu E, Cameron ID, Kurrle S, Kaambwa B, et al. Should we provide outreach rehabilitation to very old people living in nursing care facilities after a hip fracture? A randomised controlled trial. Age Ageing. 2019;48(3):373–80.
42. Beaupre LA, Magaziner JS, Jones CA, Jhangri GS, Johnston DWC, Wilson DM, et al. Rehabilitation after hip fracture for nursing home residents: a controlled feasibility trial. J Gerontol Ser A Biol Sci Med Sci. 2019;74(9):1518–25.
43. Moran L, Francis-Coad J, Patman S, Hill AM. Using a personalized DVD to prescribe an exercise program to older people post-hip fracture enhances adherence to the exercises - a feasibility study. Geriatr Nurs (NY). 2015;36(4):273–80.
44. Bischoff-Ferrari HA, Dawson-Hughes B, Platz A, Orav EJ, Stahelin HB, Willett WC, et al. Effect of high-dosage cholecalciferol and extended physiotherapy on complications after hip fracture: a randomized controlled trial. Arch Intern Med. 2010;170(9):813–20.
45. Williams CS, Tinetti ME, Kasl SV, Peduzzi PN. The role of pain in the recovery of instrumental and social functioning after hip fracture. J Aging Health. 2006;18(5):743–62.
46. McNevin NH, Wulf G, Carlson C. Effects of attentional focus, self-control, and dyad training on motor learning: implications for physical rehabilitation. Phys Ther. 2000;80(4):373–85.
47. Shea CH, Wulf G, Whitacre C. Enhancing training efficiency and effectiveness through the use of dyad training. J Mot Behav. 1999;31(2):119–25.
48. Peterson MGE, Ganz SB, Allegrante JP, Cornell CN. High-intensity exercise training following hip fracture. Top Geriatr Rehabil. 2004;20(4):273–84.
49. Allegrante JP, Peterson MG, Cornell CN, MacKenzie CR, Robbins L, Horton R, et al. Methodological challenges of multiple-component intervention: lessons learned from a randomized controlled trial of functional recovery after hip fracture. HSS J. 2007;3(1):63–70.
50. Resnick B, Hebel JR, Gruber-Baldini AL, Hicks GE, Hochberg MC, Orwig D, et al. The impact of body composition, pain and resilience on physical activity, physical function and physical performance at 2 months post hip fracture. Arch Gerontol Geriatr. 2018;76:34–40.
51. Beaupre LA, Binder EF, Cameron ID, Jones CA, Orwig D, Sherrington C, et al. Maximising functional recovery following hip fracture in frail seniors. Best Pract Res Clin Rheumatol. 2013;27(6):771–88.
52. Gruber-Baldini AL, Zimmerman S, Morrison RS, Grattan LM, Hebel JR, Dolan MM, et al. Cognitive impairment in hip fracture patients: timing of detection and longitudinal follow-up. J Am Geriatr Soc. 2003;51(9):1227–36.

53. Petrella RJ, Payne M, Myers A, Overend T, Chesworth B. Physical function and fear of falling after hip fracture rehabilitation in the elderly. Am J Phys Med Rehabil. 2000;79(2):154–60.
54. Reimers A, Laflamme L. Hip fractures among the elderly: personal and contextual social factors that matter. J Trauma. 2007;62(2):365–9.
55. Shyu YI, Liang J, Wu CC, Cheng HS, Chen MC. An interdisciplinary intervention for older Taiwanese patients after surgery for hip fracture improves health-related quality of life. BMC Musculoskelet Disord. 2010;11:225.
56. Visschedijk J, van Balen R, Hertogh C, Achterberg W. Fear of falling in patients with hip fractures: prevalence and related psychological factors. J Am Med Dir Assoc. 2013;14(3):218–20.
57. Auais M, Al-Zoubi F, Matheson A, Brown K, Magaziner J, French S. Understanding the role of social factors in recovery after hip fractures: a structured scoping review. Health Soc Care Community. 2019;27(6):1375–138.
58. Magaziner J, Simonsick EM, Kashner TM, Hebel JR, Kenzora JE. Predictors of functional recovery one year following hospital discharge for hip fracture: a prospective study. J Gerontol. 1990;45(3):M101–7.
59. Scheffers-Barnhoorn MN, van Haastregt JC, Schols JM, Kempen GI, van Balen R, Visschedijk JH, et al. A multi-component cognitive behavioural intervention for the treatment of fear of falling after HIP fracture (FIT-HIP): protocol of a randomised controlled trial. BMC Geriatr. 2017;17(1):71.
60. Kos N, Burger H, Vidmar G. Association of cognitive status with mobility and functioning after femoral neck fracture surgery in elderly patients: differences between hemiarthroplasty and internal fixation. Zdravniski Vestnik. 2013;82(3):150–7.
61. van Dortmont LM, Douw CM, van Breukelen AM, Laurens DR, Mulder PG, Wereldsma JC, et al. Outcome after hemi-arthroplasty for displaced intracapsular femoral neck fracture related to mental state. Injury. 2000;31(5):327–31.
62. Tabbarah M, Crimmins EM, Seeman TE. The relationship between cognitive and physical performance: MacArthur studies of successful aging. J Gerontol Ser A Biol Sci Med Sci. 2002;57(4):M228–35.
63. Jones CA, Jhangri GS, Feeny DH, Beaupre LA. Cognitive status at hospital admission: postoperative trajectory of functional recovery for hip fracture. J Gerontol Ser A Biol Sci Med Sci. 2015;21:21.
64. Soderqvist A, Ekstrom W, Ponzer S, Pettersson H, Cederholm T, Dalen N, et al. Prediction of mortality in elderly patients with hip fractures: a two-year prospective study of 1944 patients. Gerontology. 2009;55(5):496–504.
65. Ishidou Y, Koriyama C, Kakoi H, Setoguchi T, Nagano S, Hirotsu M, et al. Predictive factors of mortality and deterioration in performance of activities of daily living after hip fracture surgery in Kagoshima. Japan Geriatr Gerontol Int. 2016;28:28.
66. Gialanella B, Prometti P, Monguzzi V, Ferlucci C. Neuropsychiatric symptoms and rehabilitation outcomes in patients with hip fracture. Am J Phys Med Rehabil. 2014;93(7):562–9.
67. Feng L, Scherer SC, Tan BY, Chan G, Fong NP, Ng TP. Comorbid cognitive impairment and depression is a significant predictor of poor outcomes in hip fracture rehabilitation. Int Psychogeriatr. 2010;22(2):246–53.
68. Givens JL, Sanft TB, Marcantonio ER. Functional recovery after hip fracture: the combined effects of depressive symptoms, cognitive impairment, and delirium. J Am Geriatr Soc. 2008;56(6):1075–9.
69. Eastwood HD. The relationship between the severity of Alzheimer's disease and recovery of independent mobility after treatment for proximal femoral fracture. Clin Rehabil. 1995;9(4):343–6.
70. Duppils GS, Wikblad K. Cognitive function and health-related quality of life after delirium in connection with hip surgery. A six-month follow-up. Orthop Nurs. 2004;23(3):195–203.
71. Baker BR, Duckworth T, Wilkes E. Mental state and other prognostic factors in femoral fractures of the elderly. J Roy Coll Gen Pract. 1978;28(194):557–9.
72. Nightingale S, Holmes J, Mason J, House A. Psychiatric illness and mortality after hip fracture. Lancet. 2001;357(9264):1264–5.
73. Edelstein DM, Aharonoff GB, Karp A, Capla EL, Zuckerman JD, Koval KJ. Effect of postoperative delirium on outcome after hip fracture. Clin Orthop Relat Res. 2004;422:195–200.
74. Ruggiero C, Bonamassa L, Pelini L, Prioletta I, Cianferotti L, Metozzi A, et al. Early post-surgical cognitive dysfunction is a risk factor for mortality among hip fracture hospitalized older persons. Osteoporos Int. 2017;28(2):667–75.
75. Radinovic K, Markovic-Denic L, Dubljanin-Raspopovic E, Marinkovic J, Milan Z, Bumbasirevic V. Estimating the effect of incident delirium on short-term outcomes in aged hip fracture patients through propensity score analysis. Geriatr Gerontol Int. 2015;15(7):848–55.
76. Marcantonio ER, Flacker JM, Michaels M, Resnick NM. Delirium is independently associated with poor functional recovery after hip fracture. J Am Geriatr Soc. 2000;48(6):618–24.
77. Bellelli G, Mazzola P, Morandi A, Bruni A, Carnevali L, Corsi M, et al. Duration of postoperative delirium is an independent predictor of 6-month mortality in older adults after hip fracture. J Am Geriatr Soc. 2014;62(7):1335–40.
78. Mazzola P, Bellelli G, Broggini V, Anzuini A, Corsi M, Berruti D, et al. Postoperative delirium and pre-fracture disability predict 6-month mortality among the oldest old hip fracture patients. Aging-Clin Exp Res. 2015;27(1):53–60.
79. Holmes J, House A. Psychiatric illness predicts poor outcome after surgery for hip fracture: a prospective cohort study. Psychol Med. 2000;30(4):921–9.

80. Dubljanin-Raspopovic E, Markovic-Denic L, Matanovic D, Grajic M, Krstic N, Bumbasirevic M. Is pre-fracture functional status better than cognitive level in predicting short-term outcome of elderly hip fracture patients? Arch Med Sci. 2012;8(1):115–22.
81. Chang JD, Yoo JH, Reddy P, Lee SS, Hwang JH, Kim TY. Risk factors for contra-lateral hip fracture in elderly patients with previous hip fracture. Injury. 2013;44(12):1930–3.
82. Bellelli G, Frisoni GB, Turco R, Trabucchi M. Depressive symptoms combined with dementia affect 12-months survival in elderly patients after rehabilitation post-hip fracture surgery. Int J Geriatr Psychiatry. 2008;23(10):1073–7.
83. Landeiro F, Gray AM, Leal J. Delayed discharges and social isolation in countries with ageing populations: England versus Portugal. Eur Geriatric Med. 2016;7:S221.
84. Lee HB, Oldham MA, Sieber FE, Oh ES. Impact of delirium after hip fracture surgery on one-year mortality in patients with or without dementia: a case of effect modification. Am J Geriatr Psychiatry. 2017;25(3):308–15.
85. Kyziridis TC. Post-operative delirium after hip fracture treatment – a review of the current literature. Psycho-Soc Med. 2006;3:Doc01.
86. Rathbun AM, Shardell M, Orwig D, Gruber-Baldini AL, Ostir G, Hicks GE, et al. Effects of prefracture depressive illness and postfracture depressive symptoms on physical performance after hip fracture. J Am Geriatr Soc. 2016;64(11):e171–e6.
87. Rathbun AM, Shardell MD, Stuart EA, Gruber-Baldini AL, Orwig D, Ostir GV, et al. Persistence of depressive symptoms and gait speed recovery in older adults after hip fracture. Int J Geriatr Psychiatry. 2018;33(7):875–82.
88. Duignan D, Woodward Y, Daniel E, Burns A. An intervention to manage depression after hip fracture. Nurs Times. 2007;103(28):32–3.
89. Auais M, French SD, Beaupre L, Giangregorio L, Magaziner J. Identifying research priorities around psycho-cognitive and social factors for recovery from hip fractures: an international decision-making process. Injury. 2018;49(8):1466–72.
90. Sherrington C, Lord SR. Home exercise to improve strength and walking velocity after hip fracture: a randomized controlled trial. Arch Phys Med Rehabil. 1997;78(2):208–12.
91. Sherrington C, Lord SR, Herbert RD. A randomized controlled trial of weight-bearing versus non-weight-bearing exercise for improving physical ability after usual care for hip fracture. Arch Phys Med Rehabil. 2004;85(5):710–6.
92. Mangione KK, Craik RL, Tomlinson SS, Palombaro KM. Can elderly patients who have had a hip fracture perform moderate- to high-intensity exercise at home? Phys Ther. 2005;85(8):727–39.
93. Tsauo JY, Leu WS, Chen YT, Yang RS. Effects on function and quality of life of postoperative home-based physical therapy for patients with hip fracture. Arch Phys Med Rehabil. 2005;86(10):1953–7.
94. Yu-Yahiro JA, Resnick B, Orwig D, Hicks G, Magaziner J. Design and implementation of a home-based exercise program post-hip fracture: the Baltimore hip studies experience. PM R. 2009;1(4):308–18.
95. Mangione KK, Craik RL, Palombaro KM, Tomlinson SS, Hofmann MT. Home-based leg-strengthening exercise improves function 1 year after hip fracture: a randomized controlled study. J Am Geriatr Soc. 2010;58(10):1911–7.
96. Ziden L, Kreuter M, Frandin K. Long-term effects of home rehabilitation after hip fracture: 1-year follow-up of functioning, balance confidence, and health-related quality of life in elderly people. Disability Rehabil Int Multidiscipl J. 2010;32(1):18–32.
97. Orwig DL, Hochberg M, Yu-Yahiro J, Resnick B, Hawkes WG, Shardell M, et al. Delivery and outcomes of a yearlong home exercise program after hip fracture: a randomized controlled trial. Arch Intern Med. 2011;171(4):323–31.
98. Edgren J, Salpakoski A, Sihvonen SE, Portegijs E, Kallinen M, Arkela M, et al. Effects of a home-based physical rehabilitation program on physical disability after hip fracture: a randomized controlled trial. J Am Med Dir Assoc. 2015;16(4):350.e1–7.
99. Hauer K, Specht N, Schuler M, Bartsch P, Oster P. Intensive physical training in geriatric patients after severe falls and hip surgery. Age Ageing. 2002;31(1):49–57.
100. Portegijs E, Kallinen M, Rantanen T, Heinonen A, Sihvonen S, Alen M, et al. Effects of resistance training on lower-extremity impairments in older people with hip fracture. Arch Phys Med Rehabil. 2008;89(9):1667–74.
101. Singh NA, Quine S, Clemson LM, Williams EJ, Williamson DA, Stavrinos TM, et al. Effects of high-intensity progressive resistance training and targeted multidisciplinary treatment of frailty on mortality and nursing home admissions after hip fracture: a randomized controlled trial. J Am Med Dir Assoc. 2012;13(1):24–30.

MIX
Papier aus verantwortungsvollen Quellen
Paper from responsible sources
FSC® C105338

If you have any concerns about our products,
you can contact us on
ProductSafety@springernature.com

In case Publisher is established outside the EU,
the EU authorized representative is:
Springer Nature Customer Service Center GmbH
Europaplatz 3, 69115 Heidelberg, Germany

Printed by Libri Plureos GmbH
in Hamburg, Germany